Neurodevelopmental Disorders: Evaluation and Treatment

Neurodevelopmental Disorders: Evaluation and Treatment

Editor: Nolan Morales

AMERICAN
MEDICAL PUBLISHERS
www.americanmedicalpublishers.com

AMERICAN
MEDICAL PUBLISHERS
www.americanmedicalpublishers.com

Cataloging-in-Publication Data

Neurodevelopmental disorders : evaluation and treatment / edited by Nolan Morales.
p. cm.
Includes bibliographical references and index.
ISBN 979-8-88740-304-5
1. Developmental disabilities. 2. Developmental neurobiology. 3. Nervous system--Diseases.
4. Developmental disabilities--Diagnosis. 5. Developmental disabilities--Treatment.
6. Pediatric neurology. 7. Neurology. I. Morales, Nolan.
RJ506.D47 N48 2023
618.928 588--dc23

American Medical Publishers,
41 Flatbush Avenue,
1st Floor, New York,
NY 11217, USA

ISBN 979-8-88740-304-5 (Hardback)

Contents

Preface

Over the recent decade, advancements and applications have progressed exponentially. This has led to the increased interest in this field and projects are being conducted to enhance knowledge. The main objective of this book is to present some of the critical challenges and provide insights into possible solutions. This book will answer the varied questions that arise in the field and also provide an increased scope for furthering studies.

Neurodevelopmental disorders refer to a group of disorders which impact the development of the nervous system. It leads to altered brain function that may affect self-control, emotion, memory and learning ability. The effect of these disorders can be seen throughout the person's life. There are various types of neurodevelopmental disorders including fetal alcohol spectrum disorders, attention deficit hyperactivity disorder, specific learning disorders, intellectual disabilities (Ids), developmental language disorder (DLD), neurogenetic disorders, autism spectrum differences (ASD), traumatic brain injury and motor disorders. There are several causes associated with neurodevelopmental disorders such as nutritional factors, genetic and metabolic diseases, infectious diseases, toxic and environmental factors, immune disorders, social deprivation, and physical trauma. The diagnosis of these disorders can be done through examination of specific symptoms and behaviors in a child. These disorders can also be confirmed through genetic testing. This book covers in the detail the evaluation and treatment of neurodevelopmental disorders. It will help new researchers by foregrounding their knowledge in this condition.

I hope that this book, with its visionary approach, will be a valuable addition and will promote interest among readers. Each of the authors has provided their extraordinary competence in their specific fields by providing different perspectives as they come from diverse nations and regions. I thank them for their contributions.

Editor

1

Conceptual, Regulatory and Strategic Imperatives in the Early Days of EEG-Based Biomarker Validation for Neurodevelopmental Disabilities

Joshua B. Ewen[1,2,3], John A. Sweeney[4] and William Z. Potter[5]*

[1] Department of Neurology and Developmental Medicine, Kennedy Krieger Institute, Baltimore, MD, United States, [2] Department of Neurology, Johns Hopkins University School of Medicine, Baltimore, MD, United States, [3] Department of Psychological and Brain Sciences, Johns Hopkins University, Baltimore, MD, United States, [4] Department of Psychiatry, University of Cincinnati, Cincinnati, OH, United States, [5] National Institute of Mental Health, National Institutes of Health, Bethesda, MD, United States

***Correspondence:**
Joshua B. Ewen
ewen@kennedykrieger.org

Biological treatment development for syndromal neuropsychiatric conditions such as autism has seen slow progress for decades. Speeding drug discovery may result from the judicious development and application of biomarker measures of brain function to select patients for clinical trials, to confirm target engagement and to optimize drug dose. For neurodevelopmental disorders, electrophysiology (EEG) offers considerable promise because of its ability to monitor brain activity with high temporal resolution and its more ready application for pediatric populations relative to MRI. Here, we discuss conceptual/definitional issues related to biomarker development, discuss practical implementation issues, and suggest preliminary guidelines for validating EEG approaches as biomarkers with a context of use in neurodevelopmental disorder drug development.

Keywords: biomarker, EEG, validation, autism, neuropsychiatry

INTRODUCTION

Pressing needs in clinical care and concerns about low-yield clinical trials in neurodevelopmental disabilities (NDD) have increased enthusiasm for brain-based biomarkers, with particular additional challenges in neurodevelopmental disorders (NDD) (Sahin et al., 2018). The current push for biomarker development in the realm of brain disorders follows on the heels of several well-known failures in clinical trials in genetically more homogeneous disorders (Berry-Kravis et al., 2012; Hagerman et al., 2018). While there is high enthusiasm for biomarkers for NDDs, the field is just at the beginning of establishing utility of biomarkers for guiding selection of therapies and the patients most likely to benefit in clinical trials. Therefore, the aims of this paper are to help guide early-phase efforts in this area by providing a conceptual framework for planning biomarker validation research, suggestions for early phase investigation strategy and an early framework of thresholds for determining successful reliability/validation, and to explore issues specific to the use of EEG.

These trial failures have been difficult to interpret and seem to have lower-than-expected statistical power due to unpredictable responses to interventions (including placebo), which are in turn due to patient heterogeneity that has not yet been differentiated. The last few decades have made clear that there is poor correspondence across levels of analyses in behaviorally defined NDD ("degeneracy"): patients with a particular genotype may have a range of behavioral phenotypes as in Fragile X syndrome (FXS), and a single behaviorally defined diagnosis [e.g., autism spectrum disorder (ASD)] may be caused by a range of genetic alterations (e.g., Angelman, tuberous sclerosis, FXS, multiple risk loci). Situated between genotype and clinical phenotype are molecular pathways and cellular processes most relevant to the mechanism of action of pharmacological interventions—so called *intermediate phenotypes.* In behaviorally defined disorders and behavioral/cognitive therapies, the most relevant level of intermediate phenotype may be at the cognitive level (Morton, 2005). Because interventions assessed in clinical trials may be effective (or, alternatively, dangerous) for a latent sub-group within a behavioral or genetic diagnosis, there is substantial risk that a true benefit for such a sub-group could be statistically overshadowed by a null effect in most subjects (Type II error). The hope placed in biomarkers is that they can better report on the level of this treatment-linked intermediate phenotype, and thus refine inclusion/exclusion criteria or generate a stratification approach. A solid example comes from epilepsy: the clinical (behavioral) description of a seizure can be misleading in terms of choice of treatment. A generalized tonic-clonic seizure (GTC) may result either from seizure activity arising in the brain all at once, or seizure activity arising from one spot in the brain and spreading quickly across the brain; different medications are effective for each type. These two mechanism are better separated by EEG results than by clinical (behavioral) descriptions of the seizure. The EEG findings therefore, represent a treatment mechanism-relevant intermediate phenotype useful for guiding optimal clinical therapy and testing of novel agents.

Consider clinical trials in FXS, for which a seemingly promising treatment was brought forward unsuccessfully based on compelling data from a genetic animal model (Berry-Kravis et al., 2012) to appreciate how the absence of a biomarker limits the interpretation of results. In the FMR1 knock-out (KO) mouse model of FXS, metabotropic glutamate receptor type 5 (mGluR5) antagonists produce beneficial neurobiological and behavioral effects. No translational biomarker of functional brain data, such as EEG, were collected in the mice, or in the decisive clinical trial. Without a translational biomarker establishing that some desired brain effect was achieved or a clinical biomarker for stratifying individuals based on pre-treatment functional brain alterations related to mGluR5 alterations, it was impossible to conclude whether mGluR5 antagonism did anything to brain function and relate any such effect to clinical outcome. If EEG biomarker data from both the KO mice and the enrolled patients had been available, the extent to which they would have shown similar EEG alterations would have been informative (Ethridge et al., 2017; Wang et al., 2017; Lovelace et al., 2018). While is not yet clear if a pattern of EEG biomarkers reflects a mediator of the effect between mGluR5 antagonism and behavioral change, variable treatment response might be accounted for by those with a better clinical response in those who had abnormal biomarker values before treatment. This pattern may suggest a pathway for using an EEG biomarker for patient stratification or inclusion in future trials.

Further, if in humans, we were confident that the mGluR5 antagonist modified the biomarker in the same way that it did within the mouse model, industry leaders might be more willing to invest in finding out whether a meaningful clinical benefit requires longer treatment, inclusion of a specifiable subgroup of patients with the target syndrome and/or adjunctive behavioral treatment in future trials. Alternatively, no or very limited change in the EEG-based biomarker would argue against pursuing mGluR5 antagonism as a means of altering brain function, especially if there were additional data establishing that the full range of receptor occupancy of the antagonist had been explored using an appropriate positron emission tomography (PET) ligand.

These possibilities illustrate the multiple ways in which biomarkers might facilitate drug discovery programs. At a more rigorous standard, biomarkers validated as surrogate endpoints could reduce expense by identifying in early phase 2 studies the drugs unlikely to translate from mouse to human in a clinically effective manner. Imagine an EEG method that predicts or reports, with high sensitivity and specificity, successful modulation of the mGluR5 system within individuals with FXS. A conventional clinical trial using a single agent might require months of intervention before the robust behavioral or cognitive effects of the drug could be achieved. By contrast, a *sensitive,* validated marker of mGluR5 modulation could allow fast-fail testing of multiple drug candidates, eliminating those which fail to modulate mGluR5 in humans. The presence of target engagement, however, would not necessarily ensure that the compound could safely create the clinical outcomes of interest, but at least large-scale clinical trials could be focused on a biomarker determined dose range for testing drug efficiency.

While genetically homogenous disorders, such as FXS, have a "head start" in identifying mechanisms for targeted drug therapies, biomarkers can still be relevant for identifying processes to target given that behaviorally defined disorders given their often have diverse behavioral presentations indicating that factors beyond a specific genotype are at play. A theory of ASD which has been gaining traction over the last decade specifies that the behavioral phenotype results from an imbalance in inhibitory and excitatory (I/E) processes toward increased neural excitability (Rubenstein and Merzenich, 2003; Belmonte et al., 2004; Ajram et al., 2019). Belmonte et al. (2004) linked these findings with a cognitive model suggesting that decreased inhibition results in dysfunction of early attentional mechanisms and subsequent "overload" of later, capacity-limited processes. They proposed that such physiological-cognitive changes would result in a greater amplitude of event-related potentials (ERPs) captured during relevant tasks. If this could be established, one might select agents which facilitate inhibitory pathways using normalization of ERP amplitude as a read-out.

To date, successful development and validation of biomarkers has usually depend on demonstration of a relationship to some tissue pathology [e.g., plaques and tangles in Alzheimer's disease (AD)] or a robust functional measure that can be related to some pathological event (e.g., blood pressure and stroke). In the case of AD, before current biomarkers were developed, a definitive diagnosis depended on findings at autopsy. AD biomarkers, such as PET imaging and cerebro-spinal fluid (CSF) assays, are now established as sufficiently predictive of autopsy findings to serve as entry criteria in many clinical trials as well as providing a basis for new diagnostic criteria that included biomarkers (Jack et al., 2018; Veitch et al., 2019).

Advances in the mechanistic knowledge of NDD, even in the absence of known brain tissue pathologies, coupled with advances in EEG analysis technology, have raised the hope of identifying EEG-based biomarkers to increase the yield of clinical trials and ultimately enhance clinical care. The question arises as to whether EEG represents a good investment as a potential biomarker. This question is poorly posed, as EEG is a technology rather than a specific biomarker. An infinite number of parameters can be derived from the EEG signal in both task-locked and spontaneous recordings: time-domain evoked- and ERPs, spectral power, entropy, cross-frequency coupling, and a wide range of different connectivity metrics (Cohen, 2014). Each approach needs to be validated in each individual context (e.g., patient group, treatment) and will rise or fall in that context on its own merits. However, to answer the question as to whether EEG as a technology holds promise as a basis for biomarkers, one need only consider that EEG has been *the* technology *par excellence* (apart from the neurological exam and psychometric testing) for measuring CNS physiology in the clinical setting for the better part of a century. Not only clinical EEG, but somatosensory evoked potentials, motor evoked potentials, brainstem auditory evoked potentials and visual evoked potentials have had unparalleled tenure meeting the high bar of clinical validation.

The question at the current time is whether new EEG approaches will have the reproducibility (reliability) and discriminatory ability (validity) to serve a useful purpose in drug trials for NDD. In the best work to date, biomarker development and validation has taken cues from decades of experience with clinical test validation in the fields of psychometrics and clinical laboratory medicine (Lord, 1955). However, at the current stage of research progress, specific issues related to validation in the context of NDD and EEG are beginning to be grappled with. The vision is that biomarkers can fill a need for reducing uncertainty in clinical care and clinical trials. Poorly validated biomarkers, however, can be expensive and time-consuming wastes of subject and investigator time. To achieve success in biomarker development, it is important that biomarker validation proceed systematically and rigorously to establish utility/validity in the context of performing a specific function in order to be accepted by clinicians, the pharmaceutical industry, and the FDA and related agencies world-wide. With this background in mind, the primary goal of this manuscript is to identify conceptual, strategic and regulatory issues relevant to beginning the path toward valid biomarkers for behaviorally defined NDD and to propose solutions to the many obstacles to success.

Many things are regularly said about what we hope biomarkers will be able to do: that they will offer a highly specific index of one particular molecular or cognitive mechanism, that they can reframe our nosology in a more productive way, or that they will be able to transcend "squishy" outcome measures. We return to these commonly held beliefs over the course of the paper, but begin by offering a concrete definition of "biomarker" and "validation," in line with how clinical laboratory tests have long been validated. A biomarker is simply *a read-out that empirically provides an estimate of a reference test* (i.e., a previously established diagnostic determination or treatment outcome), under specific operating conditions (specific patient criteria, including age group, symptomatology and/or diagnoses; a specific intervention, where relevant; a specific function, such as prediction of response; and a specific machine and analysis pipeline). Validation establishes how good the estimate is (i.e., sensitivity and specificity. The requirements and logic of a validation study, specifically targeting EEG-based biomarkers, is covered elsewhere (Ewen and Beniczky, 2018), and necessary components *for diagnostic biomarkers* (but not other types of biomarkers relevant to clinical trials) are defined by the STARD checklist (Bossuyt et al., 2015).

A process similar to validation is *qualification,* which refers to a regulatory processes within FDA for judging the effectiveness of a set of biomarkers; it explicitly differs from validation in that qualified (and not only-validated) biomarkers need to be shown to function independently of the technology and precise procedures used (Califf, 2018; CDER Biomarker Qualification Program, 2019). The goal of the qualification process is to allow biomarkers to be used in clinical trials without regulatory endorsement of similar biomarkers individually within each new clinical trial. Validation and qualification differ in that validation occurs in the scientific literature using appropriate psychometric procedures, whereas qualification is currently achieved via consensus panels. For context, only 8 biomarker families have been qualified by FDA, and none for brain-based processes. In the case of AD, amyloid measures have not yet been qualified, despite being in widespread use.

The field has not yet progressed to the point where EEG-based biomarkers in NDD are being routinely validated, and it is informative to consider the "pre-validation" types of studies that are occurring currently (**Table 1**). We may call these studies *biomarker discovery.* Discovery includes two-groups comparisons of some physiological measure as a dependent variable, or the demonstration that a certain EEG measure correlates with a clinical measure within a patient group. Such studies do not inherently meet the rigorous requirements of validation studies for three reasons: (1) the demonstration of *group* differences in a dependent variable is a lower statistical bar than showing accurate classification at the *individual* level, (2) two-group studies often by design refine the clinical and especially the control samples, whereas validation studies face the more daunting task of classification using groups that encompass all of the real-world patient heterogeneity that will be faced by the clinical trialist or the clinician, and (3) validation studies require setting a threshold based on a "training sample" and replication in the form of a "test sample" (Ewen and Beniczky, 2018).

TABLE 1 | Types of Studies Related to Biomarker Development.

Study Type	Form	Implication
Biomarker Discovery	Two-group comparisons Correlation between physiological (EEG) measure and clinical variable Data-driven cluster identification Identification of EEG measure in which clinical group is in tail of normative distribution	*A priori* information to suggest that a physiological metric may be a promising candidate for validation
Biomarker Reliability	Test-retest measurement of biomarker read-out	Studies demonstrating poor reliability are adequate to exclude a biomarker candidate from further consideration.
Biomarker Validation	Data collection in training sample. Determination of optimal threshold. In test sample, calculation of sensitivity/specificity.	Adequately validated, a biomarker is ready for use *within the constrained context under which it was validated.*
FDA Biomarker Qualification	Similar to biomarker validation, but not limited to a single methodology or analysis pipeline	Allows the biomarker to be used in FDA studies without re-validation.
Establishing Biomarker as Tool for Measuring an Underlying Physiologic Process in Multiple Contexts	Not a study *per se*, but an accumulation of mechanistic and validation results for a single physiological metric under different contexts of use (COU), different disorders, different age groups and different therapeutic agents	Cross-linked knowledge that will allow us to propose, with some confidence, utility of the biomarker in an even greater range of applications

Another class of biomarker discovery study is data-driven identification of clusters within a particular physiological read-out (i.e., at the intermediate level of the biomarker). While such studies inherently work at the individual level and the overarching sample often contains a great deal of heterogeneity, these clusters are not of value until it has been shown that they are (1) replicable and (2) represent a clinically meaningful heterogeneity (e.g., predicting a response to a particular therapy). The empirical demonstration that data-driven clusters predict some clinically meaningful outcome is the work of validation, whereas the identification of the clusters in the first place is discovery. Efforts are underway and show promising results in neighboring fields. For example, data-driven "biotype" clusters have been identified in EEG and cognitive data in individuals with psychosis syndromes (Clementz et al., 2016). The groups were primarily differentiated using EEG data, with one group showing increased responsiveness to sensory input and increased intrinsic neurophysiological activity relative to healthy controls, and a second group showing reduced responsivity sensory input, reduced intrinsic activity and reduced cortical volumes relative to healthy controls. Inferential statistical tests, such as meaningful heterogeneity and mixture models (Anderberg, 1973; Pauler et al., 1996; Sun et al., 2018), can help establish whether these clusters are likely by chance. This step opens the door to determining whether membership in a cluster better predicts natural history and treatment responsiveness in individuals with psychosis than does clinical diagnostic categorization. In this instance, even if the EEG measure overlaps with normal functioning in some cases, and approximately 1/3 of patients do not show either pattern or difference from healthy controls on these measures, having high or low values might be predictive of response to one or another class of medications.

A related type of discovery study is one in which it is shown that some clinical group occupies the tail of a distribution of a normative sample, on some EEG metric. As with cluster analysis, these data would serve as preliminary evidence that the biomarker may index something of relevance to the clinical group, but it does not specify what the utility of this information may be. All of these biomarker discovery approaches generate potentially important motivation for biomarker validation, but they are insufficient in and of themselves.

Between biomarker discovery and biomarker validation lie *reliability studies,* which demonstrate that a particular biomarker (within a particular context) is reproducible (test-retest reliability) and insensitive to factors which we hope would not affect it, such as site or specific technologist (inter-rater reliability). Reliability studies, unlike validation studies, do not require demonstration that the biomarker candidate estimates the reference test (e.g., clinical outcome). While reliability is insufficient for validation, it is, however, *necessary:* reliability sets the mathematical ceiling for validity. Therefore a biomarker candidate can be efficiently excluded prior to a full validation study based solely on poor reliability. In a reliability study, two measurements can be take in the same day, whereas a validation study could take years to show that a biomarker measurement at the outset predicts an outcome years later. We argue it is this is the stage of development—assessment of reliability—where the field should currently have a focus of attention, both in terms of rapidly screening biomarker candidates as well as for establishing field-wide, empirically derived guidance. Some tentative proposals for steps in this direction are made in the final section of this paper.

On the other hand, going even beyond the level of knowledge required by validation studies, we also begin to imagine what it would take to develop biomarkers that are so well validated, in so many clinical groups and contexts that we can begin to understand them as a representation of a pathological mechanism, like cholesterol in heart disease or a blood sugar in diabetes mellitus. Such an outcome would require cross-linked knowledge and iterative studies (Woo et al., 2017)—both mechanistic and validation—that would transcend the "single-use" biomarker validation studies that form the core of the current discussion.

One crucial aspect this shift from discovery science to biomarker development efforts is to consider data at the individual participant rather than as group means. Biomarkers need to be applied to individuals, and their utility for some context of use needs to be established with such data to demonstrate prediction of outcome, dose optimization, etc. Data in discovery studies are rarely reported from individuals, and this limits existing literature in establishing promising parameters for consideration as targets for biomarker development in future studies. Individual data are also important for identifying cut points for decisions (increase dose, stratify for trials) and to examine distributions for a group of outliers from the range of healthy controls, or bimodality/discrete heterogeneity that would suggest subgroups that could be examined separately.

The goal of this manuscript is not to review the state-of-the-art in EEG-based biomarkers in NDD; several such reviews are in the recent literature (Wang et al., 2013; Takarae et al., 2016; Gurau et al., 2017). Our goal, rather, is twofold: in the first half, we dissect commonly held conceptual issues specific to NDD-focused and EEG-based biomarkers. Specifically, we discuss knowledge requirements for reliability and validation studies. We consider factors of heterogeneity/comorbidity, development and state/task performance.

In the second half of this manuscript, we argue for a strategic approach that includes academic, industry and governmental stakeholders (including NIH and FDA). We talk about the many significant advantages of EEG for biomarker development in NDD populations. We offer tentative reliability thresholds a promising biomarker should meet for it to be intensively studied and used for biomarker purposes. While the suggested criteria are preliminary and will evolve over time, we believe that they represent a good starting point, based on experience across fields, and highlight the need for operational standards. We argue that much research to date aiming to advance biomarkers of brain function has suffered from a lack of alignment on performance characteristics ("psychometrics") of the methods, the rare use of biomarkers in randomized clinical trials, especially in pediatric neuropsychiatry, and emphasis of grant funding on using technologies at hand to explore disease mechanisms. These latter studies often occur in the context of small single-site studies using "pure" samples with restricted recruitment criteria and novel neuroscience techniques. These studies are rarely followed by larger multi-site studies that take into account the heterogeneity and confounds encountered in typical clinical populations in order to validate measures as biomarkers for broad use. Large multisite studies can accelerate testing of a range of measures to select which provide information that is truly useful for a context of use, and to identify biologically distinct subgroups in behaviorally defined conditions. Such first steps are needed for biomarker discovery, but are insufficient toward validating biomarkers to improve clinical trials, enhance the replicability of studies of disease mechanisms and ultimately inform clinical practice for the general population. For years, the FDA has pointed out (Mullard, 2019) that consortia models are far more likely to succeed in developing data in support of biomarkers.

Criteria for Validation

As discussed above, the core of validation is the empirical demonstration that a biomarker performs its specified function at some criterion level. As such, only an empirical statistical relationship between biomarker and reference test is needed; no mechanistic knowledge is required. Indeed, some of the most widely ordered and demonstrably useful tests in the history of modern medicine are not supported by an understanding of how the test read-out relates to the pathophysiology of the disorder. The Westergren erythrocyte sedimentation rate (ESR or "sed rate") has been a widely utilized test in the care of patients with possible and actual inflammatory conditions, yet the rate at which red blood cells settle in test tubes is only indirectly related to the pathogenesis of those inflammatory conditions (**Figure 1**). We return to causal diagrams later, when envisioning sets of biomarkers that begin to transcend single applications.

While the process of EEG-based biomarker validation has been explicated elsewhere (Ewen and Beniczky, 2018), it may help to organize our thinking by considering four "ingredients": a specified EEG measure derived from the raw data; a context of use (COU), a reference test for comparison, and selection of population.

What to Measure

The EEG is a complex signal, and there is no end to the mathematical techniques that can be applied to it (Cohen, 2014). This poses the challenge of identifying which specific EEG measures and what specific behavioral paradigms from this infinite list stand the greatest chance of successfully proving valid for their intended purpose. Biomarker discovery studies, of the type laid out in the Introduction, identify potential biomarker candidates. Scientific studies of the pathogenesis of the disorder in question or the pharmacological mechanism of the proposed treatment also allow one to identify candidate biomarkers that seem most promising. Because EEG-based techniques are widely used as scientific tools in the study of NDD mechanisms both at the behavioral/cognitive and molecular/circuit levels, there is an active literature for first-stage evaluation of the most

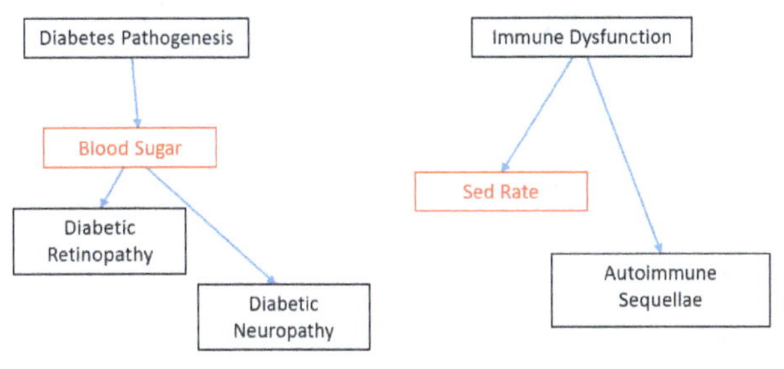

FIGURE 1 | Causal models of blood sugar used as a biomarker In diabetes and sed rate as a biomarker in autoimmune disorders. Biomarkers shown in red. Mechanistic knowledge is neither necessary nor sufficient for demonstrating validity of a biomarker candidate within a particular COU. However, because we know that blood sugar has a direct causal role on certain complications of diabetes, this knowledge opens up the reasonable possibility that blood sugar could be successfully validated as a surrogate biomarker as well as a diagnostic, pharmacodynamics/response and monitoring biomarker. By contrast, little It known about the relationship between sed rate, most used as a monitoring biomarker, and the causal path of clinical sequellae in autoimmune disorders. This absence of information does prohibit the sed rate from being validated as a diagnostic, response or monitoring biomarker; it simply means there is less *a priori* knowledge going into those validation studies.

disorder-relevant EEG measurements and paradigms that are biomarker candidates.

There may be a difference in how this step is approached in behaviorally defined disorders *vs.* genetically defined disorders, because of the "convergence point" of both the pathophysiology of the disorder as well as of therapies. Genetically defined disorders typically implicate a molecular pathway in their pathogenesis, and current-day efforts at treatment are often pharmacological, targeting the pathogenic pathway. The EEG biomarkers most tapped in an effort to specifically index these pathways tends to be low-level sensory responses, for which animal models provide extensive information about relevant neurophysiology and neurochemistry. Low-level sensory responses are biologically "closer" to molecular, cellular and circuit processes, and can also be performed on relevant animal models, facilitating direct translational application of testing and measurement procedures. A specific example and what is needed to advance it for some COU is provided later.

Behaviorally defined disorders, such as ASD, likely have multiple potential genetic, molecular and circuit deficits that all result in a more or less common cognitive deficit [though see also (Waterhouse et al., 2016)]. Because we cannot currently parse or subdivide the potential "lower level" causes, we are currently left with conceptualizing and managing the disorder on a cognitive level. The differential diagnosis (e.g., social-pragmatic language disorder, intellectual disability) is also defined at the cognitive level. The partially effective therapies for core symptoms to date are behavioral in nature, such as Applied Behavior Analysis (Lovaas, 1987). As a result, it seems reasonable that one would have the highest probability of validation success for a biomarker candidate that was designing on a cognitive intermediate phenotype, taking into account known and theorized factors about the specific disorder and intervention. The ERP paradigm involving looking at faces discussed later is an example involving observable and theorized aspects of ASD.

Task-related EEG measures have been a mainstay of experimental (cognitive) psychology and psychophysics for decades (Luck, 2014), parsing such models in both "health" and disorder. Therefore, we can leverage existing scientific tools from that literature for consideration as biomarker candidates. We are hesitant about the use of "out-of-the-box" paradigms to elicit certain ERP components *vs.* developing or selecting tools based on intended use and clinical considerations. For example, the P3 component (a/k/a P300) is elicited in oddball paradigms. Tasks can be designed, however, to elicit the P3 to specifically index stimulus discrimination effects (Patel and Azzam, 2005), expectancy effects (Wu and Zhou, 2009), contextual effects (Polich, 2007), memory recall effects (Fabiani et al., 1986), resource allocation effects (Kida et al., 2004), and processing efficiency effects (van Dinteren et al., 2014). A biomarker is more likely to be shown to be empirically valid if a task is designed that takes into account data and theory regarding the disorder under study, the cognitive endophenotype under study, as well as intended or known effects of the study therapy.

Additional EEG metrics and their corresponding constructs in neuroscience, such as cerebral connectivity (Vasa et al., 2016; O'Reilly et al., 2017), are currently under scientific investigation and could potentially serve as biomarker candidates in the future. This line of work is now widely used in the fMRI and EEG literature, but its use for biomarker purposes is largely unexplored.

Recording standards and procedures, and the analysis pipeline are also specified within this element. Multi-site studies such as the (ABC-CT) are taking the lead in developing rigorous standards. This effort follows in the footsteps of long-standing standards in clinical EEG (Sinha et al., 2016) and more recent guidelines in EEG-based research (Picton et al., 2000; Webb et al., 2015).

Context of Use

The second ingredient for validation is the COU. COU is FDA language for the specific *function* that the biomarker performs. FDA and NIH, in their "BEST" (Biomarkers, EndpointS and other Tools) collaboration (CDER Biomarker Qualification Program, 2019) define the multiple types of COU and are critical for preparation for FDA qualification (**Table 2**).

This manuscript focuses on prospective biomarkers in clinical trials. There are some preliminary efforts at diagnostic biomarkers for clinical care in NDD (Loo et al., 2013; Snyder et al., 2015; Ewen, 2016; Gloss et al., 2016). There is at least one prognostic, EEG-based biomarker used in NDD, beyond clinical EEG interpretation: infants born with a port-wine birthmark (PWB) have around a 25% probability of going on to develop the brain involvement that is definitional to Sturge-Weber syndrome (SWS). The use of a quantitative EEG metric, based on a measure validated to measure ischemia during carotid endarterectomy (van Putten et al., 2004), prognosticates which infants are at higher risk and is less expensive and invasive than using MRI (risks associated with sedation and gadolinium contrast administration) and possibly an earlier biomarker, given the rates of MRI false negatives in the first year of life (Hatfield et al., 2007; Ewen et al., 2009).

While a particular method or read-out may eventually be shown to function validly in multiple COU, a single validation study reports on performance only within a single COU.

TABLE 2 | FDA Biomarker Contexts of Use (COU).

COU	Description
Diagnostic	Concurrent biomarker that specifies whether or not an individual has a disorder/pathologic process
Monitoring	Concurrent biomarker that concurrently reflects a change in a disease or in a side effect
Safety	Concurrent biomarker that reflects presence/degree of toxicity from an exposure
Response	Prospective biomarker that reflects a response to an intervention; when highly well validated, may serve as a *surrogate endpoint* in a clinical trial
Prognostic	Prospective biomarker that predicts clinical course
Predictive	Prospective biomarker that predicts response to an intervention
Susceptibility/Risk	Prospective biomarker that reflects potential for developing or disease sensitivity to a negative outcome following an exposure

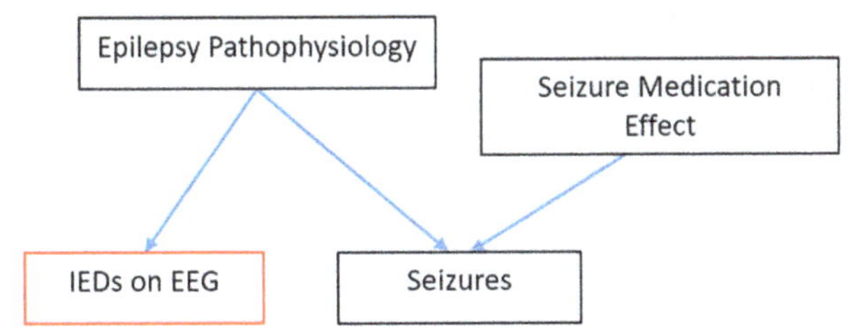

FIGURE 2 | EEG finding can be a good diagnostic biomarker while being a poor monitoring biomarker in epilepsy. In this causal model, IEDs follow from the pathophysiology that causes seizures but are upstream to the effect of seizure medications.

Successful performance in one COU does not guarantee adequate performance in another COU (**Figure 2**). For example, a valid and useful diagnostic biomarker may not be an effective response biomarker. An example from current clinical practice: if a patient is suspected of having epilepsy, we often perform an EEG to look for inter-ictal epileptiform discharges (IEDs)—spikes and sharp waves which indicate an increased likelihood that the spells are epileptic, rather than some non-epileptic "mimic." IEDs on EEG, while imperfect, are a clinically useful diagnostic biomarker. If our example patient is then diagnosed with epilepsy, the goal of treatment is to reduce or eliminate the seizures. In the process, some seizure medications also normalize the EEG (suppress IEDs), but others effectively reduce seizures without minimizing or eliminating IEDs on EEG. IEDs on EEG, then, are a good *diagnostic biomarker*, but they are a poor *monitoring biomarker* for patients treated with non-spike-suppressing anti-seizure medications.

As the field develops, we can envision biomarkers that have been validated in multiple COUs, and paired with progress in the understanding of how lower-level mechanisms produce the biomarker read-out (**Table 1**). Imagine an EEG-based biomarker that is similar to blood sugar (**Figure 1**). Blood sugar has been validated as diagnostic marker for diabetes mellitus. Because we understand how high blood sugar plays a pathogenic, causal role in the complications associated with diabetes, we can we can propose with confidence (and subsequently validate) blood sugar not only as a diagnostic biomarker, but also as a monitoring biomarker. This link would not be true if blood sugar were only a peripheral, epiphenomenological read-out. This mechanistic knowledge can also motivate novel therapeutics (e.g., those which control blood sugar) and subsequently serve as a pharmacodynamics/response biomarker or even surrogate endpoint for this new therapy. However, despite this mechanistic knowledge, sensitivity/specificity need to be calculated separately in each COU (validation). The number of EEG read-outs tightly linked to lower-level mechanisms is small. One auditory ERP paradigm is tentatively becoming linked to a LTP-like mechanism, with systematic studies that showing it is sensitive to the same experimental manipulations as LTP in mouse models (Clapp et al., 2012). If one were to conduct a clinical trial of a drug that is known to affect LTP in animal models and whose mechanism of action to benefit the patient is through modulation of LTP, then using this LTP-sensitive ERP biomarker may give at least some *a priori* confidence that the biomarker will predict or track the efficacy of the therapy.

Reference Test

The third element of the validation "equation" is a *de facto* reference test or reference standard, in the terminology of clinical test validation (Bossuyt et al., 2015). Reference standards are often referred to as representing "ground truth" or the "gold standard." A validation study outputs the sensitivity and specificity with which the biomarker ("index test") estimates the reference test. The COUs most relevant to clinical trials are the prospective COU: *prognostic* biomarkers (for enrichment in prevention trials), *predictive* biomarkers (for stratifying based on expected sensitivity to treatment), and *risk* biomarkers (for exclusion based on anticipated risk). The value added by the novel biomarker is that it reports earlier than the reference test. The reference standard may therefore be a relatively simple outcome measure, such as a clinical global impression (CGI).

It seems self-evident that sensitivity and specificity can only be calculated relative to some "gold standard." The reason we make a point of it is in response to an oft repeated hope that a novel biomarker can transcend the limitations of a noisy or subjective reference test, such as the CGI. This hope may be founded in cases where a biomarker is so well validated in multiple contexts, disorders and therapies that it is a proven, faithful representation of a particular mechanism (**Table 1**; Woo et al., 2017). However, in the case of "single-use" validation studies, it is logically impossible to demonstrate that a novel biomarker is "better" than the reference test against which it is being compared, since it is impossible to disambiguate the uncertainty associated with the novel biomarker from the uncertainty associated with the reference test; this is analogous to being unable to solve a single equation with two unknowns in algebra. Imagine if we had a EEG biomarker which was shown to predict outcome on therapy 12 months before the CGI demonstrated that outcome. There would be some individuals in whom the two tests disagreed. If we took the position that the EEG predictive biomarker were "more correct" than the "squishy" CGI, what data that is "even more true" than the CGI reference test could we even use to demonstrate this was so?

The relationship between biomarker candidates and *concurrent biomarker* reference standards is a bit more complex and will not be fully discussed here. Put briefly, the motivation for developing a new biomarker to substitute for or complement an existing concurrent reference test is because the newer biomarker is less expensive, easier to perform or is less invasive than the biomarker it will replace. Moreover, special issues pertain to reference standards for concurrent COUs specifically in behaviorally defined NDD, and diagnostic biomarkers in particular. However, it is worth mentioning that potential advances in reframing our current diagnostic paradigms to be more in line with evolving therapies could be made via predictive biomarkers. Responsiveness to Intervention (RTI) diagnostic approaches have been used in the context of academic interventions for specific learning disabilities (Ewen and Shapiro, 2008). Because a patient with a NDD may eventually be prescribed both pharmacological and behavioral/cognitive therapies, an RTI framework may be multiaxial and contain multiple, parallel frameworks, one for each of the types of therapy.

Selection of Population

The fourth element of the validation "equation" is the selection of the population to be studied (i.e., inclusion/exclusion criteria for the validation study and also patients on whom the biomarker can be validly used in clinical practice or trials). These same inclusion/exclusion criteria and sampling scheme that define the participants/patients for which the biomarker can be validly used in eventual clinical trials or clinical practice. Because we are limiting our discussion primarily to biomarkers which are validated prospectively (prognostic, predictive, and risk COUs), only one group will be recruited; considerations about appropriate comparison groups for validated biomarkers with concurrent reference standards (e.g., diagnostic COU) are not relevant here.

Heterogeneity is a potential confound in validation studies that is well recognized in the study of behaviorally defined NDD as well as across neuropsychiatry generally. Aspects of heterogeneity include ranges of severity of core features, presence/absence of non-core but highly penetrant features (e.g., motor dysfunction in ASD) and the presence of comorbidities (e.g., Axis I psychiatric comorbidities). When considering the impact of heterogeneity on biomarker validation, the first point is to restate that a particular biomarker is only valid in implementation for the inclusion/exclusion criteria under which it was validated. While mechanistic science typically seeks "pure" samples to reduce the effect of confounds, biomarkers for advancing drug discovery typically need to seek study participants with more diverse ecological heterogeneity. This heterogeneity then is "baked into" the sensitivity and specificity estimates, which are the end result of validation. Because of this, biomarker studies need to include more messy heterogeneity than projects primarily interested in disease mechanism.

It is possible, however, to improve on gross sensitivity/specificity estimates derived from binary biomarker outcomes by including additional terms in a more complex predictive model. Such terms may and generally should include age, gender, intelligence, duration of symptoms and psychiatric comorbidities in the case of NDDs; the choice of terms will depend on existing knowledge and mechanistic hypotheses about how these factors could influence the biomarker output, but machine learning can readily accommodate such data, given adequate sample size. An interaction term may be critical. Anxiety, for example, may manifest and be due to different mechanisms when co-occurring with ASD *vs.* when occurring in individuals without ASD (Rosen et al., 2018). As a consequence, if one tries to control for a psychiatric comorbidity in a NDD biomarker, it is important to study the biomarker in a 2 × 2 contrast (NDD, psychiatric diagnosis), and to use interaction terms in the predictive model. Similarly, if we hope to account for the effect of medication on the EEG dependent variable, such effects need to be studied both independently and within the context of the disorder of interest.

Certain confounds will require exclusion, such as inadequate visual, auditory or motor function to participate in the biomarker data collection (Picton et al., 2000).

Development represents a special case of a confound. We know that many both resting state EEG measures and ERPs vary over the course of development (Tome et al., 2015; Eberhard-Moscicka et al., 2016). While the inclusion/exclusion criteria define the relevant potential patients for biomarker use, *a priori* knowledge about development in neurotypical subjects may itself indicate a need to limit use of a given biomarker only to a relatively narrow age group that does not have significant changes in the EEG dependent variable, or to carefully define developmental progression prior to broad biomarker implementation.

Most biomarker dependent variables represent a measurement at a single point in time. *Monitoring COU* biomarkers, by contrast, measure changes over time. Measurements of such changes will be influenced by test-retest variability, typical developmental changes over long follow-up periods and intervention-related changes. Control measurements over a variety of time courses are necessary to quantify test-retest variability and typical developmental changes for specific COU. There is also, in principle, no reason that diagnostic biomarkers could not be defined by trajectories over time, rather than by point measurements, or that predictive biomarkers showing a small response to a brief treatment challenge could not validly predict a larger response to a longer treatment.

At the current stage of development, most EEG-based biomarker candidates for NDD have only begun to be systematically evaluated for biomarker use. Research efforts typically have focused on a specified age group, in the context of a single disorder, a single therapy (where relevant), and a single specific assay/analysis pipeline – often focused much more on mechanistic science than practical use of measurement for applied biomarker purposes. The latter requires focus on casewise data, utility for prediction or classification, and optimal thresholds for decision making. As we move toward biomarker families that index an important mechanism across multiple conditions, COUs and age groups, we may develop *normative data*. Such studies, as in the field of psychometrics, will require large, heterogeneous groups with random sampling, with sample sizes dependent on the relevant variance (reliability) and effect sizes in the groups.

Analytic Approach for Reliability and Validity

Reliability is a precondition for validity. Said another way, it is impossible to detect a meaningful change if the metric varies randomly in the absence of a substantive change of the process that is being measured. Reliability is a metric that is internal to the biomarker itself and does not need to be compared with the reference standard (in fact, the reference standard is taken to be a scalar and not a probability distribution, therefore a reference standard does not have reliability *per se*). Reliability can, however, be compared with that of other, competing biomarkers. Because measurement error and reliable effect size have an inverse relationship, smaller changes can be detected in a measure that has greater reliability. When clinicians or trialists hope that an EEG biomarker will be "less subjective" than, say, parent report, it is increased reliability that they are to a large extent seeking. Because reliability of a certain effect size is necessary for validity at that effect size, it is possible to exclude a biomarker candidate if the reliability is lower than an acceptable threshold. Specific recommendations for EEG-based biomarkers in NDD will be made in the next section.

Validity: Many of the clinical electrophysiological tests that have been used in practice for decades have had extremely high sensitivity (like 3 Hz spike-wave for absence epilepsy) or have been definitionally related to their clinical syndrome (Trisomy 21). We cannot assume that current day biomarker candidates, considered in isolation, will have such robustness for syndromal neurodevelopmental disorders, and we need statistical approaches to deal with this reality.

Most analytic approaches for validation have a pipeline of continuous data, binarized data and probabilities. Validation studies require the recruitment of two participant samples with identical inclusion/exclusion criteria: the training set and the test set. Within a training set, continuous data (e.g., ERP amplitude) is collected for subjects in each group; in the case of prospective (prognostic, predictive and risk) biomarkers, group status is assigned retrospectively (good *vs.* bad outcome). receiver operator curves (ROC) allow the break point to be set at a preferred sensitivity/specificity trade-off. The second sample, the test sample, then has the same procedures run, with the same EEG metric, same procedures, same reference standard and same inclusion/exclusion criteria. On this test sample data, the data are binarized via the threshold determined using the training sample, and the true sensitivity and specificity are computed as probabilities. These sensitivities and specificities explicate the uncertainty with which the biomarker estimates the reference standard and serve as the culmination of the validation process.

Criteria for judging minimal data quality standards for a particular set of data from a particular patient/participant to be considered "valid" also need to be explicated within the training sample stage, both from EEG data quality as well as from behavioral performance on any task under which the EEG is recorded.

Biomarkers may be judged not only by their sensitivity and specificity, but by their cost, availability, invasiveness, ease of deployment (including training requirements for staff), rate of data loss to artifact/non-compliance and ability to be tolerated by patients. These considerations can often help decide between two biomarker technologies as most likely to be most efficient for clinical and trial needs. Compared with fMRI, EEG is less sensitive to motion because the electrodes move with the head, and it is far less expensive, therefore more widely available.

State-, Performance- and Noise-Related Confounds

A variety of confounds commonly encountered in individuals with NDD and in EEG metrics can create problems of variance (reliability) and bias (specificity and subsequently validity). Cognitive electrophysiology biomarkers can be sensitive to processes that are outside the causal chain of (epiphenomenological to) the biological mechanism that is the focus of study—processes which can differ between systematically less- and more-severely affected individuals or

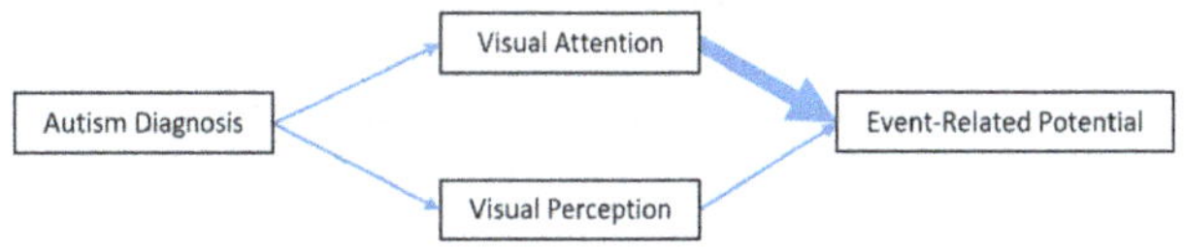

FIGURE 3 | Confounded measure intended to index visual perception. In this example relevant to a diagnostic biomarker, a specific form of Visual Perception alteration is understood to be a consequence of ASD and is intended to be indexed by the Event-Related Potential (ERP). However, Visual Attention (such as looking at the stimulus display) is both necessary for task performance and is also systematically different between the ASD group and the control group. In this example, Visual Attention has a bigger impact on the ERP dependent variably (heavy arrow) than does the Visual Perception ability, and therefore confounds the interpretation of the ERP read-out as a valid measure of Visual Perception.

treatment responders and non-responders. In the example of **Figure 3**, the ERP read-out as a valid measure of a particular visual processing mechanism is confounded by a visual attention capacity which is systematically different between groups.

There are at least three approaches to minimizing the effect of artifact and other confounds: utilizing measures insensitive to the artifact generator, using signal processing methods to remove the artifact, and controlling statistically for artifact. The optimal solution is to use electrophysiological metrics which are relatively insensitive to these confounds. For example, the mismatch negativity (MMN) ERP component is minimally sensitive to attention, whereas the P3 component is highly dependent on attention. Auditory perception does not require the orienting of sensory organs in the way that vision does, and therefore auditory tasks may be preferable when testing children who are less able to follow task instructions. EEG and magnetoencephalography (MEG) are silent, making them preferable to fMRI for auditory tasks, and especially for patients with auditory hypersensitivity.

It is critical to study these metrics explicitly in terms of their sensitivity to confounds. A poignant example comes from the fMRI literature, in which it was learned that motion artifact (Power et al., 2012) leads to spurious changes in connectivity measures, which subsequently led to a substantial portion of ASD connectivity literature being called into question (Vasa et al., 2016). Muscle artifact can be a similar issue in EEG studies. When a particular target mechanism or confound is not amenable to direct control, an alternative is to try to equate participant state during individual trials as much as possible. For example, eye tracking can be used to trigger stimulus presentation only when a participant is looking at the screen (Varcin et al., 2016). Behavioral psychological preparation and management during testing can help equate task engagement in a way that is often not directly quantifiable (Paasch et al., 2012). When the EEG biomarker is collected in the context of a psychophysical task, it may be possible to use a staircase method to equate subjects on task performance, to eliminate measured differences that may be due to performance-related mechanisms and not diagnosis-related mechanisms. Parametric studies across a wide range of task difficult are another strategy for dealing with this issue, as it allows brain activity to be modeled across a range of task performance quality.

A final method to control for state/performance confounds is to record behavioral variables during the task and to adjust statistically. In some cases, the behaviors quantified are subjective (e.g., behavioral aide impression of participant engagement); in other cases, they are objective (e.g., reaction times and error rates to the psychophysical task being recorded). Control conditions in psychophysical tasks may help in controlling statistically for confounding processes. There is an added benefit by contrasting conditions within a subject, that any within-subject error term that is common to two conditions is eliminated (Webb et al., 2015).

The number of trials excluded for behavioral (not attended, incorrect task response) and EEG-signal-quality reasons also needs to be tracked, at the very least to make a judgment about which subjects are judged to have inadequate data, invalidating the use of the biomarker for that particular testing session. The same objective criteria for excluding a subject's data need to be employed both during the biomarker validation study and when the biomarker is eventually used in clinical trials or clinical practice, which involves objective, rules-based definition of acceptable data *a priori*.

Electrophysiology signal quality may differ between groups for reasons that are not clearly known and may not be related to the processes that the biomarker is intended to index (Butler et al., 2017). Additional signal quality metrics are on the horizon. In the meanwhile, it should be pointed out that biomarker studies and mechanistic studies differ in terms of how they are impacted by unaddressed confounds. In mechanistic or treatment studies, where the end result is a binary conclusion (groups do or do not differ in a certain regard), confounds may bias toward a Type I or Type II error. In biomarker studies, the end result is not binary, but statistical measure of uncertainty (sensitivity, specificity), and uncontrolled confounds may simply result in poorer sensitivities and specificities than would otherwise be the cases (assuming random sampling). In some instances, the confounds make the biomarker. The ADHD200 competition was an attempt to discover and validate a fMRI-based diagnostic biomarker for ADHD—and the head-movement variable turned out to be the key predictor (Eloyan et al., 2012)!

Epilepsy, which has increased in recognized prevalence in ASD (Spence and Schneider, 2009; Ewen et al., 2019) and many other NDDs, presents several confounds. First, frank seizures can affect both consciousness/the ability to make volitional responses as well as the EEG tracing. One would suspect that most perceptual/cognitive/motor biomarkers would not be reliable in patients actively having seizures during the recording. The role that IEDs have in alterations of consciousness in the absence of clinical seizures is controversial (Landi et al., 2018). However, patients who have epilepsy but who are not actively seizing also have IEDs in their EEGs (Fisher and Lowenbach, 1934; Gibbs et al., 1935). The extent to which these inter-ictal EEG changes affect (bias) any particular EEG analysis method is an empiric question. Perhaps surprisingly, Key et al. were able to obtain similar ERP waveforms with a similar number of trials from controls and children with Angelman syndrome—a disorder which is known to cause extreme abnormalities of both background oscillatory activity as well as the frequent presence of IEDs, since the IEDs and oscillations are not consistently phase-locked to the stimulus and were therefore canceled out in time-locked averaging. It is probable that spectral (frequency-domain) measurements would be more affected than ERPs in Angelman syndrome. On the other hand, while working on this very manuscript, one of the authors' (JBE) labs recorded an ERP study in a participant with epilepsy who had IEDs time-locked to and apparently evoked by an auditory stimulus; these focal sharp waves confounded the ERP waveform in certain channels.

In summary, researchers and clinicians desire predictive, prognostic and risk biomarkers to provide an indication of efficacy or side effect earlier than would otherwise be possible, thus making clinical trials more efficient and potentially reframing diagnosis to an intermediate phenotype more tightly related to effective treatments. These biomarkers can also help stratify patients to increase effective power in clinical trials, using the same sample size. While few biomarker candidates are on the horizon for full validation, the simpler assessment of reliability may help cull the heard of candidates. Mechanistic knowledge is not formally required for validation but has the potential to link validated biomarkers to new COUs and can help investigators predict and mitigate certain confounds.

Developing Paths Forward for EEG-Based Biomarkers in NDDs

As noted earlier, the FDA process, which endorses some specific COU for biomarker qualification, does not have explicitly published requirements. Nor for the broader field is there alignment as to the level of evidence required to judge a biomarker as both sufficiently validated and robust to justify decision making in any interventional study. In order for a biomarker to be used as an inclusion criteria or early intermediate outcome measure, cut off points for decision making need to be specified. And when using a cut-off value in an individual for such uses one wants to have as much confidence as possible that the value truly represents a characteristic of that individual which is potentially relevant to treatment and not due to other sources of variation. In the absence of any EEG based biomarker embraced as likely to currently serve such a role, an initial step in recommending a path forward is to identify gaps in approaches taken to date.

Performance characteristics of single analyte biomarkers in a biofluid such as serum cholesterol are much more straightforward to establish—e.g., standard tube type and processing of sample prior to determination of concentration with clinical laboratory improvement amendments (CLIA) standards in place to provide confidence in reported values—than any functional EEG measure. The wide range of factors that can affect EEG data have been spelled out in the preceding section. Clinical EEG societies specify minimal technical standards (Sinha et al., 2016), and research ERP standards have been published in cognitive psychology broadly (Picton et al., 2000) and for ASD specifically (Webb et al., 2015), but these are not at the level of CLIA standards. It remains to be seen whether they are sufficient for purposes of biomarker qualification and validation or are even followed by most investigators. Given that fMRI-based biomarkers are the other major functional brain measure being pursued in syndromal CNS disorders, we refer the reader to recent reviews of the various roles of fMRI as a functional brain measure applied to drug development (Woo et al., 2017; Carmichael et al., 2018), since these highlight many parallel issues to those arising with EEG. fMRI and EEG though provide very different information. While fMRI provides whole brain coverage and far superior source resolution, the superior temporal resolution of EEG (~1000Hz *vs.* 1Hz for fMRI) provides a far better characterization of the dynamic interaction of cortical regions and latencies of brain responses, and the biological meaning of frequency information is much clearer than are oscillations in fMRI BOLD signals.

Typical gaps in EEG biomarker development efforts result from a failure to study a sufficiently large and representative slice of the population for which it is ultimately intended. Most preliminary studies of a novel biomarker candidate focus on some small (less than 25 subjects) rarified patient group accessible to a single site and a completely asymptomatic healthy-control group. As a corollary, studies in special populations at sites with staff enthusiastic about and committed to the measure may convey an overly optimistic sense of what percentage of participants can comply with the biomarker procedure and return valid data. This consideration is particularly critical in EEG-based tests for children with neurodevelopmental disabilities (NDD). Task-based EEG measures, particularly those which require behavioral responses in addition to the EEG data collection, set a higher bar for participant compliance than do spontaneous ("resting-state") metrics.

Differing EEG data-cleaning and processing pipelines are used by different investigators, and it is not clear whether these differences account for differences in reported values and biomarker utility. Variability also occurs because many EEG measures are sensitive to subject state: drowsiness/level of alertness, effortful cooperativeness and degree of relaxation—so how such variables are controlled needs to be clearly defined for reproducibility. There is also a potential impact of duration of testing, as these factors may become increasingly relevant with longer testing of NDD patients.

At its core, validation requires an evaluation of sensitivity and specificity which are in turn limited by the test-retest reliability for which precise estimates, especially across sites, requires methodologic studies. Ideally, everything relevant to having confidence in reported values should be addressed in the methods section of reports. Fundamental research is needed to investigate explicitly the impact of technical and analytical differences. While equipment manufacturer is assumed to play a far smaller role in EEG output than in fMRI, it would be helpful to know to what extent different EEG amplifiers produce meaningfully different results. Questions also arise about whether activity should be averaged over a prespecified set of electrodes to increase reproducibility, *vs.* selecting electrodes on an individual patient level (through some principled basis) in hopes of increasing SNR. Studies to consider different behavioral test paradigms and different data analytic approaches are thus a crucial part of EEG biomarker development.

In the context of these considerations, performance thresholds or targets for biomarkers likely to be adequate for use in trials and/or qualification by the FDA will need to be refined iteratively with experience. As a starting point, we propose explicit (albeit preliminary) criteria which we hope will drive forward EEG-based biomarker development for drug discovery. To illustrate why we believe that target criteria might be helpful, and to provide and critique examples of biomarker development approaches, we next consider examples from three different classes of EEG based studies—resting-state EEG, ERP to a sensory stimulus anchored in neural systems research, and ERP to a more complex stimulus derived from psychological models and clinical observations.

We start with consideration of resting state EEG studies, using a recent review of relevant published studies in ASD published between 1980–2016 (Gurau et al., 2017). Their summary is instructive with regard to what might be required to nail down an EEG measure as a biomarker at the individual level. All reviewed case-control studies reported some, but not the same, differences between ASD and control subjects. The review considered studies of potential diagnostic biomarkers and efforts to identify pathophysiologic subgroups. The greatest number of studies focused on spectral analysis as a potential diagnostic index with four out of 21 reporting a directionally similar finding as interpreted by Gurau et al. (2017). They concluded that, despite inconsistencies, some generalizations could be inferred. Significant differences in the alpha band were shown by five studies with relaxed eyes open condition. Four studies showed a decrease in absolute alpha spectral power in ASD in children of similar ages, but another showed elevated absolute alpha power in adults. Inspection of the cited studies reveal that even a common finding of "decrease in absolute spectral power" is unclear because absolute spectral power was not presented in each paper.

Specifically, selecting the only two studies among the four with supposedly common findings that included an ASD group of more than 25 subjects, one reports lower relative (not absolute) alpha power calculated from channels T3 + T6 + C3 + F4 (selected by stepwise discriminant-function analysis) (Chan et al., 2007) whereas another study used retrospective clinical recordings from a 10 year period (2001–2011) to look for differences in recordings from subjects diagnosed as ASD (children 4–8 years old). The control group was based on selecting EEGs that had been read as normal in same age children over the same period who based on chart review were free of any NDD although the reasons for EEGs having been done were not specified. This later study reported a lower ratio of posterior to anterior alpha power (Matlis et al., 2015). Relative advantages of examining absolute and relative power in a particular frequency bandwidth require empirical study.

At the current exploratory stage of the development of EEG biomarkers, investigators appear to be operating with the dual aim of discovery neuroscience and a secondary goal of finding or generating data suggestive that there might be something worth following as a biomarker. But from the vantage point of looking for biomarkers that might be informative at an individual level, for predicting something of clinical importance about a specific person, small, site-specific studies with varying analytic approaches and specific outcome measures make it difficult to select parameters to pursue for biomarker development with confidence. Developing such confidence will require multisite studies (using coordinated recruitment or at least some set of overlapping data) using common (standardized) measures that allow not only for apples to apples comparisons of results across sites but also, ideally, allowing for aggregation of data into common databases.

As an example of a systems neuroscience-based sensory ERP study, a recent study utilized an EEG measure that can applied across a genetic mouse model of a disorder and in patients with the disorder utilizing an ingenious aural chirp stimulus. To evaluate the ability of the brain to generate robust oscillatory responses across a 1–100 Hz frequency range, they evaluated neural synchronization across this range to an auditory stimulus oscillating from low to high frequency in the 1–100 Hz frequency range band. Deficits were detectable in the gamma frequency range in FXS patients (Ethridge et al., 2017) as they were later observed in fMR1 KO mice (Lovelace et al., 2018). The human study was a single site study in 17 subjects with full mutation FXS individuals (age range 13–57 of whom 4 were female) and 17 age/gender matched controls. Obviously, issues of potential age and gender effects would ultimately need to be addressed as well as what is usually required to move from a single site study in a small number of individuals to a broader population in diverse settings. Such issues will be partially resolved in the ongoing multisite NeuroNEXT study of the Novartis mGluR5 negative allosteric modulator AFQ056.

The investigators used an analytic approach including PCA-weighted un-baseline-corrected epoched single-trial data to generate single-trial power (STP) metrics which revealed decreased gamma band phase-locking to the chirp stimulus in FXS individuals. Interestingly, there were elevations of baseline gamma power in FXS *vs.* control subjects before, during and after chirp presentation as in fMR1 KO mice. This raises the question of what additional information is provided by the STP measure of the ability to synchronize neural oscillations to the frequency of the auditory stimulus relative to information provided by increased baseline gamma power from a predictive biomarker perspective, given the observed correlation between elevated baseline gamma power values and the reduced entrainment of gamma band activity to the chirp stimulus.

To advance these measures as potential biomarkers, one might begin with examining whether the two measures (baseline resting-state gamma-power and gamma-band STP to chirp) met a criteria of 90% test-retest reliability on the same day and over longer periods. A second issue is the examination of distributional characteristics of these alterations, such as whether there is a subgroup of highly deviant outliers or bimodality with discrete subgroups. This is needed to get a sense of the distribution of values at the individual level, something not provided by group-level heat-maps that displayed log power at neural oscillation frequencies over time (ms). To move from discovery science to establishing the promise and utility of the measures as biomarkers for advancing drug discovery, future studies will need to establish clinical relevance and study larger groups to reasonably estimate parameter distributions and ROC curves for the different metrics examined. Optimal electrodes to use for this work would also need to be formally determined and validated to maximize the signal to noise ratio of data in a consistent way across laboratories for individual study participants.

The third example considers ERP response to a psychological stimulus in studies of ASD. A recent meta-analysis of 23 studies (374 participants) established the finding of delayed N170 response to face stimuli in individuals with ASD (Kang et al., 2018). The N170 is a negative-going change in the ERP waveform that peaks approximately 170ms after stimulus presentation. In healthy individuals, it is larger in amplitude and shorter in latency to faces in comparison with responses to inanimate objects. As such, it is presumed to reflect neural activity associated with early-stage face processing, and believed to reflect aspects of social cognition. Overall deficits in N170 ERP amplitudes were not seen, but amplitudes were reduced in adults and those with higher cognitive ability relative to matched typically developing controls. Only 3 of the studies involved at least 25 subjects per group and the review utilized effect sizes of group differences calculated from each study. The extent to which the specific latencies or amplitudes did or did not align across studies is not addressed in the review and difficult to extract from the actual papers given differences in the details of the paradigms employed.

Neural indices of face processing are of interest as candidate biomarkers for social processes in ASD, and build on an extensive psychological literature linking face perception to social process in typically developing (TD) individuals and in ASD (Bublatzky et al., 2017; Webb et al., 2017). While overall effects are promising at the group level, potential limitations of this line of work include: (1) some non-confirming reports in the literature, (2) uncertainty about how much this deficit relates to early-stage visual system disturbances *vs.* later perceptual analysis of faces, (3) uncertainty about whether or how the effect is related to affective response to faces *vs.* a disturbance in the perceptual ability to process face information, (4) uncertainty about whether an index of this nature will separate subtypes of patients for stratification purposes or provide a dimensional/objective measure of a core behavioral trait in ASD with which the EEG measure is correlated—and therefore the additional information provided by the EEG metric, (5) the neural and cognitive implications of a delayed N170 component that is not reduced in amplitude remain to be fully elucidated, and (6) psychometric properties (reliability and validity) of the latency and amplitude measures with regard to establishing potential cut-off points at the individual level continue to be developed. Several of these issues are being addressed by the ongoing Autism Biomarkers Consortium for Clinical Trials (ABC-CT) study, a US-based multisite effort to identify biomarkers to support intervention research in autism (McPartland, 2016, 2017).

The study of N170 in ASD is rooted in psychological models and behavioral observations, and has the advantages of a relatively strong supporting literature and face-valid clinical relevance. The approach also has potential limitations, including limited potential for translational integration and limited clarity of neurobiological implications beyond localization of effect to particular areas of neocortex to be informative at a level that could provide direct rational link to drug targets. The reduced N170 latency in ASD is of interest in its own right, but the comparison to our auditory chirp example highlights the relative development, strengths and limitations of psychologically rooted and neurobiologically rooted approaches for developing EEG biomarkers for advancing drug discovery. Clarifying and maximally utilizing the relative advantages of these approaches for developing EEG biomarkers for neurodevelopmental disorders remains an important and relatively uncharted direction for future research.

What might represent a sufficient degree of standardization and what level of "assay" performance would one be looking for to rule a measure in or out as a usual biomarker for some specified COU? For any functional brain measure such as EEG, with many potential variables both as regards acquisition paradigms including number of channels and analytic approaches, the suitability of a range of approaches for different COU will require extensive evaluation. One would expect that approaches could be compared in later stage developmental efforts prior to large-scale validation. That does not mean, however, that it is not possible to specify some common practices that will allow the field to be more confident that the raw data generated at different sites does or does not replicate (same values, not simply directionally similar case-control differences). Multivariable development studies can ideally contrast distributional properties and differential utility in a COU of different EEG measures, and examine their relation to age and developmental state of the brain. This would allow for addressing questions of whether a biomarker can be informative at the individual level, which is crucial for their applied use. For that purpose, we suggest preliminary thresholds for promising biomarkers:

1. Deployable in >80% of patients administered by technician level staff outside of a CNS research center
2. Reproducible value of a specific EEG measurements within individual at ±7.5%, if tested within the same acquisition period
3. Day to day stability within an individual at ±10% in absence of change in clinical condition, treatment and environmental factors; stability week to week within ±15%
4. Evidence that different sites can achieve values in the same individual within 15% of each other (traveling subject approach) and generate mean value for a control group of 12 subjects within 10%
5. Normative data that allows for correction of data for any significant effects of age, gender, educational status or intellectual capacity that might influence measurement of an EEG biomarker

While reliability thresholds mathematically depend on effect sizes, many of these specific proposed degrees of variation of a variable within an individual reflect the experience of one of the authors (WZP) in terms of assumptions that go into powering of studies to assess the utility of potential biomarkers carried out within the Biomarkers Consortium of the Foundation of the National Institute of Health. The precise performance targets are illustrative and might be relaxed or tightened depending on the situation; the point is to have pre-specified and reasonably stringent performance targets when moving from biomarker discovery to qualification for some COU. If an EEG biomarker can meet the proposed targets, it should be relatively straightforward to determine utility in a COU with a sample size on the order of 100–200 participants.

Given the complexity of the brain, and everything that contributes to EEGs, combinations of EEG measures may ultimately achieve the most stable and useful characterization of brain function within an individual. To identify the "best" parameter combinations, approaches such as machine learning, which benefit from larger sample sizes, can help identify biomarker measures that in combination optimize practical utility. In light of the above criteria for a single biomarker, criteria that a combination is "better" should involve at least a 5% increase in, for instance, the AUC of the ROC curve for some purpose of use.

We assume that to approach meeting these criteria, which are admittedly aspirational, standardization of paradigms, analysis pipelines, electrode array size and perhaps even equipment will be required. Recently completed and ongoing studies with EEG and ERP in various neurodevelopmental and psychiatric populations as well as in healthy volunteers as measures of drug effect have generated data that will help assess whether these criteria are met under ideal research conditions. If not, the data may allow for more informed setting of criteria or argue that we search for EEG/ERP paradigms that could meet those as proposed.

We assume that later stage validation studies would necessarily be multi-site. Single site studies would be focused on biomarker discovery such as some novel ERP paradigm or resting state EEG measure. In keeping with recommendations from the FDA (Amur et al., 2015), we believe that to address criteria 1–5 at any level is best done through collaborative consortia approaches with extensive data sharing. Full transparency allows for confidence in the data and expedites the rate of uptake of any biomarker that may facilitate the development of desperately needed treatments.

Given all the considerations discussed above, it seems fair to say that biomarker development for NDDs is not nearing the end stage of well validated and regular application, but we do now see the end of the beginning phase as we move from pure discovery to planning for testing validation for application. Many small-sample studies have found promising leads, especially for EEG/ERP biomarkers both for ASD and for related single gene disorders such as FXS. Future studies will also need to examine community populations not rigorously selected for mechanistic studies in academic medical centers but recruited to characterize a disorder as it exists in the population. Secondly, biomarkers will need to be evaluated in terms of their proximity to clinical symptoms *vs.* to biological disease mechanisms. Both are important, but most approaches will have greater relevant utility for one or the other purpose. For example, one might consider ERP studies of psychological features such as emotional face viewing as a promising diagnostic biomarker for ASD, as it is likely to be common across ASD cases given its close association with social cognition, which is a defining feature of the disorder. Alternatively, a study of theta-gamma coupling at rest, a more fundamental feature of brain physiology, might be more likely to resolve syndromal heterogeneity and be linked to the selective action of particular drugs in particular individuals.

This distinction has important implications for biomarker evaluation. A biomarker useful for identifying a meaningful subgroup in a population almost by necessity would fail as a diagnostic biomarker by virtue of its low sensitivity for the condition, and a biomarker with high sensitivity likely would have limited utility for identifying subgroups within a clinical syndrome. This idea is related to the idea of degeneracy as one moves from gene to molecular biology to local circuit networks to large-scale functional networks to behavior. Biomarkers at different places along this path are likely to serve different purposes and will need to be developed and evaluated in this context. For this reason, and others, different ERP paradigms and analysis approaches to the data may be suitable for different diagnostic and predictive purposes, and need to be evaluated within the limits of their intended COU.

At a practical level, electrophysiological biomarkers will need to be evaluated for utility across the age-span, across sexes and disorders, in relation to treatment outcome to different classes of medication, and across different hardware and software analysis strategies. Given the very large amount of data provided by resting-state and task-based analyses, novel analytic and signal-processing approaches recently developed to work with the data may allow for much more information content at the individual level not possible with currently employed data analytic pipelines. Addressing such issues in scale is now a major challenge for electrophysiological biomarker development in NDDs but one that holds enormous promise. By committing to standardization of some core set of measures, the field should be able to generate a new set of EEG/ERP derived measures that will better serve various COUs for developing treatments of NDDs.

AUTHOR CONTRIBUTIONS

All authors contributed intellectually to the concepts within the manuscript, framing, writing, and editing.

FUNDING

We thank the Kennedy Krieger Institute IDDRC (U54 HD079123) for support of Dr. Ewen's effort.

ACKNOWLEDGMENTS

The authors would like to thank the organizers of the National Institute of Neurological Disorders and Stroke workshop on Biomarkers to Enable Therapeutics in Neurodevelopmental Disorders.

REFERENCES

Ajram, L. A., Pereira, A. C., Durieux, A. M. S., Velthius, H. E., Petrinovic, M. M., and Mcalonan, G. M. (2019). The contribution of [1H] magnetic resonance spectroscopy to the study of excitation-inhibition in autism. *Prog. Neuropsychopharmacol. Biol. Psychiatry* 89, 236–244. doi: 10.1016/j.pnpbp.2018.09.010

Amur, S., Lavange, L., Zineh, I., Buckman-Garner, S., and Woodcock, J. (2015). Biomarker qualification: toward a multiple stakeholder framework for biomarker development, regulatory acceptance, and utilization. *Clin. Pharmacol. Ther.* 98, 34–46. doi: 10.1002/cpt.136

Anderberg, M. R. (1973). *Cluster Analysis for Applications*. New York, NY: Academic Press.

Belmonte, M. K., Cook, E. H. Jr., Anderson, G. M., Rubenstein, J. L., Greenough, W. T., Beckel-Mitchener, A., et al. (2004). Autism as a disorder of neural information processing: directions for research and targets for therapy. *Mol. Psychiatry* 9, 646–663. doi: 10.1038/sj.mp.4001499

Berry-Kravis, E. M., Hessl, D., Rathmell, B., Zarevics, P., Cherubini, M., Walton-Bowen, K., et al. (2012). Effects of STX209 (arbaclofen) on neurobehavioral function in children and adults with fragile X syndrome: a randomized, controlled, phase 2 trial. *Sci. Transl. Med.* 4:152ra127. doi: 10.1126/scitranslmed.3004214

Bossuyt, P. M., Reitsma, J. B., Bruns, D. E., Gatsonis, C. A., Glasziou, P. P., Irwig, L., et al. (2015). STARD 2015: an updated list of essential items for reporting diagnostic accuracy studies. *BMJ* 351:h5527. doi: 10.1136/bmj.h5527

Bublatzky, F., Pittig, A., Schupp, H. T., and Alpers, G. W. (2017). Face-to-face: Perceived personal relevance amplifies face processing. *Soc. Cogn. Affect. Neurosci.* 12, 811–822. doi: 10.1093/scan/nsx001

Butler, J. S., Molholm, S., Andrade, G. N., and Foxe, J. J. (2017). An Examination of the neural unreliability thesis of autism. *Cereb. Cortex* 27, 185–200. doi: 10.1093/cercor/bhw375

Califf, R. M. (2018). Biomarker definitions and their applications. *Exp. Biol. Med.* 243, 213–221. doi: 10.1177/1535370217750088

Carmichael, O., Schwarz, A. J., Chatham, C. H., Scott, D., Turner, J. A., Upadhyay, J., et al. (2018). The role of fMRI in drug development. *Drug Discov. Today* 23, 333–348. doi: 10.1016/j.drudis.2017.11.012

CDER Biomarker Qualification Program, (2019). *Biomarker Qualification Submissions.* Available: https://www.fda.gov/drugs/cder-biomarker-qualification-program/biomarker-qualification-submissions (accessed June 5, 2019).

Chan, A. S., Sze, S. L., and Cheung, M. C. (2007). Quantitative electroencephalographic profiles for children with autistic spectrum disorder. *Neuropsychology* 21, 74–81. doi: 10.1037/0894-4105.21.1.74

Clapp, W. C., Hamm, J. P., Kirk, I. J., and Teyler, T. J. (2012). Translating long-term potentiation from animals to humans: a novel method for noninvasive assessment of cortical plasticity. *Biol. Psychiatry* 71, 496–502. doi: 10.1016/j.biopsych.2011.08.021

Clementz, B. A., Sweeney, J. A., Hamm, J. P., Ivleva, E. I., Ethridge, L. E., Pearlson, G. D., et al. (2016). Identification of distinct psychosis biotypes using brain-based biomarkers. *Am. J. Psychiatry* 173, 373–384. doi: 10.1176/appi.ajp.2015.14091200

Cohen, M. (2014). *Analyzing Neural Time Series Data: Theory and Practice.* Cambridge: MIT Press.

Eberhard-Moscicka, A. K., Jost, L. B., Fehlbaum, L. V., Pfenninger, S. E., and Maurer, U. (2016). Temporal dynamics of early visual word processing - early versus late N1 sensitivity in children and adults. *Neuropsychologia* 91, 509–518. doi: 10.1016/j.neuropsychologia.2016.09.014

Eloyan, A., Muschelli, J., Nebel, M. B., Liu, H., Han, F., Zhao, T., et al. (2012). Automated diagnoses of attention deficit hyperactive disorder using magnetic resonance imaging. *Front. Syst. Neurosci.* 6:61. doi: 10.3389/fnsys.2012.0006

Ethridge, L. E., White, S. P., Mosconi, M. W., Wang, J., Pedapati, E. V., Erickson, C. A., et al. (2017). Neural synchronization deficits linked to cortical hyper-excitability and auditory hypersensitivity in fragile X syndrome. *Mol. Autism.* 8:22. doi: 10.1186/s13229-017-0140-1

Ewen, J., Marvin, A., Law, K., and Lipkin, P. (2019). Epilepsy and autism severity: a study of 6,975 children. *Autism. Res.* doi: 10.1002/aur.2132 [Epub ahead of print].

Ewen, J. B. (2016). The eternal promise of EEG-based biomarkers: getting closer? *Neurology* 87, 2288–2289. doi: 10.1212/wnl.0000000000003275

Ewen, J. B., and Beniczky, S. (2018). "Validating biomarkers and diagnostic tests in clinical neurophysiology: developing strong experimental designs and recognizing confounds," in *Niedermeyer's Electroencephalography*, 7th Edn, eds D. L. Schomer and F. H. Lopes Da Silva (New York, NY: Oxford University Press).

Ewen, J. B., Kossoff, E. H., Crone, N. E., Lin, D. D., Lakshmanan, B. M., Ferenc, L. M., et al. (2009). Use of quantitative EEG in infants with port-wine birthmark to assess for Sturge-Weber brain involvement. *Clin. Neurophysiol.* 120, 1433–1440. doi: 10.1016/j.clinph.2009.06.005

Ewen, J. B., and Shapiro, B. K. (2008). "Specific learning disabilities," in *Developmental Disabilities in Infancy and Childhood*, 3rd Edn, ed. P. J. Accardo (Baltimore: Paul H. Brookes Publishing Co).

Fabiani, M., Karis, D., and Donchin, E. (1986). P300 and recall in an incidental memory paradigm. *Psychophysiology* 23, 298–308. doi: 10.1111/j.1469-8986.1986.tb00636.x

Fisher, M., and Lowenbach, H. (1934). Aktionsstrome des zentralnervensystems unter der einwirkung von krampfgiften. Mitteilung Strychnin und Pikrotoxin. *Arch. F. Exp. Pathol. und Pharmakol* 174, 357–382. doi: 10.1007/bf0186 4468

Gibbs, F., Davis, H., and Lennox, W. (1935). The electro-encephalogram in epilepsy and in conditions of impaired consciousness. *Arch. Neurol. Psychiatry* 34, 1133–1148.

Gloss, D., Varma, J. K., Pringsheim, T., and Nuwer, M. R. (2016). Practice advisory: the utility of EEG theta/beta power ratio in ADHD diagnosis. *Neurology* 87, 2375–2379. doi: 10.1212/wnl.0000000000003265

Gurau, O., Bosl, W. J., and Newton, C. R. (2017). How Useful Is Electroencephalography in the Diagnosis of Autism Spectrum Disorders and the Delineation of Subtypes: A Systematic Review. *Front. Psychiatry* 8:121. doi: 10.3389/fpsyt.2017.00121

Hagerman, R., Jacquemont, S., Berry-Kravis, E., Des Portes, V., Stanfield, A., Koumaras, B., et al. (2018). Mavoglurant in fragile X syndrome: results of two open-label, extension trials in adults and adolescents. *Sci. Rep.* 8:16970. doi: 10.1038/s41598-018-34978-4

Hatfield, L. A., Crone, N. E., Kossoff, E. H., Ewen, J. B., Pyzik, P. L., Lin, D. D., et al. (2007). Quantitative EEG asymmetry correlates with clinical severity in unilateral sturge-weber syndrome. *Epilepsia* 48, 191–195.

Jack, C. R. Jr., Bennett, D. A., Blennow, K., Carrillo, M. C., Dunn, B., Haeberlein, S. B., et al. (2018). NIA-AA research framework: Toward a biological definition of Alzheimer's disease. *Alzheimers Dement* 14, 535–562. doi: 10.1016/j.jalz.2018.02.018

Kang, E., Keifer, C. M., Levy, E. J., Foss-Feig, J. H., Mcpartland, J. C., and Lerner, M. D. (2018). Atypicality of the N170 event-related potential in autism spectrum disorder: a meta-analysis. *Biol. Psychiatry Cogn. Neurosci. Neuroimag.* 3, 657–666. doi: 10.1016/j.bpsc.2017.11.003

Kida, T., Nishihira, Y., Hatta, A., Wasaka, T., Tazoe, T., Sakajiri, Y., et al. (2004). Resource allocation and somatosensory P300 amplitude during dual task: effects of tracking speed and predictability of tracking direction. *Clin. Neurophysiol.* 115, 2616–2628. doi: 10.1016/j.clinph.2004.06.013

Landi, S., Petrucco, L., Sicca, F., and Ratto, G. M. (2018). Transient cognitive impairment in epilepsy. *Front. Mol. Neurosci.* 11:458. doi: 10.3389/fnmol.2018.00458

Loo, S. K., Cho, A., Hale, T. S., Mcgough, J., Mccracken, J., and Smalley, S. L. (2013). Characterization of the theta to beta ratio in ADHD: identifying potential sources of heterogeneity. *J. Atten. Disord.* 17, 384–392. doi: 10.1177/1087054712468050

Lord, F. M. (1955). Some perspectives on the attenuation paradox in test theory. *Psychol. Bull.* 52, 505–510. doi: 10.1037/h0044001

Lovaas, O. I. (1987). Behavioral treatment and normal educational and intellectual functioning in young autistic children. *J. Consult. Clin. Psychol.* 55, 3–9. doi: 10.1037//0022-006x.55.1.3

Lovelace, J. W., Ethell, I. M., Binder, D. K., and Razak, K. A. (2018). Translation-relevant EEG phenotypes in a mouse model of Fragile X Syndrome. *Neurobiol. Dis.* 115, 39–48. doi: 10.1016/j.nbd.2018.03.012

Luck, S. (2014). *An Introduction to the Event-Related Potential Technique.* Cambridge: MIT Press.

Matlis, S., Boric, K., Chu, C. J., and Kramer, M. A. (2015). Robust disruptions in electroencephalogram cortical oscillations and large-scale functional networks in autism. *BMC Neurol.* 15:97. doi: 10.1186/s12883-015-0355-8

McPartland, J. C. (2016). Considerations in biomarker development for neurodevelopmental disorders. *Curr. Opin. Neurol.* 29, 118–122. doi: 10.1097/WCO.0000000000000300

McPartland, J. C. (2017). Developing clinically practicable biomarkers for autism spectrum disorder. *J. Autism. Dev. Disord.* 47, 2935–2937. doi: 10.1007/s10803-017-3237-7

Morton, J. (2005). *Understanding Developmental Disabilities: a Causal Model Approach.* Singapore: Wiley-Blackwell.

Mullard, A. (2019). Anti-amyloid failures stack up as Alzheimer antibody flops. *Nat. Rev. Drug Discov.* doi: 10.1016/j.biopsych.2017.08.010 [Epub ahead of print].

O'Reilly, C., Lewis, J. D., and Elsabbagh, M. (2017). Is functional brain connectivity atypical in autism? a systematic review of EEG and MEG studies. *PLoS One* 12:e0175870. doi: 10.1371/journal.pone.0175870

Paasch, V., Hoosier, T. M., Accardo, J., Ewen, J. B., and Slifer, K. J. (2012). Technical tips: performing EEGs and polysomnograms on children with neurodevelopmental disabilities. *Neurodiagn. J.* 52, 333–348.

Patel, S. H., and Azzam, P. N. (2005). Characterization of N200 and P300: selected studies of the event-related potential. *Int. J. Med. Sci.* 2, 147–154. doi: 10.7150/ijms.2.147

Pauler, D. K., Escobar, M. D., Sweeney, J. A., and Greenhouse, J. (1996). Mixture models for eye-tracking data: a case study. *Stat. Med.* 15, 1365–1376. doi: 10.1002/(sici)1097-0258(19960715)15:13<1365::aid-sim232>3.0.co;2-j

Picton, T. W., Bentin, S., Berg, P., Donchin, E., Hillyard, S. A., Johnson, R., et al. (2000). Guidelines for using human event-related potentials to study cognition: recording standards and publication criteria. *Psychophysiology* 37, 127–152. doi: 10.1017/s0048577200000305

Polich, J. (2007). Updating P300: an integrative theory of P3a and P3b. *Clin. Neurophysiol.* 118, 2128–2148. doi: 10.1016/j.clinph.2007.04.019

Power, J. D., Barnes, K. A., Snyder, A. Z., Schlaggar, B. L., and Petersen, S. E. (2012). Spurious but systematic correlations in functional connectivity MRI networks arise from subject motion. *Neuroimage* 59, 2142–2154. doi: 10.1016/j.neuroimage.2011.10.018

Rosen, T. E., Mazefsky, C. A., Vasa, R. A., and Lerner, M. D. (2018). Co-occurring psychiatric conditions in autism spectrum disorder. *Int. Rev. Psychiatry* 30, 40–61. doi: 10.1080/09540261.2018.1450229

Rubenstein, J. L., and Merzenich, M. M. (2003). Model of autism: increased ratio of excitation/inhibition in key neural systems. *Genes Brain Behav.* 2, 255–267. doi: 10.1034/j.1601-183x.2003.00037.x

Sahin, M., Jones, S. R., Sweeney, J. A., Berry-Kravis, E., Connors, B. W., Ewen, J. B., et al. (2018). Discovering translational biomarkers in neurodevelopmental disorders. *Nat. Rev. Drug Discov.* 18, 235–236.

Sinha, S. R., Sullivan, L., Sabau, D., San-Juan, D., Dombrowski, K. E., Halford, J. J., et al. (2016). American clinical neurophysiology society guideline 1: minimum technical requirements for performing clinical electroencephalography. *J. Clin. Neurophysiol.* 33, 303–307. doi: 10.1097/wnp.0000000000000308

Snyder, S. M., Rugino, T. A., Hornig, M., and Stein, M. A. (2015). Integration of an EEG biomarker with a clinician's ADHD evaluation. *Brain Behav.* 5:e00330. doi: 10.1002/brb3.330

Spence, S. J., and Schneider, M. T. (2009). The role of epilepsy and epileptiform EEGs in autism spectrum disorders. *Pediatr. Res.* 65, 599–606. doi: 10.1203/PDR.0b013e31819e7168

Sun, H., Chen, Y., Huang, Q., Lui, S., Huang, X., Shi, Y., et al. (2018). Psychoradiologic utility of MR imaging for diagnosis of attention deficit hyperactivity disorder: a radiomics analysis. *Radiology* 287, 620–630. doi: 10.1148/radiol.2017170226

Takarae, Y., Sablich, S. R., White, S. P., and Sweeney, J. A. (2016). Neurophysiological hyperresponsivity to sensory input in autism spectrum disorders. *J. Neurodev. Disord.* 8:29. doi: 10.1186/s11689-016-9162-9

Tome, D., Barbosa, F., Nowak, K., and Marques-Teixeira, J. (2015). The development of the N1 and N2 components in auditory oddball paradigms: a systematic review with narrative analysis and suggested normative values. *J. Neural. Transm.* 122, 375–391. doi: 10.1007/s00702-014-1258-3 van Dinteren, R., Arns, M., Jongsma, M. L., and Kessels, R. P. (2014). P300 development across the lifespan: a systematic review and meta-analysis. *PLoS One* 9:e87347. doi: 10.1371/journal.pone.0087347

van Putten, M. J., Peters, J. M., Mulder, S. M., De Haas, J. A., Bruijninckx, C. M., and Tavy, D. L. (2004). A brain symmetry index (BSI) for online EEG monitoring in carotid endarterectomy. *Clin. Neurophysiol.* 115, 1189–1194. doi: 10.1016/j.clinph.2003.12.002

Varcin, K. J., Nelson, C. A. III, Ko, J., Sahin, M., Wu, J. Y., and Jeste, S. S. (2016). Visual evoked potentials as a readout of cortical function in infants with tuberous sclerosis complex. *J. Child. Neurol.* 31, 195–202. doi: 10.1177/0883073815587328

Vasa, R. A., Mostofsky, S. H., and Ewen, J. B. (2016). The disrupted connectivity hypothesis of autism spectrum disorders: time for the next phase in research. *Biol. Psychiatry Cogn. Neurosci. Neuroimag.* 1, 245–252. doi: 10.1016/j.bpsc.2016.02.003

Veitch, D. P., Weiner, M. W., Aisen, P. S., Beckett, L. A., Cairns, N. J., Green, R. C., et al. (2019). Understanding disease progression and improving Alzheimer's disease clinical trials: recent highlights from the alzheimer's disease neuroimaging initiative. *Alzheimers Dement* 15, 106–152. doi: 10.1016/j.jalz.2018.08.005

Wang, J., Barstein, J., Ethridge, L. E., Mosconi, M. W., Takarae, Y., and Sweeney, J. A. (2013). Resting state EEG abnormalities in autism spectrum disorders. *J. Neurodev. Disord.* 5:24. doi: 10.1186/1866-1955-5-24

Wang, J., Ethridge, L. E., Mosconi, M. W., White, S. P., Binder, D. K., Pedapati, E. V., et al. (2017). A resting EEG study of neocortical hyperexcitability and altered functional connectivity in fragile X syndrome. *J. Neurodev. Disord.* 9:11. doi: 10.1186/s11689-017-9191-z

Waterhouse, L., London, E., and Gillberg, C. (2016). ASD validity. *Rev. J. Autism. Dev. Disord.* 3:302.

Webb, S. J., Bernier, R., Henderson, H. A., Johnson, M. H., Jones, E. J., Lerner, M. D., et al. (2015). Guidelines and best practices for electrophysiological data collection, analysis and reporting in autism. *J. Autism. Dev. Disord.* 45, 425–443. doi: 10.1007/s10803-013-1916-6

Webb, S. J., Neuhaus, E., and Faja, S. (2017). Face perception and learning in autism spectrum disorders. *Q. J. Exp. Psychol.* 70, 970–986. doi: 10.1080/17470218.2016.1151059

Woo, C. W., Chang, L. J., Lindquist, M. A., and Wager, T. D. (2017). Building better biomarkers: brain models in translational neuroimaging. *Nat. Neurosci.* 20, 365–377. doi: 10.1038/nn.4478

Wu, Y., and Zhou, X. (2009). The P300 and reward valence, magnitude, and expectancy in outcome evaluation. *Brain Res.* 1286, 114–122. doi: 10.1016/j.brainres.2009.06.032

2

Age-Dependent Statistical Changes of Involuntary Head Motion Signatures Across Autism and Controls of the ABIDE Repository

*Carla Caballero[1,2], Sejal Mistry[3] and Elizabeth B. Torres[2,4,5]**

[1] Sports Research Center, Sports Sciences Department, Miguel Hernández University of Elche, Elche, Spain, [2] Department of Psychology, Rutgers, The State University of New Jersey, Piscataway, NJ, United States, [3] Department of Mathematics, Rutgers, The State University of New Jersey, Piscataway, NJ, United States, [4] Computer Science, Center for Computational Biomedicine Imaging and Modeling, Rutgers, The State University of New Jersey, Piscataway, NJ, United States, [5] Center for Cognitive Science, Rutgers, The State University of New Jersey, Piscataway, NJ, United States

Correspondence:
Elizabeth B. Torres
ebtorres@psych.rutgers.edu;
torreselizabeth248@gmail.com

Received: *25 June 2019*

The DSM-5 definition of autism spectrum disorders includes sensory issues and part of the sensory information that the brain continuously receives comes from kinesthetic reafference, in the form of self-generated motions, including those that the nervous systems produce at rest. Some of the movements that we self-generate are deliberate, while some occur spontaneously, consequentially following those that we can control. Yet, some motions occur involuntarily, largely beneath our awareness. We do not know much about involuntary motions across development, but these motions typically manifest during resting state in fMRI studies. Here we ask in a large data set from the Autism Brain Imaging Exchange repository, whether the stochastic signatures of variability in the involuntary motions of the head typically shift with age. We further ask if those motions registered from individuals with autism show a significant departure from the normative data as we examine different age groups selected at random from cross-sections of the population. We find significant shifts in statistical features of typical levels of involuntary head motions for different age groups. Further, we find that in autism these changes also manifest in non-uniform ways, and that they significantly differ from their age-matched groups. The results suggest that the levels of random involuntary motor noise are elevated in autism across age groups. This calls for the use of different age-appropriate statistical models in research that involves dynamically changing signals self-generated by the nervous systems.

Keywords: autism spectrum disorder, involuntary motions, stochastic analyses, head motion analysis, resting state – fMRI, Gamma distributed data

INTRODUCTION

The volitional control of physical movements, i.e., the control of our purposeful actions at will, and the healthy preservation of this ability, are fundamental elements to generate well-coordinated behaviors across the human lifespan. As the somatic-sensory-motor systems of human babies mature and give way to several developmental milestones, spanning from infancy to the elderly stages of our life cycle, the patterns of variability in our motions are bound to change (Torres et al., 2016b). These changes reflect the outputs of our nervous systems and can be a valuable tool to track healthy neurodevelopment and healthy aging in contrast to neurodevelopmental differences and neurodegeneration.

One of the signs of motor dysfunction that appears later in life is the abundance of undesirable involuntary motions. When a person is asked to remain still, there is (inevitably) some level of involuntary micro-motions across the body; yet if such levels are persistently high in early neurodevelopment, they can interfere with neuromotor control and forecast upcoming problems with the nervous systems. They can predict problems with action coordination and volitional control of goal directed behaviors (Torres et al., 2013a; Wu et al., 2018), but these are difficult to detect using traditional statistical analyses based on grand averaging under assumed Gaussian distribution [as explained in Torres et al. (2013a) situating autism within the broader context of Precision Medicine].

The study of evolving trends in the self-generation of undesirable involuntary motions at the periphery (Brincker and Torres, 2013), along with their variable rates of change across the human lifespan, requires age-appropriate adjustments of our statistical analyses across different aging human populations. This include for example, size-dependent (allometric) standardizations of data harnessed from different anatomies owing to different ages (Mosimann, 1970; Lleonart et al., 2000). There is, however, a paucity of studies reflecting the cross-sectional age-dependent evolution of the variability in motor patterns contributing to volitional control for neurotypicals. In the absence of such normative data to characterize patterns of motor variability in healthy early neurodevelopment and in the aging population, most statistical analyses of human behaviors are performed under a *one-size-fits-all* approach that uses parametric statistics and linear models. This treatment of the problem may prevent us from considering the non-linear complex dynamics of biorhythmic activities produced by the developing and the aging nervous systems.

While other fields have considered various non-linear models, e.g., of heart rate variability (Peng et al., 1995) and gait patterns (Raffalt et al., 2018; Caballero et al., 2019), the focus of that work has been on suitable methods to assess both long-range and short-range correlations in non-stationary and stationary systems. The data that interests us here is brief, limited by the number of frames in a scanning fMRI session, during resting state, when the person has been asked to remain still. As such, our interest focuses on the nature of the families of distributions that we could empirically derive from fluctuations of involuntary bodily motions across different age groups of the neurotypical and autistic populations. More specifically, we assess the extent to which such families of distributions may typically shift cross sectionally in the neurotypical population. Our approach contrasts with traditional approaches that make *a priori* theoretical assumptions on the nature of such distributions and tend to obfuscate our abilities to predict possible departures from normative states in pathological states of the nervous systems, where asynchronous attainment of developmental milestones abound. One such example is evidenced in research involving autism spectrum disorders (ASD).

Autism is a lifelong, highly heterogeneous, evolving condition (Lord et al., 2000; Constantino and Charman, 2016) and yet, we know very little about maturational patterns of somatic-sensory-motor signatures, critical to scaffold the volitional control of the brain over the body in motion. Understanding such differences in the peripheral input to central motor control across the population is important in more than one way. From the research standpoint, such peripheral patterns have been revealing of maturational stages and possible familial ties (Torres et al., 2013a, 2016a; Wu et al., 2018) amenable to help us further our understanding of the etiology of the condition, trace back the individual contextual and environmental features of the developmental trajectories of each person, and tailor treatments and services according to family needs, in a personalized manner. From the societal standpoint, it is important to know the ever-changing needs of the person's level of motor autonomy, to advocate for public policies that help to effectively deploy and manage resources that support the development of independent living prior to and beyond school age (**Figure 1**). Given the heterogeneity of ASD statistics (Torres et al., 2016a), there is a critical need to stratify the affected population and design interventions that are age-appropriate, personalized to the person's needs and congruent with the profound differences that define the somatic-sensory-motor profiles characterizing the autistic phenotype, e.g., (Lancaster et al., 2013; Torres et al., 2013a; Marko et al., 2015; Mosconi and Sweeney, 2015; Mosconi et al., 2015a; Sharer et al., 2015; Mahajan et al., 2016; Torres and Denisova, 2016; Chuye et al., 2018).

Designing new ways to uncover self-emergent clusters of data to stratify the heterogeneous ASD population has been rather challenging, owing this in part to the lack of access by most researchers to participants of diverse ages, and to the lack of data that is inclusive of both sexes. The advent of open access ASD and

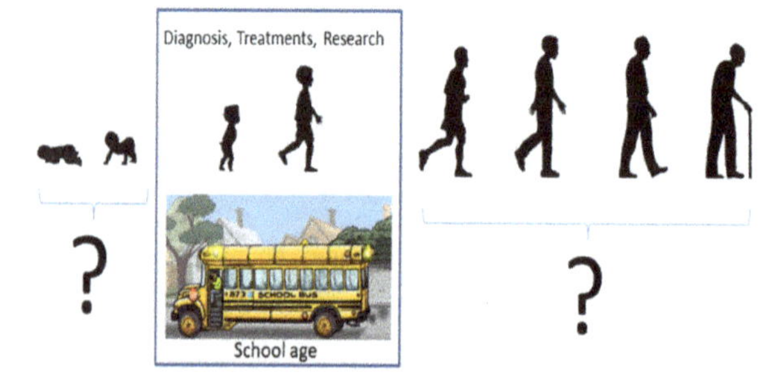

FIGURE 1 | Science has very limited knowledge of autism as a lifelong condition. Research in autism has been focused on certain age groups primarily involving children of school age. We know very little about neurodevelopment preceding autism and virtually nothing about adults. Parents ask, *"what will happen to my child when the yellow bus stops coming,"* as in the US, services taper off as children transition into adulthood (a phase that parents have coined *"falling off the cliff"*). No proper methods have been designed to study neuromotor issues of aging adults with autism, often presenting ataxia syndromes, loss of balance, frequent falls and symptoms of Parkinsonism (Starkstein et al., 2015).

typically developing (TD) data repositories addresses these issues today and enables us to explore the question of age-dependent shifts in the signatures of variability across the normative data from the neurotypical population and the population with an ASD diagnosis. One such open access databases is the Autism Brain Imaging Data Exchange (ABIDE) repository (Di Martino et al., 2014) an effort that has revealed several new features of brain organization (Alaerts et al., 2014; Ray et al., 2014; Plitt et al., 2015; Haar et al., 2016), new differentiating features of females (Torres et al., 2017) and males (Supekar and Menon, 2015; Jung et al., 2019), IQ and medication intake (Torres and Denisova, 2016) and patterns of scanner-dependent noise in the involuntary head motions (Caballero et al., 2018). This has been part of a general effort to understand neuromotor control in ASD (Ornitz, 1974; Minshew et al., 2004; Mandelbaum et al., 2006; Perry et al., 2007; Jasmin et al., 2009; Kushki et al., 2011; Donnellan et al., 2012; Torres et al., 2013a; Hannant et al., 2016). In ABIDE, it is possible to use the imaging data and extract head motions in the form of rotations and displacements (a routine step in removing motor artifacts from the images) such that the extracted involuntary head micro-motions when the person is trying to remain still, can give us a sense of the amount of volitional control that people typically have across different age groups. In turn, given that ABIDE has age- and sex- matched participants with ASD, we can interrogate the database across different age groups, to learn about age-dependent shifts in the statistics of undesirable involuntary head motions.

In this paper, we explore data in ABIDE, to characterize statistical patterns of involuntary head motions across ages, as the person is instructed to remain still and yet the data reveal undesirable involuntary head motions. We compile the imaging data to extract the patterns of head translation and rotation across each session and use these time series (waveforms) of the linear and angular speed to characterize differences in volitional control as an inevitable feature, preventing the person from remaining still at will. We ask if the stochastic signatures derived from the patterns of head motion variability differ across ages in the neurotypical population. We further ask if the participants with ASD depart from the normative signatures.

MATERIALS AND METHODS

Demographics of ABIDE I and II

All datasets included in this study are from the Autism Brain Imaging Data Exchange (ABIDE) databases: ABIDE I[1] and ABIDE II[2]. ABIDE obeys the following guideline on the use of human subject's data: "In accordance with HIPAA guidelines and 1000 Functional Connectomes Project/INDI protocols, all datasets have been anonymized, with no protected health information included."

The study includes two main comparisons:

(1) *Autism Spectrum Disorder (ASD)*, and *Typical Development (TD)*, using estimation of stochastic signatures of involuntary head micro-movements of individuals with a formal DSM-ASD (American Psychiatric Association, 2013) diagnosis of ASD and TD controls.

(2) *Ranges of age*. Each group (ASD and TD) was split in seven different groups according to their age to assess how the stochastic signature of involuntary head micro-movements evolves with growth. The ranges of age used to that end were the following: from 5 to 10 years old, from 11 to 15 years old, from 16 to 20 years old, from 21 to 25 years old, from 26 to 30 years old, from 31 to 40 years old, and from 41 to 65 years old.

Inclusion/Exclusion Criteria

This study includes all sites publicly available through ABIDE I and ABIDE II. They were comprised of 1,127 TD and 1,017 ASD. As we explained above, those groups were divided by age. **Table 1** provides the number of participants with ASD or TD are in each range of age in ABIDE dataset.

Bootstrapping Method

The analyses referring to the bootstrapping methods were previously published but we will refer to them here for simplicity.

First, we uniformly resampled all data sets to avoid temporal inconsistencies, since our focus is on fluctuations in signal amplitude. To that end, we resample all data to ensure equally spaced points for comparison across subjects and groups (outcome can be seen in **Supplementary Material** of prior work[3]). We use the MATLAB (version R2014a, The MathWorks, Inc., Natick, MA, United States) function resample which applies an antialiasing FIR low-pass filter to the time series and compensates for the delay introduced by the filter. This function resamples the input sequence, the raw head motion in our case, at P/Q times the original sample rate [see **Supplementary Table S1** of the previously published SM for more information about the resampling factors used (P and Q)].

Second, we apply uniform data length by truncating the uniformly resampled data to ensure the same length for all the time series.

Given the inconsistent group sizes extracted from the ABIDE datasets (see **Table 1**), we used a bootstrapping method previously described to ensure uniform group numbers for pairwise statistical comparisons across ages. To that end, we used random sampling with replacement and created 100 subgroups drawn from the original size group while considering the minimum number $n = 25$ at a time. These 25 randomly selected participants' data contribute to a data point in the age group of 100 participants. Their head motion time series are pooled to further create a standardized waveform, free of allometric effects from different anatomical sizes and focusing on the variability patterns relative to the overall empirically estimated mean speed amplitude expressed by the group. We chose 25 as the size to randomize because the smallest age's sub-groups size was $n = 30$. Thus, after dividing the groups by age, we extracted the 100 random sub-groups with replacement, using the same size ($n = 25$) to make up 100 group sizes from all the age's sub-groups.

[1] http://fcon_1000.projects.nitrc.org/indi/abide/abide_I.html
[2] http://fcon_1000.projects.nitrc.org/indi/abide/abide_II.html
[3] https://www.frontiersin.org/articles/10.3389/fnint.2018.00007/full

TABLE 1 | *t*-test *p*-values comparing the cumulative linear and angular excursions for ASD vs. TD in each age group (yo stands for years old).

Age group	5–10 yo	11–15 yo	16–20 yo	21–25 yo	26–30 yo	31–40 yo	41–60 yo
Cum Lin Speed	$1.00\ 10^{-12}$	$1.00\ 10^{-12}$	$1.00\ 10^{-12}$	$1.00\ 10^{-12}$	$1.00\ 10^{-12}$	$0.70\ 10^{-12}$	$1.00\ 10^{-12}$
Cum Ang Speed	$1.00\ 10^{-4}$	$1.00\ 10^{-4}$	$1.00\ 10^{-4}$	$1.00\ 10^{-4}$	$1.00\ 10^{-4}$	$0.44\ 10^{-4}$	$1.00\ 10^{-4}$

Supplementary Material Figures A4, A5 show the results from sampling without replacement.

Data Processing

Motion Extraction

Head motion patterns were extracted from imaging data during (rs) fMRI experiments. Motion extraction was performed using the Analysis of Functional NeuroImages (AFNI) software packages (Cox, 1996). Single-subject processing scripts were generated using the afni_proc.py interface[4]. Skull stripping was performed on anatomical data and functional EPI data were co-registered to anatomical images. The median was used as the EPI base in alignment. Motion parameters, 3 translational (*x*-, *y*-, and *z*-) and 3 rotational (pitch-about the *x*-axis, roll-about the *y*-axis, and yaw- about the *z*-axis), from EPI time-series registration was saved.

We note the caveat that different labs depositing data in ABIDE may use different padding to restrain/dampen head motion in general. However, each site of ABIDE has deposited data from a similar scanner and padding method for controls and autistics. We used the bootstrapping method to shuffle the fluctuations in speed amplitude and emphasize here that these fluctuations in speed amplitude that we examine are relative to an empirically estimated mean head motion speed (linear mm/s or angular rad/s). These data do not refer to the absolute value of the speed which may be differentially affected by the type of padding.

Head Excursion

To obtain the head excursions we accumulate the distance traveled per unit time (speed) and determine the pathlength of the linear displacement. We also determine the full excursion yielded by the accumulation of angular displacements. These parameters give us a sense of the net amount of physical head motion a person had while instructed to try to remain still. In both cases, we used the same number of data points for each participant, yet across those frames, each participant varied in the rate of change of displacements and their accumulation over time.

Statistical Analyses

We describe two components of the analyses of the head motions: (1) The standardized data type called micro-movement spikes, MMS and (2) the statistical platform for individualized behavioral analyses (SPIBA), both previously defined (Torres et al., 2013a) and US Patented methods publicly available[5].

In the present work, we assess the scan-by-scan speed-dependent variations in the amplitude of the linear displacement (mm/s) and in the angular rotations (rad/s) of the head relative to the empirically estimated mean of each person (personalized method) during resting-state functional magnetic resonance imaging (rs-fMRI) sessions. The analyses specifically refer to the stochastic signatures of MMS [defined in prior peer reviewed work including earlier versions of the ABIDE data and of others data sets (Torres et al., 2016a, 2017; Torres and Denisova, 2016; Caballero et al., 2018)].

Micro-Movement Spikes

The maximum amplitude of the speed (linear *mm/s* and angular *deg/s*) was obtained from the raw data extracted from the head motions (**Figure 2A**). The empirically estimated mean speed of each person was also obtained and used as reference to determine the maximal amplitude deviations from it (**Figure 2B**). The time-series of these fluctuations in maximal amplitude deviations from the empirically estimated mean provides the waveform of interest for our analyses. These are the spike trains of random fluctuations in signal amplitude (speed in this case). The fluctuations in amplitude of those spikes are normalized between [0,1] and used as continuous spike trains with amplitude values in the real domain. More generally, they are treated as an identically independent distributed (iid) continuous random process using the time series forecasting analytical framework (Hamilton, 1994), where events in the past may (or may not) accumulate evidence toward prediction of future events.

In this work, to remove allometric effects of body-size across ages in each trial we computed the normalized peak amplitude (the peak speed amplitude is divided by the sum of the peak speed amplitude and the averaged speed amplitude value comprising points between the two speed minima surrounding the local peak amplitude) (Mosimann, 1970; Lleonart et al., 2000). The normalized fluctuations define the micro-movement spikes of the original speed waveform. These are shown in **Figure 2C. Figure 2D** shows the MMS as they occurred in the original waveform, thus preserving the original number of frames. This waveform is amenable to perform other analyses (e.g., pairwise cross-coherence, pairwise cross-correlation, etc. to understand the periodic behavior of the MMS of a given biorhythm).

In the specific case of rs-fMRI data here, the data types used in this work are not the original head motions *per se*, but rather derivative information pulled out from the original time series that the head-motion extraction methods create. The commonly used methods to estimate volume-to-volume head movement from fMRI data were used here to obtain the original time series of (raw) head motion data (see section on "Materials and Methods" for head motion extraction above). Importantly ABIDE has two versions of the data sets, one which has been cleaned from artifacts and one which is raw (uncleaned). Since we are precisely interested in the continuous acquisition of head motion, we used

[4]https://afni.nimh.nih.gov/pub/dist/doc/program_help/afni_proc.py.html

[5]https://patents.google.com/patent/US10176299B2/en?inventor=Elizabeth+B.+TORRES

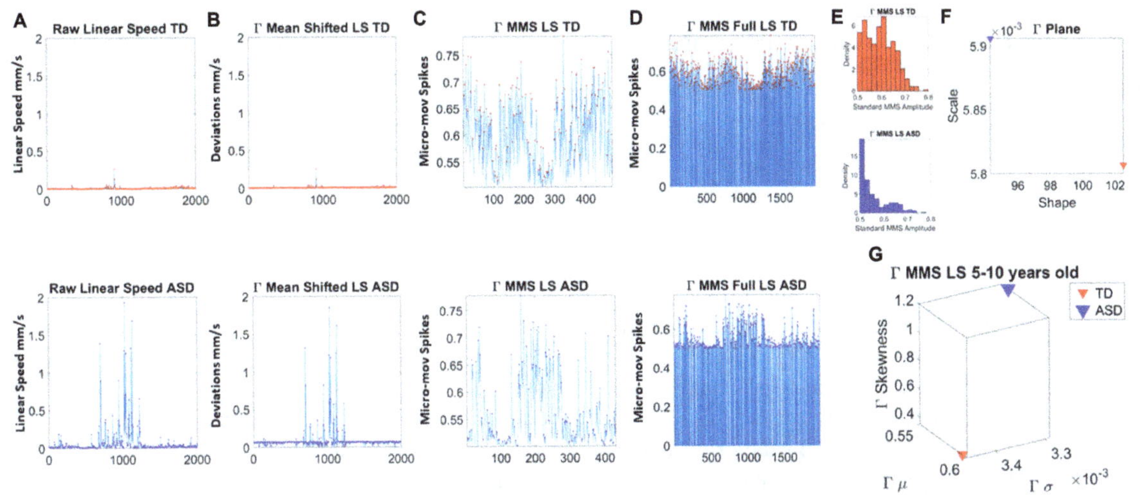

FIGURE 2 | Analytical pipeline. **(A)** Sample time series of involuntary head motion expressed as the linear speed (mm/s) derived from linear head displacements from a representative typically developing (TD) participant (top) and a representative participant with ASD (bottom) with equal number of frames for all participants. **(B)** Absolute amplitude deviations from the empirically estimated Gamma mean (empirically estimated shape × scale) amplitude. **(C)** Gamma micro-movement spikes, MMS, obtained from the deviations from the mean by normalizing the waveform to account for allometric effects. Each peak is divided by the sum of the peak value and the average value of the values comprised within the local minima adjacent to the peak (inclusive of the local minima). **(D)** All MMS embedded in the original waveform across all frames. **(E)** The MMS peaks are gathered in a frequency histogram. **(F)** The maximum likelihood estimation method is used to determine the continuous family of distributions best fitting both data sets; then the empirically estimated shape and scale values are plotted on the Gamma parameter plane. **(G)** The corresponding Gamma moments are plotted on a parameter space that includes the mean, standard deviation, skewness and kurtosis to aid visualize the signature of each participant and localize TD and ASD on these parameter spaces.

the uncleaned data sets. Note also that in an effort to reproduce our results, every publication does report to ABIDE the indexes of the data that has been used in the analyses. As such, we report to ABIDE the indexes used in this work.

To ascertain the net physical head motions across all participants, we compute the cumulative distance traveled per unit time and this gives us the path length of the linear and angular displacements (as explained above). The empirically estimated mean was obtained using the continuous Gamma family of probability distributions for every group [as in Torres and Denisova (2016), Torres et al. (2017), Caballero et al. (2018) because it gave the best fit according to maximum likelihood estimation, MLE] (see **Table 2** for information about the mean head excursion for every group).

In our prior work, the MMS generally served as input to a Gamma process under the general rubric of Poisson random process. We more specifically adapted methods from cortical spike analyses commonly used in the field of computational neuroscience, to analyze fluctuations in biorhythmic data from natural behaviors. Such data are lengthy time series of different physical units registered using different instruments. A such, they are disparate in frequency and timing, and no unifying platform existed to enable the analyses of multiple levels of neuromotor control co-registered with different instruments. We created a unitless data type amenable to combine data from different modalities (e.g., EEG in microVolts, ECG inter beat intervals in ms, EMG in volts, kinematics in m, m/s, m/s^2, rad, rad/s, rad/s^2, etc.) and paired this data type with methods to derive other parameterizations of the nervous systems output under different control regimes (voluntary, involuntary, and autonomic). These regimes are grounded on our proposed phylogenetically orderly taxonomy of neurodevelopmental maturation involving three fundamental muscle types (*skeletal muscle, smooth muscle, and cardiac muscle*) associated with specific genes and proteins that would eventually enable us to stratify heterogeneous disorders of the nervous systems using a combination of objective (digitally obtained) behavioral and genetic information. Among these disorders are Parkinson's disease, the Ataxias, Traumatic Brain Injury and Autism Spectrum Disorders, the latter being of interest in the present work.

In this paper, we specifically focus on involuntary head motions to assess the distribution fitting of the frequency histograms of the time series of their peaks for each age group. We used the stochastic characterization of fluctuations in peaks' amplitude to characterize the signature of involuntary head motions in the ASD vs. TD groups cross sectionally, across different ages. The motivation here is to estimate the spike trains' randomness and their levels of noise to signal ratio using the family of distributions best fitting the frequency histograms of the peaks accumulated from the MMS of each individual member of an age group.

We used maximum likelihood estimation, MLE to approximate the best fitting distribution encompassing all cases. To that end, we compared different families of probability distributions (e.g., the Gaussian, Lognormal, Exponential, and Gamma, although the MLE selection criterion does not penalize models with a larger number of parameters -in our case Exponential having one parameter, and other distributions two).

The motivation for these distributions came from prior work in our lab discovering the presence of the Exponential

TABLE 2 | Glass Delta and Cohen *d* values to quantify disease effect.

Age group	5–10 yo	11–15 yo	16–20 yo	21–25 yo	26–30 yo	31–40 yo	41–60 yo
Head's linear excursion (displacements)							
Glass Delta	2.76	3.24	3.17	2.34	5.44	1.32	1.17
Cohen *d*	1.30	1.80	2.28	1.68	1.71	0.59	3.53
Head's angular excursion (rotations)							
Glass Delta	2.09	2.94	3.38	2.12	2.12	0.55	4.09
Cohen *d*	1.30	1.81	2.28	1.69	1.71	0.59	3.53

distribution in biorhythms of the autistic *peripheral nervous systems* (Torres, 2011a,b). Controls up to then had been well characterized by the Lognormal family using a multiplicative random process (Ross, 1996), as heavy tailed distributions were near symmetric after log transforming the original speed data. The presence of the Exponential distribution in autistic peripheral signals prompted us to use instead an additive random process. We tried the continuous Gamma family of distributions, which includes the Exponential case when the shape parameter is 1 (as it was in Autism for linear speed peaks.) Another distribution was the Gaussian, to compare the outcome of MLE with the traditional assumption. In all cases, we estimated as well the 95% confidence intervals for the shape and for the scale parameters. The **Supplementary Material** from our prior work with ABIDE data showed the use of MLE and our finding that the continuous family of Gamma distributions was the best fit. The reader can find these explanations in detail within the **Supplementary Material** in those papers using these ABIDE sets[6].

The estimated parameters were plotted on a Gamma parameter plane, where the x-axis represents the shape parameter value and the y-axis represents the scale parameter value. **Figure 2E** shows the frequency histogram of sample data from two representative participants, while **Figure 2F** shows the sample empirically estimated Gamma parameters plotted on the Gamma parameter plane.

The Gamma scale value conveys the *noise to signal ratio* (NSR) since the Gamma mean $\mu_\Gamma = a \cdot b$ and the Gamma variance is $\sigma_\Gamma = a \cdot b^2$, thus the scale is:

$$b = \frac{\sigma_\Gamma}{\mu_\Gamma} = \frac{\cancel{a} \cdot b^{\cancel{2}}}{\cancel{a} \cdot \cancel{b}}$$

In this sense, the Gamma parameter plane allows us to infer speed-dependent processes leading to higher noise levels vs. lower noise levels. Further, since higher shape values tend toward symmetric distributions and lower values tend to be skewed distributions, with the extreme Exponential distributions at $a = 1$, we can also track processes that tend to the Exponential (memoryless, most random) vs. processes that tend toward the Gaussian distribution (more predictable at low NSR).

The scatter of points on the log–log Gamma plane uncovers a power-law relation between the shape and the dispersion of the distributions [the scale parameter or Noise-to-Signal Ratio (NSR)]. The **Supplementary Material Figure A7** (TD) and **Supplementary Material Figure A8** (ASD) show this and tabulates the fitting errors of the linear polynomial fit with the slope and intercept estimated for each age group and for the pooled data, with 95% approximated confidence intervals. We note that this linear fit is only the case upon the normalization presented here to account for allometric effects owing to different anatomical sizes across different ages. If the raw speed peaks are used instead, this power law relation does not hold. Further, other normalizations (e.g., scaling by dividing by the maximum amplitude) do not hold a power law either. In our experience the ASD data has systematically higher fitting error than the TD data.

In addition, for visualization purposes and to quantify differences in probability space, we compute the empirically estimated Gamma moments (mean along the x-axis, standard deviation along the y-axis, skewness along the z-axis and kurtosis proportional to the size of the marker). These are then plot, for each participant in each age group. **Figure 2G** shows an example for the representative TD vs. ASD participants used here to illustrate the analyses pipeline. We also plot the Gamma Probability Density Functions (PDFs) using the empirically estimated parameters.

Statistical Comparison

We used the Kruskal–Wallis non-parametric ANOVA to compare groups pairwise and report in each pairwise comparison the results for $p < 0.01$ and $p < 0.05$ in matrix form, without correction for multiple comparisons. A 7×7 matrix of 7 age groups provides the entries with p-values (see color bar in figures) and indicates the level of significance: one asterisk for $p < 0.05$ and two asterisks for $p < 0.01$. There are three such matrices, one for comparisons within the group of neurotypicals, one within the group of autistics and one comparing autistic relative to neurotypicals.

The distributions PDFs were also compared using the Kolmogorov–Smirnov test for two empirically estimated distributions and significance reported as above in matrix form. As with the non-parametric ANOVA we report p-values as entries of the matrix with one asterisk reflecting significance at 0.05, while two asterisks reflect significance at the 0.01 level.

Effect Size

In addition to the non-parametric one-way ANOVA (Kruskal–Wallis test), to assess the statistical significance of the group differences, we performed a t-test and ascertained the effect size of the differences that these comparisons yielded. To that end, we used the Cohen d test. We also used the Glass delta test, as

[6]https://www.nature.com/articles/srep37422#Sec26

the samples had equal size but significant differences in their variances. We used the head excursions [the cumulative linear (and the angular) speed] as the parameter of interest and set the neurotypical participants as the control group. The motivation for this parameter is that it is the parameter underlying the MMS computation, as they are derived from the head linear speed and the head angular speed, and we are interested in the cumulative effects over time, along these time series data.

The Cohen d test has the following formula:

$d = (M_2 - M_1)/SD_{pooled}$ where M_1 and M_2 are the means of each group,

SD_1 and SD_2 are the standard deviations of each group,

$$\text{and } SD_{pooled} = \sqrt{(SD_1^2 + SD_2^2)/2}.$$

The Glass delta test is $\Delta = (M_1 - M_2)/SD_2$ where SD_2 is the standard deviation of the control group.

We obtained these measurements for each of the 7 age-groups and within each case, compared ASD vs. TD, with TD set as the control group.

The literature (Cohen, 1992; Sawilowsky, 2003) suggests the following size effect ranges: 0.01 very small; 0.2 small; 0.5 medium; 0.8 large; 1.2 very large; and 2.0 huge.

RESULTS

Different TD Age Groups Show Different Signatures of Involuntary Head Motion Variability

The different age groups of TD participants showed differences in statistical signatures of NSR, with trend shifting downward with age. This result can be seen across all the age groups for the linear speed in **Figure 3** and for the angular speed in the **Supplementary Material Figures A1, A2** and **Supplementary Table S2.**

These differences in the involuntary head motions expressed by the linear speed extend to other Gamma parameters and moments in **Figure 3**. They reach statistical significance for all groups, as shown by **Figure 4**, ($p < 0.05$) when comparing pairwise each group. The NSR summarizing the variance to mean ratio is significantly different for some groups at the 0.01 level. All groups differ in NSR evolution at $p < 0.05$. In contrast the estimated PDF curves were only significantly different for 5-10 and 11-15 groups when comparing them to all the other groups; but the differences in PDF were not significant for the groups above 16 years of age. Comparable results for all parameters related to angular speed can be seen in **Supplementary Material Figure A1.**

Different ASD Age Groups Show Different Signatures of Involuntary Head Motion Variability

The comparisons of the age-groups with ASD also show shifting statistical signatures across ages (**Figure 5**) and they were significant at the 0.05 level for all comparisons in the NSR. This can be appreciated in **Figure 5** for the linear speed parameter and in the **Supplementary Material Figures A1–A4** for the angular speed parameter (**Supplementary Table S2**).

There Are Significant Differences Between TD and ASD Groups Across Each Age-Group

Differences between the age-dependent groups of TD and ASD can be appreciated in **Figures 4, 5**, respectively, for the linear speed. In particular, the shifts in the stochastic signatures of linear speed variability can be traced cross-sectionally across ages in the Gamma parameter space of moments, where the participants with ASD show higher variability and overall higher values of the head excursions (as quantified by the rates of linear displacements). The statistical significance of these pairwise age-group comparisons can be appreciated in the **Figure 6.** Further **Supplementary Material Figures A1, A4** show the results corresponding to the angular speed parameter reflecting the rates of fluctuations in head rotations. **Supplementary Material Figures A5, A6** further show the results for the two types of bootstrapping methods, reflecting these trends with and without replacement.

Size Effects

The t-test for head excursions based on cumulative linear speed (head translations mm/s) yielded significant differences ($p << 0.001$) when comparing ASD and TD age groups pairwise. Likewise, the t-test for head excursions based on cumulative angular speed (head rotations rad/s) yielded significant differences ($p << 0.001$) when comparing ASD and TD age groups pairwise. **Table 1** shows the p-values.

Disease Effect

For the comparison of ASD vs. TD, the size effects for the cumulative linear displacement of the head (head linear excursions) were in the range of very large to huge, with Glass Delta and Cohen d. The size effects for the cumulative angular displacements of the head (head rotational excursions) were also in the range of very large to huge, according to the Glass Delta and Cohen d, with the exception of age group 31–40 years old with a medium effect. **Table 2** shows the effect sizes per age group.

Age Effects

The pairwise comparison of age groups yielded large to huge size effects for the cumulative head excursions involving linear displacements or angular rotations. These effects are depicted in **Figure 7** as colormaps whereby each entry of the matrix represents a pairwise age group comparison.

DISCUSSION

This paper investigated age-dependent shifts in the statistical signatures of typical levels of involuntary head motions using rs-fMRI data from the ABIDE repository. We characterized the stochastic signatures of involuntary head motions as TD

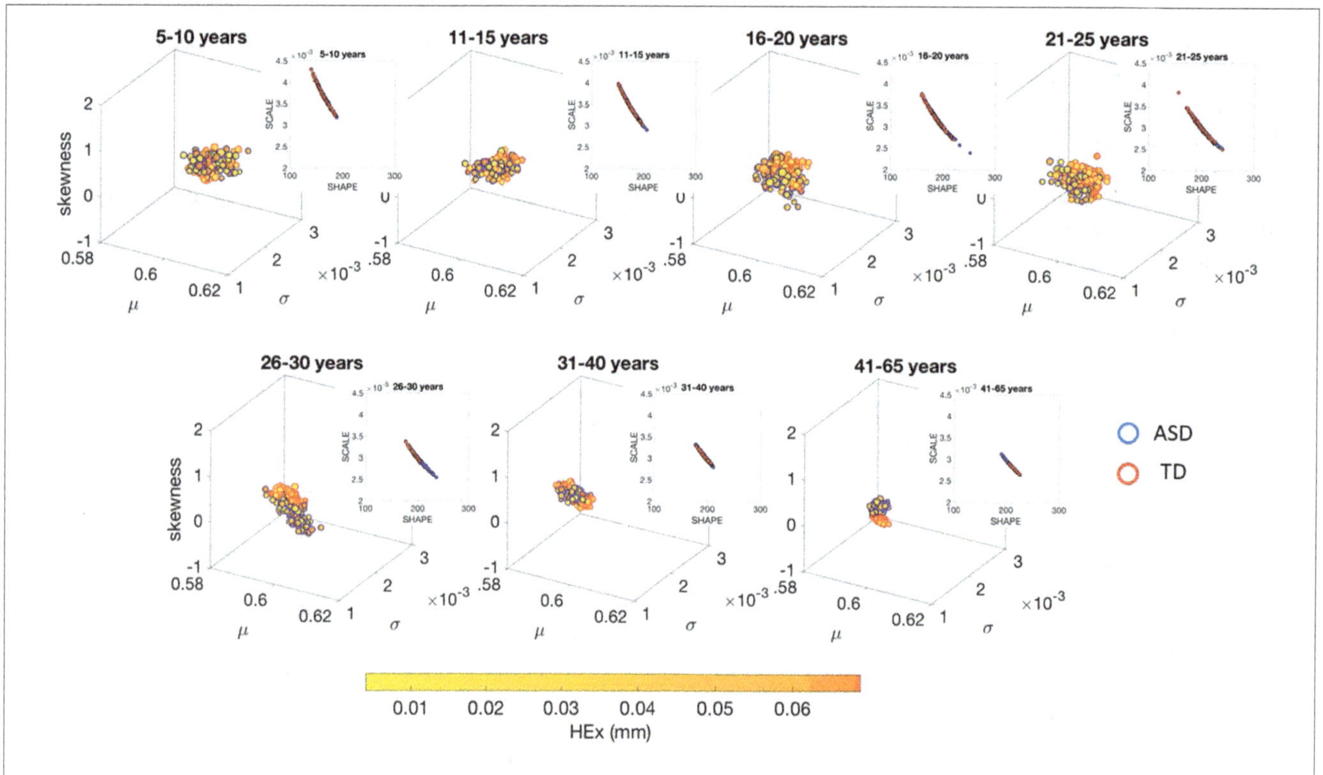

FIGURE 3 | Characterization of the shifts in age-dependent stochastic signatures derived from involuntary head motion defined by linear speed (mm/s) (as in **Figures 2A,B**) for each of the age groups under study. Each group has equal number of representative participants (100). Gamma moment parameters (mean, standard deviation and skewness are represented by the *x*-, *y*-, and *z*-axis dimensions, respectively). The size of the marker is proportional to the kurtosis (smaller being flatter probability density function and larger being peakier distributions). The color of the marker reflects the net amount of head excursion (HEx, mm) as depicted by the colorbar gradient, while the marker's edge color denotes the type of participant. Insets are the Gamma shape vs. scale parameter space, which we also show in **Supplementary Material Figures A7, A8** in log–log units for these linear speed cases for TD and ASD, respectively.

participants rested in the scanner. We uncovered age-dependent transitions in the features of empirically estimated probability distributions of the fluctuations in peak amplitudes of linear and angular speed from involuntary head motions. We also measured the departure from this normative data in different age-groups of participants with ASD. We found that from 5 to 65 years of age, there were statistically significant differences in the distribution parameters of standardized fluctuations in speed amplitude relative to normative levels. They were paired with differences in PDF skewness and differences in PDF overall shape. We quantified mostly very large to huge size effects of these differences for disorder and age effects. The findings demonstrate that it is inadequate to assume or enforce normal distributions in statistical analyses of developmental research, including autism research. Both the linear speed and the angular speed data revealed consistent results that point at high levels of speed amplitude noise in ASD, thus making it hard to forecast future from prior speed levels.

Our work strongly suggests the need to explore age-dependent variations in noise and randomness levels in ASD motor parameters and design separate, age-appropriate analyses for young children, adolescents, and older adults. In future research, we will need to more systematically explore the typical population and build records of the age-dependent rates of change in statistical parameters reflecting levels of neuromotor control, to design new non-parametric models of normative age-shifting data. Further, our results point to the importance of studying autism as a lifelong condition that changes non-uniformly, asynchronously within a given age group and dynamically as the person ages, as compared to TD controls.

The present data set offers cross-sectional information from the ASD and TD populations. These data sets are very valuable as they revealed trends in the rates of change of probability distributions derived from *involuntary* motor data as the population ages. However, to truly characterize the heterogeneous ASD, and to stratify the population into various subtypes, we will need to deploy longitudinal studies that better reflect individual differences over time. Such differences could be tracked as the person aged and received treatments. A longitudinal and dynamic characterization of neuromotor development, including voluntary purposeful, goal-directed motions will be very important to understand the evolution of motor autonomy, action planning, action generation and action adaptation in the context of the person's agency over naturalistic behaviors taking place in activities of daily life.

Some caveats of the ABIDE data sets are that there are different sampling resolutions of the scanners that different labs use. In recent work, we have characterized the types of noise

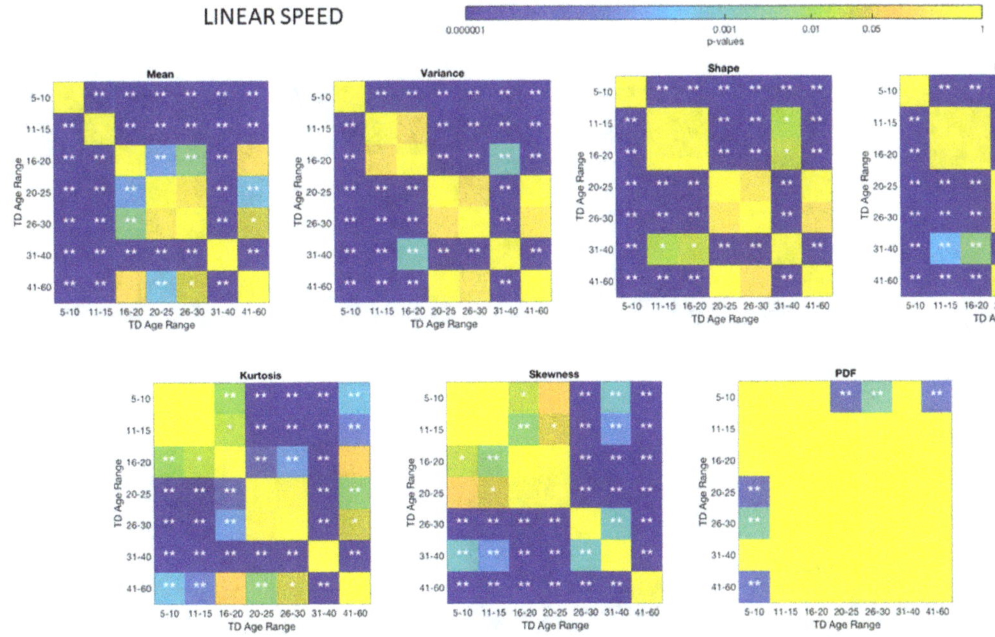

FIGURE 4 | Non–parametric ANOVA Kruskal–Wallis pairwise statistical comparison for each TD age-group for the Gamma parameters and moments, derived from the peak amplitudes of the involuntary head motions defined by the head displacements (linear speed measured in mm/s). Reported p-values are uncorrected for multiple comparisons. $^{*}p < 0.05$, $^{**}p < 0.01$.

according to sampling resolution and shown, using these same data sets, that the sampling resolution of the scanner does affect the type of noise (Caballero et al., 2018). We have also shown that the noise type can distinguish controls vs. autistic participants. Here we employed the bootstrapping technique to shuffle the speed amplitudes and randomize the possible biases that different sampling resolutions introduce. We further took care of using similar sample sizes for each age group and keeping the number of frames equal for each representative data point in the 100 set. These precautions paired with the standardization of the fluctuations deviating from an empirical estimated mean, to avoid allometric effects due to anatomical differences within a group, ensure proper comparisons. However, we also point out that breaking the groups into 5-year intervals was somewhat arbitrary, as a finer break down would have been ideal. This grouping was motivated by prior work where we were able to group medication intake and clinical scores for these groups and reveal trends across the population (Torres and Denisova, 2016). The main motivation there and here were the disparate sizes of age groups in ABIDE. We emphasize that beyond pointing out the trends in systematic shifts of probability families, we do not claim anything else. The main message of the paper is that we should not use a *one size fits all* model when performing statistical analyses, because different distributions are present in the normative groups, and in the autistic groups. Moreover, in autism, these distributions differ relative to those of controls. Levels of noise to signal ratio in these standardized waveforms systematically shift cross sectionally with aging and this reflects in a changing probability landscape that we should consider when performing our statistical analyses.

Lastly, at a different level, the results from our work are important to alert researchers, clinicians and policy makers of the shifting issues that the autistic population faces and the need for a highly flexible program that considers such shifts as the person ages. Under such profound sensory-motor differences *at the periphery* and excess of undesirable involuntary movements, it will be important to understand and characterize the types of feedback that the autistic central nervous systems are getting from the peripheral nervous systems. Once we understand these issues, we will be able to offer better support to the autistic person across all ages by leveraging sensory substitution/augmentation and noise cancelation techniques, etc. from the field of Neuroscience.

At present, autism is defined and treated as a behavioral problem reflecting issues with social interaction and communication, yet those are "*the tip of the iceberg.*" Another hidden layer of information contributing to those visible problems are these irregular micro-motions invisible to the naked eye of the diagnostician and/or the therapist. While aiming at reshaping the autistic person's behaviors to conform to social expectations without considering such intrinsic (concealed) sensory-motor issues, the current interventions used to treat autism may unintentionally create a bigger problem.

Our lab has found that in autism, under such high levels of MMS noise across the peripheral nervous systems it is difficult to develop proper motor control (Brincker and Torres, 2013). These conclusions are supported by prior work in the field of motor control (Gidley Larson et al., 2008; Haswell et al., 2009; Marko et al., 2015; Mosconi and Sweeney, 2015;

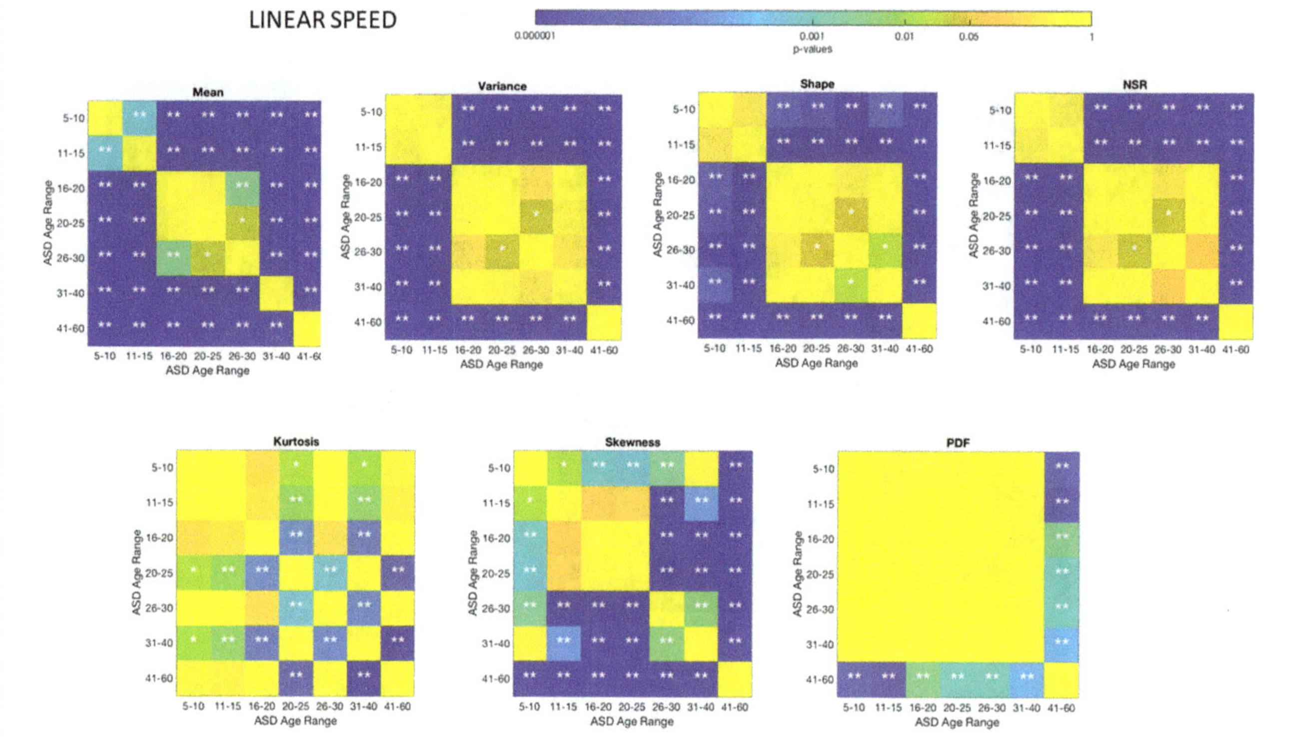

FIGURE 5 | Non-parametric ANOVA ***Kruskal–Wallis*** pairwise statistical comparison for each ASD age-group for the Gamma parameters and moments, derived from the peak amplitude of involuntary head motions defined by the head displacements (linear speed measured in mm/s). Reported **p**-values are uncorrected for multiple comparisons. $^{*}p < 0.05$ and $^{**}p < 0.01$.

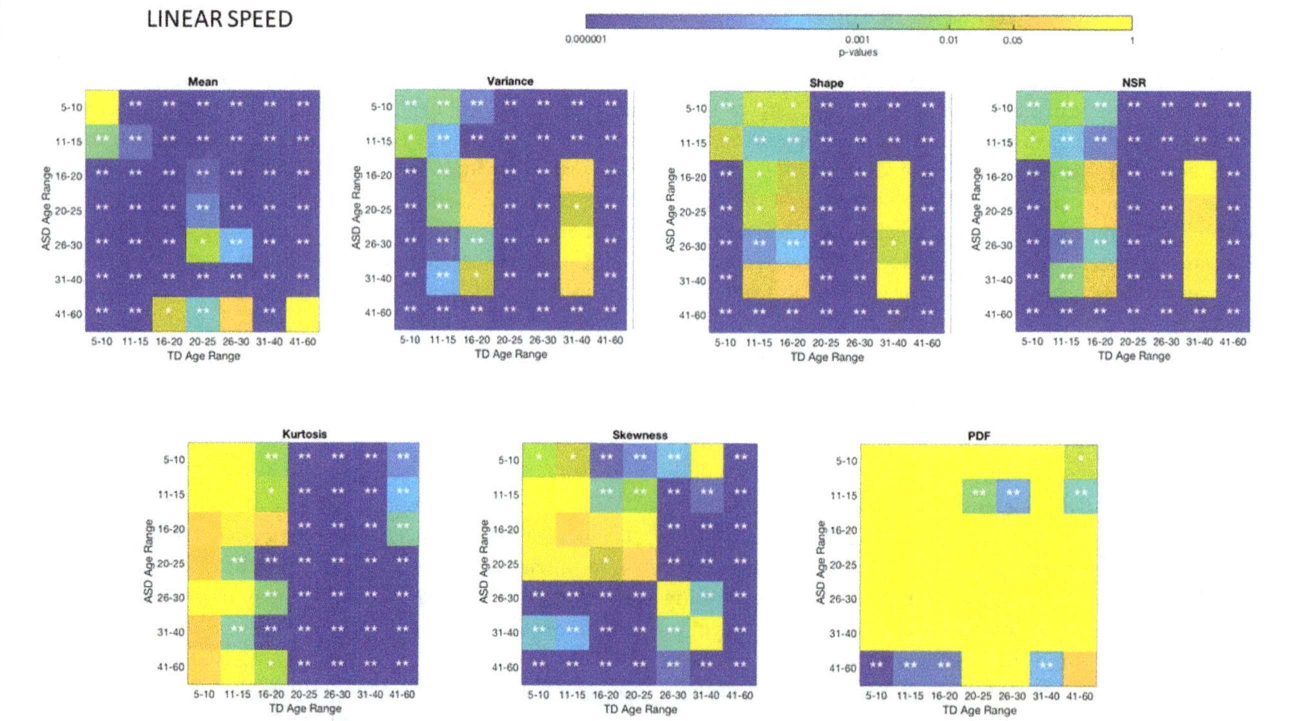

FIGURE 6 | Non-parametric ANOVA ***Kruskal–Wallis*** pairwise statistical comparison for each age-group comparing TD vs. ASD for each of the Gamma parameters and moments, derived from the peak amplitude of involuntary head motions measured by the rate of displacement (linear speed mm/s). $^{*}p < 0.05$ and $^{**}p < 0.01$.

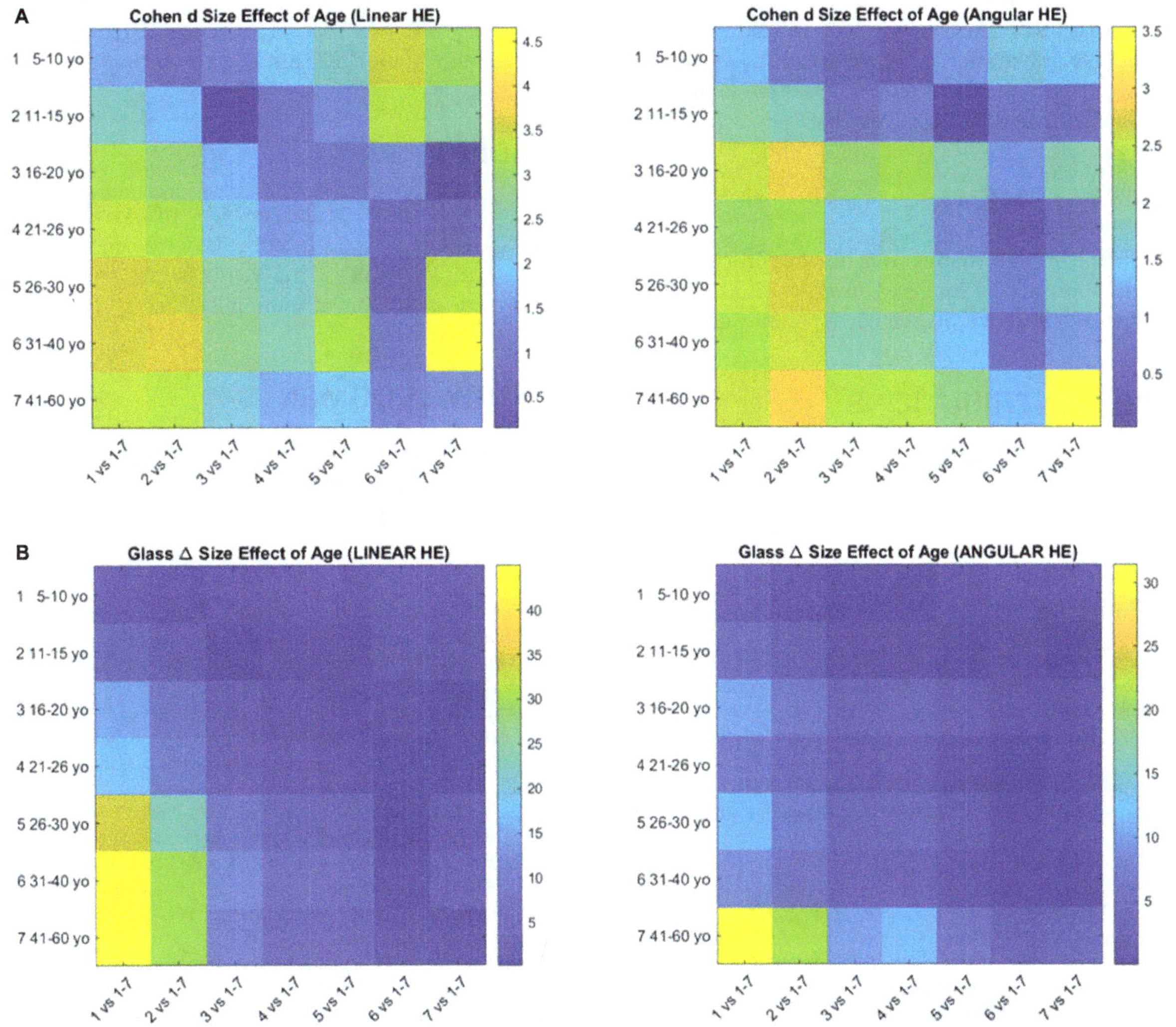

FIGURE 7 | Size effects of aging according to the Cohen's *d* **(A)** and the Glass delta **(B)** formulae applied pairwise to the age groups using the head excursion parameter derived from the cumulative linear displacements or angular rotations.

Mosconi et al., 2015a) including issues with the motor cortex (Muller et al., 2001; Theoret et al., 2005; Mostofsky et al., 2007; Floris et al., 2016; Al Sagheer et al., 2018) and the cerebellum (Mostofsky et al., 2009; Mosconi et al., 2013, 2015b). Such mounting evidence highlights the need for a better characterization of the observable behaviors defining autism in terms of underlying somatic sensory motor signatures. A neurological model (e.g., Damasio and Maurer, 1978) to explain the autistic behavioral symptoms would be more adequate to leverage the wearable sensors revolution and open a new field for *objective behavioral analyses*. Such a field would considerably help advance the neuroscience and the genetics of autism by providing new tools from AI and machine learning to automatically stratify the various subtypes of autism and guide the design of personalized treatments, accommodations and support.

One of the main features of neurotypical development is the emergence of neuromotor autonomy, which in turn depends on central control. Central control depends on the continuous peripheral feedback that kinesthetic reafferent input provides (Kandel, 2013). In neurotypical systems with intact kinesthetic feedback, mental intent matches physical action, but this is not the case in age- and sex-matched autistics (Torres et al., 2013b). This type of peripheral feedback is important for motor learning and adaptation at all levels, including socio motor behaviors, speech production via vocal apparatus and communication through pointing gestures, and gait maturation. Occupational therapists work on creating adequate support and accommodations to complete simple actions of daily living that TD individuals may take for granted, but their therapies are not always covered by medical insurance. Perhaps this type of evidence on core systemic, sensory motor differences in the autistic peripheral nervous system could help advance their programs and provide the types of objective outcome measures of treatment effectiveness that insurance companies require.

In summary, we have shown the need for new, more dynamic statistical approaches to neurodevelopment and natural aging, as well as the need to provide normative scales to measure departure from typical states in levels of motor noise, randomness and excess involuntary micro-movements in ASD.

ETHICS STATEMENT

The studies involving data sharing from human participants were reviewed and approved by Rutgers University IRB. All data in ABIDE follows IRB approval of their corresponding university.

AUTHOR CONTRIBUTIONS

Conceptualization, ET methodology, ET; software, ET, CC, SM; validation, ET, CC, SM; formal analysis, ET, CC, SM; investigation, ET, CC, SM resources, ET, CC, SM data curation, CC, SM; writing—original draft preparation, ET; writing—review and editing, ET, CC, SM; visualization, ET; supervision, ET; project administration, ET; funding acquisition, ET.

FUNDING

This work was funded by the New Jersey Governor's Council for the Medical Research and Treatments of Autism to ET and by the generosity of the Nancy Lurie Marks Family Foundation to the Rutgers Sensory Motor Integration Laboratory.

ACKNOWLEDGMENTS

We thank all the participants in the ABIDE studies and the researchers who uploaded their data to ABIDE. We thank the organizers of ABIDE.

REFERENCES

Al Sagheer, T., Haida, O., Balbous, A., Francheteau, M., Matas, E., Fernagut, P. O., et al. (2018). Motor impairments correlate with social deficits and restricted neuronal loss in an environmental model of autism. *Int. J. Neuropsychopharmacol.* 21, 871–882. doi: 10.1093/ijnp/pyy043

Alaerts, K., Woolley, D. G., Steyaert, J., Di Martino, A., Swinnen, S. P., and Wenderoth, N. (2014). Underconnectivity of the superior temporal sulcus predicts emotion recognition deficits in autism. *Soc. Cogn. Affect. Neurosci.* 9, 1589–1600. doi: 10.1093/scan/nst156

American Psychiatric Association (2013). *Diagnostic and Statistical Manual of Mental Disorders: Diagnostic and Statistical Manual of Mental Disorders, Fifth Edition.* Arlington, VA: American Psychiatric Association.

Brincker, M., and Torres, E. B. (2013). Noise from the periphery in autism. *Front. Integr. Neurosci.* 7:34. doi: 10.3389/fnint.2013.00034

Caballero, C., Davids, K., Heller, B., Wheat, J., and Moreno, F. J. (2019). Movement variability emerges in gait as adaptation to task constraints in dynamic environments. *Gait Posture* 70, 1–5. doi: 10.1016/j.gaitpost.2019.02.002

Caballero, C., Mistry, S., Vero, J., and Torres, E. B. (2018). Characterization of noise signatures of involuntary head motion in the autism brain imaging data exchange repository. *Front. Integr. Neurosci.* 12:7. doi: 10.3389/fnint.2018.00007

Chuye, L. B., Dimitri, A., Desai, A., Handelmann, C., Bae, Y., Johari, P., et al. (2018). Brain organoids: expanding our understanding of human development and disease. *Results Probl. Cell Differ.* 66, 183–206. doi: 10.1007/978-3-319-93485-3_8

Cohen, J. (1992). A power primer. *Psychol. Bull.* 112:155.

Constantino, J. N., and Charman, T. (2016). Diagnosis of autism spectrum disorder: reconciling the syndrome, its diverse origins, and variation in expression. *Lancet Neurol.* 15, 279–291. doi: 10.1016/S1474-4422(15)00151-9

Cox, R. W. (1996). AFNI: software for analysis and visualization of functional magnetic resonance neuroimages. *Comput. Biomed. Res.* 29, 162–173. doi: 10.1006/cbmr.1996.0014

Damasio, A. R., and Maurer, R. G. (1978). A neurological model for childhood autism. *Arch. Neurol.* 35, 777–786. doi: 10.1001/archneur.1978.00500360001001

Di Martino, A., Yan, C. G., Li, Q., Denio, E., Castellanos, F. X., Alaerts, K., et al. (2014). The autism brain imaging data exchange: towards a large-scale evaluation of the intrinsic brain architecture in autism. *Mol. Psychiatry* 19, 659–667. doi: 10.1038/mp.2013.78

Donnellan, A. M., Hill, D. A., and Leary, M. R. (2012). Rethinking autism: implications of sensory and movement differences for understanding and support. *Front. Integr. Neurosci.* 6:124. doi: 10.3389/fnint.2012.00124

Floris, D. L., Barber, A. D., Nebel, M. B., Martinelli, M., Lai, M. C., Crocetti, D., et al. (2016). Atypical lateralization of motor circuit functional connectivity in children with autism is associated with motor deficits. *Mol. Autism.* 7:35. doi: 10.1186/s13229-016-0096-6

Gidley Larson, J. C., Bastian, A. J., Donchin, O., Shadmehr, R., and Mostofsky, S. H. (2008). Acquisition of internal models of motor tasks in children with autism. *Brain* 131(Pt 11), 2894–2903. doi: 10.1093/brain/awn226

Haar, S., Berman, S., Behrmann, M., and Dinstein, I. (2016). Anatomical abnormalities in autism? *Cereb. Cortex* 26, 1440–1452. doi: 10.1093/cercor/bhu242

Hamilton, J. D. (1994). *Time Series Analysis.* Princeton, NJ: Princeton University Press.

Hannant, P., Tavassoli, T., and Cassidy, S. (2016). The role of sensorimotor difficulties in autism spectrum conditions. *Front. Neurol.* 7:124. doi: 10.3389/fneur.2016.00124

Haswell, C. C., Izawa, J., Dowell, L. R., Mostofsky, S. H., and Shadmehr, R. (2009). Representation of internal models of action in the autistic brain. *Nat. Neurosci.* 12, 970–972. doi: 10.1038/nn.2356

Jasmin, E., Couture, M., McKinley, P., Reid, G., Fombonne, E., and Gisel, E. (2009). Sensori-motor and daily living skills of preschool children with autism spectrum disorders. *J. Autism Dev. Disord.* 39, 231–241. doi: 10.1007/s10803-008-0617-z

Jung, M., Tu, Y., Lang, C. A., Ortiz, A., Park, J., Jorgenson, K., et al. (2019). Decreased structural connectivity and resting-state brain activity in the lateral occipital cortex is associated with social communication deficits in boys with autism spectrum disorder. *Neuroimage* 190, 205–212. doi: 10.1016/j.neuroimage.2017.09.031

Kandel, E. R. (2013). *Principles of Neural Science*, 5th Edn. New York, NY: McGraw-Hill.

Kushki, A., Chau, T., and Anagnostou, E. (2011). Handwriting difficulties in children with autism spectrum disorders: a scoping review. *J. Autism Dev. Disord.* 41, 1706–1716. doi: 10.1007/s10803-011-1206-0

Lancaster, M. A., Renner, M., Martin, C. A., Wenzel, D., Bicknell, L. S., Hurles, M. E., et al. (2013). Cerebral organoids model human brain development and microcephaly. *Nature* 501, 373–379. doi: 10.1038/nature12517

Lleonart, J., Salat, J., and Torres, G. J. (2000). Removing allometric effects of body size in morphological analysis. *J. Theor. Biol.* 205, 85–93. doi: 10.1006/jtbi.2000.2043

Lord, C., Risi, S., Lambrecht, L., Cook, E. H. Jr., Leventhal, B. L., DiLavore, P. C., et al. (2000). The autism diagnostic observation schedule-generic: a standard measure of social and communication deficits associated with the spectrum of autism. *J. Autism Dev. Disord.* 30, 205–223.

Mahajan, R., Dirlikov, B., Crocetti, D., and Mostofsky, S. H. (2016). Motor circuit anatomy in children with autism spectrum disorder with or without attention deficit hyperactivity disorder. *Autism Res.* 9, 67–81. doi: 10.1002/aur.1497

Mandelbaum, D. E., Stevens, M., Rosenberg, E., Wiznitzer, M., Steinschneider, M., Filipek, P., et al. (2006). Sensorimotor performance in school-age children with autism, developmental language disorder, or low IQ. *Dev. Med. Child Neurol.* 48, 33–39. doi: 10.1017/S0012162206000089

Marko, M. K., Crocetti, D., Hulst, T., Donchin, O., Shadmehr, R., and Mostofsky, S. H. (2015). Behavioural and neural basis of anomalous motor learning in children with autism. *Brain* 138(Pt 3), 784–797. doi: 10.1093/brain/awu394

Minshew, N. J., Sung, K., Jones, B. L., and Furman, J. M. (2004). Underdevelopment of the postural control system in autism. *Neurology* 63, 2056–2061. doi: 10.1212/01.wnl.0000145771.98657.62

Mosconi, M. W., Luna, B., Kay-Stacey, M., Nowinski, C. V., Rubin, L. H., Scudder, C., et al. (2013). Saccade adaptation abnormalities implicate dysfunction of cerebellar-dependent learning mechanisms in autism spectrum disorders (ASD). *PLoS One* 8:e63709. doi: 10.1371/journal.pone.0063709

Mosconi, M. W., Mohanty, S., Greene, R. K., Cook, E. H., Vaillancourt, D. E., and Sweeney, J. A. (2015a). Feedforward and feedback motor control abnormalities implicate cerebellar dysfunctions in autism spectrum disorder. *J. Neurosci.* 35, 2015–2025. doi: 10.1523/JNEUROSCI.2731-14.2015

Mosconi, M. W., and Sweeney, J. A. (2015). Sensorimotor dysfunctions as primary features of autism spectrum disorders. *Sci. China Life Sci.* 58, 1016–1023. doi: 10.1007/s11427-015-4894-4

Mosconi, M. W., Wang, Z., Schmitt, L. M., Tsai, P., and Sweeney, J. A. (2015b). The role of cerebellar circuitry alterations in the pathophysiology of autism spectrum disorders. *Front. Neurosci.* 9:296. doi: 10.3389/fnins.2015.00296

Mosimann, J. E. (1970). Size allometry: size and shape variables with characterizations of the lognormal and generalized gamma distributions. *J. Am. Stat. Assoc.* 65, 930–945. doi: 10.1080/01621459.1970.10481136

Mostofsky, S. H., Burgess, M. P., and Gidley Larson, J. C. (2007). Increased motor cortex white matter volume predicts motor impairment in autism. *Brain* 130(Pt 8), 2117–2122. doi: 10.1093/brain/awm129

Mostofsky, S. H., Powell, S. K., Simmonds, D. J., Goldberg, M. C., Caffo, B., and Pekar, J. J. (2009). Decreased connectivity and cerebellar activity in autism during motor task performance. *Brain* 132(Pt 9), 2413–2425. doi: 10.1093/brain/awp088

Muller, R. A., Pierce, K., Ambrose, J. B., Allen, G., and Courchesne, E. (2001). Atypical patterns of cerebral motor activation in autism: a functional magnetic resonance study. *Biol. Psychiatry* 49, 665–676. doi: 10.1016/s0006-3223(00)01004-0

Ornitz, E. M. (1974). The modulation of sensory input and motor output in autistic children. *J. Autism Child Schizophr.* 4, 197–215. doi: 10.1007/bf02115226

Peng, C. K., Havlin, S., Stanley, H. E., and Goldberger, A. L. (1995). Quantification of scaling exponents and crossover phenomena in nonstationary heartbeat time series. *Chaos* 5, 82–87. doi: 10.1063/1.166141

Perry, W., Minassian, A., Lopez, B., Maron, L., and Lincoln, A. (2007). Sensorimotor gating deficits in adults with autism. *Biol. Psychiatry* 61, 482–486. doi: 10.1016/j.biopsych.2005.09.025

Plitt, M., Barnes, K. A., and Martin, A. (2015). Functional connectivity classification of autism identifies highly predictive brain features but falls short of biomarker standards. *Neuroimage Clin.* 7, 359–366. doi: 10.1016/j.nicl.2014.12.013

Raffalt, P. C., Alkjaer, T., Brynjolfsson, B., Jorgensen, L., Bartholdy, C., and Henriksen, M. (2018). Day-to-day reliability of nonlinear methods to assess walking dynamics. *J. Biomech. Eng.* 140:124501. doi: 10.1115/1.4041044

Ray, S., Miller, M., Karalunas, S., Robertson, C., Grayson, D. S., Cary, R. P., et al. (2014). Structural and functional connectivity of the human brain in autism spectrum disorders and attention-deficit/hyperactivity disorder: a rich club-organization study. *Hum. Brain Mapp.* 35, 6032–6048. doi: 10.1002/hbm.22603

Ross, S. M. (1996). *Stochastic processes*, 2nd Edn. New York, NY: Wiley.

Sawilowsky, S. S. (2003). A different future for social and behavioral science research. *J. Mod. Appl. Stat. Methods* 2, 128–132. doi: 10.22237/jmasm/1051747860

Sharer, E., Crocetti, D., Muschelli, J., Barber, A. D., Nebel, M. B., Caffo, B. S., et al. (2015). Neural correlates of visuomotor learning in autism. *J. Child Neurol.* 30, 1877–1886. doi: 10.1177/0883073815600869

Starkstein, S., Gellar, S., Parlier, M., Payne, L., and Piven, J. (2015). High rates of parkinsonism in adults with autism. *J. Neurodev. Disord.* 7:29. doi: 10.1186/s11689-015-9125-6

Supekar, K., and Menon, V. (2015). Sex differences in structural organization of motor systems and their dissociable links with repetitive/restricted behaviors in children with autism. *Mol. Autism* 6:50. doi: 10.1186/s13229-015-0042-z

Theoret, H., Halligan, E., Kobayashi, M., Fregni, F., Tager-Flusberg, H., and Pascual-Leone, A. (2005). Impaired motor facilitation during action observation in individuals with autism spectrum disorder. *Curr. Biol.* 15, R84–R85. doi: 10.1016/j.cub.2005.01.022

Torres, E. B. (2011a). Atypical signatures of motor variability found in an individual with ASD. *Neurocase* 19, 150–165. doi: 10.1080/13554794.2011.654224

Torres, E. B. (2011b). Two classes of movements in motor control. *Exp. Brain Res.* 215, 269–283. doi: 10.1007/s00221-011-2892-8

Torres, E. B., Brincker, M., Isenhower, R. W., Yanovich, P., Stigler, K. A., Nurnberger, J. I., et al. (2013a). Autism: the micro-movement perspective. *Front. Integr. Neurosci.* 7:32. doi: 10.3389/fnint.2013.00032

Torres, E. B., and Denisova, K. (2016). Motor noise is rich signal in autism research and pharmacological treatments. *Sci. Rep.* 6, 37422. doi: 10.1038/srep37422

Torres, E. B., Isenhower, R. W., Nguyen, J., Whyatt, C., Nurnberger, J. I., Jose, J. V., et al. (2016a). Toward precision psychiatry: statistical platform for the personalized characterization of natural behaviors. *Front. Neurol.* 7:8. doi: 10.3389/fneur.2016.00008

Torres, E. B., Mistry, S., Caballero, C., and Whyatt, C. P. (2017). Stochastic signatures of involuntary head micro-movements can be used to classify females of ABIDE into different subtypes of neurodevelopmental disorders. *Front. Integr. Neurosci.* 11:10. doi: 10.3389/fnint.2017.00010

Torres, E. B., Smith, B., Mistry, S., Brincker, M., and Whyatt, C. (2016b). Neonatal diagnostics: toward dynamic growth charts of neuromotor control. *Front. Pediatr.* 4:121. doi: 10.3389/fped.2016.00121

Torres, E. B., Yanovich, P., and Metaxas, D. N. (2013b). Give spontaneity and self-discovery a chance in ASD: spontaneous peripheral limb variability as a proxy to evoke centrally driven intentional acts. *Front. Integr. Neurosci.* 7:46. doi: 10.3389/fnint.2013.00046

Wu, D., Jose, J. V., Nurnberger, J. I., and Torres, E. B. (2018). A biomarker characterizing neurodevelopment with applications in autism. *Sci. Rep.* 8:614. doi: 10.1038/s41598-017-18902-w

3

The Autism Biomarkers Consortium for Clinical Trials (ABC-CT): Scientific Context, Study Design and Progress Toward Biomarker Qualification

James C. McPartland[1], Raphael A. Bernier[2,3], Shafali S. Jeste[4], Geraldine Dawson[5], Charles A. Nelson[6,7], Katarzyna Chawarska[1], Rachel Earl[8], Susan Faja[6,7], Scott P. Johnson[4], Linmarie Sikich[5], Cynthia A. Brandt[9], James D. Dziura[9], Leon Rozenblit[10], Gerhard Hellemann[4], April R. Levin[6,7], Michael Murias[11], Adam J. Naples[1], Michael L. Platt[12], Maura Sabatos-DeVito[5], Frederick Shic[2,13], Damla Senturk[4], Catherine A. Sugar[4], Sara J. Webb[2,3] and the Autism Biomarkers Consortium for Clinical Trials*

[1] Yale Child Study Center, New Haven, CT, United States, [2] Center for Child Health, Behavior and Development, Seattle Children's Research Institute, Seattle Children's Hospital, Seattle, WA, United States, [3] Department of Psychiatry and Behavioral Sciences, University of Washington School of Medicine, Seattle, WA, United States, [4] University of California, Los Angeles, Los Angeles, CA, United States, [5] Duke Center for Autism and Brain Development, Duke University, Durham, NC, United States, [6] Boston Children's Hospital and Harvard Medical School, Boston, MA, United States, [7] Harvard University, Boston, MA, United States, [8] Center on Human Development and Disability, University of Washington, Seattle, WA, United States, [9] Yale University, New Haven, CT, United States, [10] Prometheus Research, LLC, New Haven, CT, United States, [11] Northwestern University, Chicago, IL, United States, [12] University of Pennsylvania, Philadelphia, PA, United States, [13] Department of Pediatrics, University of Washington School of Medicine, Seattle, WA, United States

***Correspondence:**
James C. McPartland
james.mcpartland@yale.edu

Clinical research in neurodevelopmental disorders remains reliant upon clinician and caregiver measures. Limitations of these approaches indicate a need for objective, quantitative, and reliable biomarkers to advance clinical research. Extant research suggests the potential utility of multiple candidate biomarkers; however, effective application of these markers in trials requires additional understanding of replicability, individual differences, and intra-individual stability over time. The Autism Biomarkers Consortium for Clinical Trials (ABC-CT) is a multi-site study designed to investigate a battery of electrophysiological (EEG) and eye-tracking (ET) indices as candidate biomarkers for autism spectrum disorder (ASD). The study complements published biomarker research through: inclusion of large, deeply phenotyped cohorts of children with ASD and typical development; a longitudinal design; a focus on well-evidenced candidate biomarkers harmonized with an independent sample; high levels of clinical, regulatory, technical, and statistical rigor; adoption of a governance structure incorporating diverse expertise in the ASD biomarker discovery and qualification process; prioritization of open science, including creation of a repository containing biomarker, clinical, and genetic data; and use of economical and scalable technologies that are applicable in developmental populations and those with special needs. The ABC-CT approach has yielded encouraging results, with one measure accepted into the FDA's Biomarker Qualification Program to date. Through these advances, the ABC-CT and other biomarker studies in progress hold promise to deliver novel tools to improve clinical trials research in ASD.

Keywords: autism spectrum disorder, biomarker, neuroscience, clinical trial methodology/study design, EEG, ERP, eye-tracking

INTRODUCTION

There are currently no validated biomarkers for use in clinical trials in autism spectrum disorder (ASD). Clinical research remains reliant upon standardized but intrinsically subjective clinician and caregiver/self-report measures. These tools have supported significant but incomplete progress in diagnosis, selection of intervention, and measurement of treatment response; however, advancement on other key objectives, such as designation of subgroups of individuals (i.e., stratification) within this heterogeneous neurodevelopmental condition, have stagnated. Notably, the most recent diagnostic taxonomy for ASD (American Psychiatric Association, 2013) discarded behaviorally defined subtypes because they were not reliable and had limited utility for treatment selection or determination of prognosis (Lord et al., 2012a). As highlighted by other articles in this collection (Ewen et al., 2019), there is a widely recognized and urgent need for biomarkers to support clinical research in ASD (McPartland, 2017). Improved understanding of biomarkers may also provide a framework to bridge understanding of mechanisms across human and animal models, in areas in which behavior may be insufficiently informative (Modi and Sahin, 2017).

This Frontiers in Neuroscience Perspective highlights the specific challenges that have impeded progress in biomarker research in ASD and presents the rationale, design, and progress of the Autism Biomarkers Consortium for Clinical Trials (ABC-CT). The ABC-CT is a multisite study specifically designed to evaluate a set of promising electrophysiological (EEG) and eye-tracking (ET) markers while addressing shortcomings of prior research and establishing a comprehensive approach to biomarker validation in ASD. Within this context, we describe the study design of the ABC-CT in terms of specific strategies implemented to address limitations of published research and to provide opportunities for enhancing understanding of ASD biomarkers. We highlight recent advances that have been made in the context of this project and describe recommended directions for future investigation.

SCIENTIFIC CONTEXT: CHALLENGES TO BIOMARKER DEVELOPMENT IN ASD

A primary factor slowing progress in biomarker development for ASD is the heterogeneity associated with the disorder. The diagnosis of ASD is based on a constellation of widely variable behaviors (American Psychiatric Association, 2013). Additional phenotypic variability is introduced by associated non-diagnostic features, such as intellectual disability, and comorbidities, such as epilepsy and attention-deficit/hyperactivity disorder. Myriad genetic, epigenetic, and environmental factors contribute to the etiology of ASD. While there is some neurobiological convergence in common neural circuits, many upstream molecular pathways lead to this disruption of network function (Jeste and Geschwind, 2014). Given that biomarker development strategies frequently focus on measurement of an identified mechanism, the challenge in ASD is significant, as candidate biological factors are selected, in large part, by purported connection to behavior rather than a clearly defined biological pathway. For example, impaired social-communication is a hallmark and universal feature of ASD, but there is neither a single neural pathway for nor standard means of quantifying social-communication. The lack of clear target mechanisms is further complicated by the dynamic and variable nature of human development. In a neurodevelopmental condition in which symptoms evolve and change throughout the lifespan, applicability of biomarkers across ages is uncertain.

Other impediments to biomarker development in ASD reflect elements of the research enterprise itself. Multiple factors, such as high costs of human subjects research and limitations on recruitment in single site studies, encourage dissemination with the minimal viable *sample size*, often permitting assessment of group discrimination or simple associations but not analysis of complex interactions or stratification. Such small studies may also be prone to generation of spurious or idiosyncratic results that are unlikely to replicate. Even in biomarker studies utilizing large samples, the task of understanding individual differences and relationships to the clinical phenotype is only possible with *deep phenotyping* of these behavioral and clinical correlates, which is resource intensive. Publication and procurement of research funding explicitly value innovation, creating a pressure to explore novel biomarkers that is, to some degree, at odds with the goal of examining the replicability and reproducibility of *well-studied biomarkers* to provide more conclusive evidence of viability. Even fewer studies include a designated *replication sample* to verify findings in an independent group.

For even the most well-studied biomarkers in ASD, there are several near universal gaps in understanding. *Methodological rigor*, such as variation among studies, is a significant and poorly understood concern. Factors such as stimulus presentation, experimental design, and variation in hardware and software could all influence biomarker measurement in unpredictable ways. For most biomarkers, it is not understood whether or how such factors contribute to observed variability in results. Few biomarker studies have included multiple sampling points in a *longitudinal design*, preventing inference regarding the stability of measurement in a person over time (i.e., test-retest reliability, developmental stability). This is critical information for the potential use of biomarkers in clinical trials.

RESPONDING TO CHALLENGES IN ASD BIOMARKER DEVELOPMENT: ABC-CT STUDY DESIGN

The scientific objectives of the ABC-CT were to evaluate a set of candidate EEG and ET biomarkers, alongside lab-based tasks, in terms of: (1) feasibility of administration in children with ASD; (2) reliability of data collection across sites; (3) construct validity of the assays (i.e., whether they manipulated neural processes as predicted in typically developing (TD) children);

Abbreviations: Co-I: Co-Investigator; NDAR: National Database for Autism Research; PD, Project Director; PI, Principal Investigator; NIH, National Institutes of Health; NIMH, National Institute of Mental Health; SPARK, Simons Powering Autism Research study; Sub, Subcontract; QA, Quality Assurance.

(4) test-retest reliability; (5) ability to discriminate children with ASD from those with TD; (6) utility for stratification into meaningful subgroups of children with ASD; (7) association with clinical phenotype; and (8) developmental stability/sensitivity to change in symptom severity. Below we describe specific elements of ABC-CT study design intended to address the aforementioned challenges for biomarker development in ASD (see sections "Study Population", "Deep Phenotyping", "Well-studied Biomarkers", "Replication Sample", "Methodological Rigor", and "Longitudinal Design"), as well as additional features of the study innovated for this purpose (see sections "Study Governance", "Formation of a Repository", and "Scalability of Biomarkers").

Study Population

A considerable strength of the ABC-CT was the administration of the selected paradigms in a large sample of children with ASD and TD. The study enrolled 280 children with ASD and 119 children with TD. Heterogeneity in the sample was considered carefully. Age range was constrained from 6 to 11 years to limit age-related confounds and to focus on an age-group in which biomarker data could be acquired reliably and validly. Presence of a known genetic syndrome or neurological condition putatively causally related to ASD or known metabolic disorder and/or mitochondrial dysfunction were exclusionary criteria. Because medication use may influence biomarker measurement, a stable regimen was required for 8 weeks prior to enrollment; all medications were allowed in order to enroll a representative sample. Cognitive ability spanned full scale IQ from 60 to 150, as assessed by the Differential Ability Scales (DAS) – 2nd Edition (Elliott, 2007), to permit evaluation of the feasibility of biomarker ascertainment procedures across a range of intellectual abilities. In this way, the sample provided strong statistical power for analyses, while constraining developmental and cognitive heterogeneity. Given the likelihood of significant developmental changes between 6 and 11 years, both chronological age and developmental level are considered in all statistical analyses.

Deep Phenotyping

An extensive phenotyping battery provided rigorous characterization, including observation, interview, and multiple perspectives (i.e., clinician and caregiver). Diagnostic characterization relied upon research gold standard instruments: DSM-5 diagnosis of ASD based on the Autism Diagnostic Observation Schedule (Lord et al., 2012b) and the Autism Diagnostic Interview-Revised (Rutter et al., 2003). Clinician administered assessments also included the DAS, 2nd Edition (Elliott, 2007), and the Vineland Adaptive Behavior Scales, 3rd Edition (Sparrow et al., 2016). Caregiver questionnaires included the Aberrant Behavior Checklist (Aman et al., 1985), the Autism Impact Measure (Kanne et al., 2014), the Pervasive Developmental Disorder Behavior Inventory (Cohen and Sudhalter, 2005), and the Social Responsiveness Scale, 2nd Edition (Constantino and Gruber, 2012). To assess clinical status, the Clinical Global Impression Scale (Guy, 1976) was employed, as this scale is widely used as an outcome measure in pharmacologic treatment studies. Finally, interventions and medications utilized both prior to and during the course of study participation were carefully recorded. The study was thus positioned to evaluate biomarkers with respect to current best practices in terms of clinical assessment.

Well-Studied Biomarkers

Candidate biomarkers were selected to measure social-communicative function or related processes, to be feasible in children with ASD across a wide range of functioning, and to be scalable for clinical trials (section "Scalability of Biomarkers"). Importantly, all biomarkers had been studied in prior research and had shown strong potential to distinguish between children with ASD and TD children or to correlate with clinical characteristics. Four EEG paradigms and five ET paradigms were included in the ABC-CT main study biomarker battery. EEG tasks included: resting state, with eyes open, acquired during viewing of abstract videos (Wang et al., 2013); N170 event-related potential (ERP) to upright human faces, compared to inverted faces and non-social stimuli (McPartland et al., 2004); ERPs to biological motion, contrasting signal between coherent and scrambled point-light animations of walking adults (Kroger et al., 2014); and visual evoked potentials, in response to presentation of phase-reversing black and white checkerboards (Siper et al., 2016). ET tasks included: activity monitoring, comparing percentage of ocular focus (POF) to human faces and heads during videos of highly structured shared activities (Shic et al., 2011); visual attention to biological motion, quantified as POF to biological motion versus scrambled and rotating point-light animations (Klin and Jones, 2008; Annaz et al., 2012); pupillary light reflex (PLR), measuring relative pupil constriction amplitude and latency in response to a flash of light (Nystrom et al., 2015); an interactive social task, measuring POF to human heads and faces during videos of two children at play (Chevallier et al., 2015); and static scenes, measuring POF to human heads and faces during images showing naturalistic scenes of children and adults (Loth et al., 2017; Ness et al., 2017).

Replication Sample

The ABC-CT coordinated study design and analyses with other networks engaged in ASD biomarker studies. For several biomarker assays (N170 ERP, ET static scenes, ET biological motion, ET PLR), acquisition paradigms were harmonized with the European Autism Interventions Multicenter Study for Developing New Medications project (EU-AIMS) (Loth et al., 2014, 2017) to permit replication in a separate sample. Likewise, data analytic teams from both groups coordinated processing pipelines and analytic strategies to ensure comparability of study results. The Janssen Autism Knowledge Engine (JAKE) (Ness et al., 2017) study applied several conceptually analogous assays (e.g., a face ERP biomarker with a different acquisition paradigm), enabling evaluation of robustness of results across different assays.

Methodological Rigor

The study design incorporated a high level of methodological rigor in terms of both clinical and biomarker data acquisition. Identical equipment was used for EEG (EGI 128 channel system) and ET (SR Research EyeLink System) data acquisition and processing at all five data collection sites; equipment was installed and tested by a central data acquisition team to ensure identical setup parameters. Detailed manuals of procedures (MOPs) were established for all biomarker paradigms and standardized protocols were adopted for data collection, processing, and analysis (Webb et al., 2020). Likewise, MOPs guided clinical data collection, and all staff underwent comprehensive training, addressing participant screening, clinical measurement, biomarker data collection procedures, data entry, and study management processes. Fidelity in procedures was maintained for clinical measurement through regular conference calls and monitoring of clinical interview reliability within and across sites. Rigor was enhanced via conduct of the study according to Good Clinical Practice standards, optimizing ABC-CT infrastructure for the conduct of clinical trials.

Longitudinal Design

The naturalistic, longitudinal design of the ABC-CT allowed for the examination of test-retest reliability and stability over time, paralleling the structure and timeline of a clinical trial. Children were assessed across three time points (Time 1: Baseline, Time 2: 6 weeks after baseline, and Time 3: 24 weeks after baseline). At each time point, clinical assessments, parent-rated measures of social impairment, independent ratings of clinical status, and the biomarker battery were completed. These time points were selected to provide information about short-term test-retest reliability (6 weeks) and developmental stability/change over a time period consistent with a potential clinical trial (24 weeks).

Study Governance

The ABC-CT adopted a complex governance structure to incorporate expertise relevant to biomarker development (see **Figure 1**). Funded through a NIH U19 collaborative agreement, the project was a public/private partnership that brought together specialists spanning academia, government agencies, and industry. Administration of the project was overseen by a Steering Committee including ABC-CT members, as well as the Program Officer and project scientists associated with the National Institute of Child Health and Human Development (NICHD), the National Institute of Neurological Disorders and Stroke (NINDS), and the National Institute of Mental Health (NIMH). The ABC-CT was designated a project of the FNIH Biomarkers Consortium, and a Biomarkers Consortium Project Team was assembled to provide additional guidance from experts from the Alzheimer's Disease Neuroimaging Initiative, drug development and neuroscience, autism biomarker projects in industry (JAKE), EU-AIMS, the Simons Foundation, and FDA scientists from the Division of Psychiatry Products. An External Advisory Board included specialists in ASD clinical trial design, an individual with ASD, a family member of individuals with ASD, neurogeneticists, and experts in the conduct of large scale ASD biomarker studies. These three groups informed study design, study conduct, interpretation of results, and preparation of biomarker qualification documentation.

Formation of a Repository

Efficient sharing of all study data was a priority for the ABC-CT. All data were uploaded to the National Database for Autism Research (NDAR, a database within the NIMH Data Archive) on a quarterly basis and made publicly available within four months of uploading (permitting time for quality assurance and control). Blood samples collected from participants and available biological parents have been shared via the NIMH Repository and Genomics Resource[1]. Through a collaboration facilitated by the FNIH Biomarkers Consortium, samples are being genotyped, creating a publicly available repository with complete clinical, biomarker, and genotypic information across the large, longitudinal sample.

Scalability of Biomarkers

Biomarker acquisition modalities utilized in the ABC-CT were selected based on their potential to yield high public health impact. Both EEG and ET are relatively economical biomarker assays, particularly within the class of neurophysiological or neurobehavioral measurements. These methods are also highly scalable and accessible, with EEG recording facilities widely available in existing health care systems, supporting efficient large-scale implementation with extant infrastructure. Though ET is not readily available in most health care settings, commercially available products can be obtained at low cost. These technologies are applicable across a developmental range (e.g., infancy though adulthood) and to individuals with neurodevelopmental conditions and intellectual disabilities.

ABC-CT PROGRESS AND FUTURE DIRECTIONS

The ABC-CT was initiated in July 2015. After a series of in-person meetings and teleconferences involving project governance, a feasibility study of 25 children with ASD and 26 TD children was conducted between December 2015 and March 2016. Based on results of the Feasibility Study, the Main Study design (described in this manuscript) was finalized (for details of review of feasibility and transition to main study, see Webb et al., 2020, sections 2.6 and 2.7). The first subject in the Main study was enrolled in October 2016, data collection was completed in May 2019, and final analyses of the complete data set are in progress, with planned dissemination in Spring 2020.

The N170 biomarker showed strong performance in terms of reliable and valid data acquisition and demonstration of predicted between-group differences at interim analyses conducted in April 2018. Based on these results, a Letter of Intent (LOI) for the *N170 latency to upright human faces* was submitted to the FDA's Center for Drug Evaluation and Research Biomarker Qualification Program (BQP) in November, 2018; the proposed context of use was identifying a biologically homogeneous subgroup within ASD to enrich clinical trials by reduction of ASD-associated heterogeneity.

[1] www.nimhgenetics.org

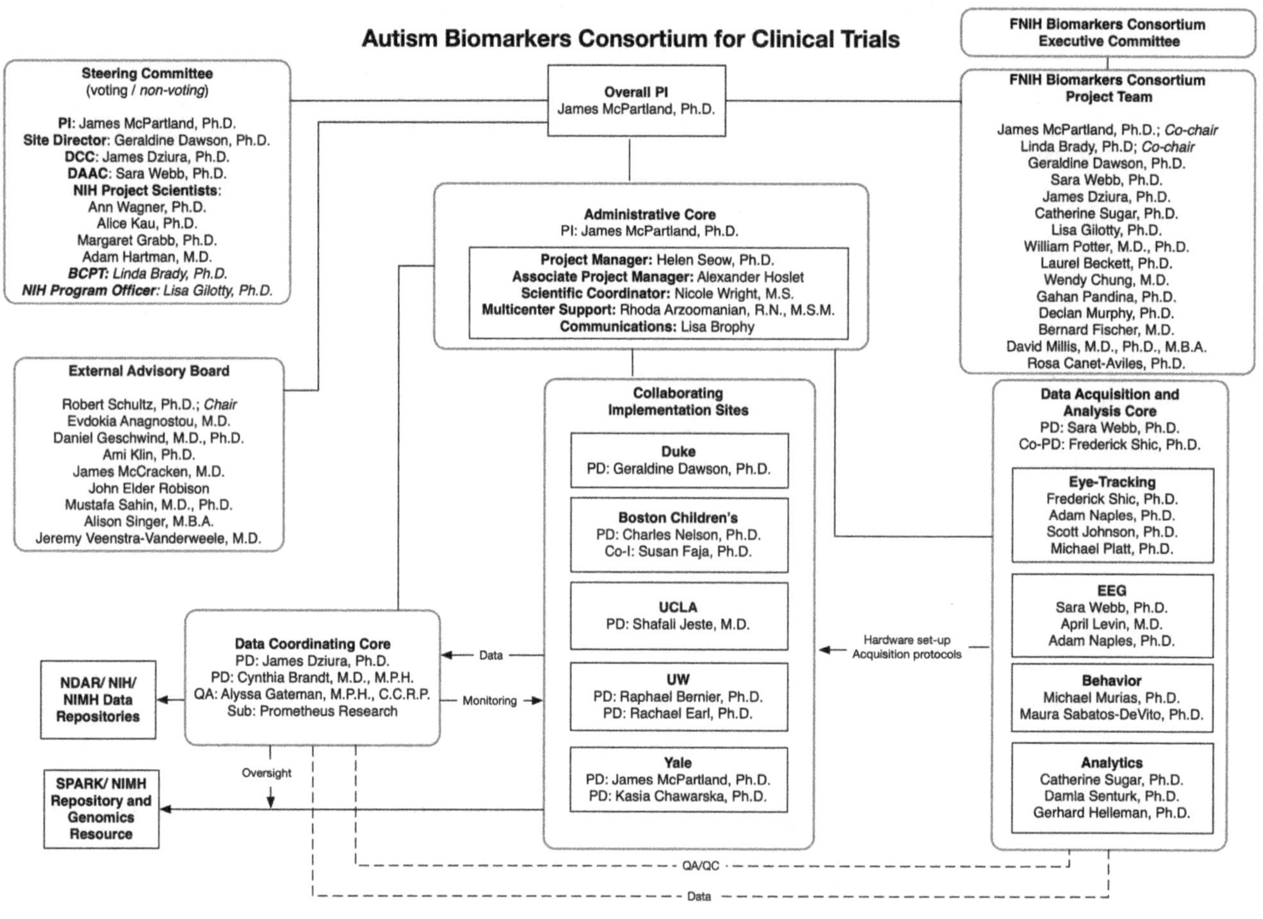

FIGURE 1 | ABC-CT organizational chart.

In May, 2019, this index was accepted into the Biomarker Qualification Program[2], marking a milestone for the field as the first biomarker for a neurodevelopmental disorder or psychiatric condition accepted into the BQP. A Biomarker Qualification Plan, the second step in the program, for the N170 is in development. In October 2019, a second LOI was submitted for the ET biomarker, *Oculomotor index of orienting to human faces*. Ongoing analyses will determine the appropriateness of other candidate biomarkers for potential submission to the BQP.

As outlined above, the ABC-CT was designed to evaluate promising biomarkers in several areas. The large sample and thorough characterization enable inference regarding group discrimination and relationships among the biomarkers, as well as evaluation of individual differences in clinical characteristics and demographic factors. The longitudinal design provides information about test-retest reliability and developmental stability over a length of time intended to align with a clinical trial; future research is needed to investigate the reliability of these biomarkers over longer periods of time. However, there are several biomarker properties that the ABC-CT was not designed to address. Because it was a naturalistic longitudinal study, without an active treatment, there is limited clinical change observed in participants during the 6 month course of the study, limiting the ability to evaluate biomarker sensitivity to change. This key objective may be addressed in future research by studies that evaluate biomarkers in the context of intervention or through naturalistic studies in younger cohorts, receiving initial diagnoses and being channeled into their first interventions, when significant progress in a six month span may be more likely. It is important to recognize that generalizability of the ABC-CT results to other populations has not yet been established; although extant research provides strong evidence of the potential utility of these biomarkers in other cohorts (e.g., younger/older children and adults, individuals with IQ below 60), studies of the scope and rigor of the ABC-CT have yet to be conducted and may be required before biomarker qualification in these groups can be pursued. The ABC-CT biomarker battery focused primarily on the visual domain because these measures were the most well-researched at the time of study design. Given the centrality of other sensory modalities (e.g., audition) to social-communication, investigation of these modalities is warranted.

[2] https://www.fda.gov/drugs/cder-biomarker-qualification-program/biomarker-qualification-submissions

CONCLUSION

The ABC-CT represents a comprehensive, collaborative approach to biomarker development in ASD. Building upon a strong foundation of prior research that has put forward candidate markers, the ABC-CT has advanced understanding by innovating in terms of study design and scope. The field of neurodevelopmental disorders has emerged as a leader within psychiatry, with the first biomarker of this nature accepted into the FDA's BQP. We move closer to a scientific reality in which clinical research may rely upon objective and sensitive biological measurements to bolster the clinical instruments on which we currently rely. The ABC-CT seeks to provide a foundation upon which novel treatments for ASD can be rigorously evaluated and that, ultimately, may lead to more effective methods for diagnosing and treating ASD.

ETHICS STATEMENT

The studies involving human participants were reviewed and approved by the Yale Institutional Review Board which served as Central Institutional Review Board for the study. Written informed consent to participate in this study was provided by the participants' legal guardian.

AUTHOR CONTRIBUTIONS

All authors made substantial contributions to the conception or design of the work or to acquisition, to analysis or interpretation of the data, to drafting or revision of the work, and provided approval for publication of the content, and agreed to be accountable for all aspects of the work in ensuring that questions related to the accuracy or integrity of any part of the work are appropriately investigated and resolved. JM, SW, SJ, and RB drafted the work.

FUNDING

Support was provided by NIMH U19 MH108206 (JM), the Autism Biomarkers Consortium for Clinical Trials.

ACKNOWLEDGMENTS

We extend gratitude to all of the families and participants who participated in this research. In addition, we thank the ABC-CT Project Management Team, the ABC-CT External Advisory Board, NIH project scientists, and colleagues from the FNIH Biomarkers Consortium.

REFERENCES

Aman, M. G., Singh, N. N., Stewart, A. W., and Field, C. J. (1985). The aberrant behavior checklist: a behavior rating scale for the assessment of treatment effects. *Am. J. Ment. Deficiency* 89, 485–491.

American Psychiatric Association (2013). *Diagnostic and Statistical Manual of Mental Disorders*, 5th Edn. Washington, D.C: American Psychiatric Association.

Annaz, D., Campbell, R., Coleman, M., Milne, E., and Swettenham, J. (2012). Young children with autism spectrum disorder do not preferentially attend to biological motion. *J. Autism Dev.Disord.* 42, 401–408. doi: 10.1007/s10803-011-1256-3

Chevallier, C., Parish-Morris, J., McVey, A., Rump, K. M., Sasson, N. J., Herrington, J. D., et al. (2015). Measuring social attention and motivation in autism spectrum disorder using eye-tracking. Stimulus type matters. *Autism Res.* 8, 620–628. doi: 10.1002/aur.1479

Cohen, I. L., and Sudhalter, V. (2005). *PDD Behavior Inventory (PDDBI)*. Lutz, FL: Psychological Assessment Resources.

Constantino, J. N., and Gruber, C. (2012). *The Social Responsiveness Scale Manual, (SRS-2)*, 2nd Edn Los Angeles: CA: Western Psychological Services.

Elliott (2007). *Differential Ability Scales:(DAS-II)*, 2nd Edn San Antonio, TX: Psychological Corporation.

Ewen, J. B., Sweeney, J. A., and Potter, W. Z. (2019). Conceptual, regulatory and strategic imperatives in the early days of EEG-Based biomarker validation for neurodevelopmental disabilities. *Front. Integr. Neurosci.* 13:45. doi: 10.3389/fnint.2019.00045

Guy, W. (1976). *ECDEU Assessment Manual for Psychopharmacology. US Department of Health, and Welfare*. Rockville, MD: National Institute of Mental Health, 76–338.

Jeste, S. S., and Geschwind, D. H. (2014). Disentangling the heterogeneity of autism spectrum disorder through genetic findings. *Nat. Rev. Neurol.* 10, 74–81. doi: 10.1038/nrneurol.2013.278

Kanne, S. M., Mazurek, M. O., Sikora, D., Bellando, J., Branum-Martin, L., Handen, B., et al. (2014). The autism impact measure (AIM): initial development of a new tool for treatment outcome measurement. *J. Autism Dev. Disord.* 44, 168–179. doi: 10.1007/s10803-013-1862-3

Klin, A., and Jones, W. (2008). Altered face scanning and impaired recognition of biological motion in a 15-month-old infant with autism. *Dev. Sci.* 11, 40–46. doi: 10.1111/j.1467-7687.2007.00608.x

Kroger, A., Bletsch, A., Krick, C., Siniatchkin, M., Jarczok, T. A., Freitag, C. M., et al. (2014). Visual event-related potentials to biological motion stimuli in autism spectrum disorders. *Soc. Cogn. Affect. Neurosci.* 9, 1214–1222. doi: 10.1093/scan/nst103

Lord, C., Petkova, E., Hus, V., Gan, W., Lu, F., Martin, D. M., et al. (2012a). A multisite study of the clinical diagnosis of different autism spectrum disorders. *Arch. Gen. Psychiatry* 69, 306–313. doi: 10.1001/archgenpsychiatry.2011.148

Lord, C., Rutter, M., DiLavore, P. C., Risi, S., Gotham, K., and Bishop, S. (2012b). *Autism Diagnostic Observation Schedule*, 2ed Edn. Torrance, CA: Western Psychological Services.

Loth, E., Charman, T., Mason, L., Tillmann, J., Jones, E. J. H. J. H., Wooldridge, C., et al. (2017). The EU-AIMS longitudinal european autism project (LEAP): design and methodologies to identify and validate stratification biomarkers for autism spectrum disorders. *Mol. Autism.* 8, 24. doi: 10.1186/s13229-017-0146-8

Loth, E., Spooren, W., Murphy, D. G., and Eu-Aims consortium, (2014). New treatment targets for autism spectrum disorders: EU-AIMS. *Lancet Psychiatry* 1, 413–415. doi: 10.1016/S2215-0366(14)00004-2

McPartland, J. (2017). Developing clinically practicable biomarkers for autism spectrum disorder. *J. Autism. Dev. Disord.* 47, 2935–2937. doi: 10.1007/s10803-017-3237-7

McPartland, J., Dawson, G., Webb, S. J., Panagiotides, H., and Carver, L. J. (2004). Event-related brain potentials reveal anomalies in temporal processing of faces in autism spectrum disorder. *J. Child Psychol. Psychiatry* 45, 1235–1245. doi: 10.1111/j.1469-7610.2004.00318.xJCPP318

Modi, M. E., and Sahin, M. (2017). Translational use of event-related potentials to assess circuit integrity in ASD. *Nat. Rev. Neurol.* 13, 160. doi: 10.1038/nrneurol.2017.15

Ness, S. L., Manyakov, N. V., Bangerter, A., Lewin, D., Jagannatha, S., Boice, M., et al. (2017). JAKE(R) multimodal data capture system: insights from an observational study of autism spectrum disorder. *Front. Neurosci.* 11:517. doi: 10.3389/fnins.2017.00517

Nystrom, P., Gredeback, G., Bolte, S., Falck-Ytter, T., and Ease team, (2015). Hypersensitive pupillary light reflex in infants at risk for autism. *Mol. Autism.* 6, 10. doi: 10.1186/s13229-015-0011-6

Rutter, M., LeCouteur, A., and Lord, C. (2003). *Autism Diagnostic Interview - Revised.* Los Angeles: Western Psychological Services.

Shic, F., Bradshaw, J., Klin, A., Scassellati, B., and Chawarska, K. (2011). Limited activity monitoring in toddlers with autism spectrum disorder. *Brain Res.* 1380, 246–254. doi: 10.1016/j.brainres.2010.11.074

Siper, P. M., Zemon, V., Gordon, J., George-Jones, J., Lurie, S., Zweifach, J., et al. (2016). Rapid and objective assessment of neural function in autism spectrum disorder using transient visual evoked potentials. *PLoS One* 11:e0164422. doi: 10.1371/journal.pone.0164422

Sparrow, S., Cicchetti, D., and Saulnier, C. A. (2016). *Vineland Adaptive Behavior Scales: Third Edition.* Bloomington: Pearson.

Wang, J., Barstein, J., Ethridge, L. E., Mosconi, M. W., Takarae, Y., and Sweeney, J. A. (2013). Resting state EEG abnormalities in autism spectrum disorders. *J. Neurodev. Disord.* 5, 24. doi: 10.1186/1866-1955-5-24

Webb, S. J., Shic, F., Murias, M., Sugar, C. A., Naples, A. J., Barney, E., et al. (2020). Biomarker acquisition and quality control for multisite studies: the autism biomarkers consortium for clinical trials. *Front. Integr. Neurosci.* 13:71. doi: 10.3389/fnint.2019.00071

4

Evoked Potentials and EEG Analysis in Rett Syndrome and Related Developmental Encephalopathies: Towards a Biomarker for Translational Research

*Joni N. Saby[1], Sarika U. Peters[2], Timothy P. L. Roberts[1,3], Charles A. Nelson[4] and Eric D. Marsh[5,6]**

[1]Lurie Family Foundations MEG Imaging Center, Department of Radiology, The Children's Hospital of Philadelphia, Philadelphia, PA, United States, [2]Department of Pediatrics, Vanderbilt University Medical Center, Nashville, TN, United States, [3]Department of Radiology, Perelman School of Medicine at the University of Pennsylvania, Philadelphia, PA, United States, [4]Laboratories of Cognitive Neuroscience, Division of Developmental Medicine, Boston Children's Hospital, Harvard Medical School, Boston, MA, United States, [5]Division of Neurology and Pediatrics, Children's Hospital of Philadelphia, Philadelphia, PA, United States, [6]Departments of Neurology and Pediatrics, Perelman School of Medicine at the University of Pennsylvania, Philadelphia, PA, United States

***Correspondence:**
Eric D. Marsh
marshe@email.chop.edu

Rett syndrome is a debilitating neurodevelopmental disorder for which no disease-modifying treatment is available. Fortunately, advances in our understanding of the genetics and pathophysiology of Rett syndrome has led to the development of promising new therapeutics for the condition. Several of these therapeutics are currently being tested in clinical trials with others likely to progress to clinical trials in the coming years. The failure of recent clinical trials for Rett syndrome and other neurodevelopmental disorders has highlighted the need for electrophysiological or other objective biological markers of treatment response to support the success of clinical trials moving forward. The purpose of this review is to describe the existing studies of electroencephalography (EEG) and evoked potentials (EPs) in Rett syndrome and discuss the open questions that must be addressed before the field can adopt these measures as surrogate endpoints in clinical trials. In addition to summarizing the human work on Rett syndrome, we also describe relevant studies with animal models and the limited research that has been carried out on Rett-related disorders, particularly methyl-CpG binding protein 2 (MECP2) duplication syndrome, CDKL5 deficiency disorder, and FOXG1 disorder.

Keywords: biomarker, Rett syndrome, developmental encephalopathy, evoked potential, EEG

INTRODUCTION

Rett syndrome is a genetic neurodevelopmental disorder that affects predominantly females. Estimated to occur in 1 of every 10,000 female births, Rett syndrome is characterized by near-normal growth and development for the first 6–18 months of life followed by a deceleration of development and loss of previously acquired skills, including spoken language and purposeful hand use (Hagberg, 1985; Neul et al., 2010). Other symptoms include stereotypic hand movements, gait apraxia, seizures, breathing abnormalities, sleep disturbances, and scoliosis, although the presence and severity of these features vary from person to person. In over 95% of cases, Rett syndrome is caused by mutations in the X-linked methyl-CpG binding protein 2 (MECP2) gene (Amir et al., 1999; Neul et al., 2014). Disease severity is largely dependent on the type of MECP2 mutation (Bebbington et al., 2008; Neul et al., 2008; Cuddapah et al., 2014), although two individuals with the same mutation can appear significantly different due to other contributing factors including genetic background and patterns of X-chromosome inactivation.

Treatment options for Rett syndrome are currently very limited. However, over the past several decades, significant progress has been made in understanding the genetic, cellular, and molecular mechanisms of the disorder (Leonard et al., 2017; Ip et al., 2018; Vashi and Justice, 2019). Advances in the understanding of the underlying pathophysiology have led to the development of new therapies, namely symptomatic pharmacologic interventions that act on the downstream cellular pathways affected in Rett syndrome, as well as gene therapy approaches that target the MECP2 gene directly. The effectiveness of these treatments in animal models of Rett syndrome has created enthusiasm within the Rett community as well as hope for a cure for the condition (van Karnebeek et al., 2016; Clarke and Abdala Sheikh, 2018). However, despite the efficacy of these treatments at the preclinical level all of the treatments that have preceded to clinical trials have so far failed to show the anticipated effects (Glaze et al., 2009, 2017; Khwaja et al., 2014; O'Leary et al., 2018).

The recurrence of failed clinical trials is not unique to Rett syndrome and has also been a point of concern for other neurodevelopmental disorders including Fragile X syndrome (Berry-Kravis et al., 2016; Erickson et al., 2017) and autism spectrum disorder (King et al., 2009; Aman et al., 2017; Veenstra-VanderWeele et al., 2017). Although a variety of factors may have contributed to the failure of these trials, one likely factor concerns the lack of sensitivity of the selected outcome measures (Jeste and Geschwind, 2016; Sahin et al., 2018). Indeed, the primary outcome measures for most extant clinical trials for neurodevelopmental disorders have been a caregiver and/or clinician impression of the child's symptoms, which are subject to placebo effects and may obscure small improvements that do not manifest clinically. Given the issue of failed trials in Rett syndrome and other neurodevelopmental disorders, it has become increasingly clear that there is an immense need for objective biological markers of central nervous system function to improve the prospects of novel therapeutics. Ideally, biomarkers or other quantitative measures would replace caregiver/clinician reports as the primary efficacy endpoints of clinical trials to provide a more sensitive measure while mitigating the subjectivity of parent or caregiver reports and may shed light on underlying neural mechanisms (Levin and Nelson, 2015).

Biomarkers of central nervous system function are typically derived from either functional magnetic resonance (MR) imaging (fMRI) or electrophysiological [electroencephalography (EEG) or magnetoencephalography] modalities. Due to the restricted nature of the MR environment and the necessity for the subject to remain still, acquiring fMRI data from participants with Rett syndrome would require sedation, which introduces a range of medical risks and precludes the possibility of examining higher-order sensory and/or cognitive processes. EEG on the other hand, is notably less constraining and allows some movement on part of the participant. Therefore, EEG can be used with individuals with Rett syndrome without requiring sedation, and thus represents a key advantage over fMRI for measuring brain activity in this population. Another fundamental benefit of EEG is its scalability due to its low cost, wide availability, relative ease of use.

EEG measures typically focus on quantifying neural responses to a repeated sensory stimulus (evoked potentials, EPs) or characterizing on-going background activity during rest or sleep (resting state). EPs can be elicited using the passive presentation of a sensory (auditory, visual, or somatosensory) stimulus, without requiring overt effort or a behavioral response on part of the participant. Similarly, resting-state EEG can be acquired from a subject while their attention is diverted by another activity such as bubbles or a silent movie. Therefore, both of these approaches can work with severely impaired populations, such as individuals with Rett syndrome.

This review aims to summarize the existing EP and EEG studies of Rett syndrome and describe how we can build on this work to begin applying EP and EEG measures as surrogate endpoints in clinical trials. We will also describe relevant EEG studies that have been conducted for related developmental encephalopathies (DEs), specifically MECP2 duplication syndrome, CDKL5 deficiency disorder (CDD), and FOXG1 disorder. Similar to children with Rett syndrome, children with MECP2 duplication syndrome, CDD, and FOXG1 disorder exhibit intellectual impairment, breathing abnormalities, apraxia, and epilepsy with a progressive postnatal onset (Paciorkowski et al., 2018). Given the overlap in symptomatology, many individuals with these disorders were frequently considered variants of Rett syndrome. However, ongoing clinical research has revealed that in addition to having unique genetic etiologies, each of these disorders has a unique set of symptoms and a characteristic clinical course that distinguish them from Rett syndrome and one another (Fehr et al., 2013; Lim et al., 2017; Paciorkowski et al., 2018). Very few EP or EEG studies have focused on MECP2 duplication syndrome, CDD, or FOXG1 disorder. This omission is likely due in part to the fact that these other disorders have only recently been recognized and the number of affected children (thus the number of potential research participants) is notably more restricted. Therefore, the present review will concentrate on Rett syndrome, although we describe findings from the other disorders when available.

In addition to describing the extant human research, we also summarize the relevant preclinical work with animal models of Rett syndrome, MECP2 duplication syndrome, CDD, and FOXG1 disorder to highlight the shared and disparate aspects of the preclinical models which are used for treatment development. We conclude with suggestions for future research, including how increased coordination between preclinical and human studies will further facilitate the identification of reliable biomarkers and ultimately, the development of effective treatments.

REVIEW OF EXISTING STUDIES

Auditory Evoked Potentials

Concerning EPs in Rett syndrome, the most thoroughly studied sensory domain has been the auditory system. Many of the early studies in this area focused exclusively on auditory brainstem responses (ABRs). The results of these studies were inconsistent, with several studies reporting normal ABRs in participants with Rett syndrome (Verma et al., 1987; Kálmánchey, 1990; Stach et al., 1994) and others reporting differences between Rett and typically developing (TD) groups (Bader et al., 1987, 1989b; Pelson and Budden, 1987; Pillion et al., 2000, 2010). The inconsistency in findings may be attributed in part to the use of small sample sizes and variability in the ages and clinical profiles of the individuals tested. Methodological differences, including the selected comparison group and use of sedation in some studies (Pelson and Budden, 1987; Pillion et al., 2000) and not others (Stach et al., 1994), may have also contributed to the mixed results (Pillion et al., 2010). When group differences were observed, they were mostly in the latency of the later aspects of the ABR, specifically wave V and the wave III-V complex, with normal values for the earlier components.

In contrast to the mixed findings on ABRs, studies that have considered the subsequent (middle and cortical) components of the auditory evoked potential (AEP) have consistently noted atypical responses in Rett syndrome, at least in a subset of participants (see **Table 1** for a summary of studies; Bader et al., 1989b; Stach et al., 1994; Stauder et al., 2006; Foxe et al., 2016). Those studies that have examined middle latency responses (MLR) have found the Pa component of the MLR to be absent or delayed in about half of the participants tested (Bader et al., 1989b; Stach et al., 1994). Both of these studies also reported atypical cortical responses at the vertex electrode, with Stach et al. reporting a complete absence of the N1 and P2 components in many participants. Bader et al., 1989b were able to identify N1 and P2 components in all of the participants enrolled in their study, although the latencies of these components were substantially delayed in several participants and as a group overall. More recent work by Foxe et al. has provided further evidence for atypical AEPs in Rett syndrome. In this study, gross differences were observed in both the timing and morphology of the late cortical response, including marked attenuation of the N1—P2 complex as compared to age-matched TD participants (Foxe et al., 2016). For example, AEP from an individual with Rett syndrome, see **Figure 1**.

In addition to examining basic AEPs, several studies attempted to examine higher-order auditory processing in Rett syndrome using the so-called "oddball" paradigm. An oddball paradigm presents an infrequent (deviant) tone randomly amongst a string of more frequent (standard) tones. In TD children and adults, the presentation of the deviant stimulus elicits an enhanced amplitude "mismatch" response in the ERP, which is presumed to reflect the detection of a change in stimulus parameters. The existing studies that have used an auditory oddball paradigm with individuals with Rett syndrome have suggested that these mismatch responses are retained in this population, yet attenuated compared to those of controls, reflecting deficits in the underlying cortical networks (Bader et al., 1989b; Stauder et al., 2006; Foxe et al., 2016). The first two studies to utilize this approach were limited by small sample sizes and statistical power but provided initial evidence for the discrimination between frequent and infrequent tones in individuals with Rett syndrome (Bader et al., 1989b; Stauder et al., 2006). Foxe et al. (2016) provided more direct evidence for auditory mismatch responses in individuals with Rett syndrome as part of their study on auditory processing in 14 girls with confirmed MECP2 mutations. Compared to age-matched TD girls, girls with Rett syndrome exhibited a delayed and prolonged mismatch response, which was interpreted as reflecting a slowing of information processing in the Rett group.

Another line of research on auditory processes in Rett syndrome has focused on electrophysiological responses to speech stimuli. While still a new area of research, existing studies of this type have suggested that EPs to speech stimuli may be useful for indexing higher-order language and cognitive processes in individuals with Rett syndrome and related DEs. The first study in this area examined changes in gamma band power in response to familiar and novel voices in children with Rett syndrome and MECP2 duplication syndrome (Peters et al., 2015). While both groups demonstrated electrophysiological evidence of discriminating between the familiar and novel voice, the relative changes in gamma power were in opposite directions, suggesting that over- vs. under-expression of the MECP2 protein has differential effects on the underlying cortical processes. In a second study, Peters et al. similarly noted differences in the electrophysiological responses of children with Rett syndrome and MECP2 duplication syndrome, in this case, to own name vs. other names (Peters et al., 2017). Children with MECP2 duplication syndrome exhibited more positive EPs for own vs. novel names and the extent of this effect was associated with a behavioral measure of adaptive functioning. No significant name discrimination effects were noted for participants with Rett syndrome. More recently, Key et al. (2019) reported more negative EPs to words vs. non-words in girls with Rett syndrome, although this effect was observed in the opposite hemisphere compared to TD controls. Within the Rett group, more typical responses were associated (at trend level) with higher scores on a behavioral measure of receptive vocabulary.

Visual Evoked Potentials

Visual evoked potentials (VEPs) can be elicited using either patterned or unpatterned "flash" visual stimuli. Initial studies of visual processes in Rett syndrome focused on flash VEPs, with inconsistent results. Whereas two studies reported normal VEPs (Verma et al., 1987; Kálmánchey, 1990), another study presented a distorted waveform and significantly delayed P1 component in participants with Rett syndrome (Bader et al., 1989b). Differences in age may have contributed to the disparate results across these studies.

Subsequent studies on VEPs in Rett syndrome have typically measured responses to patterned visual stimuli, which have less intra- and inter-subject variability and greater sensitivity than those for flash stimuli (see **Table 1** for a summary of studies). The earliest patterned stimuli study reported that the VEP waveforms

TABLE 1 | Summary of evoked potential (EP) and quantitative electroencephalography (EEG) studies of Rett syndrome and related developmental encephalopathies (DEs).

Study	*n*	Age Range	Stimuli	Main Findings
Auditory				
Stach et al. (1994)	36	2–28 years	Clicks, Tones	Normal ABR in all; Abnormal middle and late AEPs in an increasing percentage of patients
Foxe et al. (2016)	14	3–21 years	Tones (oddball)	AEP is abnormal; MMN is present but abnormal
Peters et al. (2015)	Rett: 5 MDD: 12	3–11 years	Familiar and unfamiliar voices	Greater gamma for familiar voice in MDD; Greater gamma for unfamiliar voice in Rett
Peters et al. (2017)	Rett: 9 MDD: 7	4–12 years	Familiar and unfamiliar names	Larger ERPs to own name in MDD; Larger ERPs to another name in Rett
Key et al. (2019)	11	4–12 years	Words and non-words	More negative ERP amplitude to words than non-words at right temporal sites (compared to left temporal sites in TD)
Visual				
Saunders et al. (1995)	11	4–24 years	Grating stimuli; Reversing checkerboard	Normal visual thresholds; Decreased VEP amplitude and varying latencies
LeBlanc et al. (2015)	34	22 months–8 years	Reversing checkboard	Decreased VEP amplitude; Reduced visual-spatial acuity
Boggio et al. (2016)	FOXG1: 3	17 months–22 years	Light flashes	VEPs in the normal range
Somatosensory				
Yoshikawa et al. (1991)	10	3–19 years	Median nerve stimulation	SEPs abnormal in 7; Giant SEPs in 5
Guerrini et al. (1998)	10	3–20 years	Median nerve stimulation	SEPs delayed and enlarged
Multisensory				
Verma et al. (1987)	9	2–15 years	Light flashes; Clicks; Median nerve stimulation	Normal evoked potentials in all participants
Bader et al. (1987)	6	10–22 years	Clicks; Median nerve stimulation	Abnormal SEPs in all participants; Abnormal ABR in all but one
Bader et al. (1989b)	9	10–22 years	Light flashes; Clicks	Slow and distorted VEPs; Early AEP components intact, later components delayed but variable
Kálmánchey (1990)	5	18 months–4 years	Light flashes; Clicks; Median nerve stimulation	Normally evoked potentials in all participants
Yamanouchi et al., 1993	9	2–19 years	Light flashes; Median nerve stimulation	Mechanisms of giant VEPs and SEPs in Rett differ from those of giant EPs in photosensitive progressive myoclonus epilepsy
Stauder et al. (2006)	17	2–60 years	Visual patterns; Tones (both oddball)	Prolonged and attenuated ERPs; A decline in ERP amplitude with increasing age
Quantitative EEG				
Khwaja et al. (2014)	10	2–10 years	n/a	Decreased right frontal alpha asymmetry between pre- and post-treatment with IGF-1
Ammanuel et al. (2015)	10	2–9 years	n/a	Abnormal delta power during slow-wave sleep
Fabio et al. (2016)	34	5–36 years	n/a	Changes in beta and theta power following cognitive intervention
Keogh et al. (2018)	42	1–23 years	n/a	Differential patterns of interelectrode coherence in individuals with MECP2 vs. CDKL5 mutations
Roche et al., 2019	57	23 months–10 years	n/a	Increased power in lower frequency bands, decreased power in middle-frequency bands

n—number of participants in the clinical group (Rett syndrome unless otherwise noted), MDD—MECP2 duplication disorder.

of 10 girls with Rett syndrome appeared subjectively different than those of TD children, particularly in regards to P1 amplitude and N2 latency (Saunders et al., 1995). However, these differences did not reach statistical significance, which the authors attributed to the small sample size and high level of individual variability in both the Rett and control groups.

A recent study with a relatively large sample of 34 girls with Rett syndrome detected significant differences in several aspects of the VEP of individuals with Rett syndrome compared to TD controls (LeBlanc et al., 2015), which paralleled the findings of Saunders et al. (1995). The most striking difference was attenuation of the P1 component in individuals with Rett syndrome as indexed by both N1—P1 and P1—N2 interpeak amplitudes. The Rett group also showed delays in N2 latency, as measured by absolute peak latency as well as P1—N2 time. Further analyses revealed that these effects were particularly prominent in the later stages of the disorder. Specifically, when the larger group of 34 participants was subdivided into either active- or post-regression, the most notable differences in N1—P1 amplitude and P1—N2 time was for the post-regression vs. TD groups, with participants in active-regression falling in the middle. In addition to examining basic VEPs, LeBlanc et al. (2015) also recorded VEPs to varying spatial frequency in a smaller number of participants to evaluate visual acuity in this

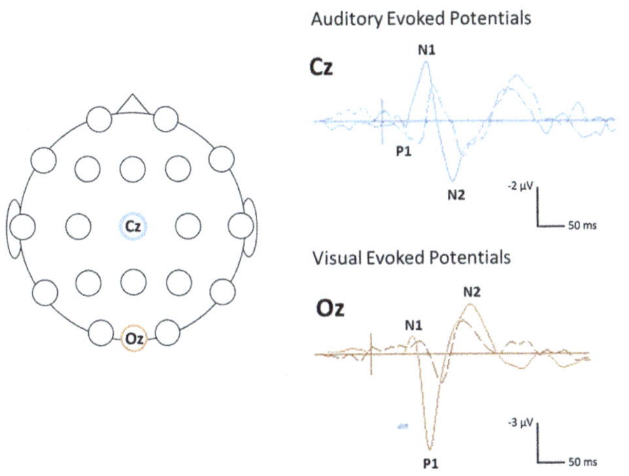

FIGURE 1 | Example of visual and auditory evoked potential (AEP) waveforms and head locations. Sample (unpublished) auditory and visual evoked potentials (AEPs/VEPs) from a 16-year-old individual with Rett syndrome (dotted line) and an age-matched typically developing (TD) control (solid line) The primary positive (P) and negative (N) components are indicated. The schematic on the left shows the location of the electrodes used for the auditory (Cz) and visual (Oz) responses. The auditory response was elicited using a 500 Hz tone. The visual response was elicited using a reversing checkerboard. Negativity is plotted up.

population. The pattern of findings indicated reduced spatial frequency sensitivity and diminished acuity in the Rett group, with a dominant spatial frequency of 0.4 cpd vs. 1.4 cpd for controls. Of note, the primary findings of diminished visual acuity and a decline in VEP amplitude with disease progression were also found in a parallel study with MECP2 deficient mice (see "Research with Animal Models" section). In addition to providing further support for the reliability of the human findings, the comparable results in mice point to the potential utility of VEPs as a biomarker, which, in an ideal case would be translatable between species (see "Discussion" section).

Only one electrophysiological study to date has considered higher-order visual processing in Rett syndrome. This study by Stauder et al. (2006) utilized an oddball design to examine how individuals with Rett syndrome process novel visual information. Compared to TD controls who demonstrated larger responses to novel vs. frequent visual stimuli, the responses for the individuals with Rett syndrome did not clearly discriminate between the two trial types. This was particularly true for older participants (15–60 years of age), who failed to show any difference for novel vs. frequent stimuli, leading the authors to conclude that individuals with Rett syndrome show a marked decline in ERP task modulation with increasing age.

Overall, the existing studies on VEPs in Rett syndrome suggest that similar to AEPs, these responses are atypical in this population, particularly when elicited using patterned visual stimuli (see **Figure 1** for a VEP from an individual with Rett syndrome). This work has further pointed to the potential influence of the clinical-stage on the VEP waveform with more atypical responses in later stages of the disorder. However, the existing studies on VEPs in Rett syndromes have been limited by small sample sizes (Verma et al., 1987; Bader et al., 1989b; Kálmánchey, 1990; Saunders et al., 1995; Stauder et al., 2006) or relatively restricted age ranges (LeBlanc et al., 2015). Therefore, additional work with larger samples and wider age ranges are needed to fully decipher the association between VEP parameters and disease progression.

Currently, it is not known how VEPs are affected in the related DEs (MECP2 duplication syndrome, CDD, or FOXG1 disorder). Preclinical studies with CDKL5- and FOXG1-mutated mice indicate that these responses are atypical in animal models of these conditions (see "Research With Animal Models" section). However, one paper reporting abnormal VEPs in FOXG1 mutated mice failed to find similar abnormalities in three human participants for whom VEPs were acquired but used different stimuli between the mice (contrast reversal) and the FOXG1 subjects (Strobe flash) tested (Boggio et al., 2016). Further work with larger samples of individuals with FOXG1 and the other syndromes will be needed to fully delineate characteristics of the VEP in these populations.

Somatosensory Evoked Potentials

Relatively less attention has been given to somatosensory processes in Rett syndrome as compared to auditory and visual processes, particularly in recent years. Overall, research in this area has indicated delayed responses and prolonged conduction times in individuals with Rett syndrome compared to normative comparison groups. Studies have reported normal latencies for the initial component following electrical stimulation of the median nerve (N9) over Erb's point in all participants, but delays in the subsequent cervical N13 and cortical N20 components in more than half of the individuals tested. In addition to delays in absolute latencies of these components, prolonged N13—N20 and N20—P30 interpeak intervals have also often been observed in a majority of individuals, further suggesting a slowing in central somatosensory pathways in Rett syndrome (Bader et al., 1987, 1989a; Kimura et al., 1992; Guerrini et al., 1998). Kimura et al. (1992) noted that these delays were most apparent in children over 9 years of age, with normal SEPs for younger children, pointing to a potential degenerative process with increasing disease duration.

In addition to noting differences in SEP latency, studies on somatosensory responses in Rett syndrome have also noted enhanced or "giant" cortical SEPs in a subset of participants (Yoshikawa et al., 1991; Yamanouchi et al., 1993; Guerrini et al., 1998). Giant SEPs are also observed with high incidence in individuals with cortical myoclonus and are presumed to reflect altered excitability within the somatosensory cortex. To better understand the pathophysiology of the enhanced SEPs in Rett syndrome, Yamanouchi et al. (1993) directly compared SEPs in nine girls with Rett syndrome with six children with progressive myoclonus epilepsy. Giant SEPs, defined as more than 3 standard deviations of the mean for age-matched controls, were observed in all of the individuals with progressive myoclonus epilepsy, but only six individuals with Rett syndrome. Another study reported giant SEPs in a similar proportion of Rett participants (Yoshikawa et al., 1991). These authors noted the individuals with giant SEPs tended to be younger (<9 years of age) and speculated that giant SEPs may be specific to earlier stages of the disorder and decline in later stages when seizures are less common. Further work with a larger sample is needed to confirm this suggestion and the associations between giant SEPs and epilepsy among individuals with Rett syndrome.

Although most studies on SEPs in Rett syndrome have reported atypical responses as compared to TD groups, two studies found no differences in the SEPs of Rett vs. control participants (Verma et al., 1987; Kálmánchey, 1990). Of note, these studies were also among the few that reported normal AEPs and VEPs in Rett syndrome. The participants were relatively young (mostly under 10 years of age) compared to the wider age ranges used in other studies. As described above, Kimura et al. (1992) specifically noted that SEPs were normal in children under 9 years of age. Together, with the findings from VEPs, these findings point to a potential decline in EPs with disease progression in Rett syndrome and reinforce the need for future work to explicitly examine how EPs change throughout the disorder. To our knowledge, no studies have been done on SEPs in MECP2 duplication syndrome, CDD, or FOXG1 disorder.

EEG Analysis

Abnormal background EEG has been considered a common feature of Rett syndrome since its initial characterization (Rett, 1966; Hagberg et al., 1983). Several articles have since described these abnormalities in detail (Niedermeyer et al., 1986; Verma et al., 1986; Glaze et al., 1987; Garofalo et al., 1988; Hagne et al., 1989; Ishizaki et al., 1989). A thorough review of this literature is beyond the scope of this article, but generally, this work has demonstrated that the most common abnormalities are diffuse slowing of the background EEG and the presence of epileptiform activity, even in individuals without a history of seizures (Niedermeyer et al., 1986; Garofalo et al., 1988; Glaze, 2002, 2005). These abnormalities tend to follow a characteristic developmental course with a pattern of largely normal EEG before regression followed by the onset of spike and sharp waves that are initially most prominent over centrotemporal regions and then become more generalized in distribution (see Glaze, 2002, 2005). These epileptiform abnormalities tend to decline in the late stages of the disorder, although the slowing of the background EEG is still apparent at this stage, particularly in the theta band over frontal-central regions.

While this literature has substantially advanced the understanding of electrophysiological abnormalities in Rett syndrome, the inferences were based primarily on visual inspection of the data. The use of resting EEG as an efficacy biomarker for clinical trials will likely require a more reproducible, quantitative approach. Few studies on resting EEG in Rett syndrome have applied quantitative EEG analysis, although these methods have been used extensively to study TD and other neurodevelopmental disorders (Saby and Marshall, 2012; Wang et al., 2013; Bick and Nelson, 2016; Heunis et al., 2016). Common approaches to quantitative analysis of resting EEG include spectral power analysis, in which the EEG signal is decomposed into component frequency bands (delta, theta, alpha, beta, and gamma) and coherence, which estimates the degree to which two areas of the brain are "networked" together by determining the similarity in neuronal oscillations between electrodes or regions.

The few studies that have applied quantitative analyses to resting EEG in Rett syndrome have provided some indication that spectral power measures are sensitive to treatment, and thus may represent a valuable objective biomarker for clinical trials. As part of the Phase-1 clinical trial on mecasermin (IGF-1) in Rett syndrome, Khwaja et al. (2014) reported a reduction in right frontal alpha asymmetry between the pre- and post-treatment period. Right frontal alpha asymmetry, which indicates greater alpha power at right vs. left frontal electrodes, has been associated with increased internalizing behaviors, including anxiety and depression (Thibodeau et al., 2006). Thus, the finding of a reduction in right frontal alpha asymmetry was considered to index a decrease in anxiety symptoms following IGF-1 treatment. This conclusion was supported by a trend-level reduction in anxiety on a standardized behavioral assessment of anxiety symptoms. Subsequently, Fabio et al. (2016) reported increased beta and decreased theta power in the resting EEG of girls with Rett syndrome following five days of cognitive training, suggesting that spectral power measures may be sensitive to even brief interventions.

Keogh et al. (2018) demonstrated that inter-electrode coherence may also prove useful as an EEG biomarker for Rett syndrome and related DEs. In this study, spectral power and inter-electrode coherence measures were calculated from the resting EEG of individuals with MECP2 and CDKL5 mutations. The results indicated no differences in spectral power between the two groups, but differing patterns of inter-electrode coherence, particularly in occipital and temporal regions. Furthermore, different patterns of inter-electrode coherence were also observed for different subgroups of individuals with MECP2 mutations, namely those with Classic Rett vs. Preserved Speech Variant, and for subgroups of individuals with epilepsy (absent, present, or treatment-resistant). No significant differences in spectral power were observed for the MECP2 vs. CDKL5 or subgroups comparisons, suggesting that inter-electrode coherence may be more specific to individual groups than power measures. Recently, Roche et al. (2019) performed EEG on 57 Rett syndrome subjects and 37 age-matched controls to conclude that EEG frequency spectral composition partially correlated with lower cognitive assessment scores. EEG power was measured and compared to controls and between active regression and post regression states with general finding of slower (higher power in the delta and theta frequencies) EEG which reached statistical significance in particular head regions (Roche et al., 2019). Finally, these authors reported that the higher log-transformed delta power was associated with lower developmental quotients.

In addition to studies of background EEG during wakefulness, there has also been an interest in EEG patterns during sleep among girls with Rett syndrome. Building on descriptive studies of EEG abnormalities during sleep in Rett syndrome, Ammanuel et al. (2015) applied quantitative EEG analyses to further characterize differences in the sleeping EEGs of girls with Rett syndrome and age-matched controls. The primary finding was that participants with Rett syndrome exhibited greater delta power during slow-wave sleep and that delta power in the Rett group did not decline overnight as it did in control participants. While these findings suggest that delta power may be useful as a biomarker for sleep dysfunction in Rett syndrome, this study lacked the power to determine how these measures related to sleep quality at the individual level.

RESEARCH WITH ANIMAL MODELS

The clinical EP and EEG studies described above, while not exhaustive, present evidence of visual, auditory, somatosensory, and resting EEG changes in Rett subjects vs. TD controls that could be used as prognostic or predictive biomarkers in the DEs. The animal literature generally supports the existing human studies, but with expected differences. As with the human studies, there are many papers on different Rett, *MECP2* duplication, *FOXG1*, and *CDKL5* mouse models, many of which study the behavioral, anatomic, molecular, and physiological changes that loss or mutation in these genes cause (Guy et al., 2001; Collins et al., 2004; Wang et al., 2012; Boggio et al., 2016). And further in line with the human studies, there are fewer animal model EP/EEG studies then there is work on the cellular and molecular biology of Rett syndrome. In agreement with the human studies, most of the research within the DEs have been done on Rett syndrome (*Mecp2* mutant) mice but with a scattering of studies on the other disorders. In all cases, much of the research has been done with EEG, followed by evoked potential studies.

There are a host of Mecp2 deficient mouse line studies and reviewing the individual findings on them is beyond the scope of this review (for review see Vashi and Justice, 2019). In almost all lines, there has been a consistent EEG finding of 5–9 Hz sharps in runs lasting 1–2 s (D'Cruz et al., 2010; Eubanks, 2017; Wither et al., 2018). These discharges have been demonstrated to decrease in frequency and content with certain drugs, mainly those that treat absence seizures in humans: valproic acid and ethosuximide (Wither et al., 2018). A few authors have shown that these discharges change with the severity of the disease in the mouse (for review see Eubanks, 2017). Detailed quantitative analysis of the EEG, by frequency measures (D'Cruz et al., 2010; McLeod et al., 2013; Colic et al., 2014) or network measures (Colic et al., 2015) have also demonstrated changes with age/severity and some which could predict response to drugs (Wither et al., 2018). The EEG findings in the *Cdkl5* mice have been normal, both in quality and quantifying frequency content (Wang et al., 2012). The Mecp2 duplication mouse line has intermittent epileptiform discharges on EEG (Collins et al., 2004). As a whole, these studies have demonstrated that the EEG mimics findings in humans and is a potential biomarker for disease course and outcome for preclinical trials.

Evoked potentials studies in Mecp2 mutant mice first showed no differences in the brain stem component of the AEP (Liao et al., 2012). These studies did show differences in the middle latency auditory and visual cortical components (Liao et al., 2012) in an exon 4 deletion mouse and subsequent studies in a missense mutation mouse showed similar findings (Goffin and Zhou, 2012). These authors also demonstrated differences in frequency coupling to the stimuli suggesting local circuit dysfunction but in different directions for the two lines (Goffin and Zhou, 2012; Liao et al., 2012). Similar increases were reported in the phase-locking factor that suggests a hyper-synchronous response to stimuli (Goffin and Zhou, 2012; Liao et al., 2012). Follow up studies by this group, demonstrated that these findings could be rescued by restoration of Mecp2 in gabaergic neurons (Goffin et al., 2014). More recent visual evoked potential studies have confirmed that there is a difference in amplitude of the VEP in *Mecp2* mice that track with disease severity and closely mirrors the human findings (see above, LeBlanc et al., 2015). A Mecp2 rat study has demonstrated that the Mecp2 mutant rats had hyperexcitable but slower responses to speech sounds across the auditory cortex. They found that the Mecp2 rats could perform consonant and vowel discrimination tasks, but this ability was impaired when the stimuli were presented with background noise. Extensive speech training improved the Mecp2 rat's performance, but differently than control rats (Engineer et al., 2015).

Studies of the AEP in *Cdkl5* mice have also demonstrated a reduction in the amplitude of the N1 and P2 responses with a change in latency of the P2 response as well as a shift in the phase-locking factor (Wang et al., 2012). Two studies by the Pizzorusso et al., first using optical blood flow imaging (Mazziotti et al., 2017; Lupori et al., 2019), then repeated with cortical EPs (Mazziotti et al., 2017), demonstrated no differences in cortical optical imaging responses at the first age tested (P25–P26), but these emerged days later (P27–P28) in *Cdkl5* mutant mice. A second study demonstrated a reduced VEP response in the mutant Cdkl5 mice at both age P28 as well as in more mature animals (P80). Other work has shown that in the Foxg1 deletion mouse line there is a reduction in visual acuity and response amplitude in visual cortex recordings in response to different visual stimuli (Boggio et al., 2016).

Together, the preclinical rodent models of the DEs present evidence for altered physiological responses that suggest both short and long-range cortical dysfunction. These findings could be used for biomarker studies for preclinical drug development along with the human EP studies described above.

DISCUSSION

Overall, this review demonstrates that EP and EEG measures are abnormal in individuals with Rett syndrome. Although limited, extant studies that have included participants with related DEs (MECP2 duplication syndrome and CDD) suggest that EPs and EEG measures are also affected in these disorders, albeit in a distinct fashion (Peters et al., 2015, 2017; Keogh et al., 2018). Studies at the preclinical level have similarly noted striking abnormalities in EP and EEG measures in animal models of these conditions (e.g., Goffin et al., 2014; Boggio et al., 2016; Mazziotti et al., 2017). The finding that electrophysiological measures are atypical in Rett syndrome and the related DEs, as well as in animal models of these disorders, suggests that these measures may have future utility as an objective marker of disease progression or treatment response. In a clinical trial, a shift in the EP/EEG waveform could indicate a response to treatment. However, several important questions must be addressed before we can translate these measures into biomarkers for clinical use.

The existing literature has identified many EP and EEG measures that appear to be affected in individuals with Rett syndrome. In the auditory domain alone, the latency and amplitude of the cortical components of the AEP response to basic tones (Bader et al., 1989b; Stach et al., 1994) as well as measures of higher-order auditory processes such as the mismatch negativity (Foxe et al., 2016) and evoked responses to speech sounds (Peters et al., 2017; Key et al., 2019) are abnormal in individual groups. Other work has shown that aspects of the VEP (LeBlanc et al., 2015), SEP (Bader et al., 1989a; Kimura et al., 1992; Guerrini et al., 1998), and resting EEG (Keogh et al., 2018; Roche et al., 2019) are also atypical. One pressing question for future work concerns which of these electrophysiological measures are the most robust and valid indicators of function and thus, represent good candidate biomarkers to pursue for qualification.

A substantial limitation of the existing work on EP/EEG measures in Rett syndrome is small sample sizes. With few exceptions (e.g., LeBlanc et al., 2015; Roche et al., 2019), existing studies in this area have typically enrolled between 5 and 15 individuals. Future research with larger samples is needed to confirm the findings from these smaller studies and importantly, elucidate how these measures relate to function. As described above, many of the extant studies noted considerable variability in the responses within the individual group, ranging from apparently normal to, in the case of EPs, completely absent responses. However, due to small Ns, most of these studies did not attempt to address the potential clinical significance of this variability. The few studies that did include brain-behavior correlations largely failed to find significant associations, likely owing to the use of small samples (Peters et al., 2015, 2017; Key et al., 2019). To precisely identify how EP and EEG measures relate to function in Rett syndrome, a study with a sufficiently large sample is needed. To fully decipher these brain-behavior associations, this sample must be not only large but also representative of the heterogeneous population of girls and women with Rett syndrome, encompassing individuals of all ages and with differing degrees of clinical severity.

In addition to a large study on Rett syndrome, more research into the related DEs (MECP2 duplication syndrome, CDD, and FOXG1 disorder) is needed. Very few EP and EEG studies have included participants with these conditions. Those that have reported different electrophysiological patterns among participants with MECP2 duplication syndrome (Peters et al., 2015, 2017) and CDD (Keogh et al., 2018) as compared to participants with Rett syndrome. Therefore, biomarkers of function for these disorders will have to be validated separately from those for Rett syndrome. Due to the low incidence of these conditions, research on these conditions type will undoubtedly require data collection at multiple sites. The most informative approach would involve applying the same methods in participants with Rett syndrome, MECP2 duplication syndrome, CDD, FOXG1 disorder, and TD controls to directly assess how EP and EEG measures in these disorders vary compared to TD and one another. An analogous study with animal models of Rett syndrome and each of the related DEs would also be extremely valuable for advancing the understanding of the similarities and differences in EP/EEG measures across these disorders.

In addressing the question of which EP/EEG measures reliably reflect function in Rett syndrome and related DEs, it is important to consider that different trials will likely require different biomarkers, depending on the nature of the treatment under study. Many of the therapeutics under development for the DEs aim to improve global functioning and reduce symptoms across a variety of domains. Others target a particular symptom such as seizures or breathing abnormalities. For trials evaluating therapeutics to improve function more generally, electrophysiological measures that are sensitive to overall neurologic functioning will be the most fitting. For trials evaluating therapeutics with more specific targets, electrophysiological measures that more specifically correlate with the severity of the symptom of interest will be more appropriate.

In addition to being sensitive to function, an ideal biomarker would also be translatable. Currently, there is a substantial divide in the outcome measures used in preclinical studies with animal models and those used in clinical trials with patient groups. Specifically, at the preclinical level, efficacy is typically assessed using animal-specific behaviors and changes at the cellular level such as increasing dendritic spine density or long-term potentiation. Considering efficacy in humans is based on caregiver or clinician impression of observable changes in function, it is not surprising that many treatments with proven efficacy in mice have failed to show similar effects in humans. If preclinical results are expected to persist in clinical trials, a more fruitful approach would be to use the same measures in animals that we do in humans. Many of the candidate EP and EEG measures described in this review are likely to be translatable in this way. For instance, LeBlanc et al. (2015) demonstrated that VEPs elicited and analyzed from mice and humans using parallel methods yield comparable results. Future studies should continue to apply the same methods with mice and humans to identify which candidate electrophysiological biomarkers are most translatable. Recently, a primate model of Rett syndrome has been generated using Talon DNA editing technology (Liu et al., 2016; Chen et al., 2017). These models recapitulate some of the features of Rett syndrome and could be excellent in-between steps from mouse to humans to test the validity of these potential biomarkers. Unfortunately, primate studies are often expensive and have limitations that could make going straight from rodent to human more feasible. Since many compounds have already proven effective at the preclinical level, future work with animal models is also needed for identifying which candidate EP and EEG measures may be the most responsive to treatment, an additional requirement for these measures to be useful as biomarkers in clinical trials.

Once candidate biomarkers are identified, it will also be necessary to understand their development. The issue of age-related changes in biomarkers is a particular challenge for biomarker discovery for neurodevelopmental disorders since most biological measures, including EPs and EEG measures, are known to change with development (McPartland, 2016; Sahin et al., 2018). It is, therefore, necessary to understand how candidate biomarkers change in the absence of treatment to more appropriately gauge improvement in the presence of an intervention. Indeed, several studies have indicated that EP measures may decline with age or disorder progression in individuals with Rett syndrome (Kimura et al., 1992; Stauder et al., 2006; LeBlanc et al., 2015). Studies will need to consider this decline when examining the effect of treatment over a long period. Furthermore, this raises the question of whether the same EP and EEG biomarkers will be valid across all ages or whether different biomarkers will be needed for individuals of different ages or in different stages of the disorder. Large studies with participants of different ages are needed to help decipher developmental changes in these measures and the degrees to which they reliably reflect neurological functioning.

Addressing these questions and validating EP/EEG biomarkers for clinical trials of Rett syndrome and related DEs will not be without challenges. Although EEG is a relatively fitting neuroimaging technique for use with individuals with profound disabilities, obtaining good-quality data from this population is often difficult and EEG artifacts arising from behavioral movement, teeth grinding, and breathing abnormalities are common (Gabard-Durnam et al., 2018). Paradigms also have to be relatively short in duration and, therefore the number of trials is often less than optimal. Another significant challenge of this work relates to the low incidence of Rett syndrome (~1 in 10,000 females) and particularly, the related DEs, which are estimated to occur in less than 1 in 100,000. For this reason, qualifying biomarkers of these disorders will require multi-site collaborations and potentially the use of large control data sets to achieve sufficiently powered samples. While multi-site research is undoubtedly beneficial for increasing power and generalizability, it also introduces a range of methodological challenges, including the need to rigorously standardize stimulus presentation and data acquisition methods. Lastly, although EPs and EEG measures have been studied in Rett syndrome and appear to have potential utility as biomarkers for efficacy endpoints in clinical trials, it should be noted that other types of biomarkers may also be useful for this purpose. This includes brain-based measures, including magnetoencephalography or transcranial magnetic stimulation, pupillometry, and sympathetic testing, as well as physiological/behavioral measures derived from wearable sensors. Although few studies to date have utilized these methods in participants with Rett syndrome (Heinen and Korinthenberg, 1996; Heinen et al., 1997; Krajnc and Zidar, 2016; Santosh et al., 2017; Artoni et al., 2019), these approaches have proven useful in biomarker research for other neurodevelopmental disorders (Roberts et al., 2010; Oberman et al., 2016; Ness et al., 2017).

CONCLUSION

Rett syndrome, MECP2 duplication syndrome, CDD, and FOXG1 disorder are severe neurodevelopmental conditions that result in life-long impairment across multiple domains of functioning. Treatment options for these disorders are currently very limited. However, promising therapeutics are now being investigated in animal models, with many of these treatments likely to proceed to clinical trials in the coming years. The success of these trials is likely to benefit from the identification of biological markers to objectively quantify neurological function in individuals with Rett syndrome and the related DEs, thus reducing the reliance on caregiver/clinician impression scales which are inherently subjective and subject to placebo effects. Various electrophysiological measures (EPs and resting EEG) are abnormal in individuals with Rett syndrome and representative animal models and thus, embody candidate biomarkers to monitor response to treatment. However, before we can apply these measures as endpoints in clinical trials, several important questions related to the functional significance, development, and progression of these biomarkers need to be addressed. Given Rett syndrome and particularly the related DEs are rare conditions, these questions will be best resolved by multi-site studies to achieve more robust and representative samples.

AUTHOR CONTRIBUTIONS

JS conceived of, wrote and edited the manuscript. EM conceived of, wrote, and was editor of the manuscript. TR, CN and SP conceived of and edited the manuscript

FUNDING

This work was supported by the Eunice Kennedy Shriver National Institute of Child Health and Human Development (U54 HD061222-15 Project 8880) and the National Institute of Mental Health (K01 MH118378 to JS).

REFERENCES

Aman, M. G., Findling, R. L., Hardan, A. Y., Hendren, R. L., Melmed, R. D., Kehinde-Nelson, O., et al. (2017). Safety and efficacy of memantine in children with autism: randomized, placebo-controlled study and open-label extension. *J. Child Adolesc. Psychopharmacol.* 27, 403–412. doi: 10.1089/cap.2015.0146

Amir, R. E., Van den Veyver, I. B., Wan, M., Tran, C. Q., Francke, U., and Zoghbi, H. Y. (1999). Rett syndrome is caused by mutations in X-linked MECP2, encoding methyl-CpG-binding protein 2. *Nat. Genet.* 23, 185–188. doi: 10.1038/13810

Ammanuel, S., Chan, W. C., Adler, D. A., Lakshamanan, B. M., Gupta, S. S., Ewen, J. B., et al. (2015). Heightened delta power during slow-wave-sleep in patients with rett syndrome associated with poor sleep efficiency. *PLoS One* 10:e0138113. doi: 10.1371/journal.pone.0138113

Artoni, P., Piffer, A., Vinci, V., LeBlanc, J., Nelson, C. A., Hensch, T. K., et al. (2019). Deep learning of spontaneous arousal fluctuations detects early cholinergic defects across neurodevelopmental mouse models and patients. *Proc. Natl. Acad. Sci. U S A* doi: 10.1073/pnas.1820847116 [Epub ahead of print].

Bader, G. G., Witt-Engerström, I., and Hagberg, B. (1987). Brain stem and spinal cord impairment in Rett syndrome: somatosensory and auditory evoked responses investigations. *Brain Dev.* 9, 517–522. doi: 10.1016/s0387-7604(87)80076-1

Bader, G. G., Witt-Engerström, I., and Hagberg, B. (1989a). Neurophysiological findings in the Rett syndrome, I: EMG, conduction velocity, EEG and somatosensory-evoked potential studies. *Brain Dev.* 11, 102–109. doi: 10.1016/s0387-7604(89)80077-4

Bader, G. G., Witt-Engerström, I., and Hagberg, B. (1989b). Neurophysiological findings in the Rett syndrome, II: visual and auditory brainstem, middle and late evoked responses. *Brain Dev.* 11, 110–114. doi: 10.1016/s0387-7604(89)80078-6

Bebbington, A., Anderson, A., Ravine, D., Fyfe, S., Pineda, M., de Klerk, N., et al. (2008). Investigating genotype-phenotype relationships in Rett syndrome using an international data set. *Neurology* 70, 868–875. doi: 10.1212/01.wnl.0000304752.50773.ec

Berry-Kravis, E., Des Portes, V., Hagerman, R., Jacquemont, S., Charles, P., Visootsak, J., et al. (2016). Mavoglurant in fragile X syndrome: results of two randomized, double-blind, placebo-controlled trials. *Sci. Transl. Med.* 8:321ra325. doi: 10.1126/scitranslmed.aab4109

Bick, J., and Nelson, C. A. (2016). Early adverse experiences and the developing brain. *Neuropsychopharmacology* 41, 177–196. doi: 10.1038/npp.2015.252

Boggio, E. M., Pancrazi, L., Gennaro, M., Lo Rizzo, C., Mari, F., Meloni, I., et al. (2016). Visual impairment in FOXG1-mutated individuals and mice. *Neuroscience* 324, 496–508. doi: 10.1016/j.neuroscience.2016.03.027

Chen, Y., Yu, J., Niu, Y., Qin, D., Liu, H., Li, G., et al. (2017). Modeling rett syndrome using TALEN-edited MECP2 mutant cynomolgus monkeys. *Cell* 169, 945.e0–955.e0. doi: 10.1016/j.cell.2017.04.035

Clarke, A. J., and Abdala Sheikh, A. P. (2018). A perspective on "cure" for Rett syndrome. *Orphanet. J. Rare Dis.* 13:44. doi: 10.1186/s13023-018-0786-6

Colic, S., Lang, M., Wither, R. G., Liang, Z., Eubanks, J. H., and Bardakjian, B. L. (2014). Characterization of HFOs in short and long duration discharges recorded from *in-vivo* MeCP2-deficient mice. *Conf. Proc. IEEE Eng. Med. Biol. Soc.* 2014, 4603–4606. doi: 10.1109/embc.2014.6944649

Colic, S., Wither, R. G., Min, L., Zhang, L., Eubanks, J. H., and Bardakjian, B. L. (2015). Support vector machines using EEG features of cross-frequency coupling can predict treatment outcome in Mecp2-deficient mice. *Conf. Proc. IEEE Eng. Med. Biol. Soc.* 2015, 5606–5609. doi: 10.1109/embc.2015.7319663

Collins, A. L., Levenson, J. M., Vilaythong, A. P., Richman, R., Armstrong, D. L., Noebels, J. L., et al. (2004). Mild overexpression of MeCP2 causes a progressive neurological disorder in mice. *Hum. Mol. Genet.* 13, 2679–2689. doi: 10.1093/hmg/ddh282

Cuddapah, V. A., Pillai, R. B., Shekar, K. V., Lane, J. B., Motil, K. J., Skinner, S. A., et al. (2014). Methyl-CpG-binding protein 2 (MECP2) mutation type is associated with disease severity in Rett syndrome. *J. Med. Genet.* 51, 152–158. doi: 10.1136/jmedgenet-2013-102113

D'Cruz, J. A., Wu, C., Zahid, T., El-Hayek, Y., Zhang, L., and Eubanks, J. H. (2010). Alterations of cortical and hippocampal EEG activity in MeCP2-deficient mice. *Neurobiol. Dis.* 38, 8–16. doi: 10.1016/j.nbd.2009.12.018

Engineer, C. T., Rahebi, K. C., Borland, M. S., Buell, E. P., Centanni, T. M., Fink, M. K., et al. (2015). Degraded neural and behavioral processing of speech sounds in a rat model of Rett syndrome. *Neurobiol. Dis.* 83, 26–34. doi: 10.1016/j.nbd.2015.08.019

Erickson, C. A., Davenport, M. H., Schaefer, T. L., Wink, L. K., Pedapati, E. V., Sweeney, J. A., et al. (2017). Fragile X targeted pharmacotherapy: lessons learned and future directions. *J. Neurodev. Disord.* 9:7. doi: 10.1186/s11689-017-9186-9

Eubanks, J. H. (2017). "Epilepsy in models of rett syndrome," in *Models of Seizures and Epilepsy: Second Edition*, eds A. Pitkänen, P. S. Buckmaster, A. S. Galanopoulou and S. L. Moshé (Toronto, ON: Elsevier Inc.), 1079–1090.

Fabio, R. A., Billeci, L., Crifaci, G., Troise, E., Tortorella, G., and Pioggia, G. (2016). Cognitive training modifies frequency EEG bands and neuropsychological measures in Rett syndrome. *Res. Dev. Disabil.* 53–54, 73–85. doi: 10.1016/j.ridd.2016.01.009

Fehr, S., Wilson, M., Downs, J., Williams, S., Murgia, A., Sartori, S., et al. (2013). The CDKL5 disorder is an independent clinical entity associated with early-onset encephalopathy. *Eur. J. Hum. Genet.* 21, 266–273. doi: 10.1038/ejhg.2012.156

Foxe, J. J., Burke, K. M., Andrade, G. N., Djukic, A., Frey, H. P., and Molholm, S. (2016). Automatic cortical representation of auditory pitch changes in Rett syndrome. *J. Neurodev. Disord.* 8:34. doi: 10.1186/s11689-016-9166-5

Gabard-Durnam, L. J., Mendez Leal, A. S., Wilkinson, C. L., and Levin, A. R. (2018). The harvard automated processing pipeline for electroencephalography (HAPPE): standardized processing software for developmental and high-artifact data. *Front. Neurosci.* 12:97. doi: 10.3389/fnins.2018.00097

Garofalo, E. A., Drury, I., and Goldstein, G. W. (1988). EEG abnormalities aid diagnosis of Rett syndrome. *Pediatr. Neurol.* 4, 350–353. doi: 10.1016/0887-8994(88)90081-1

Glaze, D. G. (2002). Neurophysiology of Rett syndrome. *Ment. Retard. Dev. Disabil. Res. Rev.* 8, 66–71. doi: 10.1002/mrdd.10024

Glaze, D. G. (2005). Neurophysiology of Rett syndrome. *J. Child Neurol.* 20, 740–746. doi: 10.1177/08830738050200090801

Glaze, D. G., Frost, J. D. Jr., Zoghbi, H. Y., and Percy, A. K. (1987). Rett's syndrome. Correlation of electroencephalographic characteristics with clinical staging. *Arch. Neurol.* 44, 1053–1056. doi: 10.1001/archneur.1987.00520220051016

Glaze, D. G., Neul, J. L., Percy, A., Feyma, T., Beisang, A., Yaroshinsky, A., et al. (2017). A double-blind, randomized, placebo-controlled clinical study of trofinetide in the treatment of rett syndrome. *Pediatr. Neurol.* 76, 37–46. doi: 10.1016/j.pediatrneurol.2017.07.002

Glaze, D. G., Percy, A. K., Motil, K. J., Lane, J. B., Isaacs, J. S., Schultz, R. J., et al. (2009). A study of the treatment of Rett syndrome with folate and betaine. *J. Child Neurol.* 24, 551–556. doi: 10.1177/0883073808327827

Goffin, D., Brodkin, E. S., Blendy, J. A., Siegel, S. J., and Zhou, Z. (2014). Cellular origins of auditory event-related potential deficits in Rett syndrome. *Nat. Neurosci.* 17, 804–806. doi: 10.1038/nn.3710

Goffin, D., and Zhou, Z. J. (2012). The neural circuit basis of Rett syndrome. *Front. Biol.* 7, 428–435. doi: 10.1007/s11515-012-1248-5

Guerrini, R., Bonanni, P., Parmeggiani, L., Santucci, M., Parmeggiani, A., and Sartucci, F. (1998). Cortical reflex myoclonus in Rett syndrome. *Ann. Neurol.* 43, 472–479. doi: 10.1002/ana.410430410

Guy, J., Hendrich, B., Holmes, M., Martin, J. E., and Bird, A. (2001). A mouse Mecp2-null mutation causes neurological symptoms that mimic Rett syndrome. *Nat. Genet.* 27, 322–326. doi: 10.1038/85899

Hagberg, B. (1985). Rett's syndrome: prevalence and impact on progressive severe mental retardation in girls. *Acta Paediatr. Scand.* 74, 405–408. doi: 10.1111/j.1651-2227.1985.tb10993.x

Hagberg, B., Aicardi, J., Dias, K., and Ramos, O. (1983). A progressive syndrome of autism, dementia, ataxia and loss of purposeful hand use in girls: Rett's syndrome: report of 35 cases. *Ann. Neurol.* 14, 471–479. doi: 10.1002/ana.410140412

Hagne, I., Witt-Engerström, I., and Hagberg, B. (1989). EEG development in Rett syndrome. A study of 30 cases. *Electroencephalogr. Clin. Neurophysiol.* 72, 1–6. doi: 10.1016/0013-4694(89)90025-4

Heinen, F., and Korinthenberg, R. (1996). Does transcranial magnetic stimulation allow early diagnosis of Rett syndrome? *Neuropediatrics* 27, 223–224. doi: 10.1055/s-2007-973794

Heinen, F., Petersen, H., Fietzek, U., Mall, V., Schulte-Mönting, J., and Korinthenberg, R. (1997). Transcranial magnetic stimulation in patients with Rett syndrome: preliminary results. *Eur. Child Adolesc. Psychiatry* 6, 61–63. doi: 10.1016/s0013-4694(97)88197-0

Heunis, T. M., Aldrich, C., and de Vries, P. J. (2016). Recent advances in resting-state electroencephalography biomarkers for autism spectrum disorder-a review of methodological and clinical challenges. *Pediatr. Neurol.* 61, 28–37. doi: 10.1016/j.pediatrneurol.2016.03.010

Ip, J. P. K., Mellios, N., and Sur, M. (2018). Rett syndrome: insights into genetic, molecular and circuit mechanisms. *Nat. Rev. Neurosci.* 19, 368–382. doi: 10.1038/s41583-018-0006-3

Ishizaki, A., Inoue, Y., Sasaki, H., and Fukuyama, Y. (1989). Longitudinal observation of electroencephalograms in the Rett syndrome. *Brain Dev.* 11, 407–412. doi: 10.1016/s0387-7604(89)80025-7

Jeste, S. S., and Geschwind, D. H. (2016). Clinical trials for neurodevelopmental disorders: at a therapeutic frontier. *Sci. Transl. Med.* 8:321fs321. doi: 10.1126/scitranslmed.aad9874

Kálmánchey, R. (1990). Evoked potentials in the Rett syndrome. *Brain Dev.* 12, 73–76. doi: 10.1016/s0387-7604(12)80181-1

Keogh, C., Pini, G., Dyer, A. H., Bigoni, S., DiMarco, P., Gemo, I., et al. (2018). Clinical and genetic Rett syndrome variants are defined by stable electrophysiological profiles. *BMC Pediatr.* 18:333. doi: 10.1186/s12887-018-1304-7

Key, A. P., Jones, D., and Peters, S. (2019). Spoken word processing in Rett syndrome: evidence from event-related potentials. *Int. J. Dev. Neurosci.* 73, 26–31. doi: 10.1016/j.ijdevneu.2019.01.001

Khwaja, O. S., Ho, E., Barnes, K. V., O'Leary, H. M., Pereira, L. M., Finkelstein, Y., et al. (2014). Safety, pharmacokinetics, and preliminary assessment of efficacy of mecasermin (recombinant human IGF-1) for the treatment of Rett syndrome. *Proc. Natl. Acad. Sci. U S A* 111, 4596–4601. doi: 10.1073/pnas.1311141111

Kimura, K., Nomura, Y., and Segawa, M. (1992). Middle and short latency somatosensory evoked potentials (SEPm, SEPs) in the Rett syndrome: chronological changes of cortical and subcortical involvements. *Brain Dev.* 14, S37–S42.

King, B. H., Hollander, E., Sikich, L., McCracken, J. T., Scahill, L., Bregman, J. D., et al. (2009). Lack of efficacy of citalopram in children with autism spectrum disorders and high levels of repetitive behavior: citalopram ineffective in children with autism. *Arch. Gen. Psychiatry* 66, 583–590. doi: 10.1001/archgenpsychiatry.2009.30

Krajnc, N., and Zidar, J. (2016). The role of transcranial magnetic stimulation in evaluation of motor cortex excitability in Rett syndrome. *Eur. J. Paediatr. Neurol.* 20, 597–603. doi: 10.1016/j.ejpn.2016.03.010

LeBlanc, J. J., DeGregorio, G., Centofante, E., Vogel-Farley, V. K., Barnes, K., Kaufmann, W. E., et al. (2015). Visual evoked potentials detect cortical processing deficits in Rett syndrome. *Ann. Neurol.* 78, 775–786. doi: 10.1002/ana.24513

Leonard, H., Cobb, S., and Downs, J. (2017). Clinical and biological progress over 50 years in Rett syndrome. *Nat. Rev. Neurol.* 13, 37–51. doi: 10.1038/nrneurol.2016.186

Levin, A. R., and Nelson, C. A. (2015). Inhibition-based biomarkers for autism spectrum disorder. *Neurotherapeutics* 12, 546–552. doi: 10.1007/s13311-015-0350-1

Liao, W., Gandal, M. J., Ehrlichman, R. S., Siegel, S. J., and Carlson, G. C. (2012). MeCP2+/− mouse model of RTT reproduces auditory phenotypes associated with Rett syndrome and replicate select EEG endophenotypes of autism spectrum disorder. *Neurobiol. Dis.* 46, 88–92. doi: 10.1016/j.nbd.2011.12.048

Lim, Z., Downs, J., Wong, K., Ellaway, C., and Leonard, H. (2017). Expanding the clinical picture of the MECP2 Duplication syndrome. *Clin. Genet.* 91, 557–563. doi: 10.1111/cge.12814

Liu, Z., Li, X., Zhang, J. T., Cai, Y. J., Cheng, T. L., Cheng, C., et al. (2016). Autism-like behaviours and germline transmission in transgenic monkeys overexpressing MeCP2. *Nature* 530, 98–102. doi: 10.1038/nature16533

Lupori, L., Sagona, G., Fuchs, C., Mazziotti, R., Stefanov, A., Putignano, E., et al. (2019). Site-specific abnormalities in the visual system of a mouse model of CDKL5 deficiency disorder. *Hum. Mol. Genet.* 28, 2851–2861. doi: 10.1093/hmg/ddz102

Mazziotti, R., Lupori, L., Sagona, G., Gennaro, M., Della Sala, G., Putignano, E., et al. (2017). Searching for biomarkers of CDKL5 disorder: early-onset visual impairment in CDKL5 mutant mice. *Hum. Mol. Genet.* 26, 2290–2298. doi: 10.1093/hmg/ddx119

McLeod, F., Ganley, R., Williams, L., Selfridge, J., Bird, A., and Cobb, S. R. (2013). Reduced seizure threshold and altered network oscillatory properties in a mouse model of Rett syndrome. *Neuroscience* 231, 195–205. doi: 10.1016/j.neuroscience.2012.11.058

McPartland, J. C. (2016). Considerations in biomarker development for neurodevelopmental disorders. *Curr. Opin. Neurol.* 29, 118–122. doi: 10.1097/wco.0000000000000300

Ness, S. L., Manyakov, N. V., Bangerter, A., Lewin, D., Jagannatha, S., Boice, M., et al. (2017). JAKE®multimodal data capture system: insights from an observational study of autism spectrum disorder. *Front. Neurosci.* 11:517. doi: 10.3389/fnins.2017.00517

Neul, J. L., Fang, P., Barrish, J., Lane, J., Caeg, E. B., Smith, E. O., et al. (2008). Specific mutations in methyl-CpG-binding protein 2 confer different severity in Rett syndrome. *Neurology* 70, 1313–1321. doi: 10.1212/01.wnl.0000291011.54508.aa

Neul, J. L., Kaufmann, W. E., Glaze, D. G., Christodoulou, J., Clarke, A. J., Bahi-Buisson, N., et al. (2010). Rett syndrome: revised diagnostic criteria and nomenclature. *Ann. Neurol.* 68, 944–950. doi: 10.1002/ana.22124

Neul, J. L., Lane, J. B., Lee, H. S., Geerts, S., Barrish, J. O., Annese, F., et al. (2014). Developmental delay in Rett syndrome: data from the natural history study. *J. Neurodev. Disord.* 6:20. doi: 10.1186/1866-1955-6-20

Niedermeyer, E., Rett, A., Renner, H., Murphy, M., and Naidu, S. (1986). Rett syndrome and the electroencephalogram. *Am. J. Med. Genet. Suppl.* 1, 195–199. doi: 10.1002/ajmg.1320250522

Oberman, L. M., Enticott, P. G., Casanova, M. F., Rotenberg, A., Pascual-Leone, A., McCracken, J. T., et al. (2016). Transcranial magnetic stimulation in autism spectrum disorder: challenges, promise, and roadmap for future research. *Autism Res.* 9, 184–203. doi: 10.1002/aur.1567

O'Leary, H. M., Kaufmann, W. E., Barnes, K. V., Rakesh, K., Kapur, K., Tarquinio, D. C., et al. (2018). Placebo-controlled crossover assessment of mecasermin for the treatment of Rett syndrome. *Ann. Clin. Transl. Neurol.* 5, 323–332. doi: 10.1002/acn3.533

Paciorkowski, A. R., Seltzer, L. E., and Neul, J. L. (2018). "Developmental encephalopathies," in *Swaiman's Pediatric Neurology Sixth Edition*, eds K. F. Swaiman, S. Ashwal, D. M. Ferriero and N. F. Schor (Philadelphia: Mosby), 242–248.

Pelson, R. O., and Budden, S. S. (1987). Auditory brainstem response findings in Rett syndrome. *Brain Dev.* 9, 514–516. doi: 10.1016/s0387-7604(87)80075-x

Peters, S. U., Gordon, R. L., and Key, A. P. (2015). Induced gamma oscillations differentiate familiar and novel voices in children with MECP2 duplication and Rett syndromes. *J. Child Neurol.* 30, 145–152. doi: 10.1177/0883073814530503

Peters, S. U., Katzenstein, A., Jones, D., and Key, A. P. (2017). Distinguishing response to names in Rett and MECP2 Duplication syndrome: an ERP study of auditory social information processing. *Brain Res.* 1675, 71–77. doi: 10.1016/j.brainres.2017.08.028

Pillion, J. P., Bibat, G., and Naidu, S. (2010). Effects of sedation on auditory brainstem response in Rett syndrome. *Pediatr. Neurol.* 42, 331–334. doi: 10.1016/j.pediatrneurol.2010.01.003

Pillion, J. P., Rawool, V. W., and Naidu, S. (2000). Auditory brainstem responses in Rett syndrome: effects of hyperventilation, seizures, and tympanometric variables. *Audiology* 39, 80–87. doi: 10.3109/00206090009073057

Rett, A. (1966). On a unusual brain atrophy syndrome in hyperammonemia in childhood. *Wien. Med. Wochenschr.* 116, 723–726.

Roberts, T. P., Khan, S. Y., Rey, M., Monroe, J. F., Cannon, K., Blaskey, L., et al. (2010). MEG detection of delayed auditory evoked responses in autism spectrum disorders: towards an imaging biomarker for autism. *Autism Res.* 3, 8–18. doi: 10.1002/aur.111

Roche, K. J., LeBlanc, J. J., Levin, A. R., O'Leary, H. M., Baczewski, L. M., and Nelson, C. A. (2019). Electroencephalographic spectral power as a marker of cortical function and disease severity in girls with Rett syndrome. *J. Neurodev. Disord.* 11:15. doi: 10.1186/s11689-019-9275-z

Saby, J. N., and Marshall, P. J. (2012). The utility of EEG band power analysis in the study of infancy and early childhood. *Dev. Neuropsychol.* 37, 253–273. doi: 10.1080/87565641.2011.614663

Sahin, M., Jones, S. R., Sweeney, J. A., Berry-Kravis, E., Connors, B. W., Ewen, J. B., et al. (2018). Discovering translational biomarkers in neurodevelopmental disorders. *Nat. Rev. Drug Discov.* doi: 10.1038/d41573-018-00010-7 [Epub ahead of print].

Santosh, P., Lievesley, K., Fiori, F., and Singh, J. (2017). Development of the tailored rett intervention and assessment longitudinal (TRIAL) database and the rett evaluation of symptoms and treatments (REST) questionnaire. *BMJ Open* 7:e015342. doi: 10.1136/bmjopen-2016-015342

Saunders, K. J., McCulloch, D. L., and Kerr, A. M. (1995). Visual function in Rett syndrome. *Dev. Med. Child Neurol.* 37, 496–504. doi: 10.1111/j.1469-8749.1995.tb12037.x

Stach, B. A., Stoner, W. R., Smith, S. L., and Jerger, J. F. (1994). Auditory evoked potentials in Rett syndrome. *J. Am. Acad. Audiol.* 5, 226–230.

Stauder, J. E., Smeets, E. E., van Mil, S. G., and Curfs, L. G. (2006). The development of visual- and auditory processing in Rett syndrome: an ERP study. *Brain Dev.* 28, 487–494. doi: 10.1016/j.braindev.2006.02.011

Thibodeau, R., Jorgensen, R. S., and Kim, S. (2006). Depression, anxiety, and resting frontal EEG asymmetry: a meta-analytic review. *J. Abnorm. Psychol.* 115, 715–729. doi: 10.1037/0021-843x.115.4.715

van Karnebeek, C. D., Bowden, K., and Berry-Kravis, E. (2016). Treatment of neurogenetic developmental conditions: from 2016 into the future. *Pediatr. Neurol.* 65, 1–13. doi: 10.1016/j.pediatrneurol.2016.07.010

Vashi, N., and Justice, M. J. (2019). Treating Rett syndrome: from mouse models to human therapies. *Mamm. Genome* 30, 90–110. doi: 10.1007/s00335-019-09793-5

Veenstra-VanderWeele, J., Cook, E. H., King, B. H., Zarevics, P., Cherubini, M., Walton-Bowen, K., et al. (2017). Arbaclofen in children and adolescents with autism spectrum disorder: a randomized, controlled, phase 2 trial. *Neuropsychopharmacology* 42, 1390–1398. doi: 10.1038/npp.2016.237

Verma, N. P., Chheda, R. L., Nigro, M. A., and Hart, Z. H. (1986). Electroencephalographic findings in Rett syndrome. *Electroencephalogr. Clin. Neurophysiol.* 64, 394–401. doi: 10.1016/0013-4694(86)90072-6

Verma, N. P., Nigro, M. A., and Hart, Z. H. (1987). Rett syndrome—a gray matter disease? Electrophysiologic evidence. *Electroencephalogr. Clin. Neurophysiol.* 67, 327–329. doi: 10.1016/0013-4694(87)90118-0

Wang, I. T., Allen, M., Goffin, D., Zhu, X., Fairless, A. H., Brodkin, E. S., et al. (2012). Loss of CDKL5 disrupts kinome profile and event-related potentials leading to autistic-like phenotypes in mice. *Proc. Natl. Acad. Sci. U S A* 109, 21516–21521. doi: 10.1073/pnas.1216988110

Wang, J., Barstein, J., Ethridge, L. E., Mosconi, M. W., Takarae, Y., and Sweeney, J. A. (2013). Resting state EEG abnormalities in autism spectrum disorders. *J. Neurodev. Disord.* 5:24. doi: 10.1186/1866-1955-5-24

Wither, R. G., Colic, S., Bardakjian, B. L., Snead, O. C. III., Zhang, L., and Eubanks, J. H. (2018). Electrographic and pharmacological characterization of a progressive epilepsy phenotype in female MeCP2-deficient mice. *Epilepsy Res.* 140, 177–183. doi: 10.1016/j.eplepsyres.2018.01.015

Yamanouchi, H., Kaga, M., and Arima, M. (1993). Abnormal cortical excitability in Rett syndrome. *Pediatr. Neurol.* 9, 202–206. doi: 10.1016/0887-8994(93)90085-q

Yoshikawa, H., Kaga, M., Suzuki, H., Sakuragawa, N., and Arima, M. (1991). Giant somatosensory evoked potentials in the Rett syndrome. *Brain Dev.* 13, 36–39. doi: 10.1016/s0387-7604(12)80295-6

5

Biomarkers Obtained by Transcranial Magnetic Stimulation of the Motor Cortex in Epilepsy

Melissa Tsuboyama [1,2], *Harper Lee Kaye* [1,2] *and Alexander Rotenberg* [1,2,3]*

[1]Neuromodulation Program, Department of Neurology, Division of Epilepsy and Clinical Neurophysiology, Boston Children's Hospital, Boston, MA, United States, [2]FM Kirby Neurobiology Center, Department of Neurology, Boston Children's Hospital, Boston, MA, United States, [3]Berenson-Allen Center for Noninvasive Brain Stimulation, Beth Israel Deaconess Medical Center, Boston, MA, United States

Correspondence:
Alexander Rotenberg
alexander.rotenberg@childrens.harvard.edu

Epilepsy is associated with numerous neurodevelopmental disorders. Transcranial magnetic stimulation (TMS) of the motor cortex coupled with electromyography (EMG) enables biomarkers that provide measures of cortical excitation and inhibition that are particularly relevant to epilepsy and related disorders. The motor threshold (MT), cortical silent period (CSP), short interval intracortical inhibition (SICI), intracortical facilitation (ICF), and long interval intracortical inhibition (LICI) are among TMS-derived metrics that are modulated by antiepileptic drugs. TMS may have a practical role in optimization of antiepileptic medication regimens, as studies demonstrate dose-dependent relationships between TMS metrics and acute medication administration. A close association between seizure freedom and normalization of cortical excitability with long-term antiepileptic drug use highlights a plausible utility of TMS in measures of anti-epileptic drug efficacy. Finally, TMS-derived biomarkers distinguish patients with various epilepsies from healthy controls and thus may enable development of disorder-specific biomarkers and therapies both within and outside of the epilepsy realm.

Keywords: biomarker (development), transcranial magnetic stimulation (TMS), epilepsy—abnormalities, classification, drug therapy, drug development and application, neuromodulation, motor cortex excitability

---

Abbreviations: TMS, transcranial magnetic stimulation; V/m, volts per meter; A/m2, ampere per meter2; T, tesla; spTMS, single-pulse TMS; ppTMS, paired-pulse TMS; rTMS, repetitive TMS; EMG, electromyography; rMT, resting motor threshold; E:I, excitation to inhibition ratio; APB, abductor pollicis brevis; ISI, inter-stimulus-interval; LTP, long-term potentiation; LTD, long-term depression; TBS, theta burst stimulation; cTBS, continuous theta burst stimulation; iTBS, intermittent theta burst stimulation; MEP, motor evoked potential; CS, corticospinal; AEDs, antiepileptic drugs; MT, motor threshold; % MO, percent machine output; aMT, active motor threshold; CSP, cortical silent period; LICI, long-interval intracortical inhibition; SICI, short-interval intracortical inhibition; CBZ, carbamazepine; LCM, lacosamide; LTG, lamotrigine; PHT, phenytoin; LEV, levetiracetam; VPA, valproate; IGE, idiopathic generalized epilepsy; TPM, topiramate; AMPA, alpha-amino-3-hydroxy-5-methy; -4-isoxazole propionic acid; KD, ketogenic diet; VNS, vagus nerve stimulator; HupA, Huperzine A; NMDAR, N-methyl-D-aspartate receptor; PTZ, pentylenetetrazole; RTG, Retigabine; PME, progressive myoclonic epilepsies; ULD, including Unverricht-Lundborg disease; LBD, Lafora body disease; MERRF, myoclonic epilepsy with ragged red fibers; PVINs, parvalbumin-positive inhibitory interneurons; DS, Dravet syndrome; (SSADH) deficiency, succinic semialdehyde dehydrogenase.

TMS BASICS AND MEASURES IN EPILEPSY

Epilepsy is among the most common neurologic disorders in childhood, and accompanies numerous neurodevelopmental disorders, particularly the autism spectrum disorders (ASDs; Levisohn, 2007; Tuchman and Rapin, 2002; Danielsson et al., 2005). For patient populations with epilepsy, biomarkers that reflect magnitudes of cortical excitation and inhibition are highly desirable as metrics of disease severity and target engagement by therapeutics. Transcranial magnetic stimulation (TMS) is a 30-year-old protocol for focal, noninvasive, electrical cortical stimulation that enables such measures across ages (Barker et al., 1985). In TMS, powerful fluctuating extracranial magnetic fields induce intracranial electrical current. When placed at the scalp, TMS induces electric current in the nearby cerebral cortex and allows for the operator to either measure or modulate focal cortical excitability.

The TMS "dose" per experiment is defined by hardware factors that affect the electromagnetic field. These include coil shape, size, electrical properties, and its placement relative to cortical structures. The stimulation parameter space also includes individual stimulus components such as pulse shape (rectangular, sinusoidal, exponential) and amplitude. The physiologic response to TMS is further determined by stimulus train parameters such as frequency, duration, inter-train interval, and the number of trains per unit time. The electric field generated by TMS is not measured *in vivo* but can be effectively modeled and represented in volts per meter (V/m). Alternatively, TMS-induced current density can be approximated in ampere per meter^2 (A/m^2; Peterchev et al., 2012).

Stimulation focality in TMS is in part governed by coil geometry. With a common type of TMS coil termed figure-of-eight, the volume of depolarized cortex with a single stimulus can be as small as 1 cm^3. When positioned over the motor cortex, TMS by a figure-of-eight coil enables selective activation of intrinsic hand muscles in the limb contralateral to the stimulated hemisphere, without co-activation of more proximal muscle groups. Such motor cortex activation can be quantified with skin surface electromyography (EMG) that records a per-stimulus motor evoked potential (MEP) which predictably reflects the magnitude of stimulation and is the main outcome measure in TMS studies of the cortical excitation:inhibition (E:I) ratio (**Figure 1**; reviewed in Kobayashi and Pascual-Leone, 2003; Frye et al., 2008).

TMS is unique among brain stimulation protocols in that it has both diagnostic and therapeutic potential. Three TMS protocols, all combined with surface EMG to measure MEP amplitude, are commonly employed to measure the cortical E:I ratio in epilepsy: (1) single-pulse TMS (spTMS); (2) paired-pulse TMS (ppTMS); and (3) repetitive TMS (rTMS). While there is appreciable device-to-device output variability of focality and magnitude of stimulation *via* TMS, the overall pulse width, and pulse shape (monophasic and biphasic) are relatively consistent across devices. Experimental devices with variable pulse width and shape are emerging, but thus to date are not widely implemented (Peterchev et al., 2011). In the most common embodiment of spTMS, the motor cortex is stimulated while muscle activation in a contralateral limb is monitored by surface EMG. spTMS, when used to determine the resting motor threshold (rMT), guides stimulation intensity in therapeutic rTMS (**Figure 2A**; Theodore, 2003; Ziemann, 2004).

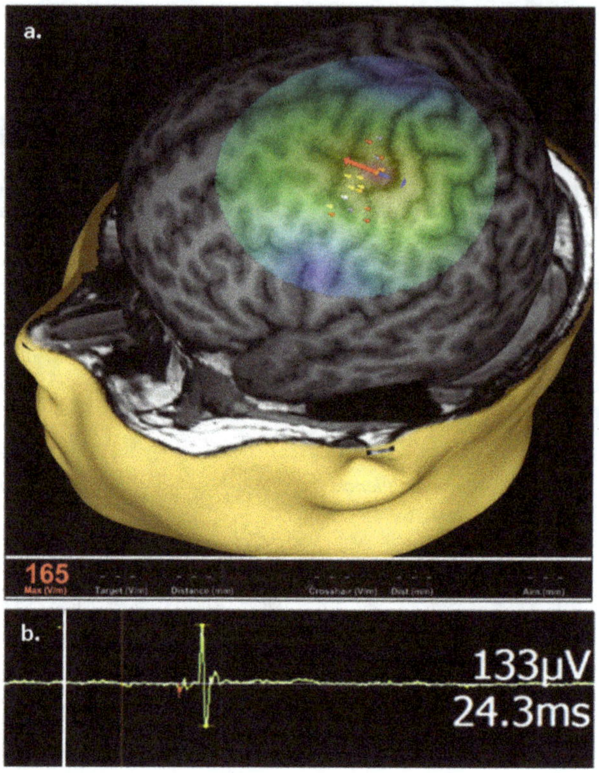

FIGURE 1 | Representative transcranial magnetic stimulation (TMS) motor cortex activation. **(A)** An approximation of stimulating electric field (e-field) induced by a single TMS pulse is displayed on a 3D reconstruction of an individual's anatomic magnetic resonance imaging (MRI), where field center is indicated by the junction between the red and blue arrows, indicating the direction of induced current, with corresponding e-field strength at the stimulation site (V/m) shown in red in the bottom left. The composite map of left hemispheric stimulation sites evoking motor evoked potentials (MEPs) of the right abductor pollicis brevis (APB) muscle, where intensity of response is color coded (heat map) from lowest (gray) to highest (white), are displayed on the cortical surface rendering. **(B)** Representative right APB MEP sample (green deflection) showing right APB resultant from left hemisphere stimulation, where the vertical line (white) corresponds to stimulus time. MEP amplitude and latency are indicated on the right.

spTMS coupled with surface EMG is also emerging as an important tool for functional topographic corticospinal tract mapping for purposes of presurgical planning (Lefaucheur and Picht, 2016; Hameed et al., 2017; Hannula and Ilmoniemi, 2017; Kaye et al., 2017b). ppTMS is an experimental technique, also delivered over the motor cortex, used to measure the cortical E:I ratio. In most common ppTMS protocols, two consecutive pulses are delivered to the hand motor region at a fixed inter-stimulus-interval (ISI) such that the MEP resultant from the second (test) stimulus is modulated by an antecedent (conditioning) stimulus. Depending on stimulus intensity and the ISI, ppTMS can reveal the magnitude of regional inhibitory or excitatory signaling

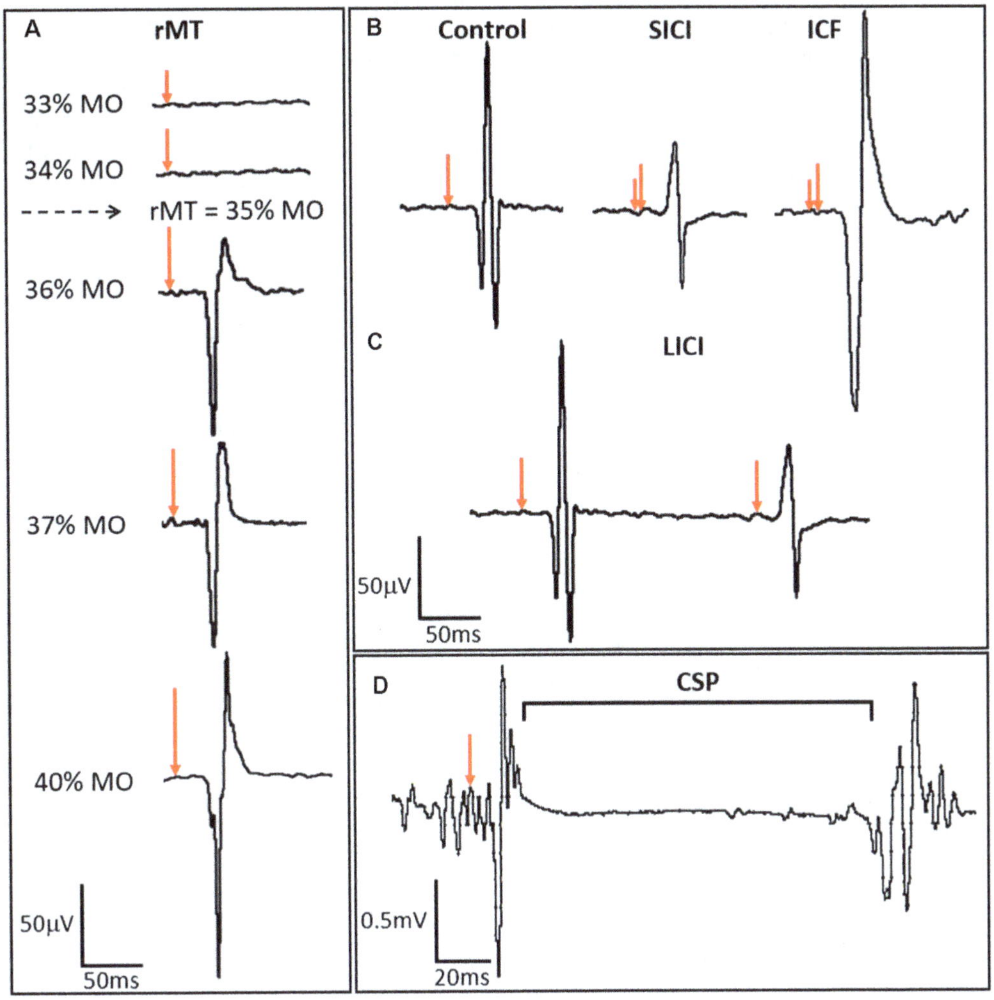

FIGURE 2 | TMS-derived metrics of motor cortex excitation and inhibition. **(A)** Resting motor threshold (rMT) for the APB muscle is calculated by identifying the minimum stimulus strength, measured in percent machine output (% MO), that evokes an MEP of a fixed amplitude (typically ≥50 μV) in the APB at rest in a majority of trials. Stimulus strength is indicated in the left panel, with resulting MEPs shown in the right panel, where red arrows indicate the time of stimulation and percent stimulator output is proportionate to the arrow length. **(B)** ppTMS paradigms where a subthreshold conditioning stimulus (short red vertical line) followed by a supra-threshold test stimulus (longer red vertical line). At short inter-stimulus-intervals (ISIs) (1–5 ms) short interval intracortical inhibition (SICI) is seen with inhibition of the test MEP by the antecedent conditioning stimulus. At longer ISIs (10–20 ms), test MEP amplitude is enhanced relative to the control MEP, such that ICF is seen. **(C)** Still longer ISIs (50–300 ms) are applied with two suprathreshold stimuli in LICI protocols where the MEP resultant from the test stimulus is predictably lower in amplitude than the preceding MEP resulting from the conditioning stimulus. In **(D)** the cortical silent period (CSP), interruption of ongoing electromyography (EMG) activity for a voluntarily contracting target muscle, occurs following single-pulse TMS (spTMS).

strength (**Figures 2B–D**; Ziemann, 2003; Dhamne et al., 2015; Hsieh et al., 2017; Damar et al., 2018).

rTMS, delivered in trains lasting minutes, is most commonly used to modulate regional cortical excitability to suppress neuropsychiatric symptoms. In the motor cortex, rTMS is commonly administered in high-frequency (>10 Hz) or low-frequency (<1 Hz) protocols aimed to enhance or suppress, respectively the MEP amplitude to provide a metric of cortical plasticity. Notably, such suppression and facilitation varies among individuals (Maeda et al., 2002). The physiologic mechanisms by which rTMS modifies cortical excitability are not completely understood but resemble well-described phenomena of use dependent long-term potentiation (LTP) and long-term depression (LTD) of excitatory synaptic strength modulated by glutamatergic and gamma-aminobutyric acid (GABA)-ergic mediators (Fitzgerald et al., 2006; Pascual-Leone et al., 2011; Pilato et al., 2012; Muller et al., 2014; Yang et al., 2014).

Patterned rTMS protocols, such as theta burst stimulation (TBS) of the motor cortex, are also used to measure cortical plasticity, where the two principal patterns of TBS are continuous theta burst stimulation (cTBS) and intermittent theta burst stimulation (iTBS). Both consist of delivery of 50 Hz pulses in bursts of three with an inter-burst interval of 200 ms, which mimic endogenous theta rhythms. As with other TMS protocols intended to produce biomarkers, TBS relies on changes in MEP amplitude as the main outcome measure. cTBS paradigms involve continuous train of TBS over a given duration, which, in typically developing individuals, result in net MEP suppression or depression of corticospinal excitability in most instances. In iTBS, a 2-s train of TBS is repeatedly delivered every 10 s, —in healthy adults, this often (though not always) leads to MEP facilitation or corticospinal excitation (Jannati et al., 2017). Mechanistically, as with conventional rTMS, TBS protocols likely engage mechanisms of glutamatergic and GABA-ergic synaptic plasticity (Huang et al., 2005; Stagg et al., 2009; Oberman et al., 2011; Mix et al., 2015; Blumberger et al., 2018).

MOTOR CORTEX TMS SAFETY IN EPILEPSY

spTMS and ppTMS are well-tolerated by subjects at the extremes of age, with only rare and mild adverse events reported among infant, child and elderly populations (Liepert et al., 2001; Eyre, 2003; Hameed et al., 2017; Kaye et al., 2017a). Several TMS devices are now FDA-cleared for use in children and adults. TMS safety and tolerability in patients with epilepsy is underscored by the growing use of neuronavigated TMS (TMS is coupled with frameless stereotaxy; **Figure 1**) as a presurgical functional mapping tool in children with developmental delay and/or epilepsy who candidates for respective epilepsy surgery (Narayana et al., 2015; Kaye et al., 2017a,b).

Specifically among children, the subjective perception of TMS seems favorable. Children who undergo TMS generally rate the experience as positive with little adverse events occurring during the sessions. Some children have even reported TMS to be more enjoyable than watching TV or going to the dentist (Garvey et al., 2001). Notably, in patients with epilepsy, per-subject risk for seizure with rTMS, spTMS or ppTMS is higher, yet is less than 3% crude per-subject risk (Schrader et al., 2004; Bae et al., 2007; Rossi et al., 2009; Pereira et al., 2016). The favorable safety profile of TMS has allowed for its use for studying cortical excitability in elderly patients with neurodegenerative disorders (Liepert et al., 2001).

TMS protocols are also available in rats, which underscores the versatility of motor cortex TMS as a protocol that is available in both clinical and preclinical arenas (Rotenberg et al., 2008; Hsieh et al., 2011; Gersner et al., 2015; Tang et al., 2016; Damar et al., 2018; Hameed et al., 2018).

TMS-DERIVED MEASURES OF CORTICAL EXCITABILITY, AND THEIR MODULATION BY ANTIEPILEPTIC DRUGS

A range of cortical excitability measures that are affected by both epilepsy and antiepileptic drugs (AEDs) can be obtained by TMS coupled with surface EMG. Motor threshold (MT) is often defined as the minimum percentage of stimulator output (% MO) that evokes an MEP of a fixed amplitude (typically >50 μV) in a target muscle either at rest (rMT) or during voluntary contraction (active motor threshold, aMT) in a majority of trials (Theodore, 2003; Ziemann et al., 2015; **Figure 2A**). The cortical silent period (CSP) is a TMS-induced interruption of activity in the EMG of the voluntarily contracting target muscle. The early segment of the CSP is related to spinal inhibition while the later segment is hypothesized to be of motor cortical origin. Short-interval intracortical inhibition (SICI) results from inhibition of the test MEP by a conditioning stimulus. This ppTMS protocol involves the application of a subthreshold conditioning stimulus and supra-threshold test stimulus at short ISIs (1–5 ms). Stimulation using a similar protocol but with longer ISIs of 10–20 ms results in intracortical facilitation (ICF; Kobayashi and Pascual-Leone, 2003; Ziemann, 2004). Long-interval intracortical inhibition (LICI) is measured using ppTMS with two supra-threshold stimuli applied at long ISIs of 50–300 ms in which the conditioning stimulus inhibits the test MEP. Such TMS-EMG parameters are summarized in **Table 1** (Rotenberg, 2018) and illustrated in **Figures 2B–D**.

rMT reflects the degree of cortical excitability which is affected by voltage-gated sodium channel blockers. Carbamazepine (CBZ), lacosamide (LCM), lamotrigine (LTG), and phenytoin (PHT), increase rMT compared to the rMT in drug-naïve patients with epilepsy and in patients without epilepsy; these changes are reversible with withdrawal of the given medication (Chen et al., 1997; Manganotti et al., 1999; Kimiskidis et al., 2005; Lee et al., 2005; Li et al., 2009; Lang et al., 2013; Ziemann et al., 2015). The effect of levetiracetam (LEV) on rMT remains uncertain, as Sohn et al. (2001) show no change in rMT with LEV administration, while Reis et al. (2004) report a significant increase in rMT in patients taking LEV (Sohn et al., 2001; Reis et al., 2004).

Notably, there is a dose-dependent relationship between rMT and certain AEDs. Lee et al. (2005) measured serial rMT and serum drug levels in healthy volunteers taking gradually increasing dosages of CBZ over 5 weeks followed by an abrupt cessation of the drug. rMT increased with increasing serum drug levels of total and free CBZ (Lee et al., 2005). In 7 of 10 patients, upon abrupt CBZ cessation, rMT remained elevated initially and then gradually returned to the baseline over several days despite the abrupt drop in serum CBZ levels. The sustained increase in rMT despite absent serum CBZ level indicates that the rMT (and perhaps other TMS-derived E:I metrics) may distinguish between drug pharmacodynamics and pharmacokinetics (Lee et al., 2005). As with CBZ, Lang et al. (2013) show a trend towards a dose-responsive effect on rMT with LCM dosages of 200 mg and 400 mg (Lang et al., 2013).

The effect a drug has on rMT can also provide information regarding its antiepileptic mechanism of action. For example, valproate (VPA) has no significant effect on rMT in healthy volunteers. VPA does increase rMT in focal epilepsies while its effect on rMT in patients with idiopathic generalized epilepsy (IGE) remains unclear as there are contradictory findings among studies (Reutens et al., 1993; Kazis et al., 2006; Li et al., 2009; Zunhammer et al., 2011; Badawy et al., 2014). Topiramate (TPM), like VPA has several mechanisms of action, including voltage gated sodium channel antagonism, but does not affect rMT while reducing ICF as its anti-epileptic properties stem primarily from inhibition of ligand-gated AMPA subtype

TABLE 1 | Transcranial magnetic stimulation-electromyography (TMS-EMG) metrics.

TMS-EMG parameter	Protocol*	Likely mechanism	Examples of change with medication
Resting motor threshold (rMT)	Single-pulse TMS: measure of stimulus strength necessary for a motor response (recorded either by visual inspection or EMG)	Cortical motor neuron voltage-gated sodium channel-mediated membrane excitability	Increased by voltage-gated sodium channel blockers (e.g., phenytoin, lacosamide) and voltage-gated potassium channel openers (e.g., retigabine)
Cortical silent period (CSP)	Single-pulse TMS: measure of pause in voluntary EMG activity after TMS	$GABA_B$-mediated and $GABA_A$-mediated motor cortex inhibition	Increased by $GABA_B$ agonists (e.g., baclofen); increased by $GABA_A$ positive allosteric modulators (e.g., lorazepam)
Short-interval intracortical inhibition (SICI)	Paired-pulse TMS: subthreshold conditioning stimulus precedes test stimulus by 1–5 ms	$GABA_A$-mediated regional cortical inhibition	Increased by $GABA_A$ positive allosteric modulators (e.g., lorazepam)
Intracortical facilitation (ICF)	Paired-pulse TMS: subthreshold conditioning stimulus precedes test stimulus by 10–20 ms	Glutamate (NMDA and AMAPA receptor types)- mediated excitation	Decreased by NMDA-type and AMPA-type glutamate receptor antagonists (e.g., memantine)
Long-interval intracortical inhibition (LICI)	Paired-pulse TMS: suprathreshold conditioning stimulus precedes test stimulus by 50–300 ms	$GABA_B$-mediated inhibition and (likely) $GABA_A$-mediated network inhibition	Increased by $GABA_B$ agonists (e.g., baclofen); increased by $GABA_A$ positive allosteric modulator (e.g., pentobarbital)

**Protocols vary slightly among laboratories; nearly always obtained from intrinsic hand muscles.*

glutamate receptors and agonist effects on some subtypes of the $GABA_A$ receptor (Angehagen et al., 2005). If VPA and TPM do not modulate the rMT, then while *in vitro* they may indeed have sodium channel blocking properties, these are not prominent *in vivo*, or in humans—thus the antiepileptic efficacy of these AEDs is less likely due to the sodium channel properties.

Antiepileptic medications also affect CSP duration, SICI, and LICI—all measures of components of GABA-ergic inhibition. CSP duration and SICI reflect motor cortical postsynaptic inhibition. ICF reflects glutamate receptor-mediated excitability that counters the inhibitory circuits reflected in SICI. $GABA_A$ receptor positive allosteric modulators such as benzodiazepines prolong short CSPs when low-intensity stimulation is used and shorten long CSPs when high-intensity stimulation is used. SICI is thought to represent fast inhibitory postsynaptic potentials (IPSPs) in corticospinal neurons mediated by $\alpha2$- or $\alpha3$-$GABA_A$ receptors. SICI is predictably enhanced by benzodiazepines and barbiturates. LICI reflects slow IPSPs mediated in part by $GABA_B$ receptors. LICI, where the long interval between pulses enables signals to propagate across multiple local and distal networks also likely reflects an aggregate inhibitory tone that is mediated by the $GABA_A$ receptor system (Hsieh et al., 2011). As expected, vigabatrin increases LICI, while there are conflicting reports on lorazepam's effect on LICI (Ziemann et al., 1996; Teo et al., 2009). In animal models, LICI is also enhanced by pentobarbital and suppressed by the $GABA_A$ receptor blocker pentylenetetrazole (PTZ; Hsieh et al., 2011).

Notably, however, tiagabine has a more complex interaction between the $GABA_A$ and $GABA_B$ receptor subtypes. Increased extracellular GABA availability in this instance results in predictable CSP prolongation and increased LICI. However, tiagabine decreases SICI which is controlled by presynaptic $GABA_B$ receptor-mediated autoinhibition of inhibitory interneurons. This contributes to the net increase in excitatory response as illustrated by the increase in ICF with tiagabine administration.

N-methyl-D-aspartate (NMDA)-receptor antagonists such as dextrorphan, the active metabolite of the prodrug dextromethorphan, and memantine, and benzodiazepines such as diazepam decrease ICF while enhancing SICI (Schwenkreis et al., 1999). **Table 2** summarizes the effects of various classes of drugs on these variables.

TMS-EMG MEASURES IN EPILEPSY PHARMACOTHERAPY

While changes in TMS parameters following acute drug administration aid in the identification of mechanisms of action of various drugs (or identify the mechanism of TMS-derived phenomena) at the receptor level, the effect of long-term administration of antiepileptic medications on these parameters may serve as a proxy for prognosticating efficacy of antiepileptic medications. A longitudinal study with 1-year follow-up illustrated a reduction in cortical excitability in patients with IGE or focal epilepsy who became seizure-free with anti-seizure medications (Badawy et al., 2010). In fact, while the rMTs were overall higher in these patients than in the control subjects without epilepsy, only the subset of patients with epilepsy who became seizure-free demonstrated an increase in rMT. These findings were independent of seizure type, seizure frequency, patient current age or age at seizure onset, and serum levels of the medication.

A subsequent study with a 3-year follow-up period compared measures of cortical inhibition and facilitation in patients with IGE or focal epilepsy, between those who remained refractory to antiepileptic drugs and those who achieved seizure freedom (Badawy et al., 2013). The mean rMT was higher in the

TABLE 2 | Antiepileptic drug effect on TMS parameters.

Class/Drug	MT	CSP	SICI	ICF	LICI	Dose-responsive?	Comments
Sodium channel							
Carbamazepine	↑	-	-	-		Yes	
Lacosamide	↑	-	-	-		Yes	
Lamotrigine	↑	-	-	-		Yes	
Oxcarbazepine	↑	-	-	-			
Phenytoin	↑	-	-	-			
Potassium channel							
Retigabine	↑		-	-	-		
XEN1101	↑					Yes	
$GABA_A$ receptor							
Diazepam	-	↓[§]	↑	↓	-		
Lorazepam	-	↑[§]	↑	↓,-	↓		Conflicting reports on effects on ICF in healthy controls and a subject with spinal cord stimulator
Tiagabine	-	↑	↓	↑	↑		
Vigabatrin	-	↑	-	↓	↑		
Calcium channel							
Gabapentin[†]	-	↑	↑	↓		No	
Pregabalin[†]	-	↑	↓	-	↑	No	
NMDA glutamate receptor							
Dextromethorphan	-	-	↑	↓			
Memantine	-	-	↑	↓			
AMPA glutamate receptor							
Perampanel	↑						
Topiramate[†]	-	-	↑	↓/-**		Yes	Dose-responsive relationship with SICI
Other							
Levetiracetam	↑, -	-	-	-			Conflicting reports on effects on MT in healthy controls
Valproic acid[†]	↑,-	-	-	-			Increased MT in IGE, no change in healthy controls

*MT, motor threshold; CSP, cortical silent period; SICI, short-interval intracortical inhibition; ICF, intracortical facilitation; LICI, long-interval intracortical facilitation; IGEm, idiopathic generalized epilepsy; [§]stimulation intensity-dependent; **trending towards decrease but not statistically significant; [†]multiple mechanisms of action; ↑ increase; ↓ decrease; - no change; blank cells, not tested; , conflicting results.*

affected hemisphere in patients with focal epilepsy compared to the unaffected hemisphere prior to initiation of anti-seizure medications. There was no difference in pre-drug treatment rMT between control patients without epilepsy and patients with IGE. Patients whose focal seizures remained refractory following initiation of one AED had an increase in rMT in the contralateral (unaffected) hemisphere such that there was no difference between the rMT in the two hemispheres. In patients who achieved seizure freedom on monotherapy, mean rMTs were higher in bilateral hemispheres in patients with IGE and patients with focal epilepsy compared to those patients who remained refractory. This pattern was maintained by the 30–36 months follow-up time-frame. Patients with refractory focal epilepsy developed a hyperexcitable contralateral hemisphere (at ISIs of 2 and 5 ms) at 30–36 months. A similar hyperexcitable response was also seen during a time of continued seizures in patients who would become seizure-free after the second medication. When those patients became seizure-free, however, there was subsequent normalization of all ISIs by the 30–36 months time frame. For the seizure-free patients in this cohort, rMT was higher than that measured in non-epilepsy controls, and SICI and LICI gradually increased to normal or near normal-values at most ISIs (Badawy et al., 2013).

These results suggest a close association between seizure freedom and normalization of TMS-derived cortical excitability metrics with prolonged AED use in patients with both focal and generalized epilepsy. Whether this effect is due to a change within the brain's predisposition to generate seizures or attributable to the cessation of continued seizure activity is unknown. However, regardless of the drug(s) used, a common effect of successful AED treatment is the restoration of normal responses to TMS.

TMS-EMG MEASURES IN NONPHARMACOLOGIC TREATMENT OF EPILEPSY

As SICI reflects the activity of intracortical inhibitory circuits, particularly that of $GABA_A$ receptor-mediated activity (Ziemann, 2004), serial SICI measurements over a given time course provide an index for GABA-mediated motor cortex inhibition (Maeda et al., 2002). Cantello et al. (2007) tested a range of TMS-derived metrics in healthy volunteers placed on the ketogenic diet (KD), to find that short-term KD (14-days) was followed by significant SICI enhancement. Notably, rMT was unchanged after KD initiation suggesting a prominent $GABA_A$

receptor contribution to the KD antiepileptic mechanism of action (Cantello et al., 2007).

Di Lazzaro et al. (2004) compared baseline TMS measures (rMT, SICI) for five patients with medically-refractory epilepsy who underwent vagus nerve stimulator (VNS) implantation. TMS measures were obtained in the stimulator-off and stimulator-on conditions. Patient rMT was higher than healthy age-matched controls but did not change with the VNS on. In contrast, SICI significantly increased when the VNS was on. As with KD, these results indicate a TMS-derived marker of target engagement, and a capacity for TMS-EMG to identify a GABAergic contributor to an antiepileptic intervention's mechanism (Di Lazzaro et al., 2004).

TMS IN THE ANTI-EPILEPTIC DRUG DEVELOPMENT PIPELINE

Changes in cortical excitability detected by ppTMS can be used in both preclinical and clinical studies to develop and assess the efficacy of novel AEDs. Huperzine A (HupA), a traditional Chinese medicine administered for treatment of epilepsy, is a naturally occurring esquiterpene alkaloid compound found in the firmoss *Huperzia serrata* that is both an acetylcholinesterase inhibitor and N-methyl-D-aspartate receptor (NMDAR) antagonist. Preclinical trials show that HupA suppresses seizures in a range of rodent epilepsy models. By ppTMS and differential pharmacology, Gersner et al. (2015) identified a potent GABAergic effect of HupA that was reflected in preserved paired-pulse inhibition of the MEP when rats were co-administered HupA and PTZ (a convulsant and GABA-A receptor blocker), and augmented LICI when HupA was administered in isolation (Gersner et al., 2015). The group concluded that at least in part the anti-seizure HupA effects may result from the enhancement of cortical GABAergic tone. These initial preclinical results justify continued preclinical and clinical investigations of HupA as a potential new anti-seizure drug compound.

Retigabine (RTG) is a newer generation drug that acts as a positive allosteric opener of KCNQ2–5 potassium channels to increase potassium efflux resulting in neuronal hyperpolarization and a decrease in neuronal excitability. In a cross-over, double-blind, placebo-controlled, randomized control trial, Ossemann et al. (2016) used single-pulse TMS with a figure-of-eight coil to measure rMT and aMT, and intensity to obtain a 1 mV peak-to-peak amplitude potential (SI1mV), and ppTMS to measure SICI, LICI, and ICF (Ossemann et al., 2016). Baseline measurements and measurements 2 h following administration of an oral dose of 400 mg RTG or placebo were obtained. RTG increased rMT, aMT, and S1mV compared to placebo, suggesting that RTG decreases neuronal excitability by increasing the resting potential as hypothesized from *in vitro* studies. However, SICI/ICF, and LICI were not significantly different between the RTG and placebo groups, suggesting that RTG does not affect intracortical inhibition (Ossemann et al., 2016).

XEN1101 is a voltage-gated potassium channel opener in the early stages of development that has shown promising preliminary data as a new antiseizure drug through the use of TMS. In a Phase 1 open-label study, spTMS was used to measure rMT in healthy control subjects taking 10 mg, 15 mg, or 20 mg of XEN1101. Premoli et al. (2019) found that 20 mg of XEN1101 decreased cortical excitability compared to the lower dosages (Premoli et al., 2019). In a subsequent double-blind, randomized, two-period crossover study, XEN1101 elevated rMT in a plasma concentration-dependent fashion. These encouraging findings support that XEN1101 reduces corticospinal and cortical excitability in a plasma concentration-dependent manner and have prompted plans for Phase 2 clinical trials.

TMS-DERIVED METRICS IN RARE EPILEPSIES

As expected, alterations in cortical inhibitory networks are also seen in various genetic and metabolic epilepsies (**Table 3**). SICI is decreased in patients with progressive myoclonic epilepsies (PME), including Unverricht-Lundborg disease (ULD), Lafora body disease (LBD), progressive myoclonic ataxia, sialidosis, and myoclonic epilepsy with ragged red fibers (MERRF). In patients with noncortical myoclonus, such as those with DYT-1 myoclonus-dystonia syndrome, SICI can be normal or mildly impaired. These findings help elucidate the pathophysiology of these diseases. For example, mutations in laforin or malin lead to formation and accumulation of neuronatin aggregates, typically found in parvalbumin-positive inhibitory interneurons (PVINs), resulting in significant reduction in and degeneration of PVINs on brain biopsy of patients with LBD. This reduction in cortical

TABLE 3 | TMS-EMG metrics in rare epilepsies.

Subjects	Findings (relative to control); Comments				
	MT	**SICI**	**ICF**	**LICI**	**CSP**
PME	-/↑ (rMT unchanged or increased; aMT increased in ULD and LBD)	↓	↓ (LBD only)	↓ (- in ULD)	-
DS	-	↓	-	-	
SSADHD	↑/- (unchanged after taurine treatment)	-/↑ (increased after taurine treatment)	↓/-(unchanged after taurine treatment)	↑/-	↓
LGS	↑	↑	↑	↑	

MT, motor threshold; SICI, short-interval intracortical inhibition; ICF, intracortical facilitation; LICI, long-interval intracortical facilitation; CSP, cortical silent period; PME, primary myoclonus epilepsies; LBD, Lafora body disease; ULD, Unverricht-Lundborg disease; DS, Dravet syndrome; SSADHD, succinic semialdehyde dehydrogenase deficiency; LGS, Lennox–Gastaut Syndrome; ↑, increase; ↓, decrease; -: no change; blank cells, not tested; results for cohort 1, results for cohort 2; /: conflicting results.

inhibition is reflected by the decreased SICI, and simultaneously illustrates the role of cortical PVINs on SICI (Rotenberg, 2018).

SICI is also reduced in SCN1A-related epilepsies such as Dravet syndrome (DS), which again reflects abnormal cortical inhibition networks, while the other TMS-derived markers of cortical excitability remain normal (Stern et al., 2017). These findings are consistent with preclinical data showing PVIN and somatostain-positive inhibitory interneuron dysfunction in murine DS models (Tai et al., 2014).

LICI abnormalities can also indicate cortical inhibitory network dysfunction, but, unlike SICI, reflect $GABA_B$ receptor activity. In patients with succinic semialdehyde dehydrogenase (SSADH) deficiency, LICI is reduced and CSP is shortened while SICI is preserved. These findings are supported by preclinical data showing $GABA_B$ receptor loss and/or dysfunction in a murine SSADH deficiency model (Rotenberg, 2018).

Additionally, rMT is increased in young patients with SSADH deficiency compared to their parents who are heterozygous for the causal pathogenic variant. However, this may be related to the age-dependent changes in rMT seen in healthy children and in patients with epilepsy (Hameed et al., 2017; Säisänen et al., 2018). Increase in rMT can also be found in several forms of cortical myoclonus, such as PME. In contrast to patients with chronic refractory IGE or those with chronic refractory FE, interictal cortical excitability is decreased in Lennox–Gastaut syndrome (LGS), where cortical excitability was lower in LGS patients. Cortical excitability was also lower in LGS when compared with healthy controls. This low cortical excitability across TMS measures thus distinguishes LGS from other medically refractory epilepsy syndromes (often showing measures of increased cortical excitability; Badawy et al., 2012).

CONCLUSION

Noninvasive stimulation of the motor cortex with TMS has practical and easily attainable implications for identification of biomarkers in epilepsy. TMS-derived metrics of E:I properties resultant from motor cortex stimulation paradigms elucidate mechanisms of action, pharmacodynamics, and pharmacokinetics of AEDs, and speak to the underlying pathophysiology of a range of epilepsy disorders. A range of established protocols and metrics are available in numerous laboratories, and can not only be deployed to measure disease severity, predict and measure response to existing treatments in epilepsy, but also aid in the identification and development of novel areas for target engagement in the treatment of an array of disorders.

AUTHOR CONTRIBUTIONS

All authors wrote and revised the manuscript, approved the final version, and agreed to be accountable for the content of the work.

FUNDING

AR is supported by the Boston Children's Hospital Translational Research Program, National Institutes of Health (NIH, NINDS NS088583), Massachusetts Life Sciences, The Assimon Family, and the Sestito Family. The content is solely the responsibility of the authors and does not necessarily represent the official views of Harvard University and its affiliated academic health care centers, National Institutes of Health, or any of the other listed granting agencies.

REFERENCES

Angehagen, M., Rönnbäck, L., Hansson, E., and Ben-Menachem, E. (2005). Topiramate reduces AMPA-induced Ca^{2+} transients and inhibits GluR1 subunit phosphorylation in astrocytes from primary cultures. *J. Neurochem.* 94, 1124–1130. doi: 10.1111/j.1471-4159.2005.03259.x

Badawy, R. A. B., Jackson, G. D., Berkovic, S. F., and MacDonell, R. A. L. (2013). Cortical excitability and refractory epilepsy: a three-year longitudinal transcranial magnetic stimulation study. *Int. J. Neural Syst.* 23:1250030. doi: 10.1142/s012906571250030x

Badawy, R. A. B., MacDonell, R. A. L., Berkovic, S. F., Newton, M. R., and Jackson, G. D. (2010). Predicting seizure control: cortical excitability and antiepileptic medication. *Ann. Neurol.* 67, 64–73. doi: 10.1002/ana.21806

Badawy, R. A. B., MacDonell, R. A. L., Vogrin, S. J., Lai, A., and Cook, M. J. (2012). Cortical excitability decreases in Lennox-Gastaut syndrome. *Epilepsia* 53, 1546–1553. doi: 10.1111/j.1528-1167.2012.03599.x

Badawy, R. A. B., Strigaro, G., and Cantello, R. (2014). TMS, cortical excitability and epilepsy: the clinical impact. *Epilepsy Res.* 108, 153–161. doi: 10.1016/j.eplepsyres.2013.11.014

Bae, E. H., Schrader, L. M., Machii, K., Alonso-Alonso, M., Riviello, J. J. Jr., Pascual-Leone, A., et al. (2007). Safety and tolerability of repetitive transcranial magnetic stimulation in patients with epilepsy: a review of the literature. *Epilepsy Behav.* 10, 521–528. doi: 10.1016/j.yebeh.2007.03.004

Barker, A. T., Jalinous, R., and Freeston, I. L. (1985). Non-invasive magnetic stimulation of human motor cortex. *Lancet* 1, 1106–1107. doi: 10.1016/s0140-6736(85)92413-4

Blumberger, D. M., Vila-Rodriguez, F., Thorpe, K. E., Feffer, K., Noda, Y., Giacobbe, P., et al. (2018). Effectiveness of theta burst versus high-frequency repetitive transcranial magnetic stimulation in patients with depression (THREE-D): a randomised non-inferiority trial. *Lancet* 391, 1683–1692. doi: 10.1016/S0140-6736(18)30295-2

Cantello, R., Varrasi, C., Tarletti, R., Cecchin, M., D'Andrea, F., Veggiotti, P., et al. (2007). Ketogenic diet: electrophysiological effects on the normal human cortex. *Epilepsia* 48, 1756–1763. doi: 10.1111/j.1528-1167.2007.01156.x

Chen, R., Samii, A., Caños, M., Wassermann, E. M., and Hallett, M. (1997). Effects of phenytoin on cortical excitability in humans. *Neurology* 49, 881–883. doi: 10.1212/wnl.49.3.881

Damar, U., Gersner, R., Johnstone, J. T., Kapur, K., Collins, S., Schachter, S., et al. (2018). Alterations in the timing of huperzine A cerebral pharmacodynamics in the acute traumatic brain injury setting. *J. Neurotrauma* 35, 393–397. doi: 10.1089/neu.2017.5258

Danielsson, S., Gillberg, I. C., Billstedt, E., Gillberg, C., and Olsson, I. (2005). Epilepsy in young adults with autism: a prospective population-based follow-up study of 120 individuals diagnosed in childhood. *Epilepsia* 46, 918–923. doi: 10.1111/j.1528-1167.2005.57504.x

Dhamne, S. C., Ekstein, D., Zhuo, Z., Gersner, R., Zurakowski, D., Loddenkemper, T., et al. (2015). Acute seizure suppression by transcranial direct current stimulation in rats. *Ann. Clin. Transl. Neurol.* 2, 843–856. doi: 10.1002/acn3.226

Di Lazzaro, V., Oliviero, A., Pilato, F., Saturno, E., Dileone, M., Meglio, M., et al. (2004). Effects of vagus nerve stimulation on cortical excitability in epileptic patients. *Neurology* 62, 2310–2312. doi: 10.1212/01.wnl.0000131743.45131.ae

Eyre, J. A. (2003). Development and plasticity of the corticospinal system in man. *Neural Plast.* 10, 93–106. doi: 10.1155/np.2003.93

Fitzgerald, P. B., Fountain, S., and Daskalakis, Z. J. (2006). A comprehensive review of the effects of rTMS on motor cortical excitability and inhibition. *Clin. Neurophysiol.* 117, 2584–2596. doi: 10.1016/j.clinph.2006.06.712

Frye, R. E., Rotenberg, A., Ousley, M., and Pascual-Leone, A. (2008). Transcranial magnetic stimulation in child neurology: current and future directions. *J. Child Neurol.* 23, 79–96. doi: 10.1177/0883073807307972

Garvey, M. A., Kaczynski, K. J., Becker, D. A., and Bartko, J. J. (2001). Subjective reactions of children to single-pulse transcranial magnetic stimulation. *J. Child Neurol.* 16, 891–894. doi: 10.1177/088307380101601205

Gersner, R., Ekstein, D., Dhamne, S. C., Schachter, S. C., and Rotenberg, A. (2015). Huperzine A prophylaxis against pentylenetetrazole-induced seizures in rats is associated with increased cortical inhibition. *Epilepsy Res.* 117, 97–103. doi: 10.1016/j.eplepsyres.2015.08.012

Hameed, M. Q., Dhamne, S. C., Gersner, R., Kaye, H. L., Oberman, L. M., Pascual-Leone, A., et al. (2017). Transcranial magnetic and direct current stimulation in children. *Curr. Neurol. Neurosci. Rep.* 17:11. doi: 10.1007/s11910-017-0719-0

Hameed, M. Q., Hsieh, T.-H., Morales-Quezada, L., Lee, H. H. C., Damar, U., MacMullin, P. C., et al. (2018). Ceftriaxone treatment preserves cortical inhibitory interneuron function *via* transient salvage of GLT-1 in a rat traumatic brain injury model. *Cereb. Cortex* doi: 10.1093/cercor/bhy328 [Epub ahead of print].

Hannula, H., and Ilmoniemi, R. J. (2017). "Basic principles of navigated TMS," in *Navigated Transcranial Magnetic Stimulation in Neurosurgery*, ed. S. M. Krieg (Cham: Springer), 3–29.

Hsieh, T.-H., Dhamne, S. C., Chen, J.-J. J., Pascual-Leone, A., Jensen, F. E., and Rotenberg, A. (2011). A new measure of cortical inhibition by mechanomyography and paired-pulse transcranial magnetic stimulation in unanesthetized rats. *J. Neurophysiol.* 107, 966–972. doi: 10.1152/jn.00690.2011

Hsieh, T. H., Lee, H. H. C., Hameed, M. Q., Pascual-Leone, A., Hensch, T. K., and Rotenberg, A. (2017). Trajectory of parvalbumin cell impairment and loss of cortical inhibition in traumatic brain injury. *Cereb. Cortex* 27, 5509–5524. doi: 10.1093/cercor/bhw318

Huang, Y.-Z., Edwards, M. J., Rounis, E., Bhatia, K. P., and Rothwell, J. C. (2005). Theta burst stimulation of the human motor cortex. *Neuron* 45, 201–206. doi: 10.1016/j.neuron.2004.12.033

Jannati, A., Block, G., Oberman, L. M., Rotenberg, A., and Pascual-Leone, A. (2017). Interindividual variability in response to continuous theta-burst stimulation in healthy adults. *Clin. Neurophysiol.* 128, 2268–2278. doi: 10.1016/j.clinph.2017.08.023

Kaye, H. L., Gersner, R., Boes, A. D., Pascual-Leone, A., and Rotenberg, A. (2017a). Persistent uncrossed corticospinal connections in patients with intractable focal epilepsy. *Epilepsy Behav.* 75, 66–71. doi: 10.1016/j.yebeh.2017.07.013

Kaye, H. L., Peters, J. M., Gersner, R., Chamberland, M., Sansevere, A., and Rotenberg, A. (2017b). Neurophysiological evidence of preserved connectivity in tuber tissue. *Epilepsy Behav. Case Rep.* 7, 64–68. doi: 10.1016/j.ebcr.2016.10.001

Kazis, D. A., Kimiskidis, V. K., Papagiannopoulos, S., Sotirakoglou, K., Divanoglou, D., Vlaikidis, N., et al. (2006). The effect of valproate on silent period and corticomotor excitability. *Epileptic Disord.* 8, 136–142.

Kimiskidis, V. K., Papagiannopoulos, S., Sotirakoglou, K., Kazis, D. A., Kazis, A., and Mills, K. R. (2005). Silent period to transcranial magnetic stimulation: construction and properties of stimulus-response curves in healthy volunteers. *Exp. Brain Res.* 163, 21–31. doi: 10.1007/s00221-004-2134-4

Kobayashi, M., and Pascual-Leone, A. (2003). Transcranial magnetic stimulation in neurology. *Lancet Neurol.* 2, 145–156. doi: 10.1016/S1474-4422(03)00321-1

Lang, N., Rothkegel, H., Peckolt, H., and Deuschl, G. (2013). Effects of lacosamide and carbamazepine on human motor cortex excitability: a double-blind, placebo-controlled transcranial magnetic stimulation study. *Seizure* 22, 726–730. doi: 10.1016/j.seizure.2013.05.010

Lee, H. W., Seo, H. J., Cohen, L. G., Bagic, A., and Theodore, W. H. (2005). Cortical excitability during prolonged antiepileptic drug treatment and drug withdrawal. *Clin. Neurophysiol.* 116, 1105–1112. doi: 10.1016/j.clinph.2004.12.004

Lefaucheur, J.-P., and Picht, T. (2016). The value of preoperative functional cortical mapping using navigated TMS. *Neurophysiol. Clin.* 46, 125–133. doi: 10.1016/j.neucli.2016.05.001

Levisohn, P. M. (2007). The autism-epilepsy connection. *Epilepsia* 48, 33–35. doi: 10.1111/j.1528-1167.2007.01399.x

Li, X., Ricci, R., Large, C. H., Anderson, B., Nahas, Z., and George, M. S. (2009). Lamotrigine and valproic acid have different effects on motorcortical neuronal excitability. *J. Neural Transm.* 116, 423–429. doi: 10.1007/s00702-009-0195-z

Liepert, J., Bär, K. J., Meske, U., and Weiller, C. (2001). Motor cortex disinhibition in Alzheimer's disease. *Clin. Neurophysiol.* 112, 1436–1441. doi: 10.1016/s1388-2457(01)00554-5

Maeda, F., Gangitano, M., Thall, M., and Pascual-Leone, A. (2002). Inter-and intra-individual variability of paired-pulse curves with transcranial magnetic stimulation (TMS). *Clin. Neurophysiol.* 113, 376–382. doi: 10.1016/s1388-2457(02)00008-1

Manganotti, P., Bongiovanni, L. G., Zanette, G., Turazzini, M., and Fiaschi, A. (1999). Cortical excitability in patients after loading doses of lamotrigine: a study with magnetic brain stimulation. *Epilepsia* 40, 316–321. doi: 10.1111/j.1528-1157.1999.tb00711.x

Mix, A., Hoppenrath, K., and Funke, K. (2015). Reduction in cortical parvalbumin expression due to intermittent theta-burst stimulation correlates with maturation of the perineuronal nets in young rats. *Dev. Neurobiol.* 75, 1–11. doi: 10.1002/dneu.22205

Muller, P. A., Dhamne, S. C., Vahabzadeh-Hagh, A. M., Pascual-Leone, A., Jensen, F. E., and Rotenberg, A. (2014). Suppression of motor cortical excitability in anesthetized rats by low frequency repetitive transcranial magnetic stimulation. *PLoS One* 9:e91065. doi: 10.1371/journal.pone.0091065

Narayana, S., Rezaie, R., McAfee, S. S., Choudhri, A. F., Babajani-Feremi, A., Fulton, S., et al. (2015). Assessing motor function in young children with transcranial magnetic stimulation. *Pediatr. Neurol.* 52, 94–103. doi: 10.1016/j.pediatrneurol.2014.08.031

Oberman, L., Edwards, D., Eldaief, M., and Pascual-Leone, A. (2011). Safety of theta burst transcranial magnetic stimulation: a systematic review of the literature. *J. Clin. Neurophysiol.* 28, 67–74. doi: 10.1097/wnp.0b013e318205135f

Ossemann, M., de Fays, K., Bihin, B., and Vandermeeren, Y. (2016). Effect of a single dose of retigabine in cortical excitability parameters: a cross-over, double-blind placebo-controlled TMS study. *Epilepsy Res.* 126, 78–82. doi: 10.1016/j.eplepsyres.2016.06.004

Pascual-Leone, A., Freitas, C., Oberman, L., Horvath, J. C., Halko, M., Eldaief, M., et al. (2011). Characterizing brain cortical plasticity and network dynamics across the age-span in health and disease with TMS-EEG and TMS-fMRI. *Brain Topogr.* 24, 302–315. doi: 10.1007/s10548-011-0196-8

Pereira, L. S., Müller, V. T., da Mota Gomes, M., Rotenberg, A., and Fregni, F. J. (2016). Safety of repetitive transcranial magnetic stimulation in patients with epilepsy: a systematic review. *Epilepsy Behav.* 57, 167–176. doi: 10.1016/j.yebeh.2016.01.015

Peterchev, A. V., Murphy, D. L., and Lisanby, S. H. (2011). Repetitive transcranial magnetic stimulator with controllable pulse parameters. *J. Neural. Eng.* 8, 1–24. doi: 10.1088/1741-2560/8/3/036016

Peterchev, A. V., Wagner, T. A., Miranda, P. C., Nitsche, M. A., Paulus, W., Lisanby, S. H., et al. (2012). Fundamentals of transcranial electric and magnetic stimulation dose: definition, selection, and reporting practices. *Brain Stimul.* 5, 435–453. doi: 10.1016/j.brs.2011.10.001

Pilato, F., Profice, P., Ranieri, F., Capone, F., Di Iorio, R., Florio, L., et al. (2012). Synaptic plasticity in neurodegenerative diseases evaluated and modulated by *in vivo* neurophysiological techniques. *Mol. Neurobiol.* 46, 563–571. doi: 10.1007/s12035-012-8302-9

Premoli, I., Beatch, G., Rossini, P., Abela, E., Posadas, K., Green, L., et al. (2019). TMS-EEG and TMS-EMG to assess the pharmacodynamic profile of a novel potassium channel opener (XEN1101) on human cortical excitability. *Brain Stimul.* 12:459. doi: 10.1016/j.brs.2018.12.494

Reis, J., Wentrup, A., Hamer, H. M., Mueller, H.-H., Knake, S., Tergau, F., et al. (2004). Levetiracetam influences human motor cortex excitability mainly by modulation of ion channel function—a TMS study. *Epilepsy Res.* 62, 41–51. doi: 10.1016/j.eplepsyres.2004.08.001

Reutens, D. C., Berkovic, S. F., Macdonell, R. A. L., and Bladin, P. F. (1993). Magnetic stimulation of the brain in generalized epilepsy: reversal of cortical hyperexcitability by anticonvulsants. *Ann. Neurol.* 34, 351–355. doi: 10.1002/ana.410340308

Rossi, S., Hallett, M., Rossini, P. M., and Pascual-Leone, A. (2009). Safety, ethical considerations, and application guidelines for the use of transcranial magnetic stimulation in clinical practice and research. *Clin. Neurophysiol.* 120, 2008–2039. doi: 10.1016/j.clinph.2009.08.016

Rotenberg, A. (2018). "Measures of cortical excitability by transcranial magnetic stimulation," in *Inherited Metabolic Epilepsies*, ed. P. L. Pearl (New York, NY: Demos), 201–206.

Rotenberg, A., Muller, P., Birnbaum, D., Harrington, M., Riviello, J. J., Pascual-Leone, A., et al. (2008). Seizure suppression by EEG-guided repetitive transcranial magnetic stimulation in the rat. *Clin. Neurophysiol.* 119, 2697–2702. doi: 10.1016/j.clinph.2008.09.003

Säisänen, L., Julkunen, P., Lakka, T., Lindi, V., Könönen, M., and Määttä, S. (2018). Development of corticospinal motor excitability and cortical silent period from mid-childhood to adulthood-a navigated TMS study. *Neurophysiol. Clin.* 48, 65–75. doi: 10.1016/j.neucli.2017.11.004

Schrader, L. M., Stern, J. M., Koski, L., Nuwer, M. R., and Engel, J. Jr. (2004). Seizure incidence during single-and paired-pulse transcranial magnetic stimulation (TMS) in individuals with epilepsy. *Clin. Neurophysiol.* 115, 2728–2737. doi: 10.1016/j.clinph.2004.06.018

Schwenkreis, P., Witscher, K., Janssen, F., Addo, A., Dertwinkel, R., Zenz, M., et al. (1999). Influence of the N-methyl-D-aspartate antagonist memantine on human motor cortex excitability. *Neurosci. Lett.* 270, 137–140. doi: 10.1016/s0304-3940(99)00492-9

Sohn, Y. H., Kaelin-Lang, A., Jung, H. Y., and Hallett, M. (2001). Effect of levetiracetam on human corticospinal excitability. *Neurology* 57, 858–863. doi: 10.1212/wnl.57.5.858

Stagg, C. J., Wylezinska, M., Matthews, P. M., Johansen-Berg, H., Jezzard, P., Rothwell, J. C., et al. (2009). Neurochemical effects of theta burst stimulation as assessed by magnetic resonance spectroscopy. *J. Neurophysiol.* 101, 2872–2877. doi: 10.1152/jn.91060.2008

Stern, W. M., Sander, J. W., Rothwell, J. C., and Sisodiya, S. M. (2017). Impaired intracortical inhibition demonstrated *in vivo* in people with Dravet syndrome. *Neurology* 88, 1659–1665. doi: 10.1212/wnl.0000000000003868

Tai, C., Abe, Y., Westenbroek, R. E., Scheuer, T., and Catterall, W. A. (2014). Impaired excitability of somatostatin-and parvalbumin-expressing cortical interneurons in a mouse model of Dravet syndrome. *Proc. Natl. Acad. Sci. U S A* 111, E3139–E3148. doi: 10.1073/pnas.1411131111

Tang, A. D., Lowe, A. S., Garrett, A. R., Woodward, R., Bennett, W., Canty, A. J., et al. (2016). Construction and evaluation of rodent-specific rTMS coils. *Front. Neural Circuits* 10:47. doi: 10.3389/fncir.2016.00047

Teo, J. T. H., Terranova, C., Swayne, O., Greenwood, R. J., and Rothwell, J. C. (2009). Differing effects of intracortical circuits on plasticity. *Exp. Brain Res.* 193, 555–563. doi: 10.1007/s00221-008-1658-4

Theodore, W. H. (2003). Transcranial magnetic stimulation in epilepsy. *Epilepsy Curr.* 3, 191–197. doi: 10.1046/j.1535-7597.2003.03607.x

Tuchman, R., and Rapin, I. (2002). Epilepsy in autism. *Lancet Neurol.* 1, 352–358. doi: 10.1016/S1474-4422(02)00160-6

Yang, X.-R., Kirton, A., Wilkes, T. C., Pradhan, S., Liu, I., Jaworska, N., et al. (2014). Glutamate alterations associated with transcranial magnetic stimulation in youth depression: a case series. *J. ECT* 30, 242–247. doi: 10.1097/YCT.0000000000000094

Ziemann, U. (2003). Pharmacology of TMS. *Suppl. Clin. Neurophysiol.* 56, 226–231. doi: 10.1016/S1567-424X(09)70226-0

Ziemann, U. (2004). TMS and drugs. *Clin. Neurophysiol.* 115, 1717–1729. doi: 10.1016/j.clinph.2004.03.006

Ziemann, U., Lönnecker, S., Steinhoff, B. J., and Paulus, W. (1996). The effect of lorazepam on the motor cortical excitability in man. *Exp. Brain Res.* 109, 127–135. doi: 10.1007/bf00228633

Ziemann, U., Reis, J., Schwenkreis, P., Rosanova, M., Strafella, A., Badawy, R., et al. (2015). TMS and drugs revisited 2014. *Clin. Neurophysiol.* 126, 1847–1868. doi: 10.1016/j.clinph.2014.08.028

Zunhammer, M., Langguth, B., Landgrebe, M., Frank, E., Müller, S., Burger, J., et al. (2011). Modulation of human motor cortex excitability by valproate. *Psychopharmacology* 215, 277–280. doi: 10.1007/s00213-010-2126-y

6

Day-to-Day Test-Retest Reliability of EEG Profiles in Children with Autism Spectrum Disorder and Typical Development

April R. Levin[1†], Adam J. Naples[2*†], Aaron Wolfe Scheffler[3], Sara J. Webb[4,5], Frederick Shic[4], Catherine A. Sugar[6,7], Michael Murias[8], Raphael A. Bernier[5], Katarzyna Chawarska[2], Geraldine Dawson[9,10,11], Susan Faja[12], Shafali Jeste[7], Charles A. Nelson[12], James C. McPartland[2]* and Damla Şentürk[6]* and the Autism Biomarkers Consortium for Clinical Trials*

[1]Department of Neurology, Boston Children's Hospital and Harvard Medical School, Boston, MA, United States, [2]Child Study Center, School of Medicine, Yale University, New Haven, CT, United States, [3]Department of Epidemiology and Biostatistics, University of California, San Francisco, San Francisco, CA, United States, [4]Center for Child Health, Behavior, and Development, Seattle Children's Research Institute, Seattle, WA, United States, [5]Department of Psychiatry and Behavioral Sciences, University of Washington, Seattle, WA, United States, [6]Department of Biostatistics, University of California, Los Angeles, Los Angeles, CA, United States, [7]Department of Psychiatry and Biobehavioral Sciences, University of California, Los Angeles, Los Angeles, CA, United States, [8]Institute for Innovations in Developmental Sciences, Northwestern University, Chicago, IL, United States, [9]Duke Institute for Brain Sciences, Duke University, Durham, NC, United States, [10]Duke Center for Autism and Brain Development, Duke University, Durham, NC, United States, [11]Department of Psychiatry and Behavioral Sciences, Duke University, Durham, NC, United States, [12]Laboratory of Cognitive Neuroscience, Division of Developmental Medicine, Boston Children's Hospital, Harvard Medical School, Boston, MA, United States

***Correspondence:**
April R. Levin
april.levin@childrens.harvard.edu
Adam J. Naples
adam.naples@yale.edu
Damla Şentürk
dsenturk@ucla.edu
James C. McPartland
james.mcpartland@yale.edu

†These authors have contributed equally to this work and share first authorship

Biomarker development is currently a high priority in neurodevelopmental disorder research. For many types of biomarkers (particularly biomarkers of diagnosis), reliability over short periods is critically important. In the field of autism spectrum disorder (ASD), resting electroencephalography (EEG) power spectral densities (PSD) are well-studied for their potential as biomarkers. Classically, such data have been decomposed into pre-specified frequency bands (e.g., delta, theta, alpha, beta, and gamma). Recent technical advances, such as the Fitting Oscillations and One-Over-F (FOOOF) algorithm, allow for targeted characterization of the features that naturally emerge within an EEG PSD, permitting a more detailed characterization of the frequency band-agnostic shape of each individual's EEG PSD. Here, using two resting EEGs collected a median of 6 days apart from 22 children with ASD and 25 typically developing (TD) controls during the Feasibility Visit of the Autism Biomarkers Consortium for Clinical Trials, we estimate test-retest reliability based on the characterization of the PSD shape in two ways: (1) Using the FOOOF algorithm we estimate six parameters (offset, slope, number of peaks, and amplitude, center frequency and bandwidth of the largest alpha peak) that characterize the shape of the EEG PSD; and (2) using nonparametric functional data analyses, we decompose the shape of the EEG PSD into a reduced set of basis functions that characterize individual power spectrum shapes. We show that individuals exhibit idiosyncratic PSD signatures that are stable over recording sessions using both characterizations. Our data show that EEG activity from a brief 2-min recording provides an efficient window into characterizing brain activity at the single-subject level with desirable psychometric characteristics that persist across different analytical decomposition methods. This is a necessary step towards analytical validation of biomarkers based on the EEG PSD and provides insights into parameters of the PSD that offer short-term reliability (and thus promise as potential biomarkers of trait or diagnosis) vs. those that are more variable over the short term (and thus may index state or other rapidly dynamic measures of brain function). Future research should address the longer-term stability of the PSD, for purposes such as monitoring development or response to treatment.

Keywords: EEG, autism, autism spectrum disorder, test-retest, power, FOOOF, reliability

INTRODUCTION

The development of translational biomarkers is a crucial step towards clinical trial readiness for neurodevelopmental disorders such as autism spectrum disorder (ASD; Sahin et al., 2018). The recent failure of several promising clinical trials (Krueger et al., 2017; Berry-Kravis et al., 2018) underscores the importance of biomarker development, and the need for a range of biomarkers serving a range of purposes. For example, a diagnostic biomarker can confirm the presence or absence of a disorder, or identify individuals with a biologically-defined subtype thereof (FDA-NIH Biomarker Working Group, 2016), to guide patient selection for clinical trials. A monitoring biomarker can serially assess the status of a disorder (FDA-NIH Biomarker Working Group, 2016), and thus measure the response to medical therapies or other exposures. The ideal properties of a given biomarker thus depend largely on its context of use. For example, a diagnostic biomarker should not change significantly over a given time window if the biology of the disorder it is indexing has not changed. On the other hand, a monitoring biomarker should change over time in a manner that reflects the biological impact of a medical treatment.

One of the most promising imaging tools for biomarker development in neurodevelopmental disorders is electroencephalography (EEG). EEG is an index of the neural networks that bridge genotype to phenotype across a variety of ages, disorders, and species, and thus offers substantial promise for the development of scalable biomarkers that are relevant to the brain mechanisms underlying ASD (Port et al., 2014; Jeste et al., 2015). Within EEG, the power spectral density (PSD), which represents the contributions of oscillations at various frequencies to the EEG, offers both diagnostic and monitoring potential. For example, among children with ASD compared to typical development, there is evidence that the resting PSD shows (at a group level) higher power in the low (delta, theta) and high (beta, gamma) frequency bands and lower power in the middle (alpha) frequency bands (Wang et al., 2013). This suggests the potential utility of some aspects of the PSD as a diagnostic biomarker for autism. Moreover, EEG is a measure of cortical activity and is thus fundamentally dynamic; it changes throughout development, across awake and asleep states, and in response to pharmacological treatment. This suggests that there may be aspects of the PSD that offer potential in other categories of biomarker development (e.g., monitoring or response biomarkers).

Thus, to inform the development of biomarkers using EEG-based measures, it is necessary to evaluate the reliability of the PSD within an individual over brief time intervals, as well as across development and in response to various therapies. This is of particular importance in ASD, given the suggestion that intra-individual variability in brain activity may itself be an endophenotype of ASD (David et al., 2016). Different features of the PSD may exhibit different measurement properties, with some parameters reflecting more transient or "state-like" properties of brain activity and others reflecting more stable "trait-like" interindividual differences. To begin this process, in the present study, we focus on test-retest reliability of the PSD and specific parameters thereof over a short time window (median of 6 days) during which one would not expect significant changes in underlying diagnosis, developmental changes are minimal, no new treatments are given, and EEG is collected under identical conditions.

Prior studies in healthy adults have demonstrated good to excellent test-retest reliability for certain features of the PSD. EEG power for mid-range frequencies (theta, alpha, and beta, as opposed to delta and gamma; Ip et al., 2018) and relative power (as opposed to absolute power; Salinsky et al., 1991) have shown correlation coefficients >0.8 for EEG sessions a few weeks apart; this is in the range of test-retest correlations for commonly used tests of cognitive ability (Elliott, 2007; Canivez and Watkins, 1999). Methodological advances in EEG pre-processing, such as a robust reference to average and wavelet independent component analysis which act to attenuate the effects of data collection artifact, improve test-retest reliability in higher frequency bands such as beta and gamma (Suarez-Revelo et al., 2016). However, the reliability of these features in children with or without neurodevelopmental disabilities remains unmeasured.

Notably, traditional methods of characterizing the PSD rely on measuring power within a particular frequency band, which conflates important aspects of underlying EEG activity. First, the EEG PSD typically contains a series of periodic oscillations atop an aperiodic background activity in which the power decreases as frequency (f) increases, leading to a consistent $1/f^{\alpha}$ distribution to the PSD, with the exponent α determining the slope of this background activity. This aperiodic activity, and the offset thereof, may reflect crucial mechanistic underpinnings of brain activity (He et al., 2010), such as tonic excitation/inhibition balance or total spiking activity of underlying neural populations respectively (Haller et al., 2018). The influence of this background activity on the measurement of oscillatory activity is partially (though not completely) eliminated using techniques such as normalization or log transform of the PSD. Second, *a priori* assumptions about the frequency bands wherein oscillations occur may compromise accurate measurement and fail to capture the meaningful variation of these oscillations. For example, averaging power in the predefined alpha range (e.g., 8–13 Hz) removes information about the peak alpha frequency in a given individual; however, the exact location of this alpha peak is well known to change with age and cognitive status (Angelakis et al., 2004; Grandy et al., 2013) and can even occur outside of the 8–13 Hz range. Because oscillations rarely span the exact range specified in a frequency band, their activity can be inadvertently included in neighboring frequency bands if they are wide or shifted. Finally, in cases where a periodic oscillation has a narrow bandwidth or is nonexistent with a prespecified frequency band, measurement of activity in that band will predominantly reflect the aperiodic activity. For these reasons, it is useful to characterize the EEG as a unique profile, with parameterization informed by the shape of each individual's PSD rather than piecemeal averages across distinct frequency bands.

As of October 2019, ClinicalTrials.gov reported 315 currently recruiting studies collecting EEG data and of those 102 were recruiting pediatric populations. Given the extent of this ongoing research, addressing how best to characterize the profile of the EEG PSD and determine its reliability and stability over time, particularly in clinical and developmental populations, is both important and timely. Such work forms an important foundation on which to base future research, and provides critical information to contextualize current findings.

In this study, we, therefore, explore the test-retest reliability of the profile of the EEG PSD in children with ASD and typical development (TD) over EEG recordings conducted within a short (~6 days) time-span. We applied two approaches to characterizing the profile of the PSD: (1) parametric model-based decomposition of the PSD into offset, slope, and oscillatory peaks using the Fitting Oscillations and One-Over-F (FOOOF) algorithm (Haller et al., 2018); and (2) nonparametric functional data analysis, which identifies a small set of principal component functions that combine to describe the shape of the power spectrum. We hypothesized that these complementary approaches would exhibit high levels of short-term test-retest reliability. In this way, we demonstrate the utility of resting EEG PSD shape, and some specific parameters thereof, as stable biomarkers of cortical activity over short time windows.

MATERIALS AND METHODS

These data were collected as part of the ongoing Autism Biomarkers Consortium for Clinical Trials (ABC-CT[1]; McPartland, 2016). Details of the ABC-CT data acquisition are reported elsewhere (Webb et al., 2019; McPartland et al., 2020). The objective of the ABC-CT is to evaluate a set of electrophysiological (EEG), eye-tracking, and behavioral measures for use in clinical trials for ASD. The ABC-CT began with a "Feasibility Study," which included the participants described below and involved two EEGs separated by a short window of time (median 6 days) as described below. The ABC-CT then moved on to the "Main Study," which included a larger number of participants, with EEGs separated by longer windows of time (6 weeks, and then 6 months). Only the data from the "Feasibility Study" is included here, as the focus of this manuscript is on the shorter-term test-retest reliability of the EEG PSD; this type of information (two EEGs separated by a few days) was not collected in the "Main Study." This study was carried out following the recommendations of the central Institutional Review Board at Yale University, with written informed consent from a parent or legal guardian and assent from each child before their participation in the study.

Participants

Fifty-one participants (25 with ASD, 26 with TD), were enrolled in the feasibility phase of the ABC-CT. Inclusion criteria included age 4–11 years, IQ 50–150 (as assessed by the Differential Ability Scales–2nd Edition), and participant and their parent/guardian must be English speaking. Exclusion criteria included a known genetic or neurological syndrome, metabolic disorder, mitochondrial dysfunction, significant sensory and/or motor impairment not correctable by a hearing aid or glasses/contact lenses, and history of significant prenatal/perinatal/birth injury, neonatal brain damage, or epilepsy. All participants (and at least one biological parent, if accompanying the child to the visit) were required to participate in a blood draw. Medication was not exclusionary, but participants were required to have been stable for 8 weeks on a current medication regimen. Additionally, environmental circumstances likely to account for ASD (e.g., severe nutritional or psychological deprivation) were exclusionary in the ASD group. In the TD group, additional exclusionary criteria included an active psychiatric disorder, a historical diagnosis of ASD, or a sibling with ASD.

Group characteristics are presented in **Table 1**. Groups differed significantly on age ($t_{(45)} = 2.3$, $p = 0.025$) and IQ ($t_{(45)} = 4.6$, $p < 0.001$). One participant with ASD and 3 participants with TD were left-handed. The "Feasibility Study Visit" consisted of two EEGs on two separate days (termed here "Day 1" and "Day 2"), separated by a short window of time (range 1–22 days, median 6 days) during this phase. Participants were characterized using rigorous autism diagnostic standardized measures [Autism Diagnostic Observation Schedule, 2nd edition (ADOS-2; Lord et al., 2001), Autism Diagnostic Interview-Revised (ADI-R; Lord et al., 1994),

[1] www.asdbiomarkers.org

TABLE 1 | Participant sex, age, and IQ by diagnostic group.

Group	*N* (N female)	Mean Age (Y)	Min. Age (Y)	Max. Age (Y)	Mean IQ (SD)
ASD	24 (5)	8.0*	4.42	11.4	93 (18.2)*
TD	26 (9)	6.6	4.01	11.4	114 (9.4)

Indicates measures that differ by group, as described in the text.

and Diagnostic and Statistical Manual of Mental Disorders (DSM-5) criteria (American Psychiatric Association, 2013)] by research-reliable clinicians (Webb et al., 2019), and cognitive measures [Differential Ability Scales 2nd edition (DAS-II; Elliott, 2007)].

EEG Protocol

In the feasibility phase of the ABC-CT, EEG acquisition included six paradigms (Webb et al., 2019), with "Resting EEG eyes open during calm viewing" of silent, chromatic digital videos (similar to screensavers) collected twice on two separate days. Video stimuli consisted of six 30 s non-social abstract videos purchased from Shutterstock, which were presented to the participant in random order in three blocks of 1 min on each day (Webb et al., 2018). The videos were played forward for 15 s and then reversed for the following 15 s. To allow for counterbalancing of the methods used in the ABC-CT (Eye Tracking and EEG), at screening, participants were stratified based on variables that could be assessed by phone to include group (ASD/TD), biological sex (male/female), age (split at 8 years 6 months), and cognitive ability (ASD only, assessed in person by a trained clinician at first visit). Half of the participants received eye-tracking first at each visit and the other half received EEG first.

Data were collected at five different sites. All sites had a high-density EEG acquisition system (Philips Neuro, Eugene, OR, USA), including either Net Amps 300 (Boston Children's Hospital, University of California Los Angeles, University of Washington, and Yale University) or Net Amps 400 amplifiers (Duke University). All sites used the 128 electrode HydroCel Geodesic Sensor Nets, applied according to Philips Neuro/Electrical Geodesics, Inc. standards. Four of the five sites removed electrodes 125–128, which are positioned on the participant's face, from the EEG caps to the tolerability of wearing the cap. Appropriate EEG acquisition protocols and software (500 Hz sampling rate, MFF file format, onset recording of amplifier and impedance calibrations) were provided to each site. EPrime 2.0 (Psychological Software Tools, Sharpsburg, PA, USA) was used for experimental control. The coordinating site reviewed and provided feedback on the net application, adherence to administration protocol, and data quality for every session. Sites conducted regular monthly checks of equipment function.

One participant with ASD refused to wear the net; EEG data was therefore available on 24 ASD and 26 TD participants. After the preprocessing described below, EEG from one additional ASD participant was excluded from the parametric and nonparametric data analyses due to having a substantially lower number of observed segments than the rest of the sample (61 segments vs. an average of 91 segments) and only 1 day of EEG recording. Thus, in total, there was usable data on at least 1 day from 23 ASD and 26 TD participants (N: $Duke_{ASD}$ = 4; $Duke_{TD}$ = 5; BCH_{TD} = 5; BCH_{ASD} = 5; $Yale_{TD}$ = 5; $Yale_{ASD}$ = 5; UW_{TD} = 5; UW_{ASD} = 5; $UCLA_{TD}$ = 6; $UCLA_{ASD}$ = 5). Data on one ASD and one TD participant were recorded only on day 1. There was thus usable data on both days from 22 ASD and 25 TD participants (of note, **Table 1** includes data on all participants who had EEG data available on at least 1 day, and not just those who contributed 2 days of EEG; this is because the mixed-effects models described below can still make use of the data from participants who contributed just 1 day of EEG).

Preprocessing of the EEG

Processing of the raw EEG data was done using the Harvard Automated Processing Pipeline for Electroencephalography (HAPPE; Gabard-Durnam et al., 2018) embedded within the Batch EEG Automated Processing Platform (BEAPP; Levin et al., 2018). In brief, data were 1 Hz high pass and 100 Hz low pass filtered, downsampled to 250 Hz, and run through the HAPPE module including a selection of 18 channels corresponding to the 10-20 system channels (excluding Cz, as data were originally collected in reference to Cz), 60 Hz electrical line noise removal, bad channel rejection, wavelet-enhanced thresholding, independent component analysis with automated component rejection (Winkler et al., 2011, 2014), automated segment rejection, interpolation of bad channels, and re-referencing to average (Of note, the selection of 18 channels from the full 128-channels is necessary to generate a robust signal decomposition using independent component analysis, given the short length of the EEG recording. Details of how to determine an appropriate number of channels included in an independent component analysis decomposition are provided elsewhere; Gabard-Durnam et al., 2018; Levin et al., 2018). Data were then segmented into two-second segments, and the PSD was calculated *via* multitaper spectral analysis (Thomson, 1982; Babadi and Brown, 2014) using three tapers. The PSD was estimated for each participant and electrode by averaging the PSDs of artifact-free segments. Scalp-wide spectral densities were obtained by averaging spectral densities across the 18 electrodes for each subject on each day. Parametric analyses were based on absolute power, whereas nonparametric analyses were based on relative power.

Parametric Decomposition of Periodic and Aperiodic Activity

In order to characterize periodic and aperiodic features of the PSD profile, we used the Fitting Oscillations and One-Over-F (FOOOF) algorithm (Haller et al., 2018). The algorithm

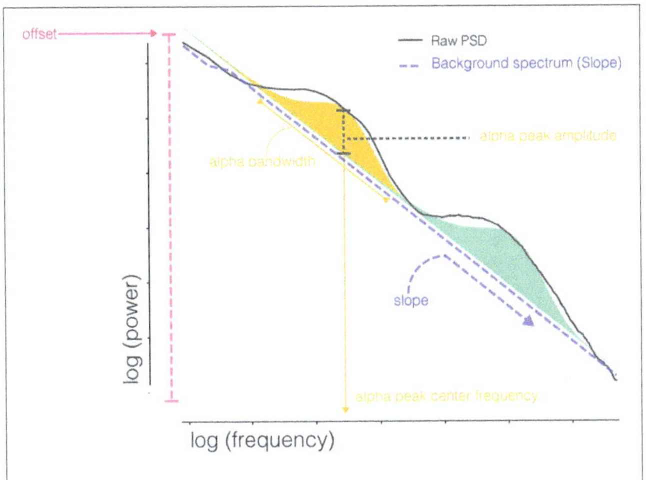

FIGURE 1 | Parameters extracted from FOOOF decomposition of the power spectral densities (PSD). FOOOF models individual oscillatory peaks atop the PSD and estimates the slope and offset of aperiodic activity below those peaks. Shaded regions (blue and orange) indicate distinct oscillatory peaks identified by model fitting.

operates by removing an aperiodic slope (**Figure 1**) from the absolute PSD in the semilog-power space (linear frequencies and logged power), which is fully characterized by offset and slope terms. After removing the aperiodic component, the spectral density contains periodic oscillatory peaks that are modeled as a finite sum of Gaussians. Each Gaussian peak is defined by its amplitude, center frequency, and bandwidth (defined as two standard deviations of the fitted Gaussian). Thus, the PSD profile, including both the aperiodic background and periodic oscillations, can be fully parameterized by the following parameters: offset, slope, number of peaks (Gaussians), and the center frequency, amplitude, and bandwidth for each peak. These scalar features are then available for analysis across recording sessions using standard statistical techniques. The FOOOF model parameters were chosen by visually inspecting model fit across a range of parameters, blind to participant group and recording session, and selecting those which best captured oscillatory peaks across all of the recordings. A single parameter set was selected for all recordings. Specifically, the bandwidth of oscillatory peaks ranged between 1 and 10 Hz, and the minimum peak height (to be included in the fit) was 1.85 standard deviations above the aperiodic background activity.

Since the number of total peaks identified on each spectral density varied across subjects and days, for comparison purposes across consecutive days we first considered the agreement of the location [in terms of frequency band, i.e., delta (2–4 Hz), theta (4–6 Hz), low alpha (6–9 Hz), high alpha (9–13 Hz), beta (13–30 Hz), and gamma (30–55 Hz)] of the peak with the largest amplitude between days. For comparison of the largest peak features (center frequency, amplitude, and bandwidth), we then considered the largest peak in the entire alpha band for stability of results and ease of comparison between diagnostic groups. This allowed characterization of each scalp-wide spectral density by six FOOOF parameters: offset, slope, number of peaks, and (for the largest peak in the alpha range) center frequency, amplitude, and bandwidth. The agreement of these six FOOOF parameters across the 2 days for each diagnostic group was evaluated using the intraclass correlation coefficient (the ratio of between-person variance to total variance; ICC; Donner and Koval, 1980). Age-adjusted and IQ-adjusted ICCs are also presented, by adding these variables as predictors in the mixed-effects model. ICC values less than 0.40 are considered poor, between 0.40 and 0.59 fair, between 0.60 and 0.74 good, and between 0.75 and 1.00 excellent (Cicchetti, 1994). For all reported ICC values, bootstrap based on resampling subjects with replacement was used for forming percentile confidence intervals (CIs). Bootstrap methods yield more reliable inference in small samples (bootstrap CIs were based on 200 resampled data sets).

Nonparametric Analysis of the Relative Spectral Density *via* Functional Data Analysis

Scalp-wide relative spectral densities were obtained by averaging relative spectral densities across electrodes for each subject observed on each day. The agreement in relative spectral density across days for both electrode-specific and scalp-wide relative spectral densities was computed by functional ICC within each diagnostic group. Since a trend of lower functional ICC was observed for the most peripheral electrodes [electrodes 9 (FP2), 22 (FP1), 45 (T3), 70 (O1), 83 (O2) and 108 (T4)] across diagnostic groups, a sensitivity analysis was also run through the functional ICC of the scalp-wide relative spectral densities excluding these six electrodes. Computation of functional ICC follows a functional ANOVA decomposition of the data within each diagnostic group with days as the within-subject factor. Functional ICC is the functional analog of the intra-class correlation in standard mixed-effects models. It corresponds to the ratio of the between-subject variability to total variance (between + within) similar to ICC but estimates variance parameters using functional data analysis techniques. Hence it can be interpreted as the intra-subject correlation of the entire relative spectral density across days, as opposed to the ICC for the FOOOF parameters which refer to the stability of certain features of the spectral density (but not the spectral density in its entirety). The functional ANOVA model is fit using a multilevel functional principal component decomposition (Di et al., 2009) which entails estimation of the subject- and day-level eigenvalues and eigenfunctions that enrich interpretations by allowing us to connect the nonparametric functional data analysis to results from the parametric analysis *via* FOOOF. For all reported functional ICC values, bootstrap percentile CIs were formed based on 200 resampled data sets based on resampling from subjects with replacement.

RESULTS

Age, sex, and IQ for study participants are in **Table 1**.

The power spectrum of each individual on day 1 and day 2 is plotted in **Figure 2**. Within participants, PSD shapes exhibit visual similarity across separate recording sessions.

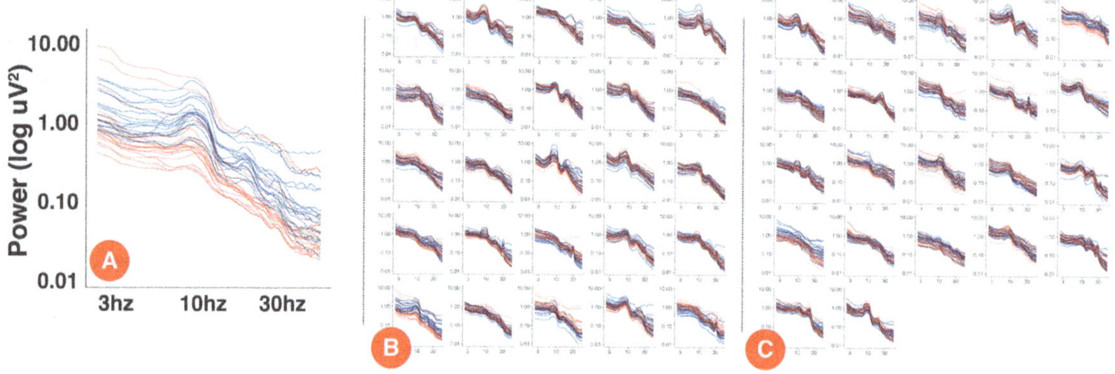

FIGURE 2 | PSDs for each session by participant. Panel **(A)** displays an expanded, single participant, PSD with the log-10 axis labels. Each electrode is a single line. Day one PSDs are shown in blue and day 2 PSDs are shown in red. Panels **(B)** and **(C)** show individual PSDs for TD **(B)** and ASD **(C)** participants. Each smaller figure is data from a single participant.

Data quality metrics output from HAPPE (Gabard-Durnam et al., 2018) are described in **Table 2**. Overall, data quality was high across groups.

Parametric Analysis of the Absolute Power Spectral Density *via* FOOOF

The location of the dominant peak (i.e., the peak with the greatest amplitude according to the FOOOF algorithm) from both days is provided in **Table 3** for both diagnostic groups. The dominant peak occurred most frequently in the high alpha frequency band in the ASD group and low alpha frequency band in the TD group. Across days, while the dominant peak stayed within the alpha band (low and high alpha) mostly for the TD group, it stayed more broadly within the alpha-beta range in the ASD group.

The estimated ICCs along with their bootstrap CIs for an agreement of the six FOOOF parameters derived from scalp-wide absolute PSD across the two experimental days are provided in **Table 4** for both diagnostic groups. Among offset, slope, and number of peaks, offset yielded consistently fair agreement in both groups [TD 0.484 95% CI (0.004, 0.775); ASD 0.525 95% CI (0.167, 0.806)], with slope between the 2 days showing poor agreement in the TD group (0.284 95% CI (0, 0.674) but good agreement in the ASD group [0.699 95% CI (0.527, 0.815)]. Among the three FOOOF parameters describing the largest alpha peak, amplitude had the highest ICC in both groups [TD 0.862 95% CI (0.729, 0.939); ASD 0.828 95% CI (0.664, 0.926)], followed by center frequency [TD 0.700 95% CI (0.437, 0.862); ASD 0.619 95% CI (0.342, 0.852)], and bandwidth [TD 0.424 95% CI (0.028, 0.696); ASD 0.340 95% CI (0.034, 0.727)]. While the agreement of the largest alpha peak amplitude was high in both groups, agreement in the peak frequency was slightly higher in the TD group than the ASD group. In the sensitivity analysis, when the analysis was repeated on FOOOF parameters derived after the exclusion of the six peripheral electrodes, these results remained unchanged. Age-adjusted ICC values (**Supplementary Table S1**) are notable predominantly for a decrease in the ICC of the center frequency of the alpha peak (as compared to unadjusted ICC values). This decrease is larger in the TD group than the ASD group. The TD group also shows a decrease in ICC of the alpha bandwidth when adjusting for age. IQ-adjusted ICC values (**Supplementary Table S2**) remain largely unchanged from unadjusted ICC values.

Nonparametric Analysis of the Relative Power Spectral Density *via* Functional Data Analysis

The estimated functional ICC for the scalp-wide relative spectral density was excellent in both groups, though higher in the TD group than the ASD group [TD 0.858 95% CI (0.748, 0.926); ASD 0.807 95% CI (0.650, 0.914)]. The estimated functional ICC for each of the 18 electrodes and their 95% bootstrap CIs are shown by diagnostic group in **Figure 3**. While the average electrode-specific ICC in the TD group is approximately equal to that of the ASD group, there is greater variation in the functional ICC among electrodes in the TD group (both higher and lower values of the functional ICC) compared to the ASD group. In the sensitivity analysis, the estimated scalp-wide functional ICC for both diagnostic groups was slightly higher when the six peripheral electrodes are excluded [TD 0.874 95% CI (0.741, 0.931); ASD 0.815 95% CI (0.712, 0.913)], though the magnitude of difference between the two diagnostic groups was unchanged.

The functional ANOVA model captures individual deviations from the mean scalp-wide relative spectral density over the 2 days by partitioning the total variance into participant- and day-level variation. Participant-level variation captures the variation among participants whereas day-level variation captures the variation within a subject across days. Within each level of variation, ordered curves known as eigenfunctions identify which portions of the frequency domain account for the most variation by placing more magnitude at these locations. The two estimated leading participant- and day-level

TABLE 2 | Data quality measures, based on HAPPE metrics.

Group	Day	Good Channels (%)	# of EEG segments retained	Rejected components (%)	EEG variance retained (%)	Mean retained artifact probability	Median retained artifact probability
ASD	1	95.4 (3.4)	90.7 (1.8)	29 (11)	70.2 (17.1)	0.08 (0.03)	0.03 (0.02)
	2	95.9 (3.9)	90.7 (1.8)	30 (12)	70.6 (15.8)	0.08 (0.03)	0.02 (0.02)
TD	1	97.4 (3.8)	90.8 (1.7)	18 (10)	82.5 (13.2)	0.05 (0.02)	0.01 (0.01)
	2	97.1 (3.8)	90.9 (1.7)	19 (10)	80.2 (15.2)	0.06 (0.04)	0.02 (0.02)

Data are reported as mean (SD). EEG segments are 2 s long.

TABLE 3 | The location of the dominant peak in day 1 (rows) vs. day 2 (columns) among the TD and ASD groups.

Day 1/2	Low_Alpha	High_Alpha	Beta	Gamma
TD				
Low_Alpha	6	6	0	0
High_Alpha	5	3	0	1
Beta	1	1	0	0
Gamma	1	0	0	1
ASD				
Low_Alpha	2	2	1	0
High_Alpha	2	4	3	0
Beta	2	3	1	0
Gamma	0	1	1	0

Values indicate the number of participants with a given combination of dominant peak locations across days.

TABLE 4 | The estimated intraclass correlation coefficients (ICCs) and their 95% bootstrap CI for the six FOOOF parameters for each diagnostic group.

FOOOF Parameter	TD	ASD
Offset	0.484 (0.004, 0.775)	0.525 (0.167, 0.806)
Slope	0.284 (0, 0.674)	0.699 (0.527, 0.815)
Number of peaks	0.021 (0, 0.571)	0.226 (0.003, 0.609)
Largest alpha peak: Center Frequency	0.700 (0.437, 0.862)	0.619 (0.342, 0.852)
Largest alpha peak: Amplitude	0.862 (0.729, 0.939)	0.828 (0.664, 0.926)
Largest alpha peak: Bandwidth	0.424 (0.028, 0.696)	0.340 (0.034, 0.727)

eigenfunctions for both diagnostic groups are shown in **Figure 4**. We restrict our discussion to the first two participant-level eigenfunctions, since combined they explain at least 60% of the total variation in both groups. We include the first 2 day-level eigenfunctions for completeness. The first participant-level eigenfunction for both groups displays that most variation in the data is explained by the variation in the amplitude of the alpha peak (with maximal variation at approximately 9 Hz), explaining similar total variation for the TD group (48% total variance explained) and the ASD group (43% total variance explained). While the first participant-level eigenfunction highlights variation in the amplitude of the largest peak, the second participant-level eigenfunction highlights the variation in the frequency (location) of the largest peak, where TD participants show the largest variation in the low and high alpha band (24% total variance explained) and ASD participants show it in high alpha and beta relative power (18% variance explained). These findings are consistent with the locations of

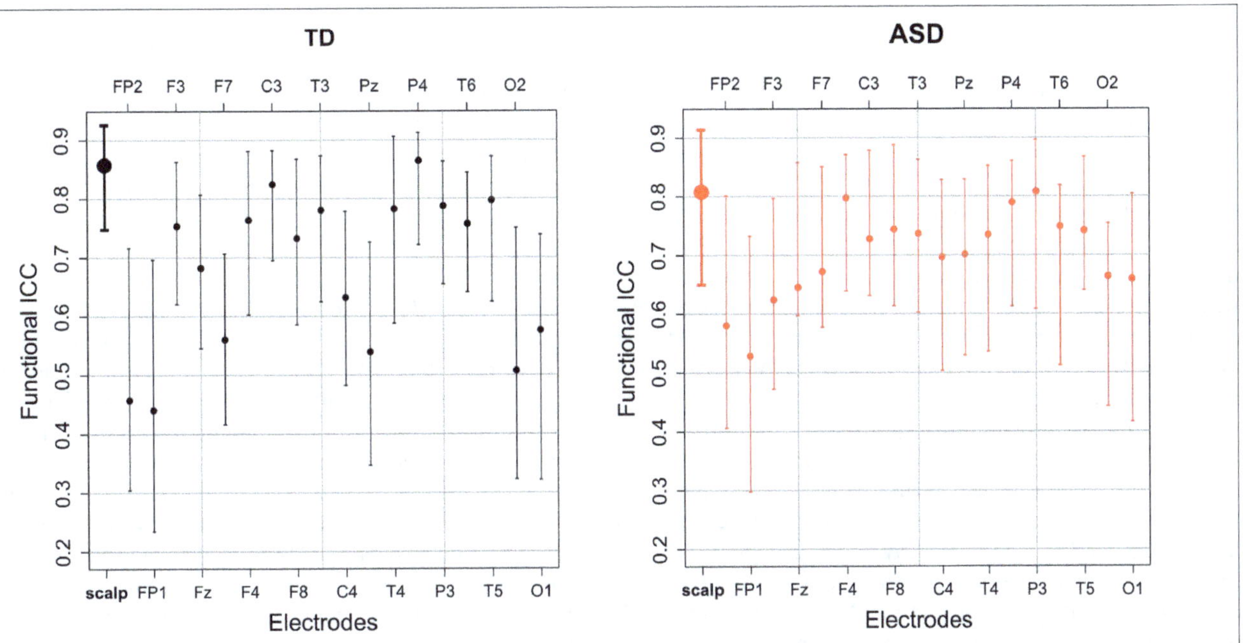

FIGURE 3 | The estimated scalp-wide (bold) and electrode-specific functional intraclass correlations and their 95% bootstrap CI by diagnostic group.

the largest peak summarized in **Table 3** across days for the two groups. While the first day-level eigenfunction highlights across day variability in alpha and beta relative power, the second eigenfunction highlights across day variability in the location of the largest peak (between high and low alpha for TD, and between high alpha and beta for ASD) similar to the second participant-level eigenfunction. The fact that most of the variation is explained by the participant-level eigenfunctions (compared to day-level eigenfunctions) supports our interpretation that most of the variation in the data is variation across subjects and there is less variability within a subject across days. Also, participants maintain stable alpha peaks across experimental days, both in terms of peak frequency and amplitude, consistent with the high ICCs reported in **Table 4** for alpha peak amplitude and frequency in the two groups in the FOOOF analysis.

DISCUSSION

In this manuscript, we examine the test-retest reliability of the EEG power spectral density in children with ASD and TD. EEG power-based measures are currently being evaluated and employed as biomarkers in a variety of neurodevelopmental and psychiatric disorders, and analytical validation (including understanding the test-retest reliability of these measures) is an important early step in the biomarker development process (Micheel and Ball, 2010).

Overall, our findings demonstrate excellent test-retest reliability for scalp-wide EEG profiles. This high test-retest reliability reflects the overall stability of the EEG power spectrum over relatively short time windows (a few days). For the development of diagnostic biomarkers, this reliability is crucial—we would not expect the fundamental biology of the brain to change over several days without intervention, and therefore biomarkers indexing brain function for diagnostic purposes should not change significantly over this period.

On the other hand, there are scenarios in which we would not expect (or want) aspects of the EEG power spectrum to remain stable. For example, while markers of phenotypic traits may remain stable, markers of state and other modifiable factors (e.g., epileptiform activity) may vary over short periods. For example, changes in the emotional state during testing, and attention to the stimuli, may lead to changes in EEG power that reflect true physiologic changes in brain function over even short time windows. Similarly, scarce epileptiform activity may occur in some of a participant's EEG recordings but not others. While the ABC-CT does not involve a specific intervention, this concept will become particularly relevant when treatments target a specific modifiable factor (e.g., psychotropic medications which may modify state; spike suppressing anti-epileptic medications which may modify epileptiform activity). Identifying the parameters of the EEG PSD that predominantly reflect stable factors (e.g., traits), and separately those that predominantly reflect modifiable factors (e.g., state, mood, attention, and epileptiform activity), while beyond the scope of the study described here, will allow us to harness the wealth of information available from EEG recordings to develop a range of biomarker types in future studies. This concept will be crucial for clinical trials as well. For example, monitoring biomarkers will ideally remain relatively stable when treatment is not given, but show a significant change in response to targeted medical and behavioral treatments.

The high test-retest reliability for EEG profiles is present in both TD and ASD groups, though reliability was higher overall in the TD group (ICC 0.858) than the ASD group (ICC 0.807). This is consistent with prior findings suggesting more variable neural activity in ASD compared to TD (David et al., 2016) and may suggest that reliability, in addition to providing important information for biomarker development, may in and of itself represent a potential biomarker. Notably, higher neural variability may reflect (or provoke) more variable emotional states during testing and more variable attention to the stimuli. Such factors are often found to be clinically more variable among children with ASD. Notably, there is also a decrease in ICC of the alpha peak frequency when adjusted for age. This is likely related to the fact that alpha peak frequency typically increases with age; therefore, adjustment for age will absorb some of the across-subject variations, thus making the ratio of across-subject variation to total variation (ICC) decrease. The larger decrease of alpha peak frequency ICC in the TD group with age adjustment may reflect a stronger tendency for alpha peak frequency to increase with age in the TD group as compared to the ASD group; this tendency has been previously described (Edgar et al., 2019). The decrease in alpha bandwidth ICC in the TD group with age adjustment may reflect a similar tendency; however, to our knowledge alpha bandwidth has not been extensively studied in the past, and thus this may be an interesting direction for future studies.

Because the EEG PSD captures a range of parameters, it is important to consider specifically which of those parameters have high short-term test-retest reliability (and thus offer the potential for diagnostic biomarker development), vs. those with low short-term test-retest reliability (potentially reflecting state, attention or perhaps noise). Our findings suggest that within the PSD, a relatively small set of parameters is largely responsible for capturing the fingerprint-like quality of each individual's EEG. FOOOF-based parameterization suggests that the alpha peak is particularly useful for individualizing the power spectrum. Within the alpha peak, amplitude offers particular promise in this regard, although the center frequency of the alpha peak also provides strong reliability within individuals. Here, it is particularly notable that the frequency of alpha is often considered to be an individual trait (changing only gradually with age and other factors but otherwise remaining relatively stable in most cases), whereas alpha amplitude varies more with the state. For example, the posterior dominant rhythm tends to arise when the eyes are closed and is suppressed with eye-opening; similarly, mu rhythms over the motor cortex are suppressed by imagining or engaging in motor tasks. However, our findings suggest that in the context of the environment in which EEGs were collected in the ABC-CT (watching a silent, screen-saver type videos), alpha amplitude remains quite stable—even more so, in fact, than alpha frequency.

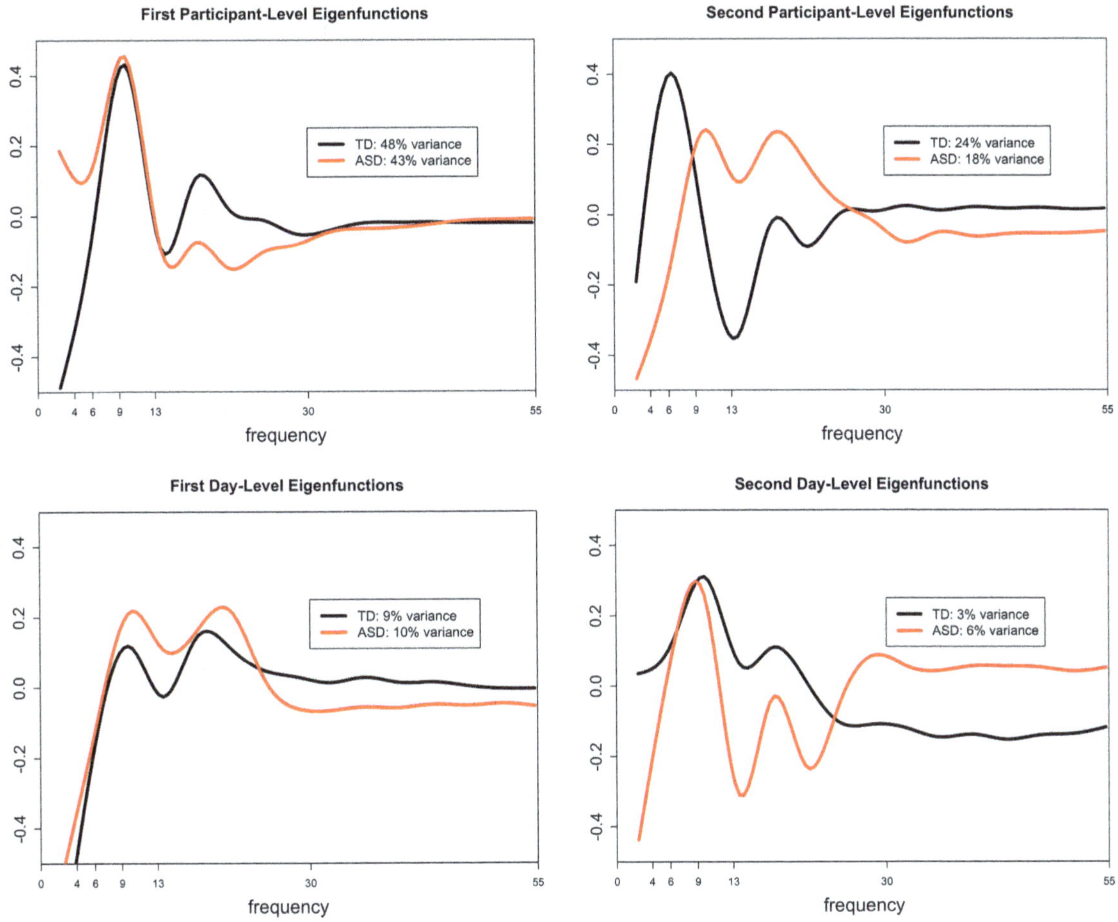

FIGURE 4 | The estimated first and second leading eigenfunctions for the participant-level variation (top row) and day-level variation (bottom row) for each diagnostic group. The total variation explained by each component is included in the legend.

For the slope of the power spectrum as measured by FOOOF, ICC was good in the ASD group but poor in the TD group. This suggests that slope (at least as measured by FOOOF with the parameters used here) is unstable across sessions in the TD group. One possible explanation for this is that the TD group may be more sensitive to session effects (e.g., due to habituation, adaptation, or learning) than the ASD group, and this is being reflected in the slope. It is also possible that the older mean age or lower mean IQ of the ASD group, rather than TD or ASD status *per se*, contributed to this difference. An alternative explanation, supported by a visual review of **Figure 2**, is that there is very little inter-individual variability in the PSD slope among the TD group; therefore, intra-individual reliability (across days) cannot be much higher than inter-individual reliability (across participants) in the TD group, because inter-individual reliability is high to begin with. In the ASD group, which may be more heterogeneous given the wide variety of genetic and other underlying factors that lead to ASD, the inter-individual variability in slope is higher. In this case, similarly strong intra-individual reliability in the TD and ASD groups would lead to a higher ICC in the ASD group, because of the higher inter-individual variability in this group.

Importantly, the eigenfunctions which best characterized PSD shape exhibited the most variance at relatively low frequencies (4–13 hz), corresponding to overall offsets of the PSD and in the theta to alpha range of the EEG, aligning with the parametric findings from FOOOF and highlighting the import of this frequency range for characterizing stable interindividual differences in brain activity. This finding, combined with the tendency for a variance to be explained by activity at slightly higher frequencies in the ASD group (alpha-beta) than TD participants (predominantly alpha), may help to explain the higher estimated ICC for offset and slope in the ASD group compared to TD. Because the slope and offset terms in FOOOF are fit in the semilog-power space, these parameters are sensitive to power dynamics at higher frequencies, which are often of lower magnitude.

For the nonparametric analyses of relative power, reliability in both groups improves with the removal of peripheral electrodes. Notably, because peripheral electrodes are closer than central electrodes to many non-brain-based sources of detected activity (e.g., muscle and eye movements), they are often more susceptible to artifact than more central electrodes. This suggests (perhaps reassuringly) that brain-based findings, more so than artifact-based findings, remain stable across EEG sessions within an individual. On the other hand, for the parametric analyses of absolute power, the removal of peripheral electrodes does not improve reliability. This may be because the majority of parameters identified by FOOOF are not significantly affected by an artifact in peripheral electrodes, raising the possibility that FOOOF is less susceptible to artifact contamination than nonparametric analyses; this may be further studied in future work.

Nonparametric analyses otherwise reveal complementary results to the parametric analyses. Parametric analyses reveal excellent ICC for the amplitude of the largest alpha peak and good ICC for the frequency of the largest alpha peak. This is true in both the ASD and TD groups, though the ICC in the TD group is slightly higher than that in the ASD group for both of these parameters. Similarly, nonparametric analyses highlight alpha amplitude as capturing the majority of variance for the participant-level spectral densities, followed by alpha frequency. This is again true in both the ASD and TD groups, though slightly more variance is captured by the first two eigenfunctions in the TD as compared to the ASD group. Parametric functions also demonstrate that the dominant peak tended to stay within the alpha band for the TD group, but tended to stay more broadly in the range of both the alpha and beta bands for the ASD group. Similarly, nonparametric functions demonstrate that the TD participants show the largest variation in the alpha band, whereas ASD participants show variation in alpha but also extending into beta.

Nonparametric functional data analysis and FOOOF thus provide convergent and complementary approaches to characterizing the PSD. Nonparametric functional data analysis characterizes PSD shape accurately and with a small number of principal functions yielding high levels of reliability. However, it relies on "learning" these functions based on the current data set and thus yields different principal functions based on the input data, as we see here between our diagnostic groups. Additionally, the resulting functions need careful interpretation to ground their relationship with brain activity. Conversely, FOOOF estimates require more parameters to characterize the PSD. However, fitting these parameters does not depend on the presence of other members of the data set (although the algorithm fitting settings can indirectly force information sharing among power spectra). Also, the interpretation of FOOOF parameters is more direct. FOOOF explicitly attempts to separate biophysically meaningful model parameters such as slope, offset, and oscillatory peaks.

It is important to note the specific questions that the present study is designed to answer. First, the two testing days for each individual took place within approximately a week. While this suggests promise for biomarker development in trials where EEG-based findings are expected to change over very short periods, many pharmacological interventions aim to change neural activity over the longer term (weeks, months, or longer). Examining test-retest stability of the EEG power spectrum over these longer periods is part of ongoing analyses for the ABC-CT main study, which will include 6 weeks and 6-month follow-up recordings. Additionally, here we report only test-retest reliability for a single set of EEG measures, all based on the power spectrum. EEG is a rich source of information beyond that which can be captured in the power spectrum, in both the time domain and the frequency domain. As future studies suggest additional EEG-based measurements that may offer promise for biomarker developments, the test-retest reliability of the measurements will need to be explicitly evaluated. Finally, the data presented here specifically evaluates ICC and group variability thereof (ASD vs. TD); however, our sample size was not large enough to compare ICC across sites. Other analyses relevant to the EEG power (e.g., comparing power, rather than ICC thereof, across groups) are underway for the larger "Main Study" of ABC-CT but are beyond the scope of the data presented here.

Developing biomarkers for ASD and other neurodevelopmental disorders remains a high priority in the field, given the potential benefits, biomarkers offer for clinical trials, diagnostics, and monitoring (Krueger et al., 2017). While future studies will continue to assess which measurements (in EEG and otherwise) offer the most promise as potential biomarkers of various types, our findings of high short-term test-retest reliability of the EEG power spectral density are a crucial step towards ensuring that potential biomarkers meet necessary criteria for validation.

ETHICS STATEMENT

The studies involving human participants were reviewed and approved by central Institutional Review Board at Yale University. Written informed consent to participate in this study was provided by the participants' parent/legal guardian.

AUTHOR CONTRIBUTIONS

AL, AN, AS, SW, FS, CS, MM, RB, KC, GD, SF, SJ, CN, JM, and DŞ made substantial contributions to the conception or design of the ABC-CT and provided critical revisions related to the important intellectual content. AL, AN, AS, and DŞ contributed to the analysis of the data described in this manuscript. AL, AN, AS, SW, and DŞ contributed to the drafting of this manuscript. All named authors read and provided approval for publication of the content.

FUNDING

Support for this project was provided by the Autism Biomarkers Consortium for Clinical Trials (NIMH U19 MH108206; McPartland) and National Institute of General Medical Sciences (R01 GM111378-01A1; DŞ and CS).

ACKNOWLEDGMENTS

A special thanks to all of the families and participants who joined with us in this effort. Also, we thank our external advisor board, NIH scientific partners, and the FNIH Biomarkers Consortium. Additional important contributions were provided by members of the ABC-CT consortium including Heather Borland and Megha Santhosh, who were responsible for EEG acquisition including EEG experimental and pipeline programming, site training and initiation, and quality control.

REFERENCES

American Psychiatric Association. (2013). *Diagnostic and Statistical Manual of Mental Disorders, 5th Edition.* Arlington, VA: American Psychiatric Publishing, Inc.

Angelakis, E., Lubar, J. F., Stathopoulou, S., and Kounios, J. (2004). Peak α frequency: an electroencephalographic measure of cognitive preparedness. *Clin. Neurophysiol.* 115, 887–897. doi: 10.1016/j.clinph.2003.11.034

Babadi, B., and Brown, E. N. (2014). A review of multitaper spectral analysis. *IEEE Trans. Biomed. Eng.* 61, 1555–1564. doi: 10.1109/TBME.2014.2311996

Berry-Kravis, E. M., Lindemann, L., Jønch, A. E., Apostol, G., Bear, M. F., Carpenter, R. L., et al. (2018). Drug development for neurodevelopmental disorders: lessons learned from fragile X syndrome. *Nat. Rev. Drug Discov.* 17, 280–298. doi: 10.1038/nrd.2017.221

Canivez, G. L., and Watkins, M. W. (1999). Long-term stability of the wechsler intelligence scale for children-third edition among demographic subgroups: gender, race/ethnicity, and age. *J. Psychoeduc. Assess.* 17, 300–313. doi: 10.1177/073428299901700401

Cicchetti, D. V. (1994). Guidelines, criteria, and rules of thumb for evaluating normed and standardized assessment instruments in psychology. *Psychol. Assess.* 6, 284–290. doi: 10.1037/1040-3590.6.4.284

David, N., Schneider, T. R., Peiker, I., Al-Jawahiri, R., Engel, A. K., and Milne, E. (2016). Variability of cortical oscillation patterns: a possible endophenotype in autism spectrum disorders? *Neurosci. Biobehav. Rev.* 71, 590–600. doi: 10.1016/j.neubiorev.2016.09.031

Di, C. Z., Crainiceanu, C. M., Caffo, B. S., and Punjabi, N. M. (2009). Multilevel functional principal component analysis. *Ann. Appl. Stat.* 3, 458–488. doi: 10.1214/08-AOAS206

Donner, A., and Koval, J. J. (1980). The estimation of intraclass correlation in the analysis of family data. *Biometrics* 36, 19–25. doi: 10.2307/2530491

Edgar, J. C., Dipiero, M., McBride, E., Green, H. L., Berman, J., Ku, M., et al. (2019). Abnormal maturation of the resting-state peak α frequency in children with autism spectrum disorder. *Hum. Brain Mapp.* 40, 3288–3298. doi: 10.1002/hbm.24598

Elliott, C. D. (2007). *Differential Ability Scales-II (DAS-II).* San Antonio, TX: Psychological Corporation.

FDA-NIH Biomarker Working Group. (2016). *BEST (Biomarkers, Endpoints, and Other Tools) Resource.* Silver Spring, MD: Food and Drug Administration (US). Available online at: https://www.ncbi.nlm.nih.gov/books/NBK326791/?report=classic.

Gabard-Durnam, L. J., Mendez Leal, A. S., Wilkinson, C. L., and Levin, A. R. (2018). The harvard automated processing pipeline for electroencephalography (HAPPE): standardized processing software for developmental and high-artifact data. *Front. Neurosci.* 12:97. doi: 10.3389/fnins.2018.00097

Grandy, T. H., Werkle-Bergner, M., Chicherio, C., Schmiedek, F., Lövdén, M., and Lindenberger, U. (2013). Peak individual α frequency qualifies as a stable neurophysiological trait marker in healthy younger and older adults. *Psychophysiology* 50, 570–582. doi: 10.1111/psyp.12043

Haller, M., Donoghue, T., Peterson, E., Varma, P., Sebastian, P., Gao, R., et al. (2018). Parameterizing neural power spectra. *bioRxiv* [Preprint]. doi: 10.1101/299859

He, B. J., Zempel, J. M., Snyder, A. Z., and Raichle, M. E. (2010). The temporal structures and functional significance of scale-free brain activity. *Neuron* 66, 353–369. doi: 10.1016/j.neuron.2010.04.020

Ip, C. T., Ganz, M., Ozenne, B., Sluth, L. B., Gram, M., Viardot, G., et al. (2018). Pre-intervention test-retest reliability of EEG and ERP over four recording intervals. *Int. J. Psychophysiol.* 134, 30–43. doi: 10.1016/j.ijpsycho.2018.09.007

Jeste, S. S., Frohlich, J., and Loo, S. K. (2015). Electrophysiological biomarkers of diagnosis and outcome in neurodevelopmental disorders. *Curr. Opin. Neurol.* 28, 110–116. doi: 10.1097/wco.0000000000000181

Krueger, D. A., Sadhwani, A., Byars, A. W., de Vries, P. J., Franz, D. N., Whittemore, V. H., et al. (2017). Everolimus for treatment of tuberous sclerosis complex-associated neuropsychiatric disorders. *Ann. Clin. Transl. Neurol.* 4, 877–887. doi: 10.1002/acn3.494

Levin, A. R., Méndez Leal, A. S., Gabard-Durnam, L. J., and O'Leary, H. M. (2018). BEAPP: the batch electroencephalography automated processing platform. *Front. Neurosci.* 12:513. doi: 10.3389/fnins.2018.00513

Lord, C., Rutter, M., DiLavore, P. C., and Risi, S. (2001). *Autism Diagnostic Observation Schedule (ADOS).* Los Angeles, CA: Western Psychological Services.

Lord, C., Rutter, M., and Le Couteur, A. (1994). Autism Diagnostic Interview-Revised: a revised version of a diagnostic interview for caregivers of individuals with possible pervasive developmental disorders. *J. Autism Dev. Disord.* 24, 659–685. doi: 10.1007/bf02172145

McPartland, J. C. (2016). Considerations in biomarker development for neurodevelopmental disorders. *Curr. Opin. Neurol.* 29, 118–122. doi: 10.1097/wco.0000000000000300

McPartland, J. C., Bernier, R. A., Jeste, S. S., Dawson, G., Nelson, C. A., Chawarska, K., et al. (2020). The autism biomarkers consortium for clinical trials (ABC-CT): scientific context, study design, and progress towards biomarker qualification. *Front. Integr. Neurosci.* 14:16. doi: 10.3389/fnint.2020.00016

Micheel, C. M., and Ball, J. R. (2010). *Evaluation of Biomarkers and Surrogate Endpoints in Chronic Disease.* Washington, DC: National Academies Press.

Port, R. G., Gandal, M. J., Roberts, T. P. L., Siegel, S. J., and Carlson, G. C. (2014). Convergence of circuit dysfunction in ASD: a common bridge between diverse genetic and environmental risk factors and common clinical electrophysiology. *Front. Cell. Neurosci.* 8:414. doi: 10.3389/fncel.2014.00414

Sahin, M., Jones, S. R., Sweeney, J. A., Berry-Kravis, E., Connors, B. W., Ewen, J. B., et al. (2018). Discovering translational biomarkers in neurodevelopmental disorders. *Nat. Rev. Drug Discov.* doi: 10.1038/d41573-018-00010-7 [Epub ahead of print].

Salinsky, M. C., Oken, B. S., and Morehead, L. (1991). Test-retest reliability in EEG frequency analysis. *Electroencephalogr. Clin. Neurophysiol.* 79, 382–392. doi: 10.1016/0013-4694(91)90203-g

Suarez-Revelo, J., Ochoa-Gomez, J., and Duque-Grajales, J. (2016). Improving test-retest reliability of quantitative electroencephalography using different preprocessing approaches. *Conf. Proc. IEEE Eng. Med. Biol. Soc.* 2016, 961–964. doi: 10.1109/embc.2016.7590861

Thomson, D. J. (1982). Spectrum estimation and harmonic analysis. *Proc. IEEE* 70, 1055–1096. doi: 10.1109/proc.1982.12433

Wang, J., Barstein, J., Ethridge, L. E., Mosconi, M. W., Takarae, Y., and Sweeney, J. A. (2013). Resting state EEG abnormalities in autism spectrum disorders. *J. Neurodev. Disord.* 5:24. doi: 10.1186/1866-1955-5-24

Webb, S. J., Borland, H., Santhosh, M., Naples, A., Levin, A. R., Bernier, R., et al. (2018). *Data Acquisition and Analytic Core EEG Main Study Manual of Operations Version 2.2* Seattle, WA.

Webb, S. J., Shic, F., Murias, M., Sugar, C. A., Naples, A. J., Barney, E., et al. (2019). Biomarker acquisition and quality control for multisite studies: the autism biomarkers consortium for clinical trials. *Front. Integr. Neurosci.* 13:71. doi: 10.3389/fnint.2019.00071

Winkler, I., Brandl, S., Horn, F., Waldburger, E., Allefeld, C., and Tangermann, M. (2014). Robust artifactual independent component classification for BCI practitioners. *J. Neural Eng.* 11:035013. doi: 10.1088/1741-2560/11/3/035013

7

Biomarker Acquisition and Quality Control for Multi-Site Studies: The Autism Biomarkers Consortium for Clinical Trials

Sara Jane Webb[1,2], Frederick Shic[1,3], Michael Murias[4], Catherine A. Sugar[5,6,7], Adam J. Naples[8], Erin Barney[1], Heather Borland[1], Gerhard Hellemann[6], Scott Johnson[6], Minah Kim[1], April R. Levin[9,10], Maura Sabatos-DeVito[4], Megha Santhosh[1], Damla Senturk[5,7], James Dziura[8], Raphael A. Bernier[1,2,11], Katarzyna Chawarska[8], Geraldine Dawson[4], Susan Faja[10,12], Shafali Jeste[6,13], James McPartland[8]* and the Autism Biomarkers Consortium for Clinical Trials*

[1] Center on Child Health, Behavior, and Development, Seattle Children's Research Institute, Seattle, WA, United States, [2] Department of Psychiatry and Behavioral Sciences, University of Washington School of Medicine, Seattle, WA, United States, [3] Department of Pediatrics, University of Washington School of Medicine, Seattle, WA, United States, [4] Duke Center for Autism and Brain Development, Duke University, Durham, NC, United States, [5] Department of Biostatistics, University of California, Los Angeles, Los Angeles, CA, United States, [6] Department of Psychiatry and Biobehavioral Sciences, University of California, Los Angeles, Los Angeles, CA, United States, [7] Department of Statistics, University of California, Los Angeles, Los Angeles, CA, United States, [8] Yale Child Study Center, Yale University, New Haven, CT, United States, [9] Department of Neurology, Boston Children's Hospital, Boston, MA, United States, [10] Harvard Medical School, Harvard University, Boston, MA, United States, [11] Center on Human Development and Disability, University of Washington, Seattle, WA, United States, [12] Department of Pediatrics, Boston Children's Hospital, Boston, MA, United States, [13] Department of Neurology, University of California, Los Angeles, Los Angeles, CA, United States

***Correspondence:**
Sara Jane Webb
sjwebb@uw.edu
James McPartland
james.mcpartland@yale.edu

The objective of the Autism Biomarkers Consortium for Clinical Trials (ABC-CT) is to evaluate a set of lab-based behavioral video tracking (VT), electroencephalography (EEG), and eye tracking (ET) measures for use in clinical trials with children with autism spectrum disorder (ASD). Within the larger organizational structure of the ABC-CT, the Data Acquisition and Analytic Core (DAAC) oversees the standardization of VT, EEG, and ET data acquisition, data processing, and data analysis. This includes designing and documenting data acquisition and analytic protocols and manuals; facilitating site training in acquisition; data acquisition quality control (QC); derivation and validation of dependent variables (DVs); and analytic deliverables including preparation of data for submission to the National Database for Autism Research (NDAR). To oversee consistent application of scientific standards and methodological rigor for data acquisition, processing, and analytics, we developed standard operating procedures that reflect the logistical needs of multi-site research, and the need for well-articulated, transparent processes that can be implemented in future clinical trials. This report details the methodology of the ABC-CT related to acquisition and QC in our Feasibility and Main Study phases. Based on our acquisition metrics from a preplanned interim analysis, we report high levels of acquisition success utilizing VT, EEG, and ET experiments in a relatively large sample of children with ASD and typical development (TD), with data acquired across multiple sites and use of a manualized training and acquisition protocol.

Keywords: autism spectrum disorder, biomarkers, clinical trial methods, guidelines, EEG, eye tracking, video tracking

INTRODUCTION

To develop more targeted diagnostic and treatment methods to improve outcomes in autism spectrum disorder (ASD) (Loth et al., 2016), the scientific field must address the current lack of reliable and sensitive objective measures that inform treatment target engagement or subgroup identification (Jeste et al., 2015; McPartland, 2017; Sahin et al., 2018; Ewen et al., 2019). The Autism Biomarkers Consortium for Clinical Trials (ABC-CT[1]) was created to advance biomarker validation for eventual use in clinical trials for children with ASD with a number of potential contexts of use, including reduction of heterogeneity of samples via stratification, potential for indication of early efficacy or demonstration of target engagement, and outcome measurement (McPartland, 2016). The ABC-CT is a response to the RFA-MH-15-800 U19 Consortium on Biomarker and Outcome Measures of Social Impairment for use in Clinical Trials in ASD. To this end, the ABC-CT consortium (McPartland et al., 2019) is evaluating behavioral video tracking (VT), electroencephalography (EEG), and eye tracking (ET) as indices of *social communication* for potential use in ASD clinical trials—as social communication is one of the core targets for pharmacological and behavioral interventions (e.g., Lerner et al., 2012; Anagnostou, 2018).

In this report, we articulate the standard operating protocols developed by the ABC-CT Data Acquisition and Analytic Core (DAAC) related to: (1) the design and implementation of multi-site experimental protocols and (2) the quality control (QC) processes related to rigorous, scientifically valid, and replicable procedures used for data acquisition. Unlike a traditional theoretical or empirical paper describing clinical findings (which will be described in a companion manuscript), we focus on methods of acquisition and the rationale for these choices—addressing the question "can a biomarker be measured accurately?" (Institute of Medicine (US) Committee on Qualification of Biomarkers and Surrogate Endpoints in Chronic Disease, 2010; Amur et al., 2015). To oversee consistent application of scientific standards and methodological rigor for data acquisition, processing, and analytics, we developed standards of work that reflect the logistics of multi-site research, and the need for well-articulated, transparent processes that can be implemented by the scientific community in future clinical trials of children with ASD and other neurodevelopmental disorders. As these processes often reflect the internal workings of a study or laboratory, but are critical for replication and/or use in future clinical trials, full transparency of these processes is critical when considering the potential for broad implementation.

PROTOCOL

The ABC-CT study was conducted in two phases: a Feasibility phase and a Main study phase. The Feasibility Study (see section "Feasibility Study" for details) was conducted to address whether or not the methods could be successfully implemented for the participant group across the five sites consistently in a small sample (n = 50, 50% ASD). After review of results from the Feasibility Study, the Main Study battery was developed with a goal of 275 participants [n = 200 ASD; n = 75 typical development (TD); aged 6–11 years], each observed at three timepoints (Time 1 = baseline, Time 2 = 6 weeks, Time 3 = 6 months) (and as specified in the RFA-MH-15-800). Data were evaluated at the interim point in the Main Study, at which approximately 50% of participants had been enrolled and completed the first and second timepoint. (Sample characteristics from the Main Study Interim Sample are presented in **Supplementary Material**).

Four principles guided the work of the ABC-CT across both phases: First, the study was conducted in partnership between the scientific key personnel and the NIH scientific and program officers, the FNIH Biomarkers Consortium, and an external advisory board. Second, all work was performed in accordance with Good Clinical Practice regulatory standards (FDA, 2019). Third, the data were acquired by clinical sites separate from both data management and data analytic teams. Fourth, the domains of assessment (see section "Domains") included clinical characterization of the participants (both ASD and TD), automated behavioral assessments, EEG, and ET.

Domains

Clinical Characterization

The sample of participants was characterized using autism diagnostic standardized measures, including the Autism Diagnostic Observation Schedule, 2nd Edition (Lord et al., 2012) and the Autism Diagnostic Interview - Revised (Rutter et al., 2003) (ADI-R). Participant behaviors were quantified in the following domains: Social communication; verbal and non-verbal ability; physical, medical, and psychological conditions; and psychotropic medications. All information was collected from both the participants with ASD and a TD control group (see **Supplementary Material** for the interim sample characteristics).

To allow for counterbalancing of the methods and experiments, at screening, participants were stratified based on variables that could be assessed by phone to include group (ASD/TD), biological sex (male/female), age (split at 8 years 6 months), and functioning (ASD only). Of note, pre-visit functioning for the Feasibility Study was identified based on response to the ADI-R question assessing functional language (Rutter et al., 2003); at Main Study, functioning was split based on a report of a full scale IQ above or below 80. These factors were used to create four stratification groups, which then directed the counterbalancing protocol. For Feasibility, this included method order (**Table 1**) and experiment order (**Tables 2, 3**); for Main Study, method order was fixed (**Table 1** "Main Study Order") but experimental order was randomized within method (**Tables 2, 3**).

Behavioral Video Tracking of Child Behavior

The parent–child context is critical to children's development and is often the target of early intervention models for children with ASD (e.g., Dawson et al., 2010; Kasari et al., 2010; Estes et al., 2014). Currently, it is standard practice to manually code children's behaviors in the context of child play tasks. Such work is labor intensive, time consuming, prone to human error and subjectivity, and thus infeasible for large clinical

[1] www.asdbiomarkers.org

TABLE 1 | Acquisition methodology protocol order for Feasibility and Main Study.

	Feasibility Order-A	Feasibility Order-B	Feasibility Order-C	Feasibility Order-D	Main Study Order
Day 1	Behavior	Behavior	Behavior	Behavior	Behavior
	VT	VT	VT	VT	VT
	ET	ET	EEG	EEG	ET
	EEG	EEG	ET	ET	
Day 2	Behavior	Behavior	Behavior	Behavior	EEG
	ET	EEG	ET	EEG	ET
	EEG	ET	EEG	ET	

Key: VT = video tracking, ET = eye tracking.

TABLE 2 | Acquisition experiment Order-A within EEG for Feasibility and Main Study.

	Day 1	Day 2
EEG Feasibility	Set 1	Set 2
	1. Resting eyes open	1. Resting eyes open
	2. EU-AIMS faces	2. Biomotion
	3. VEP	3. Emotion faces
		4. Social/non-social dynamic
EEG Main Study	No day 1 EEG	Day 2
		1. Resting eyes open
		2. ABC-CT faces
		3. VEP
		4. Biomotion

trials. As a goal of the ABC-CT is to develop objective, reliable measures of social behavior that do not rely on parent report or clinical judgment, we implemented a behavioral protocol and post-acquisition automatic quantification of child motion and location via VT with the Noldus EthoVision XT (EVXT) 11.5 software (Sabatos-DeVito et al., 2019). We implemented EVXT as a potential objective, standardized, quantitative, and scalable measure of social approach in ASD in the context of a parent–child interaction (Cohen et al., 2014).

For the ABC-CT, VT was used to provide automated measures of voluntary physical approach-withdrawal toward a social partner (the parent) in the context of a parent–child free play (PCFP) session (see **Figure 1** for an example of child physical movement). In both the Feasibility and Main Study, the PCFP included a standard room setup (furniture, module-based toy kit, and parent placement) that allowed for the child to move about the environment and engage in solitary, interactive, or social play. During the PCFP, the parent sat in a chair, readily available for interaction if and when approached by the child, while the child freely explored the room and available toys. The location of the toys and parent in relation to the ceiling-mounted Noldus camera allowed for tracking of child location, including time and frequency of interaction in various regions of interest (Sabatos-DeVito et al., 2018).

EEG

Scalp electrophysiological recordings are a non-invasive method of measuring the brain's electrical activity. EEG does not require the participant to produce motor or verbal responses and can be collected from experimental paradigms requiring no overt response. The methodology can thus be used across the lifespan and with participants who have limited cognitive or communicative abilities. It also offers opportunities for translational research across species. Despite strong theoretical and methodological arguments for the use of EEG in understanding the neural correlates of autism (Jeste et al., 2015; Loth et al., 2017; McPartland, 2017), the

TABLE 3 | Acquisition experiment order (A) within ET for Feasibility and Main Study for day 1 (left) and day 2 (right).

	Day 1	Day 2
ET Feasibility	1. Pupillary light reflex	1. Pupillary light reflex
	2. Spontaneous social orienting	2. Dynamic scenes
	3. Pupillary light reflex	3. Pupillary light reflex
	4. Gap overlap	4. Social interactive
	5. Pupillary light reflex	5. Pupillary light reflex
	6. Gap overlap	6. Social interactive
	7. Biological motion preference	7. Pupillary light reflex
	8. Pupillary light reflex	8. Activity monitoring
	9. Biological motion preference	9. Pupillary light reflex
	10. Dynamic scenes	10. Activity monitoring
	11. Pupillary light reflex	11. Pupillary light reflex
	12. Social interactive	12. Visual search/static scenes
	13. Pupillary light reflex	13. Pupillary light reflex
	14. Social interactive	14. Visual search/static scenes
	15. Pupillary light reflex	15. Biological motion preference
	16. Activity monitoring	16. Pupillary light reflex
	17. Pupillary light reflex	17. Biological motion preference
	18. Activity monitoring	18. Gap overlap
	19. Pupillary light reflex	19. Pupillary light reflex
		20. Gap overlap
ET Main Study	1. Pupillary light reflex	1. Pupillary light reflex
	2. Activity monitoring	2. Social interactive
	3. Pupillary light reflex	3. Pupillary light reflex
	4. Activity monitoring	4. Social interactive
	5. Pupillary light reflex	5. Pupillary light reflex
	6. Biological motion preference	6. Visual search/static scenes
	7. Pupillary light reflex	7. Pupillary light reflex
	8. Biological motion preference	8. Visual search/static scenes
	9. Pupillary light reflex	9. Pupillary light reflex
	10. Social interactive	10. Activity monitoring
	11. Pupillary light reflex	11. Pupillary light reflex
	12. Social interactive	12. Activity monitoring
	13. Pupillary light reflex	13. Pupillary light reflex
	14. Visual search/static scenes	14. Biological motion preference
	15. Pupillary light reflex	15. Pupillary light reflex
	16. Visual search/static scenes	16. Biological motion preference
	17. Pupillary light reflex	17. Pupillary light reflex

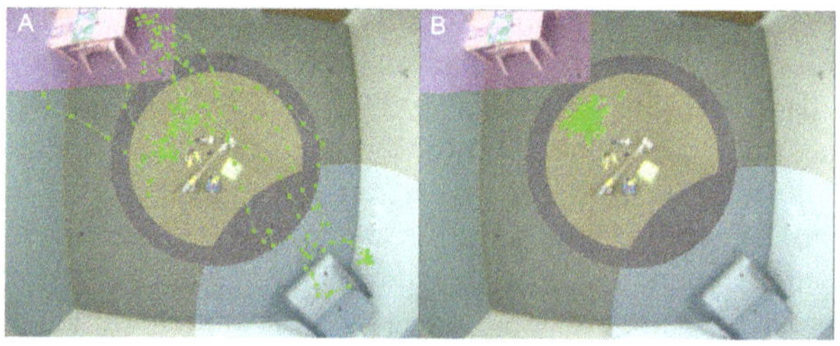

FIGURE 1 | Video tracking of child physical movement. Room setup for PCFP with overlay of video tracking of movement of child 1 **(A)** and 2 **(B)**.

practice of collecting, processing, and evaluating EEG data is complex, particularly when data acquisition involves children or those with developmental or cognitive disabilities. Descriptions of basic methodology can be found in a number of published texts and guidelines (Pivik et al., 1993; Picton et al., 2000) and specifically related to use in ASD (Webb et al., 2015).

In the ABC-CT, EEG acquisition included six paradigms addressing basic brain functioning as well as social ability and understanding. The six experiments in the Feasibility Study were reduced to four in the Main Study (Webb et al., 2018): (1) Resting EEG eyes open during calm viewing of digital videos (similar to screensavers). (2) Event-related responses to upright and inverted faces compared to upright houses, targeting early stage attention and perception of social information. [Note: in the Feasibility Study this paradigm was the same as that employed in the EU-AIMS protocol (Loth et al., 2017) but an additional object stimulus condition was included, which then was also implemented in phase 2 of the EU-Aims protocol. For the Main Study, the paradigm was altered to utilize a pre-stimulus fixation crosshair as in Webb et al. (2012), while the EU-AIMS version utilized a pre-stimulus object icon.] (3) Event-related responses to biological motion ("biomotion"), investigating the responses to coherent and scrambled point light animation of adult male walkers (Naples, Webb, et al., in development); and (4) visual evoked potentials (VEPs) elicited by an alternating black and white checkerboard (1 Hz) to assess functional integrity of the afferent visual pathway and basic visual processing (LeBlanc et al., 2015). The two experiments included in Feasibility but excluded from Main Study were: (5) event-related response to fear and neutral facial expressions (Dawson et al., 2004) and (6) EEG to social and non-social dynamic videos (Jones et al., 2015, 2016), which is included in the EU-AIMS battery.

Eye Tracking

Remote video oculographic ET uses a video of participant's eyes to determine point of regard (POR) on a computer screen, with this video also often allowing for a measure of pupil diameter (Shic, 2013). This POR is considered a proxy for visual attention in practical, real-world situations and is associated both with the cognitive information processing of attended-to locations as well as the motivational process involved in selection of PORs (Kowler, 1990). Modern ET relies primarily upon video oculographic techniques which (as compared to other ET techniques, such as scleral coils) are non-invasive, highly tolerable, robust to movement, and can provide quantitative data on looking patterns at less than a degree of visual angle and with millisecond timing (Duchowski, 2007; Holmqvist et al., 2011; Shic, 2016). In autism research, the use of ET has matured, expanded, and seen widespread adoption over the past decade, and may offer a feasible early-efficacy biomarker in clinical trials (Dawson et al., 2012; Murias et al., 2017).

The ABC-CT ET included nine paradigms in Feasibility, reduced to five in the Main Study: (1) activity monitoring, which includes both static images and dynamic videos of two adult actors playing with children's toys while gazing at each other or at their shared activity (Shic et al., 2011; Umbricht et al., 2017; Del Valle Rubido et al., 2018). (2) Biological motion preference, where two point-light displays are shown on either side of the screen, one displaying biological motion and one displaying a control condition of rotating or scrambled dots (Annaz et al., 2011; Umbricht et al., 2017; Del Valle Rubido et al., 2018). (3) Pupillary light reflex, in which a dark screen with a small fixation animation at the center is shown, then replaced briefly by a white screen, followed by the same dark screen with animation (Nyström et al., 2015). This task was interleaved between blocks of all other paradigms and came from the EU-AIMS protocol (Loth et al., 2017). (4) Social interactive, where children play with toys either together or separately with no sound (Chevallier et al., 2015) and (5) static scenes (SS), which included photographs of adults and children engaged in social activities. This task came from the EU-AIMS protocol. Included in Feasibility only were: (6) Dynamic naturalistic scenes, in which two, 4-min videos were shown (one on each day) that drew from clips of live-action movies (adapted from Rice et al., 2012). (7) Gap overlap, in which an animation was shown at the center of the screen and then a peripheral stimulus was displayed while the central stimulus was on screen (overlap condition), immediately after the central stimulus left the screen (baseline condition), or after the central stimulus left the screen (gap condition) (Elsabbagh et al., 2013a). (8) Spontaneous social orienting, which involved an actress speaking directly to the camera while conducting an activity and directing the participant's attention to various toys (Chawarska et al., 2012) and (9) visual search, in which five images were displayed in a circle for the participant to free view (Sasson et al., 2011; Elsabbagh et al., 2013b). Note that visual search trials were interleaved with SS trials, as in the EU-AIMS protocol. To preserve the structure of the task, visual search trials were left in the Main Study protocol but were not prioritized in analysis.

Equipment and General Experimental Structure

VT

Video data of interpersonal interaction were collected with an overhead color CCD IP camera with a wide-angle lens mounted in the center of the room and recorded using Noldus Media Recorder 3.0 software. A second side camera video with audio was added in the Main Study in order to enhance quality review of overhead recordings. The PCFP protocol was standardized including positioning of furniture, parent seating and behavior suggestions, and arrangement of child toys on the floor and on a table (Sabatos-DeVito et al., 2018). All sites utilized the same toys for the PCFP. Sites transferred collected data (overhead camera.avi file, side camera video recording) to a subject specific folder, compressed the folder, and then transferred the folder to a computer with internet access to the DCC database. The VT session log was entered via online data capture.

EEG

Each experiment was standardized (Borland et al., 2018) to start with a welcome screen, direction screen, general directions ["please sit still and watch the (insert stimulus)"] and start directions. Site specific seating distance modifications were used to ensure standard visual angle. All introduction screens included both text and audio. Experimenters were provided with additional sample language to support child understanding and compliance in regard to the method, order, and behavioral expectations.

Experiments were divided into blocks of about ~2 min to facilitate participant attention, engagement, and compliance. Pauses or "rest time" occurred between blocks; the goal was to have block breaks of less than 2 min. Experiments were not allowed to be re-run or conducted out of order. The projected time for the EEG battery in the Main Study was 16.0 min, with no breaks; at Interim, the average actual run time (from time of start of first experiment, to end of last experiment) was 24.44 min (SD 7.1) suggesting greater use of break periods than seen in Feasibility.

As shown in **Figures 2A–F**, all sites had an EGI 128 channel EEG acquisition system, including both 300 and 400 amps, the 128 electrode EGI HydroCel Geodesic Sensor Nets (applied according to EGI standards), Logitech Z320 Speakers, Cedrus StimTracker (for visual presentation timing), and a monitor (Dell P2314H 23" resolution 1920 × 1080, Main Study) (Webb et al., 2018). Appropriate Net Station acquisition setups (1000 Hz sampling rate, 0.1–200 Hz filter, EGI MFF file format, onset recording of amplifier and impedance calibrations) were provided to each site. EPrime 2.0 was used for experimental control; a master experiment was created and then modifications from that master were made based on site differences. Experimental versions were tracked and acquisition files were verified to make sure the correct versions were implemented. Sites transferred collected data (EEG raw MFF file, session log, E-Prime data file) to a subject specific folder, compressed, and then transferred to the DCC database. The EEG session log was entered via online data capture.

Eye Tracking

All sites collected ET data using SR Research Eyelink 1000 Plus binocular remote eye trackers at 500 Hz (in EDF file format) with 24″ Dell monitors for display (1920 × 1200 pixels) (Naples et al., 2018; Shic et al., 2018). Each participant was required to wear a target sticker on their forehead to allow the eye tracker to locate their eyes (**Figure 3A**). This sticker also allowed the computer to determine child-to-monitor distance. Participants were positioned at 650 mm from the ET camera at the start of each session. ET sessions had both an experimenter running the computers and a behavioral assistant sitting with the child to support them throughout the task if needed (**Figure 3D**). Experiments were presented in an integrated delivery system programmed in Neurobehavioral Stimulus Presentation version 18.1 that included an initial video to ease participant setup (including participant positioning and ET calibration), delivery of core experimental paradigms, embedded periodic ET calibration/validation routines, and the incorporation of routines to allow for experimenter-triggered breaks for behavioral management. Paradigm blocks lasted 1–4 min each and were interleaved to combat fatigue. The projected total time of the experiments was 15 min; average actual run time (including setup, calibration, to end of the experiment set) was 18.2 min (SD 2.3).

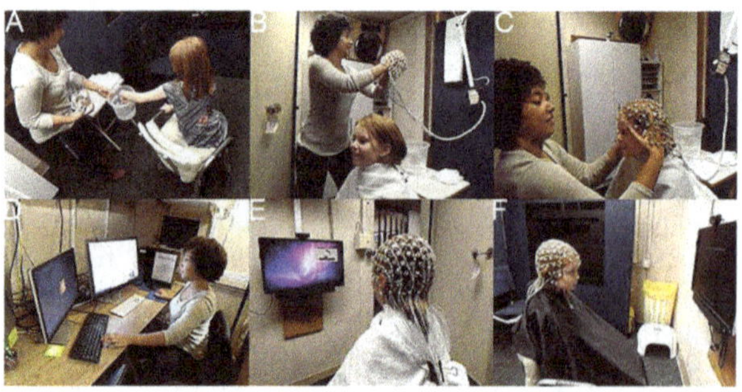

FIGURE 2 | EEG session. **(A)** Participant exploring the EEG equipment; **(B)** preparing for the net; **(C)** net placement; **(D)** experimenter setup for monitoring experiment, data, and child attention; **(E)** child watching video while setup is finalized; and **(F)** child attending to instruction screen for experiment. Written consent was obtained from the adult experimenter and the parents of the child shown; the child provided assent.

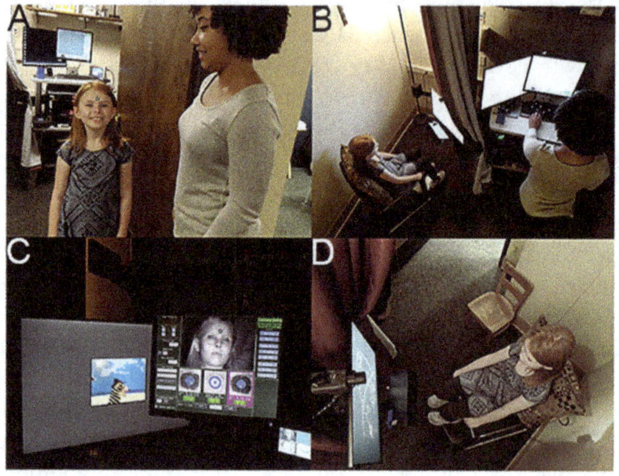

FIGURE 3 | ET session. **(A)** Preparing to enter ET room and ET sticker placement; **(B)** overhead view of room with participant and experimenter; **(C)** experimenter setup for monitoring experiment, data, and child attention; and **(D)** child attention to experiment. Written consent was obtained from the adult experimenter and the parents of the child shown in the images; the child provided assent.

A Python script with a user interface was created to help sites compress the ET output files and video files that could then be transferred to the DCC database. The ET Run Logs were entered directly into the online database.

Environment and Supports

Overall, the environment was to be free of distractions that might impede, interrupt, or alter performance differentially by child or site. Fixed characteristics of the sites' data collection environments were taken into consideration in the design of the equipment and the analytic pipelines. These characteristics were tracked in the acquisition protocols and monitored during QC review. When alterations had to be made to the environment based on child characteristics that prohibited the use of the standard environment, this was noted as a protocol deviation on the methodology log. Note, we did have sites that changed room locations between Feasibility and Main Study—this occurred due to new spaces becoming available that better accommodated the participants and the equipment and was not done because of specific concerns with the rooms *per se*.

A number of physical (booster chairs, footstools, tables), social (social scripts or videos), and behavioral supports (visual schedules) were identified to facilitate individual child performance and were deemed not to interfere with the acquisition parameters or the psychological constructs being assessed. Questions about allowed supports were addressed during training and via the weekly coordinator call. These were noted in the logs, but not identified as a protocol deviation.

VT

Environmental effects were most obvious for the VT protocol in which room size and layout could not be made physically identical across sites. Detailed measurements of the room size, positioning of furniture, and PCFP items were created and each site was expected to maintain within-site standardization. The VT Manual of Operations (Sabatos-DeVito et al., 2018) details room variations, scaling procedures to standardize regions of interest, and their implications for abstraction of child positioning and movement in the EVXT software.

EEG

For EEG, because all site rooms had different lighting setups (type of lights, location in relation to participant/monitor), and concern about participant reaction to dark/dim lighting, we conducted all sessions in full room light. Due to room layout, the location of the behavioral assistant (who facilitated child compliance) differed by site but was standardized within a site. Sites were instructed to send monthly pictures of their lab setup to check compliance for room layout, including subject to monitor distance (for visual angle).

Eye Tracking

For ET, the equipment and acquisition setup was developed for installation on a cart or fixed location (see **Figure 3**). Behavioral assistants were allowed to be on either side of the child or behind on a case-by-case basis at each site. Ambient room lighting during sessions was monitored (via a light meter) and sites were instructed to keep the lighting dim but not completely dark. Before each session, sites were instructed to test the sound levels of their speakers using a test tone and an external sound meter. Sound was set at 65 dB. Sites were asked not to adjust sound or lighting during a session.

Training

Training was provided by the DAAC via in-person site visits, online training, regular weekly phone calls, and written documents. All sites were at academic institutions, directed by PIs with extensive history of training in these methodologies, and thus, a decision was made to maintain staffing and basic training responsibilities with the site PI. The DAAC provided some general acquisition training, but focused primarily on the methodology for the ABC-CT protocol. For example, training in EGI net placement was done within the lab but training on the net placement scoring system was done by the DAAC trainer.

To be "certified" as collection staff, all personnel had to complete requirements at their institution (including human subjects training) and their PI's current lab training protocol. Then the staff members received in-person training either with a DAAC acquisition lead or the onsite trainer, reviewed all written documents, and provided two to five protocol evaluation files for DAAC to review that demonstrated competence in acquiring valid data. New staff also had the first five sessions with participants (for each methodology) intensively reviewed by DAAC staff. Written feedback was provided to the staff member acquiring the data, site method lead, and PI. Feedback was provided during protocol evaluation training and during ongoing intensive review. This was manualized (Barney et al., 2018; Sabatos-DeVito et al., 2018; Santhosh et al., 2018). The DAAC conducted method-based meetings bi-weekly to review feedback reports and current site acquisition validity. Any significant issues identified by the DAAC were addressed via re-training at the Site. The DAAC acquisition lead attended the ABC-CT weekly coordinator call to answer questions and provide feedback related to acquisition. Site staff turnover was also monitored by the DAAC. Transition of the on-site trainer, more than 50% of acquisition staff, or request by PI triggered an on-site visit for training.

Experimenter Roles and Interactions

The protocol "with child in room," essentially the running of the experimental battery, was manualized so that each child experienced the same steps from the time upon entry into the lab space until departure. This included scripted language and actions. As one of our main analytic aims was to assess test–retest validity of our biomarker dependent variables (DVs), eliminating individual session variability was a key principle.

Because of variability in age of participants (6 years 0 month to 11 years 11 months) and functioning level (full scale IQ 60–150), pre-testing participant familiarization was not standardized and was left to individual decisions between the lead clinician, acquisition experimenter, and parent. The setup order as well as within methodology experimental order was not allowed to be altered, again because of concerns about how protocol modifications might impact test–retest validity. Thus, variability in changing order, or "moving" a method to a stand-alone session was not allowed. It is possible that utilizing a fixed acquisition protocol order lowered rates of acquisition for later tasks in children that might have been more fatigued by the battery or may have been able to succeed with more familiarization.

Correct identification of no data or poor data was deemed to be of high priority for sites during acquisition for two reasons: First, acquisition rates were critically important for sites to set subject flow and update enrollment targets. Second, site monitoring and feedback included establishing when no or poor data resulted from valid participant interactions (e.g., the session was run correctly but the child did not have the behavioral skills to comply with the method) versus quality of experimenter interactions (e.g., the experimenter made decisions that did not support collection of valid data).

Staff monitoring of child behavior for data validity occurred through two main methods: (1) Monitoring and coding behavior online during the experiment and (2) logging child behavior per method per experiment per block on a standard form. For monitoring online, ET and EEG experiments were coded such that non-attention or non-compliance could be recorded (via a keypress) in the raw data recording. This allowed for tracking of behavior moment-to-moment.

Acquisition staff utilized a methodology-specific session log, which included child characteristics (e.g., description of child for video-log identity matching, child head size), session characteristics (e.g., start time, child positioning, distance to monitor, staff location, parent presence), and method-specific details that might impact post-acquisition processing (e.g., EEG-net fit impacting signal acquisition; VT-presence of red in room interfering with person tracking; ET-ambient room light levels that could impact pupil size). For logging of general behaviors, several drafts of the logs were attempted, with the final reflecting the balance between time of staff to log behaviors during an active session and the types of information needed to aid in post-processing decisions.

Brief directions for staff were also included in the logs to provide reminders for key actions or events necessary for valid data (e.g., "Lights on"; "Check Flags"). Experimental staff also reported the number of trials attended, validity of each block of trials (data questionable, poor/no data, did not run), pauses (yes/no), and any additional notes to quantify child behavior during acquisition. After experiment completion, the staff marked overall behavioral data quality by experiment, including attention and affect, and identified the presence of other types of error (equipment, experimenter). Copies of the logs are available within the Acquisition Protocol documents (Barney et al., 2018; Borland et al., 2018; Sabatos-DeVito et al., 2018).

VT

All VT sessions were video recorded utilizing a standardized system (ceiling mounted Basler GigE IP camera with Pylon software interface to Noldus Media Recorder 3.0) and a second wall-mounted standalone side camera audio/video recording system (pre-existing at each site). The examiner at each site read standardized instructions describing the PCFP session. The camera operator sat in an adjacent room monitoring the Noldus and side camera recordings for QC and protocol compliance during the session. The camera operator informed the examiner of any compliance problems or deviations during the session.

EEG

All EEG sessions were videotaped, with video time locked to the NetStation recording. In our two-staff acquisition protocol, the experimenter monitored the acquisition computers, incoming EEG activity, and participant behavior via a real-time video embedded in the NetStation recording (**Figure 2**). The behavioral assistant, sitting next to the child, provided direction, prompts, and other supports to the child as manualized. The experimenter also coded child non-attention or other off-task behaviors via a keyboard response, which inserted a marker into the EPrime file and transferred to the NetStation EEG recording for file markup. At block breaks and end of experiment, the staff were presented (within the display) the number of attended trials.

ET

All ET sessions were videotaped and multiplexed onto a four-screen display that showed the participant, the Stimulus Presentation screen, and the ET Host screen, with the fourth screen left blank. The date and time was overlaid on top of this video and recording started before the child entered the room. In our two-staff setup, the experimenter monitored the stimulus presentation, tracking of the eye, and participant behavior via the four-screen display. The behavioral assistant, seated near the child, provided direction, prompts, and other supports to the child as manualized. The experimenter manually accepted each calibration point while the child was looking at it and could repeat points as necessary. The experimenter also had the ability to insert breaks or re-calibrations into the paradigms based on the data quality and the child's needs using keyboard presses. Verbal re-directions, provided by the behavioral assistant to the child, were coded by the experimenter using keyboard presses. The use of these keyboard shortcuts was manualized in the protocol.

Feasibility Study

The Feasibility phase included 51 participants (n = 26 ASD; n = 25 TD) aged 4–11 years. For Feasibility, we specifically addressed whether or not the methods and experiments could be successfully acquired for the participant groups. The sites were directed to each enroll 10 participants, five ASD and five TD. Sites were not directed to target enrollment by other characteristics due to the limited time window for this phase of the study. Across the Feasibility Study, we enrolled 73% male, 61% "older" (8–11 years sample), all with some verbal language.

Because feasibility of acquisition was a key outcome metric, we counterbalanced the method order (**Table 1**). Our initial biomarker battery included a one visit (or timepoint), two-day protocol with behavioral measures, EEG, and ET on both days. The PCFP with VT occurred in conjunction with the Autism Diagnostic Observation Schedule (day 1). EEG and ET occurred on both days 1 and 2.

Between days 1 and 2, the family took home the language environment analysis (LENA) system's digital language processor (DLP) to record language use in the home. LENA is an automated system that analyzes recorded speech and other sounds in the natural home environment (Xu et al., 2009) and has been used to explore the language environment of children with ASD and TD (Warren et al., 2010).

For EEG, the experiments were divided into two sets with the method order randomized (**Table 2**). In terms of task ordering, the only experiment that was fixed was the EEG resting eyes open experiment, which occurred on both days in the first position.

The projected time of the EEG experiments (from time of start of first experiment, to end of last experiment) for Set 1 was 12.5 min and for Set 2 was 13.5, not including breaks. During Feasibility, the mean actual run time was for Set 1 was 13.0 min (SD 6.8), and Set 2 was 15.0 min (SD 6.9).

For ET, the experiments also were divided across 2 days (see **Table 2**). Most paradigms were split into two blocks that were broken up by a Pupillary Light Reflex trial, with the exception of the longer videos (Spontaneous Social Orienting and Dynamic Naturalistic Scenes). The ET experiments were counterbalanced across four orders (e.g., **Table 3**, Order A) and experiments were interleaved to reduce fatigue and boredom. During Feasibility, the total projected time of the experiments (including setup, calibration, to end of the experiment set) over 2 days was 22 min; mean actual run time was 25.9 min (SD 3.3).

Note: Results from the Feasibility Study have not been published but were presented both at internal meetings with our advisory board and to the FNIH Biomarkers Consortium; based on investigator interest, some results were presented at scientific conferences and are available via the ABC-CT website.

MAIN STUDY ACQUISITION

After review of results from the Feasibility Study, including review from NIH scientific and program officers, our external advisory board, and the FNIH Biomarkers Consortium, an overall decision was made that the battery was potentially burdensome for the child/family and that analytic interpretations could be confounded by the large number of derived result comparisons. To identify which measures were to be removed from the protocol, we first focused on feasibility using acquisition rates, protocol violation rates, and feedback from site coordinators. Second, we examined group discrimination (ASD versus TD), and reviewed our DVs for those that had $F \geq 1.9$, which would reflect a power of 80%, and a potential significant result with our planned main study sample size. Third, we then examined redundancy in construct and DV between experiments. Fourth, we considered theoretical and practical barriers to eventual biomarker deployment in our target population in the context of clinical trials.

To this end, we made the following changes: (1) We discontinued use of the LENA system. LENA acquisition was poor in our Feasibility Study, with low return rates of the DLP (41% failure to return at day 2), and only 68% of recording sessions passed QC review. (2) We maintained the PCFP VT despite 91% of sessions reported as containing protocol deviations, with the majority reflecting failure to adhere to the standard room layout. We identified this as modifiable and revised the site initiation and training for the PCFP/VT. We also added a no-go criteria at the interim analysis for this paradigm. (3) We reduced the EEG acquisition to 1 day as site feedback identified high burden of netting participants twice within a timepoint. We also reduced the battery to four experiments (**Table 2**). While all experiments had good rates of usable data, emotion faces was removed because it had a lower acquisition rates (82%), did not discriminate groups (ASD versus TD: $F = 1.3$ for N170 amplitude to fear faces), and the potential for construct redundancy (e.g., early stage face processing) and DV redundancy (e.g., P1 and N170 ERP components) with the faces experiment. Although social/non-social dynamic had good acquisition rates (92%), we removed it from the battery as there were concerns with the appropriateness of content (nursery rhymes) for our age group and DV redundancy (e.g., power across the frequency spectrum) with the resting EEG experiment. (4) We maintained the acquisition of ET on both days but reduced the battery to five experiments (e.g., **Table 3**). As all nine experiments had acquisition rates > 94%, we focused on discrimination and redundancy to guide this removal decision. We eliminated the gap-overlap task because it did not discriminate groups. As the other tasks showed group discrimination, we rank ordered them based on effect size and retained SS, social interactive, and activity monitoring. PLR was maintained as a metric of basic visual system integrity. Visual search was maintained because it was acquired interleaved with SS and there was concern that construct validity would be disrupted by removing it. Dynamic naturalistic scenes and spontaneous social orienting performed well on all metrics but were removed due to concerns about the general use of the stimuli (e.g., copyright concerns for future dissemination and age appropriateness, respectively).

For each biomarker methodology in the Main Study, detailed acquisition protocols and manuals of operations were created to serve as the technical record, training manual, and protocol for acquisition (Naples et al., 2018; Sabatos-DeVito et al., 2018; Shic et al., 2018; Webb et al., 2018). These served as the primary training documents for the Site staff to guide data acquisition and addressed counterbalancing, experimental acquisition, equipment and setup, protocol when the child was present, site staff roles, and data logs.

Data Storage and Security

Each site had their own IRB and HIPAA compliant local storage and backup systems for VT, EEG, and ET data. All clinical and (bio)marker data were entered into the Data Coordinating Center database RexDB informatics platform[2] (Prometheus Inc.), including the transfer of the large VT, EEG, and ET data files. Data uploaded from the sites was done through this secure system. Access was limited to authorized personnel and monitored by the project management team and the DCC. Sites did not have access to the data of other sites; and only the DCC and DAAC had access to the full study data. QC review for correct stratification order was checked using grouping characteristics provided at screening (age group, diagnosis group, sex, and functioning). All review of participant data (VT, EEG, and ET files) was done blinded to participant (clinical and cognitive) characteristics except for site and date.

Quality Control

The DAAC received all raw (bio)marker data files from the DCC, conducted QC checks on data acquisition, provided

[2] https://www.rexdb.org

feedback to sites, and then implemented experiment-specific pipelines (which transformed the raw data VT, EEG, and ET to NDAR-compatible formats and then to the analytic pipelines for derived results). For QC, two versions were identified: Basic and Intensive. All files received basic review within 5 business days, which included evaluation of acquisition characteristics that were required for establishing validity (e.g., ET calibration; EEG net placement). For intensive review, videos were additionally checked for adherence to the protocol as well as less tangible qualities such as child–staff rapport. All files designated for intensive review were completed within 3 business days and written feedback was provided to the sites. For acquisition during the Feasibility Study, 100% of files received intensive QC review by the DAAC staff. For Main Study, the first 10 files from each site for the Main Study received intensive review. After these Main Study participants, a centralized list of participants was created with the data from every fifth child enrolled (by site and stratification group) being assigned to intensive review across modalities (that is, the same child received intensive review for VT, EEG, and ET and for all three timepoints) and the remaining participants received basic review. QC metrics were entered into the database for tracking and reporting. Quarterly reports were provided documenting percent of files that had been quality controlled, and percent valid. We have been able to maintain our feedback timeline for 94% of files.

Of note, acquisition QC is different than validity of derived results (i.e., a valid DV). The acquisition QC reflected adherence to the protocol and the ability of the participant to engage in the method acquisition for a minimum amount of time. As provision of either EEG *or* ET data was required to be maintained in the study, it was thus important to set a required minimum value of data that could quickly be accessed and communicated back to the sites to update recruitment goals. It was not deemed feasible to provide sites with information as to DV inclusion (i.e., did the participant have enough valid data to use in analysis) within the time frame needed to support recruitment. Moreover, balancing the need to have some amount of validly acquired data to proceed but also not requiring valid DVs, allowed us to compare characteristics of participants who might be included versus excluded if a specific biomarker was required for enrollment in a future clinical trial.

VT

Video tracking data quality was maintained by (1) confirmation of successful automated tracking of each child and (2) visual review of each recording (Sabatos-DeVito et al., 2018). Possible interference with tracking included objects of color similar to the child's shirt, child not wearing the designated color for tracking, child's shirt obscured from the overhead camera (e.g., hiding behind or under furniture, standing in a location not captured by the overhead camera), parent seating or interference, and furniture placement. Post session, acquisition was deemed valid if the child's movement was successfully automatically processed. All files received review to confirm compliance with the PCFP protocol.

EEG

Post-session, acquisition QC was deemed valid if the participant had average or excellent EEG cap placement (both as reported by the site and validated via images of the participant), had completed 50% (out of 3 × 1 min blocks) of the EEG Resting State experiment (from the EEG logs), and if the EEG recording file was readable with the expected experimental markers (Santhosh et al., 2018). Additional factors were reviewed such as naming of the file, implementation of the counterbalance order, electrode impedances and signal quality, and protocol deviations. During intensive review, the full log was compared to the video recording and the EEG signal for congruence, electrode signal across the whole recording was reviewed, and the behavioral support was evaluated.

ET

Post-session, acquisition QC included confirmation that ET files were readable with the expected stimulus markers and that at least three of 16 blocks (20%) had data (Barney et al., 2018). Additional factors were reviewed such as file naming, valid on-screen looking percentage, calibration error, valid trials per paradigm, proper counterbalance order implementation, session duration, and appropriateness of keyboard shortcuts for recalibration and breaks. During intensive review, the full ET Run Log was reviewed alongside the video recording to ensure that the protocol was being followed and that appropriate behavioral supports were being utilized.

Acquisition Results

All methods were attempted with all participants and valid acquisition of either ET or EEG at Time 1 was required to continue in the protocol. Given high rates of acquisition for the Feasibility Study, we focus on the Main Study interim results, which included 161 ASD and 64 TD participants enrolled between October 7, 2016 and December 1, 2017. In planning our interim report timeline, we pre-identified the date at which approximately 50% of the sample would have provided valid derived results for Time 1 and Time 2 based on a prespecified attrition rate (20%) and data loss rate (30%). (Note, as reported in the **Supplementary Material**, our attrition rate in the interim sample was only 2%.).

As identified in **Table 4**, acquisition rates at the interim analysis are based on inclusion in the study and provision of data that passed our QC criteria (section "Data Storage and Security"). Collapsing across Time 1 and Time 2, we had 100% valid acquisition for ET reflecting the low behavioral demands of the protocol and the rigor of the equipment hardware and software setup. VT valid acquisition was also high (96%) and the EEG session acquisition validity was 95–96%. We also tracked protocol deviations to identify when data were acquired in a non-standard manner but the deviations did not impact the ability to process the data using the analytic pipelines.

Dependent Variable Specification

As part of the pre-specification of our Interim Analysis Plan, each method specified a primary experiment and primary and secondary DVs. Consideration focused on: Construct validity,

TABLE 4 | Acquisition quality control rates for VT, ET, and EEG for Feasibility, and Main Study Time 1 and Time 2 at Interim analyses.

QC table	VT			ET			EEG		
	F	MS T1	MS T2	F	MS T1	MS T2	F	MS T1	MS T2
N	51	225	224	51	225	225	51	225	225
Acquire	51	225	224	51	225	225	51	222	222
Pass QC	50	216	215	50	225	225	50	216	215
%	98%	96%	96%	98%	100%	100%	98%	96%	95%
Protocol deviations	49 = 98%	40 = 18.5%	48 = 22.3%	5 = 10%	21 = 9.3%	22 = 9.8%	4 = 7.8%	35 = 16%	19 = 9%

Key: F = Feasibility, MS = Main Study, T1 = Time 1; T2 = Time 2/ + 6 weeks.

TABLE 5 | Main Study Interim Time 1 VT and EEG experiments: percent of the children contributing valid data and test–retest reliability ICCs.

	VT PCFP, latency to approach periphery	EEG resting, slope	ERP faces, upright face N170 latency	ERP VEP, checkerboard P1 amplitude	ERP biomotion, biological motion N2 amplitude
Percent of the children who provided a valid primary dependent variable value					
Total	94%	91%	80%	81%	59%
ASD	94%	89%	74%	80%	55%
TD	92%	97%	92%	86%	69%
Test–retest reliability (T1 to T2) ICC					
Total	0.14	0.82	0.68	0.73	0.03
ASD	0.11	0.83	0.66	0.68	−0.09
TD	0.21	0.83	0.66	0.80	0.21

that is, did the experiment elicit the intended processes? And group discrimination, that is, were there mean differences in the biomarker variables at Time 1 between the ASD and TD groups? The primary experiments/primary DVs included the (1) EEG resting eyes open experiment with slope of the power spectrum (over the whole head); (2) ERP ABC-CT faces with the N170 latency to the upright faces at the posterior right region of interest; (3) ET composite which included the average percent looking to heads for activity monitoring, social interactive, and SS; and (4) VT latency to approach the periphery. Primary variables for each of the experiments are listed in the header row for **Tables 5, 6.**

Analysis Plan

One of the key principles of the Main Study Interim Analysis Plan was to ensure that all study processes were on track, potentially identifying issues that would result in changes to the protocols or recruitment strategies. As noted in our QC analytics, rates of valid acquisition across the three methods (VT, EEG, and ET) were high across the sites, highlighting the success of our development, training, and acquisition protocols. Second, and of importance to our final study goals, the interim analysis provided preliminary identification of the DVs that might have the best potential to serve as (bio)markers in clinical trials, both in terms of their core acquisition and psychometric properties and their utility for discrimination. Thus, our Interim analysis plan also focused on the rates of acquisition of our pre-specified primary and secondary DVs. That is, if a participant provided validly acquired data, we then examined the rates for which that raw data resulted in a valid dv value.

Biomarker (Dependent Variable) Acquisition

To be considered a valid biomarker, several key characteristics were deemed critical. First, the marker needed to demonstrate high acquisition rates across sites and across key demographic/clinical factors, including age, gender, and functional level. We proposed that an acquisition disparity of less than 20% between subgroups would suggest that a biomarker could be used broadly within a sample of children with ASD. Disparities of greater than 20% in acquisition rates and valid DV rates would suggest that the biomarker would not be appropriate for broad clinical trials, particularly as an inclusion requirement or primary outcome. As seen in **Tables 5, 6**, we provide the rates for our pre-specified primary DVs for each experiment, for our Time 1 Interim sample by group. Both ET (**Table 6**) and VT (**Table 5**) demonstrated high rates of valid abstraction of the primary variables; that is, data "loss" during post acquisition processing was low.

Electroencephalography showed significantly greater data loss when comparing acquisition rates to DV abstraction (compare **Table 4** with **Table 5**). There were general concerns for abstraction rates of the primary variables for the ABC-CT (ERP) Biomotion Experiment, with overall lower rates of signal acquisition in both groups, making it problematic for use broadly. We also noted a significant decrease in valid DV rates within the ASD group with participants with IQ ≤ 70 ($n = 17$) for two of the ERP Experiments (ABC-CT Faces 35%, Biomotion 29%) and all experiments had a > -20% difference in inclusion rate for between ASD IQ > 70 compared to ASD IQ $\leq$ 70. ERP visual experiments, in general, require fixed visual attention to the screen and thus are "harder" for participants with attention deficits. While it is possible that alternate protocols

TABLE 6 | Main Study Interim Time 1 ET experiments: percent of the children contributing valid data and test–retest reliability ICCs.

	ET composite, % Heads	Activity monitoring, % Heads	Social interactive, % Social	Static scenes, % Face	Biological motion, % Affective	Pupillary light reflex, latency to max constriction
Percent of the children who provided a valid primary dependent variable value						
Total	98%	100%	99%	100%	99%	96%
ASD	97%	100%	99%	100%	99%	96%
TD	100%	100%	100%	100%	100%	98%
Test–retest reliability (T1 to T2) ICC						
Total	0.83	0.85	0.54	0.53	0.32	0.73
ASD	0.79	0.79	0.35	0.54	0.36	0.69
TD	0.83	0.83	0.13	0.42	0.23	0.82

Composite = activity monitoring, social interactive, static scenes. % = percentage of time spent attending to a specific region of interest within an image or condition.

would improve rates of attended/artifact free trials, clinical trial protocols would need to consider the relation between child characteristics and provision of data.

Biomarker (Dependent Variable) Distribution

Our second set of validity characteristics focused on the statistical properties of the candidate biomarker variables. We proposed that the biomarker values must demonstrate appropriate distributional properties, such as absence of severe non-normality, skew (values < 2, with checking for values$\neq 0$), kurtosis (values < 3, with checking for values$\neq 0$), floor/ceiling effects, and zero inflation. Floor and ceiling effects may suggest that the variable fails to cover the range of the construct; while zero inflation may suggest that the experiment manipulation failed to evoke the behavior of interest. Note that consideration of the distributional properties was done in parallel with confirmation of construct validity. For example, one goal of a potential stratification biomarker might be to identify a process that differs in the TD and ASD group. In this case, the variable of interest may show a distribution with substantial regions of non-overlap or a different probability concentration; correspondingly, the presence of distributional issues in the ASD group but not the TD group could represent an important signal and hence would not be disqualifying. Variables that exhibit multi-modality may also indicate a natural separation into subgroups. Further, potential outliers may be indicators of a separate underlying (pathophysiological) process.

At interim, all of our EEG and ET variables demonstrated adequate distribution. However, for the VT analyses and as discussed in Murias et al. (2019), the data for PCFP *latency to approach periphery* showed a significant number of participants had a valid minimum (0 s) or maximum (360 s) value, reflecting that some participants began the PCFP in the periphery region, while others never moved into the periphery region of the room, preferring to play in the activity regions (table or center) or near the caregiver. In **Figure 1A**, the child moved between caregiver, central toys and table; while in **Figure 1B**, the child remained only near the central toys. It is important to note that the VT itself worked reliably; instead it is the interaction with the construct of interest (child approach behaviors during the PCFP) that demonstrated limitations. Thus, because there were concerns both about the distribution of this variable and the construct as operationalized, it was deemed to have failed the go/no-go criteria.

Biomarker (Dependent Variable) Test–Retest Reliability

Third, the biomarker must show moderate test-retest reliability in the TD control group. This was based on an expectation of no (meaningful development or environment/treatment related) change over a 6-week (Time 1 to Time 2) period in the TD group. While we did analyze test–retest reliability in the ASD group, we did not pre-specify a required value for evaluation of the biomarker as we did not require that participants maintain treatment stability after enrollment into the study. For example, we would expect that participants with ASD might experience changes in treatment service availability (i.e., therapist vacation or start of school year) or potential need for medication adjustment.

To assess test–retest in both groups, we used intra-class correlations (ICCs) using mixed models with a random score/fixed rater structure and the absolute agreement metric. This provides a version of the correlation accounting for potential mean drift. For test–retest reliability, we pre-specified that, at Interim and for the TD group, excellent rates of test–retest would be represented by ICC of > 0.75, with adequate as 0.50–0.74, and concerns at <0.50. As shown in **Table 5**, the VT variable had distributional concerns and showed poor test–retest reliability. For EEG, values were adequate for three of the four primary variables. The Biomotion N2 amplitude to biological motion proved concerning. For the ET composite variable (which combines the primary DV from the activity monitoring, social interactive, and SS), the ICC value was excellent, and performed better than any of the individual variables. It also should be noted, that contrary to prediction, some of the ET experiments and primary variables had lower ICC values in the TD than ASD group (although they were not statistically compared). This may reflect the "artificial" nature of the social stimuli and their development as experiments that address autism specific social *disability*.

As part of the Main Study Analysis, a priority will be understanding the variables that impact test–retest reliability. Specifically, we will address how the interaction between the diagnostic groups and other demographic characteristics (e.g., age, sex, functioning) impacts test–retest as this may inform subgroups for which measures may be more appropriate in clinical trials. Second, we will identify the extent to which clinical change in symptoms or in (behavioral or medication) interventions may impact the DVs of interest. Differences in a change versus no change group, even at a global level may inform us of which biomarkers are more malleable. Third, we will examine the extent to which measurement acquisition variability influences test-retest values. To address this, we will examine (1) variables that may be modifiable within the protocol such as time of day of assessment; (2) variables that may be addressed through post-acquisition processing such as within-child matching of percent valid-included data; and (3) variables that may be difficult to address in a clinical trial such as changes in child non-compliance. Of importance for clinical trials, is the extent to which the primary DVs are "fragile" in ways that can neither be addressed in the protocol nor corrected for (or normalized) in interpretation of the values, making it difficult to identify change related to treatment effects.

LIMITATIONS

Because acquisition metrics are central to understanding how VT, EEG, and ET biomarkers might work in a future trial, it was equally important to understand who could *and* could not provide valid data, and thus we fixed aspects of the protocol and limited site variability that may have disadvantaged individual participant performance. For example, we did not allow for multiple testing attempts or alteration of protocol order. For some children with ASD, a longer phase of exposures to the equipment or environment may facilitate comfort and compliance. As well, task order was fixed such that an individual experimenter could not reduce the burden of the number, length, or types of paradigms for a child. For the EEG battery, sensory sensitivities (to the net) and focused visual attention might limit the length of time the child could engage with the equipment or the task. Given the specificity of treatment targets, we might expect that a smaller set of methods and experiments would be employed in a clinical trial, reducing the burden on the participant and the experimental teams. We suggest that similar types of QC metrics be applied, however, to ensure that any variability in performance is not due to site implementation.

Second, while we allowed sites individual flexibility in preparing the participant for tasks and using the individual's support tools, we did limit some types of engagement around the protocol. For example, language describing the tasks and stimuli was prescribed and we did not allow for modifications to the environment. We also did not allow for modifications such as reducing the number of measures per visit or allowing multiple visit attempts. It is possible alternative individual modifications could have been considered that would have benefited acquisition while preserving the integrity of the task (Webb et al., 2015). While some environmental changes (like ambient lighting) are known to impact performance on certain measures (e.g., pupillary light response), there are others where the impact is less clear. The difficulty of teasing apart the impact of individual modifications and the resulting performance is that we might expect that children that are the most impaired are not only most likely to need modifications to the protocol but also the most likely to have outlier or atypical responses. Thus, differentiating whether or not the responses are related to the individual's phenotype or to the modifications will require additional study.

Third, all ABC-CT sites had significant experience collecting behavioral, EEG, and ET data for research purposes and all site PIs had > 10 years of experience with the specific EEG hardware and software employed in this protocol. Thus, sites entered the study with a demonstrated track record in acquisition, analytics, and dissemination. In addition to the ABC-CT, two other large efforts are addressing the issue of "translational neuroimaging" with the goal of improving clinical trial measurement; both the EU-AIMS LEAP (e.g., Loth et al., 2017) and Janssen Autism Knowledge Engine (JAKE) study (e.g., Ness et al., 2017). In contrast to our protocol, EU-AIMS LEAP has greater site variability in equipment and populations included, while JAKE was specifically designed to allow acquisition to occur in clinical environments. The contrast of results from these will provide insight into standardization requirements. Regardless, with novice sites, it would be expected that a longer training or feasibility phase might be needed to address experience. The use of formalized QC feedback, delivered with 3–5 days of acquisition, also supports early identification of protocol drift or need for re-training.

Fourth, within the scope of this report, we have focused on our acquisition protocol and acquisition QC metrics. All three methods detailed also have extensive post-acquisition processing pipelines wherein the raw data are transformed into analyzable DVs. These protocols will also be detailed in manuals that will be available to the scientific community. The reliability of our results is not only contingent on acquisition procedures but also the definitions of artifact and signal that are implemented in post-acquisition data pipelines. These details will be included in our empirical papers and discussed in relation to their impact on our conclusions.

CONCLUSION

Based on the preliminary acquisition metrics, experiments that utilize VT, EEG, and ET in a sample of children with ASD can be acquired across multiple academic laboratories utilizing a well specified, manualized standard training and acquisition protocol with significant success. Our ABC-CT protocol for successful acquisition includes development and utilization of standardized equipment and experiments; on-site training and consistent, regular contact between acquisition leads and experimenters; and manualized QC and feedback. Our Interim Analyses stressed the importance of validity of acquisition, including equivalent functioning across site and participant characteristics, distributional properties, and test–retest validity as these are critical in evaluating the suitability of a biomarker for use in a clinical trial context. Final analyses with the full Main Study sample will offer the opportunity to explore discrimination, factors that impact test–retest reliability, clinical and behavioral correlates, supervised stratification, multivariate biotypes, and naturalistic illness trajectories. Ultimately, preliminary clinical trials will be required to validate candidate biomarkers for context of use and acquisition metrics (FDA-NIH Biomarker Working Group, 2016). Overall, our ABC-CT protocol demonstrates a successful framework for the analytic validation of potential (bio)markers for use in autism and other neurodevelopmental disorders. The next step will be to move to qualification and utilization (Institute of Medicine (US) Committee on Qualification of Biomarkers and Surrogate Endpoints in Chronic Disease, 2010).

ETHICS STATEMENT

This study was carried out in accordance with the recommendations of "Yale University Institutional Review Board" with written informed consent from parents of all child participants. All parents gave written informed consent in accordance with the Declaration of Helsinki. The protocol was approved by the "Yale University Human Subjects Committee."

AUTHOR CONTRIBUTIONS

All named authors made substantial contributions to the conception or design of the work and read and provided approval for publication of the content. SW, FS, MM, AN, EB, MK, MS-D, MS, and DS contributed to the drafting of the work. SW, FS, MM, AN, EB, MK, MS-D, MK, AL, MS, DS, RB, KC, GD, and JM provided critical revisions related to the important intellectual content.

FUNDING

Support was provided by the U19 Consortium on Biomarker and Outcome Measures of Social Impairment for use in Clinical Trials in Autism Spectrum Disorder (ABC-CT) NIMH U19 MH108206 (JM).

ACKNOWLEDGMENTS

A special thanks to all of the families and participants who join with us in this effort. In addition, we thank our external advisory board, NIH scientific partners, and the FNIH Biomarkers Consortium. Additional important contributions were provided by members of the ABC-CT consortium including: Adham Atyabi Ph.D., Madeline Aubertine, Carter Carlos, Shou-An A. Chang, Scott Compton, Kelsey Dommer, Alyssa Gateman, Simone Hasselmo, Bailey Heit, Toni Howell, Ann Harris, Kathryn Hutchins, Julie Holub, Beibin Li, Samantha Major, Samuel Marsan, Takumi McAllister, Andriana S. Méndez Leal, Lisa Nanamaker, Charles A. Nelson, Helen Seow, Dylan Stahl, and Andrew Yuan. We refer to a number of experiments as well as support documents detailing our standard operation procedures and manuals of operation for the ABC-CT Feasibility phase and Main Study phase; these documents can be accessed by request from the principal investigator (james.mcpartland@yale.edu) and additional project information can be found via our website https://medicine.yale.edu/ycci/researchers/autism/.

REFERENCES

Amur, S., LaVange, L., Zineh, I., Garner, S. B., and Woodcock, J. (2015). Biomarker qualification: toward a multiple stakeholder framework for biomarker development, regulatory acceptance, and utilization. *Clin. Pharmacol. Ther.* 98, 34–46. doi: 10.1002/cpt.136

Anagnostou, E. (2018). Clinical trials in autism spectrum disorder: evidence, challenges and future directions. *Curr. Opin. Neurol.* 31, 119–125. doi: 10.1097/WCO.0000000000000542

Annaz, D., Campbell, R., Coleman, M., Milne, E., and Swettenham, J. (2011). Young children with autism spectrum disorder do not preferentially attend to biological motion. *J. Autism Dev .Disord.* 42, 401–408. doi: 10.1007/s10803-011-1256-3

Barney, E., Naples, A. J., Chang, S. A., Li, B., McAllister, T., Kim, M., et al. (2018). *ABC-CT Data Acquisition and Analytic Core ET Main Study Quality Control Manual, Version 1.3*, 1st Edn.

Borland, H., Santhosh, M., Naples, A., Levin, A. R., Bernier, R., Dawson, G., et al. (2018). *ABC-CT Data Acquisition and Analytic Core EEG Main Study Acquisition Protocol, Version 2.4*, 2nd Edn.

Chawarska, K., Macari, S., and Shic, F. (2012). Context modulates attention to social scenes in toddlers with autism. *J. Child Psychol. Psychiatry* 53, 903–913. doi: 10.1111/j.1469-7610.2012.02538.x

Chevallier, C., Parish-Morris, J., McVey, A., Rump, K. M., Sasson, N. J., Herrington, J. D., et al. (2015). Measuring social attention and motivation in autism spectrum disorder using eye-tracking: stimulus type matters. *Autism Res.* 8, 620–628. doi: 10.1002/aur.1479

Cohen, I. L., Gardner, J. M., Karmel, B. Z., and Kim, S.-Y. (2014). Rating scale measures are associated with Noldus EthoVision-XT video tracking of behaviors of children on the autism spectrum. *Mol. Autism* 5, 1–16. doi: 10.1186/2040-2392-5-15

Dawson, G., Bernier, R., and Ring, R. H. (2012). Social attention: a possible early indicator of efficacy in autism clinical trials. *J. Psychoeduc. Assess.* 4:11. doi: 10.1186/1866-1955-4-11

Dawson, G., Rogers, S., Munson, J., Smith, M., Winter, J., Greenson, J., et al. (2010). Randomized, controlled trial of an intervention for toddlers with autism: the Early Start Denver Model. *Pediatrics* 125, e17–e23. doi: 10.1542/peds.2009-0958

Dawson, G., Webb, S. J., Carver, L., Panagiotides, H., and McPartland, J. (2004). Young children with autism show atypical brain responses to fearful versus neutral facial expressions of emotion. *Dev. Sci.* 7, 340–359. doi: 10.1111/j.1467-7687.2004.00352.x

Del Valle Rubido, M., McCracken, J. T., Hollander, E., Shic, F., Noeldeke, J., Boak, L., et al. (2018). In search of biomarkers for autism spectrum disorder. *Autism Res.* 11, 1567–1579. doi: 10.1002/aur.2026

Duchowski, A. T. (2007). *Eye Tracking Methodology*. Berlin: Springer.

Elsabbagh, M., Fernandes, J., Webb, S. J., Dawson, G., Charman, T., Johnson, M. H., et al. (2013a). Disengagement of visual attention in infancy is associated with emerging autism in toddlerhood. *Biol. Psychiatry* 74, 189–194. doi: 10.1016/j.biopsych.2012.11.030

Elsabbagh, M., Gliga, T., Pickles, A., Hudry, K., Charman, T., Johnson, M. H., et al. (2013b). The development of face orienting mechanisms in infants at-risk for autism. *Behav. Brain Res.* 251, 147–154. doi: 10.1016/j.bbr.2012.07.030

Estes, A., Vismara, L., Mercado, C., Fitzpatrick, A., Elder, L., Greenson, J., et al. (2014). The impact of parent-delivered intervention on parents of very young children with autism. *J. Autism Dev. Disord.* 44, 353–365. doi: 10.1007/s10803-013-1874-z

Ewen, J. B., Sweeney, J. A., and Potter, W. Z. (2019). Conceptual, regulatory and strategic imperatives in the early days of eeg-based biomarker validation for neurodevelopmental disabilities. *Front. Integr. Neurosci.* 13:45. doi: 10.3389/fnint.2019.00045

FDA (2019). *Draft Guidance Documents: Good Clinical Practice.* Maryland: FDA.

FDA-NIH Biomarker Working Group (2016). *BEST (Biomarkers, EndpointS, and other Tools) Resource.* Maryland: FDA.

Holmqvist, K., Andrà, C., Lindström, P., Arzarello, F., Ferrara, F., Robutti, O., et al. (2011). A method for quantifying focused versus overview behavior in AOI sequences. *Behav. Res. Methods* 43, 987–998. doi: 10.3758/s13428-011-0104-x

Institute of Medicine (US) Committee on Qualification of Biomarkers and Surrogate Endpoints in Chronic Disease (2010). *Evaluation of Biomarkers and Surrogate Endpoints in Chronic Disease.* Washington, DC: National Academies Press.

Jeste, S. S., Frohlich, J., and Loo, S. K. (2015). Electrophysiological biomarkers of diagnosis and outcome in neurodevelopmental disorders. *Curr. Opin. Neurol.* 28, 110–116. doi: 10.1097/WCO.0000000000000181

Jones, E. J. H., Venema, K., Earl, R., Lowy, R., Barnes, K., Estes, A., et al. (2016). Reduced engagement with social stimuli in 6-month-old infants with later autism spectrum disorder: a longitudinal prospective study of infants at high familial risk. *J. Neurodev. Disord.* 8:7. doi: 10.1186/s11689-016-9139-8

Jones, E. J. H., Venema, K., Lowy, R., Earl, R. K., and Webb, S. J. (2015). Developmental changes in infant brain activity during naturalistic social experiences. *Dev. Psychobiol.* 57, 842–853. doi: 10.1002/dev.21336

Kasari, C., Gulsrud, A. C., Wong, C., Kwon, S., and Locke, J. (2010). Randomized controlled caregiver mediated joint engagement intervention for toddlers with autism. *J. Autism Dev. Disord.* 40, 1045–1056. doi: 10.1007/s10803-010-0955-5

Kowler, E. (1990). The role of visual and cognitive processes in the control of eye movement. *Rev. Oculomot. Res.* 4, 1–70.

LeBlanc, J. J., DeGregorio, G., Centofante, E., Vogel-Farley, V. K., Barnes, K., Kaufmann, W. E., et al. (2015). Visual evoked potentials detect cortical processing deficits in Rett syndrome. *Ann. Neurol.* 78, 775–786. doi: 10.1002/ana.24513

Lerner, M. D., White, S. W., and McPartland, J. C. (2012). Mechanisms of change in psychosocial interventions for autism spectrum disorders. *Dialogues Clin. Neurosci.* 14, 307–318.

Lord, C., Rutter, M., DiLavore, P. C., Risi, S., Gotham, K., and Bishop, S. (2012). *Autism Diagnostic Observation Schedule*, 2nd Edn, Torrance, CA: Western Psychological Services.

Loth, E., Charman, T., Mason, L., Tillmann, J., Jones, E. J. H., Wooldridge, C., et al. (2017). The EU-AIMS longitudinal european autism project (LEAP): design and methodologies to identify and validate stratification biomarkers for autism spectrum disorders. *Mol. Autism* 8:24. doi: 10.1186/s13229-017-0146-8

Loth, E., Murphy, D. G., and Spooren, W. (2016). Defining precision medicine approaches to autism spectrum disorders: concepts and challenges. *Front. Psychiatry* 7:188. doi: 10.3389/fpsyt.2016.00188

McPartland, J., Bernier, R., Jeste, S., Dawson, G., Nelson, C., Chawarska, K., et al. (2019). The Autism Biomarkers Consortium for Clinical Trials (ABC-CT): scientific context, study design, and progress towards biomarker qualification. *medRxiv.* doi: 10.1101/2019.12.18.1901454

McPartland, J. C. (2016). Considerations in biomarker development for neurodevelopmental disorders. *Curr. Opin. Neurol.* 29, 118–122. doi: 10.1097/WCO.0000000000000300

McPartland, J. C. (2017). Developing clinically practicable biomarkers for autism spectrum disorder. *J. Autism Dev. Disord.* 47, 2935–2937. doi: 10.1007/s10803-017-3237-7

Murias, M., Major, S., Davlantis, K., Franz, L., Harris, A., Rardin, B., et al. (2017). Validation of eye-tracking measures of social attention as a potential biomarker for autism clinical trials. *Autism Res.* 19, 622–629. doi: 10.1002/aur.1894

Murias, M., Sabatos-Devito, M. G., Sugar, C. A., Sugar, C., Hellemann, G., Webb, S. J., et al. (2019). "ABC-CT lab based measures - video tracking". *Paper Presented at the ABC-CT Annual Meeting*, Boston, MA.

Naples, A., Barney, E., Chang, S. A., Li, B., McAllister, T., Kim, M., et al. (2018). *ABC-CT Data Acquisition and Analytic Core ET Main Study Acquisition Protocol, Version 4.9*, 4 Edn.

Ness, S. L., Manyakov, N. V., Bangerter, A., Lewin, D., Jagannatha, S., Boice, M., et al. (2017). JAKE® multimodal data capture system: insights from an observational study of autism spectrum disorder. *Front. Neurosci.* 11:517. doi: 10.3389/fnins.2017.00517

Nyström, P., Gredebäck, G., Bölte, S., and Falck-Ytter, T. (2015). Hypersensitive pupillary light reflex in infants at risk for autism. *Mol. Autism* 6:10. doi: 10.1186/s13229-015-0011-6

Picton, T. W., Bentin, S., Berg, P., Donchin, E., Hillyard, S. A., Johnson, R., et al. (2000). Guidelines for using human event-related potentials to study cognition: recording standards and publication criteria. *Psychophysiology* 37, 127–152. doi: 10.1017/s0048577200000305

Pivik, R. T., Broughton, R. J., Coppola, R., Davidson, R. J., Fox, N., and Nuwer, M. R. (1993). Guidelines for the recording and quantitative analysis of electroencephalographic activity in research contexts. *Psychophysiology* 30, 547–558. doi: 10.1111/j.1469-8986.1993.tb02081.x

Rice, K., Moriuchi, J. M., Jones, W., and Klin, A. (2012). Parsing heterogeneity in autism spectrum disorders: visual scanning of dynamic social scenes in school-aged children. *J. Am. Acad. Child Adolesc. Psychiatry* 51, 238–248. doi: 10.1016/j.jaac.2011.12.017

Rutter, M., Le Couteur, A., and Lord, C. (2003). *ADI-R: Autism Diagnostic Interview–Revised: Manual.* Los Angeles, CA: Western Psychological Services.

Sabatos-DeVito, M., Howell, T., Murias, M., Bernier, R., Chawarska, K., Dawson, G., et al. (2018). *Data Acquisition and Analytic Core ABC-CT Main Study: Automated Tracking of Parent-Child Free Play Derived Results Manual.* Durham NC.

Sabatos-DeVito, M., Murias, M., Dawson, G., Howell, T., Yuan, A., Marsan, S., et al. (2019). Methodological considerations in the use of Noldus EthoVision XT video tracking of children with autism in multi-site studies. *Biol. Psychol.* 146:107712. doi: 10.1016/j.biopsycho.2019.05.012

Sahin, M., Jones, S. R., Sweeney, J. A., Berry-Kravis, E., Connors, B. W., Ewen, J. B., et al. (2018). Discovering translational biomarkers in neurodevelopmental disorders. *Nat. Rev. Drug Discov.* 18, 235–236. doi: 10.1038/d41573-018-00010-7

Santhosh, M., Borland, H., Naples, A., Levin, A. R., Chang, S. A., Hasselmo, S., et al. (2018). *Data Acquisition and Analytic Core ABC-CT Main Study: EEG Pre-Processing Quality Control Manual, Version 1.2*, 1st Edn.

Sasson, N. J., Elison, J. T., Turner-Brown, L. M., Dichter, G. S., and Bodfish, J. W. (2011). Brief report: circumscribed attention in young children with autism. *J. Autism Dev. Disord.* 41, 242–247. doi: 10.1007/s10803-010-1038-3

Shic, F. (2013). *Eye-Tracking. In Encyclopedia of Autism Spectrum Disorders* (New York, NY: Springer), 1208–1213.

Shic, F. (2016). Eye tracking as a behavioral biomarker for psychiatric conditions: the road ahead. *JAAC* 55, 267–268. doi: 10.1016/j.jaac.2016.02.002

Shic, F., Bradshaw, J., Klin, A., Scassellati, B., and Chawarska, K. (2011). Limited activity monitoring in toddlers with autism spectrum disorder. *Brain Res.* 1380, 246–254. doi: 10.1016/j.brainres.2010.11.074

Shic, F., Naples, A., Barney, E., Chang, S. A., Li, B., McAllister, T., et al. (2018). *ABC-CT Data Acquisition and Analytic Core ET Main Study Manual of Operations, Version 4.8*, 4 Edn.

Umbricht, D., Del Valle Rubido, M., Hollander, E., McCracken, J. T., Shic, F., Scahill, L., et al. (2017). A single dose, randomized, controlled proof-of-mechanism study of a novel vasopressin 1a receptor antagonist

(RG7713) in high-functioning adults with autism spectrum disorder. *Neuropsychopharmacology* 42, 1914–1923. doi: 10.1038/npp.2016.232

Warren, S. F., Gilkerson, J., Richards, J. A., Oller, D. K., Xu, D., Yapanel, U., et al. (2010). What automated vocal analysis reveals about the vocal production and language learning environment of young children with autism. *J. Autism Dev. Disord.* 40, 555–569. doi: 10.1007/s10803-009-0902-5

Webb, S. J., Bernier, R., Henderson, H. A., Johnson, M. H., Jones, E. J. H., Lerner, M. D., et al. (2015). Guidelines and best practices for electrophysiological data collection, analysis and reporting in autism. *J. Autism Dev. Disord.* 45, 425–443. doi: 10.1007/s10803-013-1916-6

Webb, S. J., Borland, H., Santhosh, M., Naples, A., Levin, A. R., Bernier, R., et al. (2018). *ABC-CT Data Acquisition and Analytic Core EEG Main Study Manual of Operations, Version 2.2*, 2nd Edn.

Webb, S. J., Merkle, K., Murias, M., Richards, T., Aylward, E., and Dawson, G. (2012). ERP responses differentiate inverted but not upright face processing in adults with ASD. *Soc. Cogn. Affect. Neurosci.* 7, 578–587. doi: 10.1093/scan/nsp002

Xu, D., Yapanel, U., and Boulder, S. G. (2009). *Reliability of the LENA Language Environment Analysis System in Young Children's Natural Home Environment*. Boulder: LENA Foundation.

8

Precision Sensorimotor Control in Aging FMR1 Gene Premutation Carriers

*Walker S. McKinney[1], Zheng Wang[2], Shannon Kelly[1], Pravin Khemani[3], Su Lui[4], Stormi P. White[5] and Matthew W. Mosconi[1]**

[1] Clinical Child Psychology Program, Life Span Institute and Kansas Center for Autism Research and Training (K-CART), University of Kansas, Lawrence, KS, United States, [2] Department of Occupational Therapy, University of Florida, Gainesville, FL, United States, [3] Department of Neurology, Swedish Neuroscience Institute, Seattle, WA, United States, [4] Department of Radiology, Huaxi Magnetic Resonance Research Center, West China Hospital of Sichuan University, Chengdu, China, [5] Department of Pediatrics, Marcus Autism Center, Emory University School of Medicine, Atlanta, GA, United States

***Correspondence:**
Matthew W. Mosconi
mosconi@ku.edu

Background: Individuals with premutation alleles of the *FMR1* gene are at risk of developing fragile X-associated tremor/ataxia syndrome (FXTAS), a neurodegenerative condition affecting sensorimotor function. Information on quantitative symptom traits associated with aging in premutation carriers is needed to clarify neurodegenerative processes contributing to FXTAS.

Materials and Methods: 26 *FMR1* premutation carriers ages 44–77 years and 31 age-matched healthy controls completed rapid (2 s) and sustained (8 s) visually guided precision gripping tasks. Individuals pressed at multiple force levels to determine the impact of increasing the difficulty of sensorimotor actions on precision behavior. During initial pressing, reaction time, the rate at which individuals increased their force, the duration of pressing, and force accuracy were measured. During sustained gripping, the complexity of the force time series, force variability, and mean force were examined. During relaxation, the rate at which individuals decreased their force was measured. We also examined the relationships between visuomotor behavior and cytosine-guanine-guanine (CGG) repeat length and clinically rated FXTAS symptoms.

Results: Relative to controls, premutation carriers showed reduced rates of initial force generation during rapid motor actions and longer durations of their initial pressing with their dominant hand. During sustained force, premutation carriers demonstrated reduced force complexity, though this effect was specific to younger premutation carries during dominant hand pressing and was more severe for younger relative to older premutation carriers at low and medium force levels. Increased reaction time and lower sustained force complexity each were associated with greater CGG repeat length for premutation carriers. Increased reaction time and increased sustained force variability were associated with more severe clinically rated FXTAS symptoms.

Conclusion: Overall our findings suggest multiple sensorimotor processes are disrupted in aging premutation carriers, including initial force control guided by feedforward mechanisms and sustained sensorimotor behaviors guided by sensory feedback control processes. Results indicating that sensorimotor issues in aging premutation carriers relate to both greater CGG repeat length and clinically rated FXTAS symptoms suggest that quantitative tests of precision sensorimotor ability may serve as key targets for monitoring FXTAS risk and progression.

Keywords: fragile X-associated tremor/ataxia syndrome, FMR1 premutation, sensorimotor, precision grip, neurodegeneration, bradykinesia, dysmetria

BACKGROUND

Fragile X syndrome is the most common heritable form of intellectual disability, and it is caused by "full" mutations of the *FMR1* gene consisting of >200 cytosine-guanine-guanine (CGG) repeats (Kremer et al., 1991). Premutations of the *FMR1* gene involving 55–200 CGG repeats also confer risk for multiple subclinical issues as well as medical, psychiatric, and neurodegenerative conditions (Lozano et al., 2014) including fragile X-associated tremor/ataxia syndrome (FXTAS). FXTAS is a neurodegenerative disease in which patients present with a variety of sensorimotor, cognitive, psychiatric and medical issues, as well as cerebellar and cortical degeneration typically beginning at ages 50–70 years (Brunberg et al., 2002; Jacquemont et al., 2003). The defining clinical symptoms of FXTAS include intention tremor, gait ataxia, and Parkinsonism (Hagerman et al., 2001; Jacquemont et al., 2003; Leehey et al., 2007; Juncos et al., 2011), though some patients also demonstrate cognitive decline and psychiatric issues (Grigsby et al., 2008). Pathology of the middle cerebellar peduncle (MCP sign), cerebral atrophy, and intranuclear inclusions also are associated with FXTAS (Brunberg et al., 2002; Greco et al., 2006). Still, symptom presentation is highly variable across patients, and objective, quantitative tools are needed to identify aging premutation carriers most at risk of developing FXTAS, track disease progression, and determine neurobiological mechanisms (Jacquemont et al., 2004; Leehey et al., 2007).

Prior quantitative studies have indicated that premutation carriers with FXTAS and elderly, asymptomatic premutation carriers each show sensorimotor issues. For example, FXTAS patients show increased postural sway relative to healthy aging individuals (Aguilar et al., 2008), while aging premutation carriers with and without FXTAS each show postural sway during standing that is associated with greater CGG repeat length (Kraan et al., 2013; O'Keefe et al., 2015; Wang et al., 2019). Studies of fine motor abilities critical to everyday activities have indicated that asymptomatic *FMR1* premutation carriers (Shickman et al., 2018) and FXTAS patients (Schneider et al., 2012) show reduced motor speed. Park et al. (2019) also reported increased force variability during sustained finger abduction implicating feedback processes involved in reactively adjusting ongoing precision motor behaviors in response to sensory error information. Importantly, Shickman et al. (2018) documented that more severe fine motor issues were associated with greater CGG repeat length in asymptomatic aging premutation carries, suggesting fine motor deficits may covary with FXTAS risk. While these studies indicate tests of fine motor control may be useful for quantifying clinical and subclinical issues in aging premutation carriers, precise and translational measurements that comprehensively assess multiple sensorimotor processes, including the initiation, maintenance, and termination of behavior, are needed to define affected systems, clarify neurobiological mechanisms of FXTAS, and monitor both disease risk and progression.

One candidate approach for characterizing multiple sensorimotor processes in premutation carriers is studying visually guided precision gripping. Precision gripping is important for many daily living activities (e.g., writing, grasping objects), and multiple studies have documented atypical precision gripping behavior in neurodevelopmental (Mosconi et al., 2015; Wang et al., 2015) and neurodegenerative conditions that affects patients' quality of life (Vaillancourt et al., 2001a,c). Further, the neural bases of visually guided precision gripping have been studied extensively suggesting that clarifying spared and affected processes may help identify key brain mechanisms associated with different clinical conditions (Ehrsson et al., 2000; Kuhtz-Buschbeck et al., 2008; Prodoehl et al., 2009; Neely et al., 2013). During precision gripping, individuals initiate a "rise phase" in which they rapidly increase their force output to reach a target level. Due to afferent delays of sensory feedback information, initial pressing is guided by internal action plans and often results in initial dysmetria (e.g., overshooting at lower force levels; undershooting at higher force levels), especially during rapid compared to longer duration actions (Desmurget et al., 1999; Potter et al., 2006; Wang et al., 2015). During a subsequent "sustained phase," individuals reactively adjust motor output to match their target and maintain a more constant level of force integrating feedforward and sensory feedback processes. Increases in sustained force variability and reductions in force complexity each implicate failures in the ability to dynamically and reactively adjust precision motor output in response to sensory feedback (Vaillancourt et al., 2001b; Chu and Sanger, 2009). At the end of precision gripping actions, participants engage in a "relaxation phase" in which they rapidly release their grip force by terminating motor unit firing within agonist muscles supporting gripping (e.g., first dorsal interosseus) and initiating antagonist motor unit firing.

In the present study, we systematically assessed rise, sustained, and relaxation phases of visually guided precision gripping in *FMR1* premutation carriers ages 44–77 years. Our primary goal was to comprehensively characterize precision sensorimotor behaviors in aging *FMR1* premutation carriers as the extent to which initial, sustained, and relaxation phase behaviors are impacted has not yet been assessed. Both rapid and sustained actions were tested in order to determine the differential impact of *FMR1* premutations on sensorimotor feedforward and feedback processes. During rapid sensorimotor tasks, greater demands are placed on feedforward systems responsible for the accuracy and rapid execution of initial motor plans (Ghez et al., 1991). During sustained sensorimotor action, the integrity of sensorimotor feedback processes responsible for the online translation of sensory error information into corrective motor action is tested (Desmurget and Grafton, 2000; Vaillancourt et al., 2003). We also assessed sensorimotor behavior across multiple force levels, allowing us to assess the effect of increased task requirements on precision sensorimotor behavior. By examining a large age range, we were able to determine whether visually guided precision gripping issues were more prominent at relatively earlier stages of aging suggesting that they may be prodromal markers of degeneration, or whether they may become more prominent later suggesting decline at advanced ages. Gripping was tested across both hands to determine if neurodegenerative processes associated with aging in *FMR1* premutation carriers may be lateralized as previously suggested (Przybyla et al., 2011; Raw et al., 2012). We also examined the relationship between sensorimotor outcomes, FXTAS clinical symptoms, and CGG repeat length to determine the utility of our measures for characterizing sensorimotor deterioration associated with the severity of and risk for FXTAS.

MATERIALS AND METHODS

Participants

Twenty-six premutation carriers and 31 healthy controls completed sensorimotor testing (**Table 1**). Controls and carriers did not differ on age, sex ratio, or handedness. No premutation carriers had an existing diagnosis of any neurological disorder, nor did they self-report any motor (e.g., gait ataxia, intention tremor) or memory issues. Controls were excluded for current or past neurodegenerative, neurological, or major psychiatric disorders (e.g., schizophrenia, bipolar disorder). Controls also were excluded for a family history of fragile X syndrome or intellectual/developmental disabilities in first- or second-degree relatives. Participants were excluded if they reported any neurological or musculoskeletal disorder that could cause atypical sensorimotor functioning or a history of medications known to affect sensorimotor functioning, including antipsychotics, stimulants, or benzodiazepines (Reilly et al., 2008).

FMR1 premutation carriers were identified through local fragile X clinics and postings on local and national fragile X association LISTSERVs. Control participants were recruited through community advertisements. This study was carried out in accordance with the recommendations of and was approved by the University of Texas Southwestern Medical Center Institutional Review Board. All subjects provided written informed consent after a complete description of the study in accordance with the Declaration of Helsinki.

Neurological Evaluations

FMR1 premutation carriers completed a clinical exam by a neurologist with expertise in movement control in aging (PK). The clinical exam included administration of the International Cooperative Ataxia Rating Scale (Trouillas et al., 1997). The ICARS is comprised of 19 sections examining postural and gait disturbances, ataxia, dysarthria, and oculomotor behavior. Higher scores indicate more severe neuromotor issues. The ICARS has been validated previously for diagnosis of ataxia in patients with focal cerebellar lesions (Schoch et al., 2007), hereditary spinocerebellar and Friedrich's ataxia (Schmitz-Hubsch et al., 2006). Nine premutation carriers did not complete the clinical evaluation due to scheduling difficulties. For the 17 premutation carriers who completed the clinical visit, ICARS scores are presented in **Table 1**.

Sensorimotor Testing

Participants completed two tests of sensorimotor behavior differentiated by the trial duration and inter-trial interval ("rapid" trials included 2 s of pressing alternating with 2 s of rest, and "sustained" trials included 8 s of pressing alternating with 8 s of rest). For both tests, stimuli were presented on a 102 cm (40 inches) Samsung LCD monitor with a resolution of 1366 × 768 and a 120 Hz refresh rate. Participants were tested in a darkened room while seated 52 cm from the display monitor with their

TABLE 1 | Demographic and clinical characteristics.

	Controls (n = 31)	Premutation carriers (n = 26)	t	p
Age (years)	53 (10)	57 (9)	−1.39	0.169
Age range (years)	40–73	44–77	–	–
Sex (% male)†	39%	23%	1.60†	0.206
Handedness (% right)†	90%	96%	0.74†	0.391
FSIQ	109 (13)	99 (12)	2.93	0.005**
Dominant hand MVC	87 (28)	77 (23)	1.42	0.161
Non-dominant hand MVC	84 (32)	82 (27)	0.24	0.811
ICARS total score	–	5 (5)	–	–
ICARS total range	–	0–19	–	–
CGG repeat length	–	82 (17)	–	–
CGG repeat length range	–	55–110	–	–

*FSIQ: full-scale IQ; ICARS: International Cooperative Ataxia Rating Scale; CGG: cytosine-guanine-guanine. Variables are presented as: mean (SD); **$p < 0.01$; †chi-square statistic; a group by hand interaction of MVC is reported in* ***Table 2****.*

elbow at 90° and their forearm resting in a relaxed position on a custom-made arm brace. The arm brace was clamped to a table to keep the participant's arm position stable throughout testing (**Figure 1**). The participant's hand was pronated and lay flat with digits comfortably extended. Participants used their thumb and index finger to press against two opposing precision load cells (ELFF-B4-100N; Entran) 1.27 cm in diameter secured to a custom grip device attached to the arm brace. A Coulbourn (V72-25) resistive bridge strain amplifier received analog signal from the load cells. Data were sampled at 200 Hz with a 16-bit analog-to-digital converter (DI-720; DATAQ Instruments) and converted to Newton of force using a calibration factor derived from known weights before the study (Mosconi et al., 2015).

Procedures

Before testing, each participant's maximum voluntary contraction (MVC) was calculated separately for each hand using the average of the maximum force output during three trials in which participants pressed as hard as they could for 3 s.

During sensorimotor testing, participants viewed a horizontal white force bar that moved upward with increased force and downward with decreased force and a static target bar that was red during rest and turned green to cue the participant to begin pressing at the beginning of each trial (**Figure 2**). Participants received two instructions: (1) press the load cells as quickly as possible when the red target bar turns green, and (2) keep pressing so that the force bar stays as steady as possible at the level of the green target bar. These instructions were identical for the two versions of the task described below.

"Rapid" (2 s) and "sustained" (8 s) trials were administered at 15, 45, and 85% of each individual's MVC. During the rapid test, two blocks of five trials were presented for each hand at each force level (2 hands × 3 force levels × 2 blocks × 5 trials = 60 rapid trials). Each 2 s rapid trial alternated with 2 s rest periods. A 15 s rest block was provided after each block of trials. During the sustained test, participants completed two blocks of three trials for each hand at each force level (2 hands × 3 force levels × 2 blocks × 3 trials = 36 sustained trials). Eight seconds trials were followed by 8 s rest periods, and each block was separated by 15 s of rest. For both tests, the same hand was never tested on consecutive blocks. The order of force levels was randomized across blocks. The order of the two experiments was randomly assigned to each participant. Participants self-reported their dominant hand.

Sensorimotor Data Processing

Force traces for each trial were low-pass filtered via a double-pass 4th-order Butterworth filter at a cutoff of 15 Hz in MATLAB. Data were analyzed using custom MATLAB scripts previously developed by our lab (Wang et al., 2015).

Data from three distinct phases were analyzed. During the initial *rise* phase in which individuals pressed on the load cells to reach the target level, we examined reaction time, peak rate of force increase (i.e., the maximum value of the first derivative of the force trace), the duration of the period in which individuals increased their force, and the accuracy of their initial force output. The onset of the rise phase was calculated as the time at which the rate of force increase first exceeded 5% of the peak rate of force increase and remained above this level for at least 100 ms (Grafton and Tunik, 2011; Wang et al., 2015). Reaction time was calculated as the difference between rise phase onset and the appearance of the start cue. The rise phase offset was calculated as the time-point when the rate of force increase fell below 5% of the peak rate of force increase, and the force level was within 90–110% of the mean force of the sustained phase (Wang et al., 2015). The peak rate of force increase was defined as the maximum value of the first derivative of the force trace. Rise phase duration was then calculated as the difference between

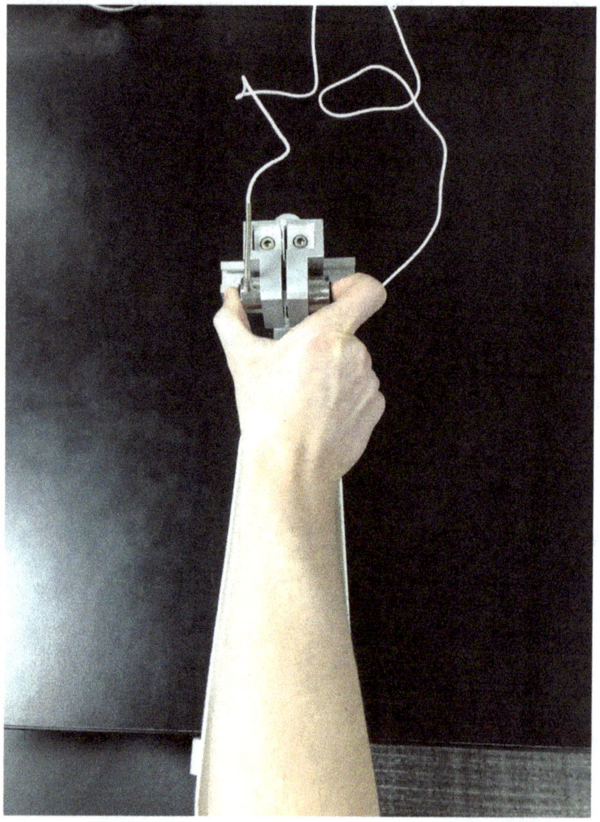

FIGURE 1 | The custom-made arm brace and load cells for precision grip testing. Participants pressed with their thumb and forefinger against two precision load cells while viewing two horizontal bars displayed vertically on the screen.

FIGURE 2 | Sensorimotor test stimuli. Participants pressed when the red bar turned green in order to move the white bar up to the target green bar. They were instructed to maintain their force level at the level of the green bar as steadily as possible.

the rise phase offset and rise phase onset. Rate of force increase and duration of initial force output were analyzed relative to rise phase force output to account for differences in force kinetics attributable to differences in force amplitude. Force accuracy for the rise phase was calculated as the force at rise offset divided by the target force (i.e., Rise Accuracy = $\frac{(F_{rise})}{(F_{target})}$). Values below 1 represent an undershooting of the target force and values above 1 reflect overshooting of the target force. An accuracy score of 1 indicates perfect accuracy. The entire rise phase was excluded if participants began gripping before the start cue, or if they returned to baseline prior to reaching 90% of the target force. Rise phase data for both the rapid and sustained tasks were analyzed within the same model to allow for the analysis of task effects (i.e., rapid vs. sustained). Consistent with prior studies, participants were expected to show faster reaction times, more rapid increases in force, shorter rise phase duration and reduced accuracy during rapid compared to sustained actions (Wang et al., 2015).

To determine the extent to which participants could maintain a constant level of force using visual feedback, the *sustained* phase was examined and defined as the period following rise phase offset and prior to the appearance of the stop cue. Due to the brief duration of rapid trials, the sustained phase was only examined during 8 s trials. The mean force of the time series was calculated to determine individuals' ability to complete the task. The variability of the force time series was calculated using the following procedures: first, force data were linearly detrended to account for systematic changes in mean force over the course of the trial (e.g., data drift). Second, the within-trial standard deviation (SD) of the force time series was calculated. To examine the time-dependent structure of the time series, the approximate entropy (ApEn) was calculated for each trial (Slifkin and Newell, 1999; Vaillancourt et al., 2001b). ApEn returns a value between 0 and 2, reflecting the predictability of future values in a time series based on previous values. For example, a sine wave has accurate short- and long-term predictability, corresponding to an ApEn value near 0. High irregularity of the data, reflective of the independence of each force value, returns an ApEn near 2. The algorithm and parameter settings for these calculations ($m = 2$; $r = 0.2 \times$ SD of the signal) were identical to previous work (Vaillancourt and Newell, 2000). Sustained phase variables were excluded if fewer than 4 s of data were available or if participants returned to baseline for more than 1 s (e.g., a > 1 s dip of the force signal).

In order to determine the rate at which individuals released force at the end of trials, the *relaxation* phase also was examined. The onset of the relaxation phase was defined as the first point following the stop cue (target bar turned red) at which velocity (i.e., rate of change of force) went below 5% of the peak velocity and remained at that level or below for at least 100 ms. The offset of the relaxation phase was defined as the first point at which velocity rose back above 5% of the peak relaxation velocity. We examined the rate of force decrease during the relaxation phase. The peak rate of force decrease was identified as the minimum value of the first derivative of the force trace following the stop cue. To control for differences in force level prior to force release, the rate of force decrease was examined relative to force amplitude prior to relaxation. Rate of force relaxation was not examined if the participant released force prior to the stop cue. Relaxation phase data was examined for both the rapid and sustained tasks in the same model.

CGG Repeat Count

All premutation carriers provided blood samples to confirm premutation status. *FMR1* CGG repeat count was quantified using molecular testing conducted at Dr. Elizabeth Berry-Kravis' Molecular Diagnostic Laboratory at Rush University. Genomic DNA was isolated from peripheral blood leukocytes samples. The *FMR1* polymerase chain reaction (PCR) test with quantification of allele-specific CGG repeat count was performed using commercially available kits (Asuragen, Inc., Austin, TX, United States). For women, CGG repeat analyses reflect the longest CGG repeat of the two alleles.

Cognitive Measures

Cognitive functioning was assessed using the abbreviated battery of the Stanford-Binet Intelligence Scales, Fifth Edition (SB-5) including non-verbal fluid reasoning and verbal knowledge subsections (Roid, 2003). One participant did not complete the SB-5 because they were not fluent in English. Healthy controls had significantly higher full-scale IQs (M = 109.3, SD = 12.8) than premutation carriers (M = 99.5, SD = 12.1), $t(54) = 2.93, p < 0.01$, though IQ was in the average range for both groups (**Table 1**).

Statistical Analyses

To determine whether sensorimotor ability differed according to premutation carrier status, linear multilevel mixed effect (MLM) analyses were conducted (Bates et al., 2015; Koller, 2016). This approach allows for the simultaneous analysis of within- and between-subject fixed effects while allowing within-subject factors to differ for each participant as random effects. This approach also allows for the analysis of interactions within the repeated measures design including participants with missing data (e.g., failed to complete dominant hand trials at 85% MVC) without listwise deletion of that participant. Task (rapid vs. sustained) and condition effects (percent MVC, hand) were identified as level 1 predictors and subject effects (group, age) were identified as level 2 predictors. Random variance components for the intercept (subject) also were analyzed. To maintain relatively parsimonious models, five-way interactions were not analyzed. Initial models included all two-, three-, and four-way interactions, after which variables and interactions were removed and model fit was compared between the previous and current models using a likelihood ratio test. Only variables which significantly ($p < 0.05$) improved model fit were incorporated into final models. Non-normally distributed variables were log-transformed. Final models used robust linear mixed effect modeling to provide more stringent fixed effect estimates and standard errors while reducing the impact of outliers (Pinheiro et al., 2001). Due to concerns with Type 1 error when interpreting robust estimates with traditional p-value cut-offs, we followed best practice guidelines and significant results are reported if $|t| \geq 1.96$ (Luke, 2017). Age was centered for all models, and each categorical predictor was dummy coded with the following conditions serving as baseline references: healthy controls, 15% MVC, dominant hand, rapid (2 s) task. Based on these references, the intercept for each model was interpreted as the predicted value of the dependent outcome for an average aged (54.87 years) healthy control during the 15% MVC dominant hand rapid task. Predicted values are then obtained by adding the relevant fixed effect and interaction estimates. Main effect and interaction effect results are reported relative to baseline reference values. Due to the MVC manipulation having three levels, MVC percent main and interaction effects are presented separately for 45 and 85% MVC relative to the 15% MVC reference condition. Significant task and age effects are reported followed by group and group interaction effects. Mixed effect modeling was conducted using the *robustlmm* and *lmer* packages within R version 3.6.0 (Bates et al., 2015; Koller, 2016).

Due to the non-normal distribution of CGG repeat length and ICARS scores, the relationships between sensorimotor outcomes, ICARS scores, and CGG repeat length were examined using Spearman's rank-order correlations. Linear regression was used to determine if total ICARS scores were related to age, CGG repeat length, or the interaction of age and CGG repeat length. Due to the large number of correlations that were performed, only results with $p < 0.01$ were interpreted as significant. Correlational and regression analyses were conducted using IBM SPSS Statistics 25.

RESULTS

Maximum Voluntary Contraction

Relative to controls, premutation carriers showed a greater difference between their dominant and non-dominant hand MVC (**Figure 3** and **Tables 1, 2**; group × hand: $\beta = 7.16$, $SE = 3.47$, $p = 0.039$, partial $R^2 = 0.010$). MVC was not related to age ($\beta = -2.01$, $SE = 4.00$, $p = 0.616$, partial $R^2 = 0.029$), and the relationship between age and MVC did not differ between groups (group × age: $\beta = 6.47$, $SE = 6.28$, $p = 0.303$, partial $R^2 = 0.055$).

Rise Phase

Reaction Time

Participants showed shorter reaction times during the rapid task relative to the sustained task (**Table 3**; $\beta = 0.14$, $SE = 0.02$, $p < 0.001$, partial $R^2 = 0.050$). Reaction time increased with increases in target MVC percent (15% vs. 45% MVC: $\beta = 0.10$, $SE = 0.02$, $p < 0.001$, partial $R^2 = 0.015$; 15% vs. 85% MVC: $\beta = 0.17$, $SE = 0.02$, $p < 0.001$, partial $R^2 = 0.036$) and age ($\beta = 0.10$, $SE = 0.04$, $p = 0.014$, partial $R^2 = 0.074$).

No significant group differences or group interactions were identified for reaction time.

Rate of Force Increase

Participants demonstrated a higher rate of force increase during the rapid compared to the sustained task (**Table 3**; $\beta = -0.16$, $SE = 0.04$, $p < 0.001$, partial $R^2 = 0.015$). After controlling for target amplitude (i.e., force level at the end of the rise phase), rate of force increase also was reduced at higher compared to lower MVC target levels (15% vs. 45% MVC: $\beta = -0.22$, $SE = 0.04$, $p < 0.001$, partial $R^2 = 0.050$; 15% vs. 85% MVC: $\beta = -0.34$, $SE = 0.04$, $p < 0.001$, partial $R^2 = 0.104$). Rate of force increase was greater with the non-dominant compared to the dominant hand ($\beta = 0.10$, $SE = 0.02$, $p < 0.001$, partial $R^2 = 0.025$) and slowed with age ($\beta = -0.07$, $SE = 0.03$, $p = 0.042$, partial $R^2 = 0.049$).

Premutation carriers showed a reduced rate of force increase relative to controls during the rapid but not the sustained task (**Figure 4**; group × task: $\beta = 0.13$, $SE = 0.04$, $p = 0.004$, partial $R^2 = 0.009$).

Rise Phase Duration

For all participants, rise phase duration was greater during the rapid compared to the sustained task (**Table 4**; $\beta = -0.31$, $SE = 0.02$, $p < 0.001$, partial $R^2 = 0.214$) and was increased at higher compared to lower MVC target levels (15% vs. 45% MVC: $\beta = -1.04$, $SE = 0.02$, $p < 0.001$, partial $R^2 = 0.680$; 15% vs. 85% MVC: $\beta = -1.59$, $SE = 0.02$, $p < 0.001$, partial $R^2 = 0.831$).

Relative to controls, premutation carriers showed longer rise phase durations, but only for their dominant hand (**Figure 5**; group × hand: $\beta = -0.12$, $SE = 0.04$, $p = 0.001$, partial $R^2 = 0.011$).

Rise Phase Accuracy

Across tasks, participants overshot target force levels at 15% MVC ($M = 1.05$; $SD = 0.14$), showed greater accuracy at 45% MVC ($M = 0.99$; $SD = 0.04$), and then undershot target force level at 85% MVC ($M = 0.96$; $SD = 0.05$). During the rapid task, participants demonstrated greater levels of overshooting compared to the sustained task at 15% MVC ($\beta = -0.02$, $SE = 0.01$, $p = 0.001$, partial $R^2 = 0.039$) but similar accuracy at 45% (15% vs. 45% MVC × task: $\beta = 0.01$, $SE = 0.01$, $p = 0.150$, partial $R^2 = 0.016$) and 85% MVC (15% vs. 85% MVC × task: $\beta = 0.02$, $SE = 0.01$, $p = 0.062$, partial $R^2 = 0.017$).

There were no significant group differences or group interactions for rise phase accuracy.

Sustained Phase

ApEn

Participants demonstrated reduced ApEn at higher compared to lower target force levels (**Table 5**; 15% vs. 45% MVC: $\beta = -0.06$, $SE = 0.02$, $p < 0.001$, partial $R^2 = 0.136$; 15% vs. 85% MVC: $\beta = -0.13$, $SE = 0.02$, $p < 0.001$, partial $R^2 = 0.026$).

Premutation carriers showed reduced ApEn relative to controls, and this group difference varied as a function of age and target force level (**Figure 6**; group × age × 15% vs. 45% MVC: $\beta = -0.001$, $SE = 0.0$, $p = 0.960$, partial $R^2 < 0.001$; group × age × 15% vs. 85% MVC: $\beta = -0.06$, $SE = 0.02$, $p = 0.008$, partial $R^2 = 0.010$). Reduced ApEn in premutation carriers relative to controls was more severe at younger ages during the 15 and 45% MVC conditions but not for the 85% MVC condition. Premutation carriers also showed reduced ApEn that varied as a function of age and hand (**Figure 7**; group × hand × age: $\beta = -0.05$, $SE = 0.02$, $p = 0.011$, partial

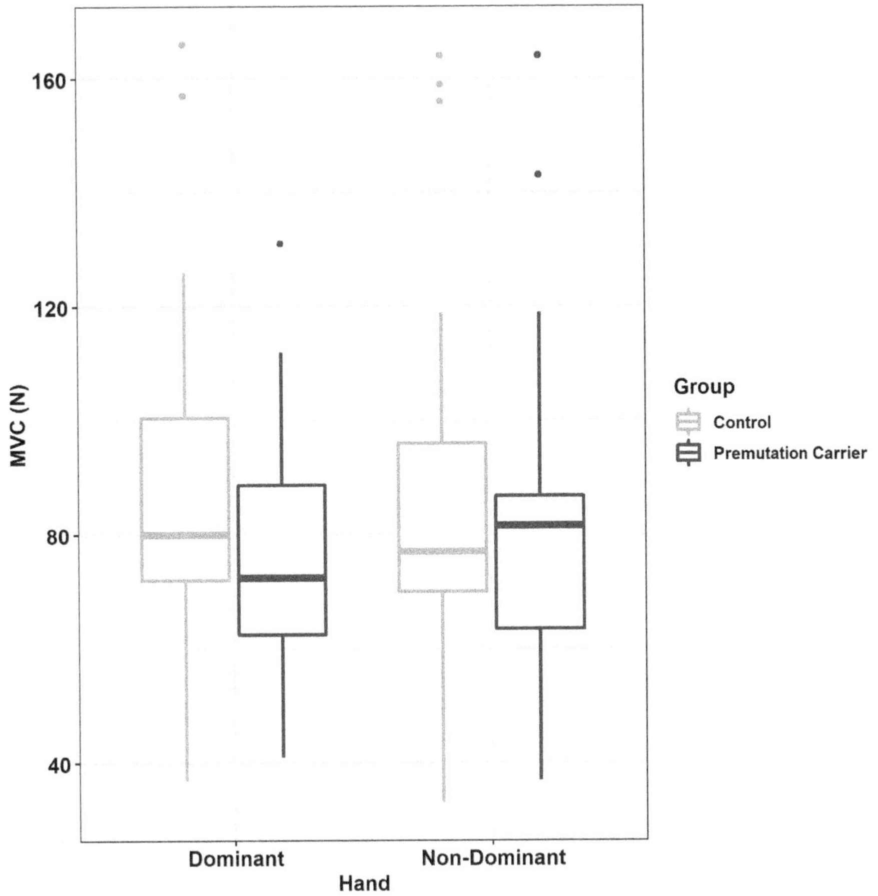

FIGURE 3 | Maximum voluntary contract (MVC) as a function of group and hand. Relative to controls, premutation carriers showed a greater difference between their dominant and non-dominant hand MVC.

TABLE 2 | Best fitting multilevel models for subject MVC.

	Fixed effect estimates	Estimate (SE)	*t*	Partial R^2
MVC	Level 1 variables			
	Intercept	83.93 (4.20)	19.96*	–
	Hand	−3.59 (2.34)	−1.53	0.003
	Level 2 variables			
	Group	−8.30 (6.23)	−1.33	0.031
	Interaction variables			
	Group × hand	7.16 (3.46)	2.07*	0.010
	Random effect variances	**Variance (SD)**		
	Level 1 residual (ε_{it})	80.68 (8.98)	–	–
	Level 2 intercept (μ_{0i})	440.24 (20.98)	–	–

**p* < 0.05 using the t-as-z approach; MVC: maximum voluntary contraction; partial R^2 reflects the proportion of residual variation accounted for by the fixed effect when added to the same model without the fixed effect.*

R^2 = 0.010). Specifically, premutation carriers showed reduced ApEn across age for the non-dominant hand, but this effect was more severe at younger ages relative to older ages for the dominant hand.

Force SD

Force SD scaled with target MVC level (**Table 5**; 15% vs. 45% MVC: $\beta = 0.09$, $SE = 0.06$, $p < 0.001$, partial $R^2 = 0.250$; 15% vs. 85% MVC: $\beta = 2.00$, $SE = 0.06$, $p < 0.001$, partial $R^2 = 0.631$).

TABLE 3 | Best fitting multilevel models for reaction time and rise phase rate of force increase.

	Fixed effect estimates	Estimate (SE)	t	Partial R^2
Reaction time	Level 1 variables			
	Intercept	−1.08 (0.04)	−24.01*	–
	15% vs. 45% MVC	0.10 (0.02)	4.62*	0.015
	15% vs. 85% MVC	0.17 (0.02)	7.65*	0.036
	Task	0.14 (0.02)	7.97*	0.050
	Level 2 variables			
	Age	0.10 (0.04)	2.47*	0.074
	Random effect variances	**Variance (SD)**		
	Level 1 residual (ε_{it})	0.05 (0.22)	–	–
	Level 2 intercept (μ_{0i})	0.09 (0.30)	–	–
	Fixed effect estimates	**Estimate (SE)**	***t***	**Partial R^2**
Rate of force increase	Level 1 variables			
	Intercept (15% MVC)	1.70 (0.05)	31.53*	–
	15% vs. 45% MVC	−0.22 (0.04)	−6.03*	0.050
	15% vs. 85% MVC	−0.34 (0.04)	−9.14*	0.104
	Hand	0.10 (0.02)	4.43*	0.025
	Task	−0.16 (0.04)	−3.79*	0.015
	Level 2 variables			
	Group	−0.13 (0.07)	−1.86	0.025
	Age	−0.07 (0.03)	−2.03*	0.049
	Interaction variables			
	Group × task	0.13 (0.04)	2.91*	0.010
	15% vs. 45% MVC × task	−0.11 (0.05)	−2.17*	0.008
	15% vs. 85% MVC × task	−0.13 (0.05)	−2.39*	0.009
	Random effect variances	**Variance (SD)**		
	Level 1 residual (ε_{it})	0.07 (0.27)	–	–
	Level 2 intercept (μ_{0i})	0.05 (0.23)	–	–

$p < 0.05$ using the t-as-z approach; MVC: maximum voluntary contraction; partial R^2 reflects the proportion of residual variation accounted for by the fixed effect when added to the same model without the fixed effect.

There were no significant group differences or group interactions for force SD.

Mean Force

Mean sustained force scaled with target MVC level (**Table 5**; 15% vs. 45% MVC: β = 1.08, SE = 0.01, $p < 0.001$, partial R^2 = 0.677; 15% vs. 85% MVC: β = 1.68, SE = 0.01, $p < 0.001$, partial R^2 = 0.840) and was reduced in the non-dominant relative to the dominant hand (β = −0.05, SE = 0.01, $p < 0.001$, partial R^2 = 0.004).

Compared to controls, premutation carriers demonstrated lower mean force with their dominant hand only (group × hand: β = 0.08, SE = 0.02, $p < 0.001$, partial R^2 = 0.007).

Relaxation Phase

Rate of Force Decrease

During the relaxation phase, participants decreased their force level more slowly during higher relative to lower target force levels (15% vs. 45% MVC: β = −0.10, SE = 0.01, $p < 0.001$, partial R^2 = 0.079; 15% vs. 85% MVC: β = −0.19, SE = 0.01, $p < 0.001$, partial R^2 = 0.219) and during rapid compared to sustained force trials (β = −0.071, SE = 0.01, $p < 0.001$, partial R^2 = 0.065).

There were no significant group differences or group interactions for rate of force decrease.

Sensorimotor Behavior and Clinical/Demographic Outcomes

Age

Increased age was significantly associated with more severe ICARS rated FXTAS symptoms ($F(1,15)$ = 9.858, p = 0.007, R^2 = 0.397). CGG repeat length was not associated with FXTAS symptoms ($F\Delta(1,14)$ = 1.891, p = 0.191, $R^2\Delta$ = 0.072).

CGG Repeat Length

Greater CGG repeat length was associated with reduced dominant hand ApEn in the 45% MVC condition (**Figure 8A** and **Table 6**; ρ = −0.529, p = 0.009). Greater CGG repeat length also was associated with increased dominant hand reaction time during the rapid task at 15% MVC (ρ = 0.543, p = 0.007). No other sensorimotor variables were associated with CGG repeat length.

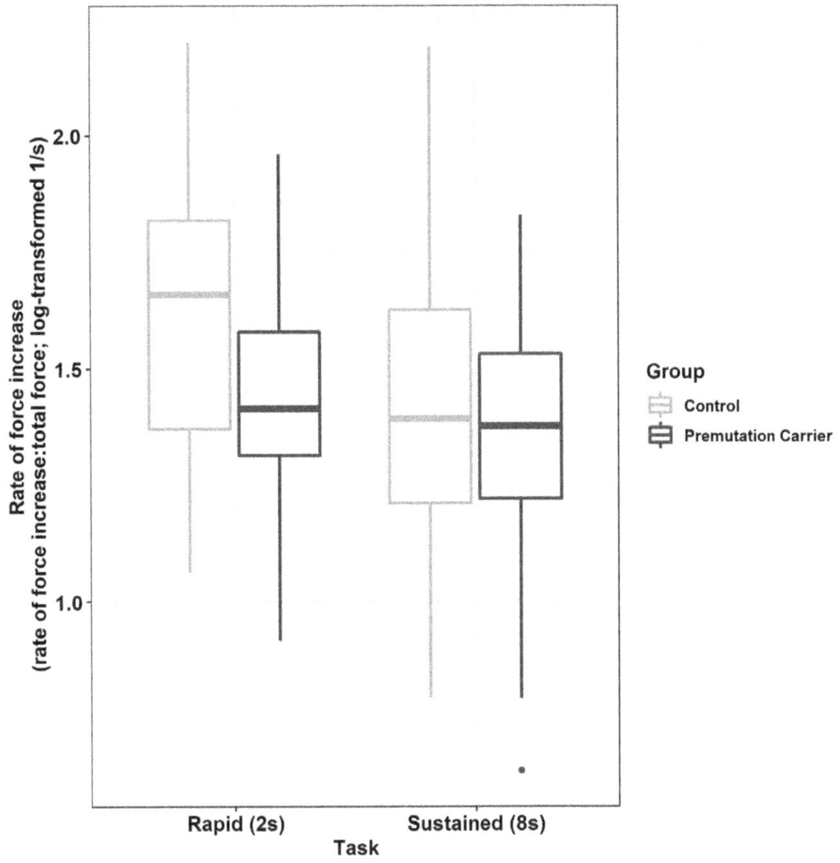

FIGURE 4 | Peak rate of force increase (relative to initial force output) as a function of group and task. Relative to controls, premutation carriers show a reduced rate of force increase during rapid pressing.

Clinical Symptoms

More severe FXTAS symptoms were associated with greater reaction times during the rapid task in the dominant hand 45% MVC condition (**Figure 8B** and **Table 7**; $\rho = 0.700$, $p = 0.002$), dominant hand 85% MVC condition ($\rho = 0.665$, $p = 0.005$), and non-dominant hand 85% MVC condition ($\rho = 0.674$, $p = 0.003$). More severe FXTAS symptoms also were associated with greater reaction times during the dominant hand 15% MVC condition of the sustained task ($\rho = 0.612$, $p = 0.009$). More severe ICARS scores were associated with higher force SD during the non-dominant hand 45% MVC condition (**Figure 8C**; $\rho = 0.663$, $p = 0.004$).

DISCUSSION

Despite sensorimotor impairments being central to the diagnosis of FXTAS, few studies have quantified precision sensorimotor behaviors in aging *FMR1* premutation carriers. Here, we examined multiple distinct component processes of precision sensorimotor behavior in aging premutation carriers in order to identify both spared and affected systems. Four key findings are documented. First, dominant hand strength was reduced relative to non-dominant hand strength in premutation carriers implicating atypical lateralized degeneration of neuromuscular systems in aging carriers of *FMR1* premutation alleles. Second, aging premutation carriers demonstrated a reduced ability to rapidly increase force during precision gripping suggesting alterations in feedforward sensorimotor control systems. Third, younger premutation carriers demonstrated reduced complexity of their sustained force output (i.e., ApEn), suggesting the ability to dynamically adjust motor output in response to sensory feedback may be impacted, especially during initial stages of aging during which premutation carriers first become vulnerable to FXTAS-associated deterioration. Last, multiple impairments of sensorimotor behavior were associated with CGG repeat length and clinically rated neuromotor issues in premutation carriers indicating that select precision measures of sensorimotor behavior may covary with FXTAS risk or progression.

Reduced MVC in Aging *FMR1* Premutation Allele Carriers

Although premutation carriers and healthy controls did not differ on overall strength (i.e., MVC) or mean force output, premutation carriers showed a greater difference between their dominant and non-dominant hand MVC and mean force relative to controls. It is possible that premutation carriers show

TABLE 4 | Best fitting multilevel models for rise phase duration and accuracy.

	Fixed effect estimates	**Estimate (SE)**	***t***	**Partial R^2**
Rise phase duration	Level 1 variables			
	Intercept	−2.43 (0.06)	−38.86*	–
	15% vs. 45% MVC	−1.04 (0.02)	−46.72*	0.680
	15% vs. 85% MVC	−1.59 (0.02)	−71.98*	0.831
	Hand	0.04 (0.02)	1.64	0.002
	Task	−0.31 (0.02)	−17.11*	0.214
	Level 2 variables			
	Group	0.15 (0.09)	1.62	0.025
	Interaction variables			
	Group × hand	−0.12 (0.04)	−3.28*	0.011
	Random effect variances	**Variance (SD)**		
	Level 1 residual (ε_{it})	0.05 (0.23)	–	–
	Level 2 intercept (μ_{0i})	0.10 (0.32)	–	–
	Fixed effect estimates	**Estimate (SE)**	***t***	**Partial R^2**
Rise accuracy	Level 1 variables			
	Intercept (15% MVC)	1.04 (0.45 × 10^{-2})	232.14*	–
	15% vs. 45% MVC	−0.04 (0.01)	−7.22*	0.076
	15% vs. 85% MVC	−0.07 (0.01)	−12.66*	0.144
	Task	−0.02 (0.01)	−3.29*	0.039
	Interaction variables			
	15% vs. 45% MVC × task	0.01 (0.01)	1.44	0.016
	15% vs. 85% MVC × task	0.02 (0.01)	1.86	0.017
	Random effect variances	**Variance (SD)**		
	Level 1 residual (ε_{it})	0.18 × 10^{-2} (0.04)	–	–
	Level 2 intercept (μ_{0i})	0.01 × 10^{-2} (0.01)	–	–

**$p < 0.05$ using the t-as-z approach; MVC: maximum voluntary contraction; Partial R^2 reflects the proportion of residual variation accounted for by the fixed effect when added to the same model without the fixed effect.*

degeneration of neuromuscular systems as suggested by previous findings documenting reduced motor unit firing rates (Park et al., 2019). Findings that MVC reductions in premutation carriers may be more prominent in the dominant relative to the non-dominant hand suggest that neuromotor deterioration may be lateralized initially during aging or during initial stages of FXTAS. Few studies have examined lateralization of sensorimotor behavior in aging FMR1 premutation carriers or patients with FXTAS, but longitudinal studies tracking neuromuscular strength across both dominant and non-dominant hands are warranted.

Rapid Force Production in Aging *FMR1* Premutation Allele Carriers

Reduced rates and increased durations of initial force output in aging premutation carriers together suggest impairment in the ability to rapidly increase force during precision sensorimotor actions. These findings likely are not attributable to diminished overall force output as we controlled for the overall amount of individuals' force generation. Instead, premutation carriers appear to have a reduced ability to rapidly generate force, suggesting that the bradykinesia associated with FXTAS (Niu et al., 2014) may be evident in some asymptomatic aging premutation carriers during actions that require rapid increases in force. Similar reductions in initial force production also have been reported in studies of Parkinson's disease suggesting basal ganglia circuit functions may be affected during aging in *FMR1* premutation carriers (Stelmach and Worringham, 1988; Fellows et al., 1998). This hypothesis is supported by studies highlighting increased iron deposition in neuronal and glial cells in putamen nuclei of FXTAS patients (Ariza et al., 2017) and case studies documenting pre- and post-synaptic nigrostriatal dysfunction (Zuhlke et al., 2004; Scaglione et al., 2008; Healy et al., 2009). Our findings also could reflect peripheral alterations. As suggested by our findings of increased lateralization of MVC in premutation carriers, atypical recruitment of motor neurons during voluntary muscle contractions is possible (Rose and McGill, 2005; Wang et al., 2017; Park et al., 2019). For example, a previous study has documented slower nerve conduction velocities and F-wave latencies in male premutation carriers with and without FXTAS (Soontarapornchai et al., 2008). EMG abnormalities, including reduced motor unit firing rates, have been reported in premutation carriers and FXTAS patients, indicating that difficulties generating force also may stem from

TABLE 5 | Best fitting multilevel models for sustained phase variables.

	Fixed effect estimates	Estimate (SE)	t	Partial R^2
ApEn	Level 1 variables			
	Intercept	0.51 (0.02)	30.06*	–
	15% vs. 45% MVC	−0.05 (0.02)	−3.63*	0.136
	15% vs. 85% MVC	−0.13 (0.02)	−8.47*	0.026
	Hand	−0.01 (0.01)	−0.51	0.001
	Level 2 variables			
	Group	−0.03 (0.03)	−1.22	0.004
	Age	−0.01 (0.02)	−0.74	0.002
	Interaction variables			
	Group × 15% vs. 45% MVC	0.03×10^{-2} (0.02)	0.01	<0.001
	Group × 15% vs. 85% MVC	0.03 (0.02)	1.28	0.002
	Group × hand	−0.01 (0.02)	−0.46	0.001
	Group × age	0.05 (0.03)	1.95	0.014
	15% vs. 45% MVC × age	−0.01 (0.01)	−0.90	0.002
	15% vs. 85% MVC × age	0.02 (0.01)	1.36	0.003
	Hand × age	0.03 (0.01)	2.26*	0.011
	Group × hand × age	−0.05 (0.02)	−2.54*	0.010
	Group × age × 15% vs. 45% MVC	-0.12×10^{-2} (0.02)	−0.05	<0.001
	Group × age × 15% vs. 85% MVC	−0.06 (0.02)	−2.67*	0.010
	Random effect variances	**Variance (SD)**		
	Level 1 residual (ε_{it})	0.01 (0.08)	–	–
	Level 2 intercept (μ_{0i})	0.38×10^{-2} (0.06)	–	–
	Fixed effect estimates	**Estimate (SE)**	t	**Partial R^2**
Force SD	Level 1 Variables			
	Intercept (15% MVC)	−1.17 (0.06)	−18.46*	–
	15% vs. 45% MVC	0.09 (0.06)	15.55*	0.250
	15% vs. 85% MVC	2.00 (0.06)	33.71*	0.631
	Random effect variances	**Variance (SD)**		
	Level 1 residual (ε_{it})	0.01 (0.08)	–	–
	Level 2 intercept (μ_{0i})	0.33×10^{-2} (0.06)	–	–
	Fixed effect estimates	**Estimate (SE)**	t	**Partial R^2**
Mean force	Level 1 variables			
	Intercept	2.53 (0.05)	47.52*	-
	15% vs. 45% MVC	1.07 (0.01)	83.75*	0.677
	15% vs. 85% MVC	1.68 (0.01)	131.09*	0.840
	Hand	−0.05 (0.01)	−3.41*	0.004
	Level 2 variables			
	Group	−0.10 (0.08)	−1.28	0.015
	Interaction variables			
	Group × hand	0.08 (0.02)	3.91*	0.007
	Random effect variances	**Variance (SD)**		
	Level 1 residual (ε_{it})	0.01 (0.28)	–	–
	Level 2 intercept (μ_{0i})	0.08 (0.28)	–	–

$p < 0.05$ using the t-as-z approach; MVC: maximum voluntary contraction; Partial R^2 reflects the proportion of residual variation accounted for by the fixed effect when added to the same model without the fixed effect.

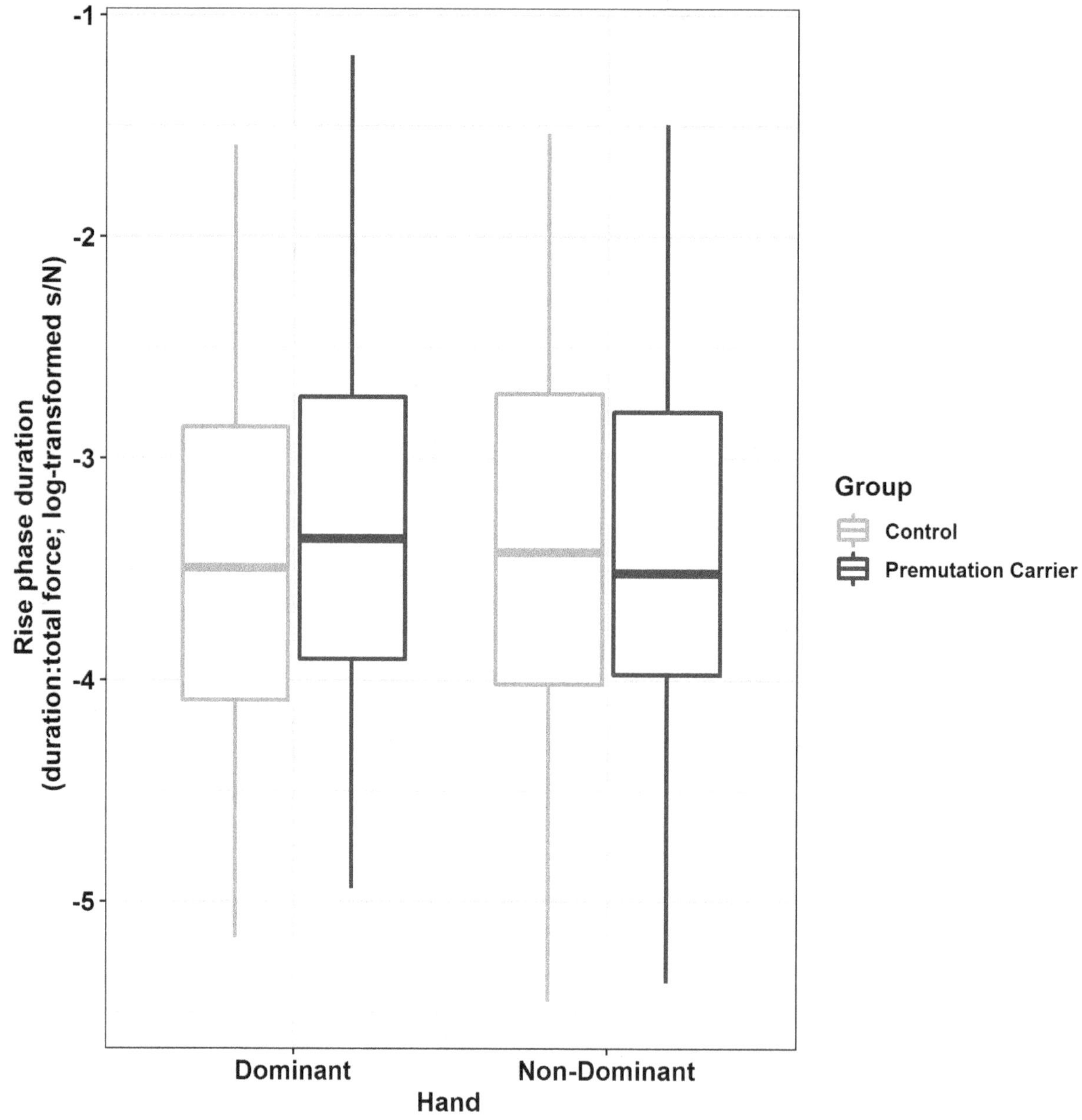

FIGURE 5 | Rise phase duration (relative to initial force output) as a function of group and hand. Relative to controls, premutation carriers showed an increased time to reach target force levels when using their dominant hand but not their non-dominant hand.

alterations at the neuromuscular level including reduced rates of motor unit recruitment (Lechpammer et al., 2017; Bravo et al., 2018; Park et al., 2019).

Sustained Sensorimotor Control in Aging *FMR1* Premutation Allele Carriers

During sustained force contractions, *FMR1* premutation carriers showed lower time series complexity (reduced ApEn), especially at lower force levels and at younger ages, reflecting a reduced ability to dynamically adjust force output in response to sensory feedback. Increased complexity of force output is adaptive and reflects individuals' ability to integrate multiple sensory feedback and feedforward processes and update internal action representations that guide the precision of sensorimotor output during sustained behavior. Lower complexity suggests reduced integration of these distinct processes and reduced ability to update precision sensorimotor behavior to meet task demands. Our finding that the severity of ApEn reductions in premutation carriers is relatively similar in magnitude across ages for the non-dominant hand, but more prominent at younger ages for the dominant hand indicates that deterioration of sustained sensorimotor behavior may be lateralized in aging premutation carriers. More specifically, our results suggest that healthy

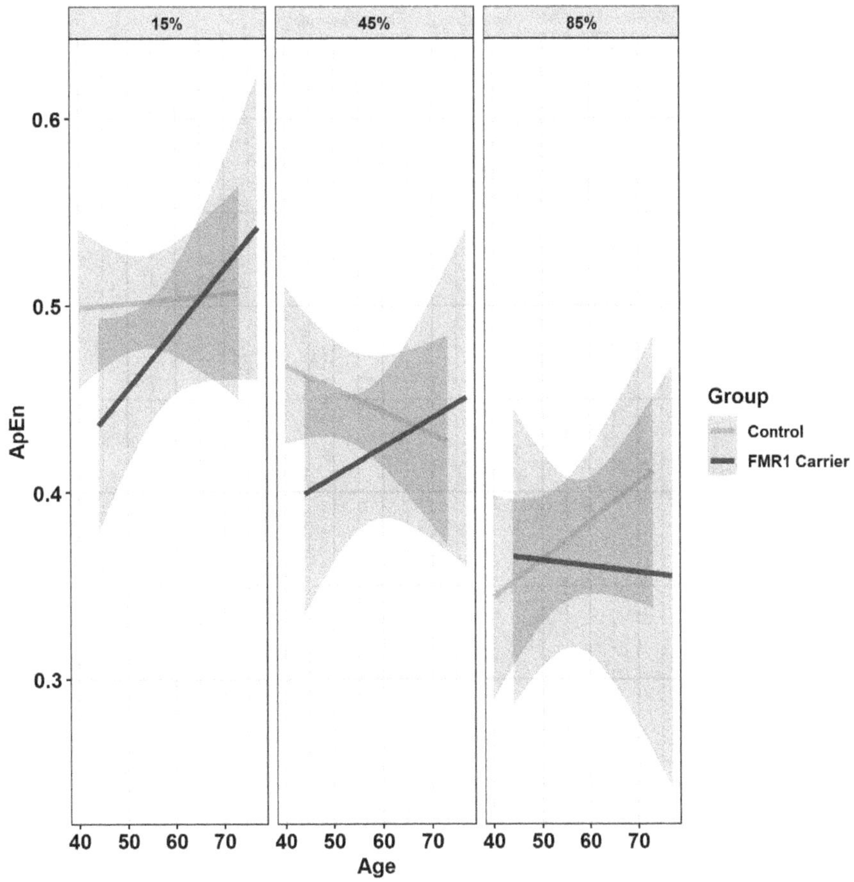

FIGURE 6 | Approximate entropy (ApEn; i.e., force complexity) as a function of group,% MVC, and age (linear fit with 95% confidence intervals). During the 15% and 45% MVC conditions, younger premutation carriers demonstrated reduced force complexity relative to controls, while premutation carriers and controls showed similar levels of force complexity across age at 85% MVC.

controls show worsening of their sustained force control as they age, whereas the opposite pattern is true for premutation carriers when using the dominant hand. We postulate that older premutation carriers in our sample who currently report being asymptomatic may be less affected by aging effects of *FMR1* premutation alleles and less likely to develop FXTAS than the younger individuals in our sample who are beginning to age into the period of adulthood during which they are most likely to develop FXTAS symptoms. This hypothesis is supported by evidence that FXTAS prevalence decreases during late adulthood reflecting increased FXTAS-related mortality rates and reduced likelihood of FXTAS onset during elderly years (Rodriguez-Revenga et al., 2009). Our finding that reduced force complexity in premutation carriers is more severe at lower force levels indicates that deficits in sustained sensorimotor behaviors likely impact multiple tasks of daily living (e.g., lifting a glass of water) but may not manifest during more strenuous activities involving higher levels of isometric force.

Reduced complexity of the time-dependent structure of force oscillations in younger premutation carriers may reflect a reduced number of neural oscillators (Vaillancourt et al., 2001b). Neural oscillators within the central nervous system each generate rhythmic output. Corticomotor neurons demonstrate preferred discharge frequencies, and so the use of a larger number of neural oscillators to generate motor output would result in greater complexity of motor output as each neural oscillator contributes output of a different frequency (McAuley and Marsden, 2000). Likewise, fewer neural oscillators generating motor output would result in the reduced variability of motor output timing consistent with a less complex and more rhythmic force output (McAuley and Marsden, 2000; Vaillancourt et al., 2001b). Our findings of reduced ApEn in younger premutation carriers thus implicate atypical integration of neural oscillators that may contribute to increased rates of tremor (Homberg et al., 1987). ApEn measurements during sustained sensorimotor behavior hold promise for determining mechanisms contributing to tremor in FXTAS, and as surrogate biomarkers useful for clinical trials targeting tremor in patients (Hagerman et al., 2012). These findings also may be consistent with our recent study documenting greater sustained force variability in aging *FMR1* premutation carriers during finger abduction (Park et al., 2019). While we did not find evidence for atypical variability in premutation carriers in the present study, we did find that greater force variability was associated with more severe FXTAS

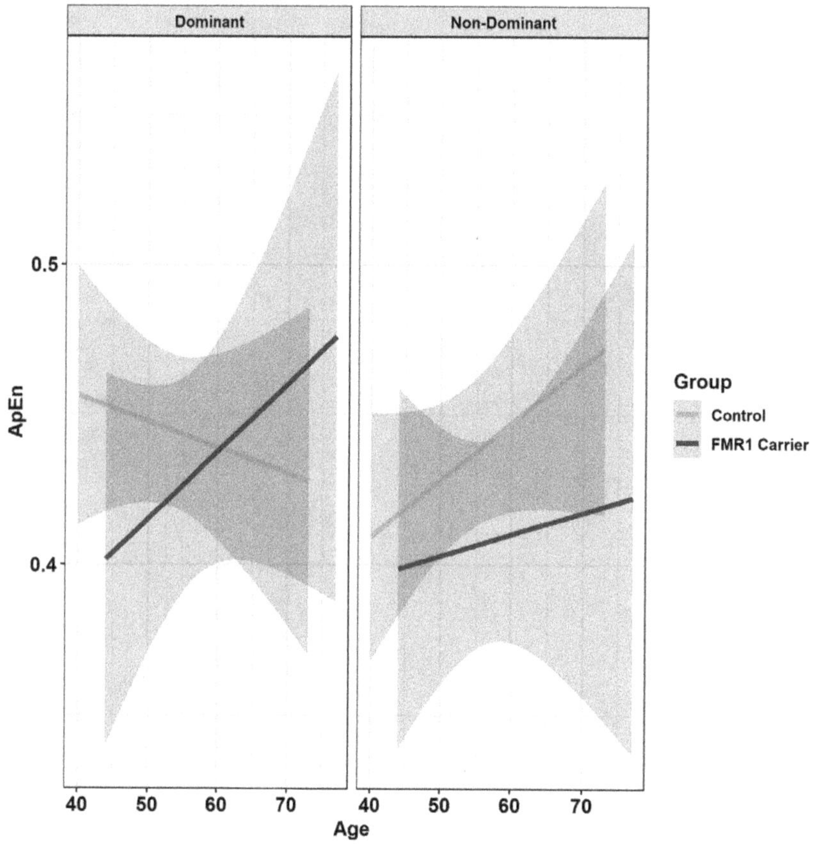

FIGURE 7 | Approximate entropy (ApEn; i.e., force complexity) as a function of group,% MVC, and age (linear fit with 95% confidence intervals). Younger premutation carriers demonstrated reduced force complexity compared to controls when using their non-dominant hand, but premutation carriers only showed reduced force complexity compared to controls at younger but not older ages when using their non-dominant hand.

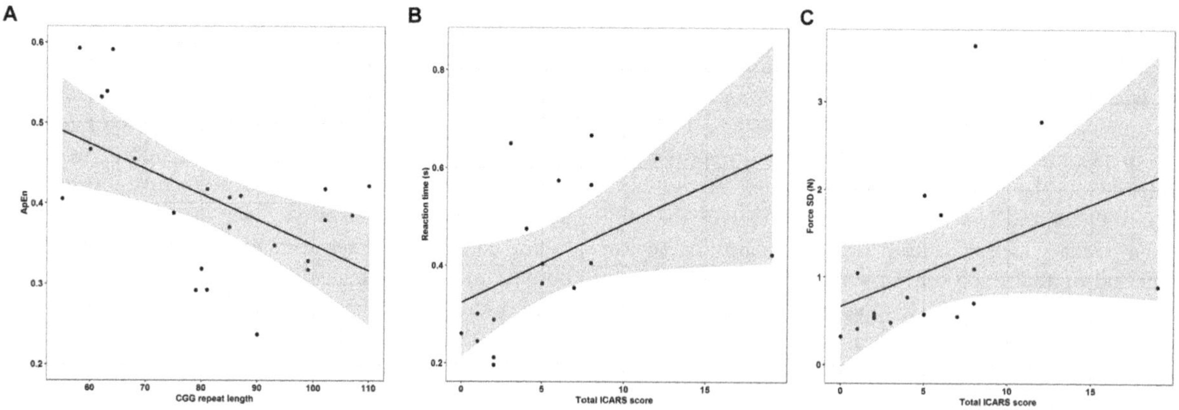

FIGURE 8 | (A) CGG repeat length is associated with reduced dominant hand approximate entropy (ApEn) at 45% MVC. Error bars represent 95% CI of a linear fit. **(B)** Increased ICARS rated FXTAS symptoms are associated with longer reaction times (data shown is from rapid test dominant hand trials at 45% MVC). Error bars represent 95% CI of a linear fit. **(C)** Increased ICARS rated FXTAS symptoms are associated with increased force variability (force SD) during the non-dominant hand 45% MVC condition. Error bars represent 95% CI of a linear fit.

symptoms suggesting that sustained sensorimotor dysmetria may be present in aging premutation carriers who are showing or beginning to show disease-related clinical issues. Ultimately, due to the relatively small effect sizes of ApEn interactions, it will be important to systematically assess sustained sensorimotor control targeting premutation carriers at the younger age range of our sample (i.e., 45–60 years) and in relation to FXTAS symptoms over time to determine the power of our

TABLE 6 | Correlational analyses of CGG and sensorimotor outcomes (Spearman ρ values).

		2 s ("Rapid")			8 s ("Sustained")		
		MVC level			MVC level		
	Dependent variable	**15%**	**45%**	**85%**	**15%**	**45%**	**85%**
Dominant hand	Rise phase reaction time	0.54**	0.37	0.26	0.44*	0.12	0.23
	Rate of force increase	0.10	0.14	0.15	−0.13	0.04	−0.10
	Rise phase duration	0.21	0.13	0.11	0.02	0.12	0.07
	Rise phase accuracy	−0.09	−0.08	−0.28	0.02	−0.05	−0.01
	ApEn	–	–	–	−0.33	−0.53**	−0.45*
	Force SD	–	–	–	0.22	0.19	0.32
	Mean force	–	–	–	−0.11	−0.13	−0.16
	Rate of force relaxation	−0.17	−0.01	−0.08	−0.27	0.12	0.14
Non-dominant Hand	Rise phase reaction time	0.30	0.38	0.40	0.46*	0.36	0.45*
	Rate of force increase	−0.09	0.02	−0.19	0.09	−0.22	−0.37
	Rise phase duration	0.30×10^{-2}	0.06	0.15	0.39	0.35	0.34
	Rise phase accuracy	0.17	0.40	−0.07	0.29	0.27	−0.25
	ApEn	–	–	–	−0.39	−0.45*	−0.38
	Force SD	–	–	–	0.35	0.18	0.08
	Mean force	–	–	–	−0.09	−0.10	−0.07
	Rate of force relaxation	0.11	0.07	0.22	−0.10	−0.17	0.24

*MVC: maximum voluntary contraction; CGG: cytosine-guanine-guanine; *$p < 0.05$; **$p < 0.01$. Rates of force relaxation are negative values, and so positive correlations indicate that an increase in CGG repeat length is associated with slower (i.e., less negative) rates of force relaxation.*

TABLE 7 | Correlational analyses of total ICARS scores and sensorimotor outcomes (Spearman ρ values).

		2 s ("Rapid")			8 s ("Sustained")		
		MVC level			MVC level		
	Dependent variable	**15%**	**45%**	**85%**	**15%**	**45%**	**85%**
Dominant hand	Rise phase reaction time	0.52*	0.70**	0.67**	0.61**	0.18	0.34
	Rate of force increase	0.09	0.11	0.30	−0.09	−0.16	0.11
	Rise phase duration	−0.05	−0.11	−0.09	−0.21	0.07	0.09
	Rise phase accuracy	−0.21	−0.04	−0.23	−0.11	0.12	−0.42
	ApEn	–	–	–	−0.18	0.02	−0.20
	Force SD	–	–	–	0.22	0.40	0.41
	Mean force	–	–	–	0.14	0.08	0.09
	Rate of force relaxation	−0.39	−0.43	−0.44	−0.27	−0.16	−0.10
Non-dominant hand	Rise phase reaction time	0.46	0.52*	0.67**	0.37	0.44	0.25
	Rate of force increase	−0.11	−0.04	−0.07	−0.22	−0.05	−0.09
	Rise phase duration	−0.22	−0.13	−0.19	-0.20×10^{-2}	0.13	-0.20×10^{-2}
	Rise phase accuracy	−0.10	0.19	0.03	−0.04	0.22	−0.43
	ApEn	–	–	–	−0.40	−0.17	−0.38
	Force SD	–	–	–	0.34	0.66**	0.58*
	Mean force	–	–	–	0.09	0.14	0.11
	Rate of force relaxation	−0.34	−0.03	0.02	0.12	−0.01	0.38

*MVC: maximum voluntary contraction; ICARS: International Cooperative Ataxia Rating Scale; *$p < 0.05$; **$p < 0.01$. Rates of force relaxation are negative values, and so positive correlations indicate that an increase in CGG repeat length is associated with slower (i.e., less negative) rates of force relaxation.*

objective measures of sensorimotor behavior to track FXTAS progression and risk.

Sensorimotor Behavior and FXTAS Symptoms

In addition to identifying multiple sensorimotor behavioral alterations in aging *FMR1* premutation carriers, we also document multiple relationships between sensorimotor behavior and clinical symptoms of FXTAS. We found that increased reaction time and increased force variability each were associated with more severe clinically rated neuromotor issues in premutation carriers suggesting that quantifiable deficits in precision sensorimotor behaviors may be part of the aging process in *FMR1* premutation carriers, or that these issues may reflect early indicators of neurodegeneration associated with FXTAS. Our findings that slower reaction times across multiple task conditions (e.g., target force level, task length, hand) are associated with more severe clinical symptoms provide evidence that initial motor preparation and planning processes may deteriorate as part of the progression of FXTAS. Degeneration of premotor responses in individuals showing clinical signs of FXTAS may result from degeneration of motor fiber tracts that limits rapid processing of sensory information and generation of action plans (Greco et al., 2006; Wang et al., 2013). Our finding that greater force variability is associated with more severe FXTAS symptoms in premutation carriers indicates that a reduced ability to precisely maintain a steady motor output in response to sensory feedback information may track with developing symptoms in premutation carriers. Increased sustained force variability also is consistent with known neuropathological indicators of FXTAS. As individuals sustain a constant level of force using visual feedback, visual input is translated into motor corrections through parietal-ponto-cerebellar pathways. The MCP serves as the primary white matter input pathway relaying parietal-ponto visual feedback information to cerebellar circuits that encode reactive motor corrections to cortex (Stein and Glickstein, 1992). Degeneration of the MCP, reflected as hyperintensities on T2-weighted scans, is symptomatic of FXTAS and may contribute to both greater sensorimotor variability and FXTAS clinical symptoms (Jacquemont et al., 2003).

Based on prior studies showing that greater CGG repeat length among premutation carriers increases risk for FXTAS (Tassone et al., 2007), our finding that reduced ApEn was related to increased CGG repeat length in premutation carriers also suggests that sustained sensorimotor behavioral issues may covary with disease risk. From a more mechanistic perspective, greater CGG repeat length in the premutation range contributes to increased mRNA transcript, sequestration of proteins, and intranuclear inclusions (Greco et al., 2006; Li and Jin, 2012). These inclusions have been documented in pontine and cerebellar cells in the majority of cases studied to date (Greco et al., 2006; Ariza et al., 2016), suggesting that greater CGG repeat length compromises ponto-cerebellar functions. The atypical sensorimotor behaviors identified in this study are consistent with this model and may serve as objective biobehavioral targets useful for understanding pathophysiological processes associated with FXTAS and quantifying clinically relevant changes in aging premutation carriers.

Limitations

Several limitations of the present study should be acknowledged. First, larger samples of FXTAS patients and asymptomatic premutation carriers are needed to examine variability in sensorimotor behavior during aging and determine disease-specific markers. Longitudinal samples are needed to track disease onset and progression and clarify the extent to which objective measures of sensorimotor precision may track with disease course. Second, it will be important to include movement disorder comparison groups in future studies of aging premutation carriers to determine the specificity of our sensorimotor markers to *FMR1* premutation carriers, though we propose that the next critical step is to determine the specificity of key sensorimotor issues to symptomatic compared to asymptomatic *FMR1* premutation carriers so that disease presence can be reliably identified in aging individuals who test positive for premutation alleles. Third, our sample consisted primarily of females who are at reduced risk for FXTAS relative to males. Despite 75% of our sample being female, we established multiple sensorimotor issues in aging premutation carriers and identified multiple participants, both male and female, showing FXTAS symptoms. Inclusion of females in FXTAS studies is warranted, though larger samples that allow for direct comparisons of sensorimotor behavior in aging males and females are needed. Fourth, while we report behavioral findings in relation to CGG repeat length, measures of mRNA, methylation ratios, and FMR protein are important for clarifying how aberrant neurobiological processes contribute to FXTAS risk or prodromal symptoms. Last, as with many hypothesis generating studies, the relatively small effect sizes of some of our group interactions highlight the need for replication. Still, our findings identify multiple sensorimotor targets and highlight important task conditions and demographic features that can be focused upon (e.g., increased sampling of middle-aged carriers) to characterize neurodegenerative processes associated with *FMR1* premutation alleles and FXTAS.

CONCLUSION

Our results identify multiple precision sensorimotor issues in aging *FMR1* premutation carriers and indicate that select sensorimotor alterations track with FXTAS symptom severity. Together, these findings suggest that subclinical deficits of precision sensorimotor behavior may be detectable prior to the onset of FXTAS and serve as objective targets for tracking disease risk and monitoring disease progression.

ETHICS STATEMENT

This study was carried out in accordance with the recommendations of the University of Texas Southwestern Medical Center Institutional Review Board with written informed consent from all subjects. All subjects gave written informed consent in accordance with the Declaration of Helsinki. The protocol was approved by the University of Texas Southwestern Medical Center Institutional Review Board.

AUTHOR CONTRIBUTIONS

MM was responsible for the conception and design of the study. PK and SW performed the clinical evaluations for *FMR1* premutation carriers. SL provided the radiological evaluations of the T2 scan images for premutation carriers. MM, ZW, and SW collected the behavioral data. ZW wrote the MATLAB scoring programs for the data analyses. MM, WM, and SK scored the raw data, performed the statistical analyses, and interpreted the results. WM and MM drafted and edited the manuscript. All authors approved the final version of the manuscript.

FUNDING

A Once Upon a Time Foundation award provided funds for the study design, data collection, and data analysis. U54 HD090216 provided support for WM and MM during the data analysis and interpretation.

ACKNOWLEDGMENTS

The authors thank the participants for their time and effort in participating in the study. The authors also thank Dr. Kandace Fleming at the Life Span Institute, University of Kansas for her significant assistance and consultation in the construction and interpretation of the statistical models.

REFERENCES

Aguilar, D., Sigford, K. E., Soontarapornchai, K., Nguyen, D. V., Adams, P. E., Yuhas, J. M., et al. (2008). A quantitative assessment of tremor and ataxia in FMR1 premutation carriers using CATSYS. *Am. J. Med. Genet. A* 146A, 629–635. doi: 10.1002/ajmg.a.32211

Ariza, J., Rogers, H., Hartvigsen, A., Snell, M., Dill, M., Judd, D., et al. (2017). Iron accumulation and dysregulation in the putamen in fragile X-associated tremor/ataxia syndrome. *Mov. Disord.* 32, 585–591. doi: 10.1002/mds.26902

Ariza, J., Rogers, H., Monterrubio, A., Reyes-Miranda, A., Hagerman, P. J., and Martinez-Cerdeno, V. (2016). A majority of FXTAS cases present with intranuclear inclusions within purkinje cells. *Cerebellum* 15, 546–551. doi: 10.1007/s12311-016-0776-y

Bates, D., Machler, M., Bolker, B. M., and Walker, S. C. (2015). Fitting linear mixed-effects models using lme4. *J. Stat. Softw.* 67, 1–48.

Bravo, G. A., Fernandez-Carril, J. M., Lopez-Zuazo, I., Izquierdo, A. Y., Abrol, T., and Alsinaidi, O. (2018). A novel clinical phenotype of fragile X-associated tremor/ataxia syndrome. *Mov. Disord. Clin. Pract.* 5, 430–432. doi: 10.1002/mdc3.12637

Brunberg, J. A., Jacquemont, S., Hagerman, R. J., Berry-Kravis, E. M., Grigsby, J., Leehey, M. A., et al. (2002). Fragile X premutation carriers: characteristic MR imaging findings of adult male patients with progressive cerebellar and cognitive dysfunction. *AJNR Am. J. Neuroradiol.* 23, 1757–1766.

Chu, W. T., and Sanger, T. D. (2009). Force variability during isometric biceps contraction in children with secondary dystonia due to cerebral palsy. *Mov. Disord.* 24, 1299–1305. doi: 10.1002/mds.22573

Desmurget, M., Epstein, C. M., Turner, R. S., Prablanc, C., Alexander, G. E., and Grafton, S. T. (1999). Role of the posterior parietal cortex in updating reaching movements to a visual target. *Nat. Neurosci.* 2, 563–567. doi: 10.1038/9219

Desmurget, M., and Grafton, S. (2000). Forward modeling allows feedback control for fast reaching movements. *Trends Cogn. Sci.* 4, 423–431. doi: 10.1016/s1364-6613(00)01537-0

Ehrsson, H. H., Fagergren, A., Jonsson, T., Westling, G., Johansson, R. S., and Forssberg, H. (2000). Cortical activity in precision- versus power-grip tasks: an fMRI study. *J. Neurophysiol.* 83, 528–536. doi: 10.1152/jn.2000.83.1.528

Fellows, S. J., Noth, J., and Schwarz, M. (1998). Precision grip and Parkinson's disease. *Brain* 121(Pt 9), 1771–1784. doi: 10.1093/brain/121.9.1771

Ghez, C., Hening, W., and Gordon, J. (1991). Organization of voluntary movement. *Curr. Opin. Neurobiol.* 1, 664–671. doi: 10.1016/S0959-4388(05)80046-7

Grafton, S. T., and Tunik, E. (2011). Human basal ganglia and the dynamic control of force during on-line corrections. *J. Neurosci.* 31, 1600–1605. doi: 10.1523/Jneurosci.3301-10.2011

Greco, C. M., Berman, R. F., Martin, R. M., Tassone, F., Schwartz, P. H., Chang, A., et al. (2006). Neuropathology of fragile X-associated tremor/ataxia syndrome (FXTAS). *Brain* 129(Pt 1), 243–255. doi: 10.1093/brain/awh683

Grigsby, J., Brega, A. G., Engle, K., Leehey, M. A., Hagerman, R. J., Tassone, F., et al. (2008). Cognitive profile of fragile X premutation carriers with and without fragile X-associated tremor/ataxia syndrome. *Neuropsychology* 22, 48–60. doi: 10.1037/0894-4105.22.1.48

Hagerman, R. J., Leehey, M., Heinrichs, W., Tassone, F., Wilson, R., Hills, J., et al. (2001). Intention tremor, parkinsonism, and generalized brain atrophy in male carriers of fragile X. *Neurology* 57, 127–130. doi: 10.1212/WNL.57.1.127

Hagerman, R. J., Pak, J. S., Ortigas, M., Olichnew, J., Frysinger, R., Harrison, M., et al. (2012). Case series: deep brain stimulation in patients with FXTAS. *Brain Disord. Ther.* 1:104. doi: 10.4172/2168-975X.1000104

Healy, D. G., Bressman, S., Dickson, J., Silveira-Moriyama, L., Schneider, S. A., Sullivan, S. S., et al. (2009). Evidence for pre and postsynaptic nigrostriatal dysfunction in the fragile X tremor-ataxia syndrome. *Mov. Disord.* 24, 1245–1247. doi: 10.1002/mds.22267

Homberg, V., Hefter, H., Reiners, K., and Freund, H. J. (1987). Differential effects of changes in mechanical limb properties on physiological and pathological tremor. *J. Neurol. Neurosurg. Psychiatry* 50, 568–579. doi: 10.1136/jnnp.50.5.568

Jacquemont, S., Hagerman, R. J., Leehey, M., Grigsby, J., Zhang, L., Brunberg, J. A., et al. (2003). Fragile X premutation tremor/ataxia syndrome: molecular, clinical, and neuroimaging correlates. *Am. J. Hum. Genet.* 72, 869–878. doi: 10.1086/374321

Jacquemont, S., Hagerman, R. J., Leehey, M. A., Hall, D. A., Levine, R. A., Brunberg, J. A., et al. (2004). Penetrance of the fragile X-associated tremor/ataxia syndrome in a premutation carrier population. *JAMA* 291, 460–469. doi: 10.1001/jama.291.4.460

Juncos, J. L., Lazarus, J. T., Graves-Allen, E., Shubeck, L., Rusin, M., Novak, G., et al. (2011). New clinical findings in the fragile X-associated tremor ataxia syndrome (FXTAS). *Neurogenetics* 12, 123–135. doi: 10.1007/s10048-010-0270-5

Koller, M. (2016). robustlmm: an R package for robust estimation of linear mixed-effects models. *J. Stat. Softw.* 75, 1–24. doi: 10.18637/jss.v075.i06

Kraan, C. M., Hocking, D. R., Georgiou-Karistianis, N., Metcalfe, S. A., Archibald, A. D., Fielding, J., et al. (2013). Cognitive-motor interference during postural control indicates at-risk cerebellar profiles in females with the FMR1 premutation. *Behav. Brain Res.* 253, 329–336. doi: 10.1016/j.bbr.2013.07.033

Kremer, E. J., Yu, S., Pritchard, M., Nagaraja, R., Heitz, D., Lynch, M., et al. (1991). Isolation of a human DNA sequence which spans the fragile X. *Am. J. Hum. Genet.* 49, 656–661.

Kuhtz-Buschbeck, J. P., Gilster, R., Wolff, S., Ulmer, S., Siebner, H., and Jansen, O. (2008). Brain activity is similar during precision and power gripping with light force: an fMRI study. *Neuroimage* 40, 1469–1481. doi: 10.1016/j.neuroimage.2008.01.037

Lechpammer, M., Cerdeno, V. M., Hunsaker, M. R., Hah, M., Gonzales, H., Tisch, S., et al. (2017). Concomitant occurrence of FXTAS and clinically defined sporadic inclusion body myositis: report of two cases. *Croat. Med. J.* 58, 310–315. doi: 10.3325/cmj.2017.58.310

Leehey, M. A., Berry-Kravis, E., Min, S. J., Hall, D. A., Rice, C. D., Zhang, L., et al. (2007). Progression of tremor and ataxia in male carriers of the FMR1 premutation. *Mov. Disord.* 22, 203–206. doi: 10.1002/mds.21252

Li, Y., and Jin, P. (2012). RNA-mediated neurodegeneration in fragile X-associated tremor/ataxia syndrome. *Brain Res.* 1462, 112–117. doi: 10.1016/j.brainres.2012.02.057

Lozano, R., Rosero, C. A., and Hagerman, R. J. (2014). Fragile X spectrum disorders. *Intractable Rare Dis. Res.* 3, 134–146. doi: 10.5582/irdr.2014.01022

Luke, S. G. (2017). Evaluating significance in linear mixed-effects models in R. *Behav. Res. Methods* 49, 1494–1502. doi: 10.3758/s13428-016-0809-y

McAuley, J. H., and Marsden, C. D. (2000). Physiological and pathological tremors and rhythmic central motor control. *Brain* 123(Pt 8), 1545–1567. doi: 10.1093/brain/123.8.1545

Mosconi, M. W., Mohanty, S., Greene, R. K., Cook, E. H., Vaillancourt, D. E., and Sweeney, J. A. (2015). Feedforward and feedback motor control abnormalities implicate cerebellar dysfunctions in autism spectrum disorder. *J. Neurosci.* 35, 2015–2025. doi: 10.1523/JNEUROSCI.2731-14.2015

Neely, K. A., Coombes, S. A., Planetta, P. J., and Vaillancourt, D. E. (2013). Segregated and overlapping neural circuits exist for the production of static and dynamic precision grip force. *Hum. Brain. Mapp.* 34, 698–712. doi: 10.1002/hbm.21467

Niu, Y. Q., Yang, J. C., Hall, D. A., Leehey, M. A., Tassone, F., Olichney, J. M., et al. (2014). Parkinsonism in fragile X-associated tremor/ataxia syndrome (FXTAS): revisited. *Parkinsonism Relat. Disord.* 20, 456–459. doi: 10.1016/j.parkreldis.2014.01.006

O'Keefe, J. A., Robertson-Dick, E., Dunn, E. J., Li, Y., Deng, Y., Fiutko, A. N., et al. (2015). Characterization and early detection of balance deficits in fragile X premutation carriers with and without fragile X-associated tremor/ataxia syndrome (FXTAS). *Cerebellum* 14, 650–662. doi: 10.1007/s12311-015-0659-7

Park, S. H., Wang, Z., McKinney, W., Khemani, P., Lui, S., Christou, E. A., et al. (2019). Functional motor control deficits in older FMR1 premutation carriers. *Exp. Brain Res.* 237, 2269–2278. doi: 10.1007/s00221-019-05566-3

Pinheiro, J. C., Liu, C. H., and Wu, Y. N. (2001). Efficient algorithms for robust estimation in linear mixed-effects models using the multivariate t distribution. *J. Comput. Graph. Stat.* 10, 249–276. doi: 10.1198/10618600152628059

Potter, N. L., Kent, R. D., Lindstrom, M. J., and Lazarus, J. A. (2006). Power and precision grip force control in three-to-five-year-old children: velocity control precedes amplitude control in development. *Exp. Brain Res.* 172, 246–260. doi: 10.1007/s00221-005-0322-5

Prodoehl, J., Corcos, D. M., and Vaillancourt, D. E. (2009). Basal ganglia mechanisms underlying precision grip force control. *Neurosci. Biobehav. Rev.* 33, 900–908. doi: 10.1016/j.neubiorev.2009.03.004

Przybyla, A., Haaland, K. Y., Bagesteiro, L. B., and Sainburg, R. L. (2011). Motor asymmetry reduction in older adults. *Neurosci. Lett.* 489, 99–104. doi: 10.1016/j.neulet.2010.11.074

Raw, R. K., Wilkie, R. M., Culmer, P. R., and Mon-Williams, M. (2012). Reduced motor asymmetry in older adults when manually tracing paths. *Exp. Brain Res.* 217, 35–41. doi: 10.1007/s00221-011-2971-x

Reilly, J. L., Lencer, R., Bishop, J. R., Keedy, S., and Sweeney, J. A. (2008). Pharmacological treatment effects on eye movement control. *Brain Cogn.* 68, 415–435. doi: 10.1016/j.bandc.2008.08.026

Rodriguez-Revenga, L., Madrigal, I., Pagonabarraga, J., Xuncla, M., Badenas, C., Kulisevsky, J., et al. (2009). Penetrance of FMR1 premutation associated pathologies in fragile X syndrome families. *Eur. J. Hum. Genet.* 17, 1359–1362. doi: 10.1038/ejhg.2009.51

Roid, G. H. (2003). *Stanford-Binet Intelligence Scales, Fifth Edition: Technical Manual.* Itasca, IL: Riverside Publishing.

Rose, J., and McGill, K. C. (2005). Neuromuscular activation and motor-unit firing characteristics in cerebral palsy. *Dev. Med. Child Neurol.* 47, 329–336. doi: 10.1017/S0012162205000629

Scaglione, C., Ginestroni, A., Vella, A., Dotti, M. T., Nave, R. D., Rizzo, G., et al. (2008). MRI and SPECT of midbrain and striatal degeneration in fragile X-associated tremor/ataxia syndrome. *J. Neurol.* 255, 144–146. doi: 10.1007/s00415-007-0711-8

Schmitz-Hubsch, T., Tezenas du Montcel, S., Baliko, L., Boesch, S., Bonato, S., Fancellu, R., et al. (2006). Reliability and validity of the international cooperative ataxia rating scale: a study in 156 spinocerebellar ataxia patients. *Mov. Disord.* 21, 699–704. doi: 10.1002/mds.20781

Schneider, A., Ballinger, E., Chavez, A., Tassone, F., Hagerman, R. J., and Hessl, D. (2012). Prepulse inhibition in patients with fragile X-associated tremor ataxia syndrome. *Neurobiol. Aging* 33, 1045–1053. doi: 10.1016/j.neurobiolaging.2010.09.002

Schoch, B., Regel, J. P., Frings, M., Gerwig, M., Maschke, M., Neuhauser, M., et al. (2007). Reliability and validity of ICARS in focal cerebellar lesions. *Mov. Disord.* 22, 2162–2169. doi: 10.1002/mds.21543

Shickman, R., Famula, J., Tassone, F., Leehey, M., Ferrer, E., Rivera, S. M., et al. (2018). Age- and CGG repeat-related slowing of manual movement in fragile X carriers: a prodrome of fragile X-associated tremor ataxia syndrome? *Mov. Disord.* 33, 628–636. doi: 10.1002/mds.27314

Slifkin, A., and Newell, K. M. (1999). Noise, information transmission, and force variability. *J. Exp. Psychol. Hum. Percept. Perform.* 25, 837–851. doi: 10.1037/0096-1523.25.3.837

Soontarapornchai, K., Maselli, R., Fenton-Farrell, G., Tassone, F., Hagerman, P. J., Hessl, D., et al. (2008). Abnormal nerve conduction features in fragile X premutation carriers. *Arch. Neurol.* 65, 495–498.doi:10.1001/archneur.65.4.495

Stein, J. F., and Glickstein, M. (1992). Role of the cerebellum in visual guidance of movement. *Physiol. Rev.* 72, 967–1017. doi: 10.1152/physrev.1992.72.4.967

Stelmach, G. E., and Worringham, C. J. (1988). The preparation and production of isometric force in Parkinson's disease. *Neuropsychologia* 26, 93–103. doi: 10.1016/0028-3932(88)90033-4

Tassone, F., Adams, J., Berry-Kravis, E. M., Cohen, S. S., Brusco, A., Leehey, M. A., et al. (2007). CGG repeat length correlates with age of onset of motor signs of the fragile X-associated tremor/ataxia syndrome (FXTAS). *Am. J. Med. Genet. B Neuropsychiatr. Genet.* 144B, 566–569. doi: 10.1002/ajmg.b.30482

Trouillas, P., Takayanagi, T., Hallett, M., Currier, R. D., Subramony, S. H., Wessel, K., et al. (1997). International Cooperative Ataxia Rating Scale for pharmacological assessment of the cerebellar syndrome. The ataxia neuropharmacology committee of the world federation of neurology. *J. Neurol. Sci.* 145, 205–211. doi: 10.1016/S0022-510X(96)00231-6

Vaillancourt, D. E., and Newell, K. M. (2000). Amplitude changes in the 8-12, 20-25, and 40 Hz oscillations in finger tremor. *Clin. Neurophysiol.* 111, 1792–1801. doi: 10.1016/S1388-2457(00)00378-3

Vaillancourt, D. E., Slifkin, A. B., and Newell, K. M. (2001a). Intermittency in the visual control of force in Parkinson's disease. *Exp. Brain Res.* 138, 118–127. doi: 10.1007/s002210100699

Vaillancourt, D. E., Slifkin, A. B., and Newell, K. M. (2001b). Regularity of force tremor in Parkinson's disease. *Clin. Neurophysiol.* 112, 1594–1603. doi: 10.1016/S1388-2457(01)00593-4

Vaillancourt, D. E., Slifkin, A. B., and Newell, K. M. (2001c). Visual control of isometric force in Parkinson's disease. *Neuropsychologia* 39, 1410–1418. doi: 10.1016/S0028-3932(01)00061-6

Vaillancourt, D. E., Thulborn, K. R., and Corcos, D. M. (2003). Neural basis for the processes that underlie visually guided and internally guided force control in humans. *J. Neurophysiol.* 90, 3330–3340. doi: 10.1152/jn.00394.2003

Wang, J. Y., Hessl, D., Schneider, A., Tassone, F., Hagerman, R. J., and Rivera, S. M. (2013). Fragile X-associated tremor/ataxia syndrome: influence of the FMR1 gene on motor fiber tracts in males with normal and premutation alleles. *JAMA Neurol.* 70, 1022–1029. doi: 10.1001/jamaneurol.2013.2934

Wang, Z., Khemani, P., Schmitt, L. M., Lui, S., and Mosconi, M. W. (2019). Static and dynamic postural control deficits in aging fragile X mental retardation 1 (FMR1) gene premutation carriers. *J. Neurodev. Disord.* 11:2. doi: 10.1186/s11689-018-9261-x

Wang, Z., Kwon, M., Mohanty, S., Schmitt, L. M., White, S. P., Christou, E. A., et al. (2017). Increased force variability is associated with altered modulation of the motorneuron pool activity in autism spectrum disorder (ASD). *Int. J. Mol. Sci.* 18:E698. doi: 10.3390/ijms18040698

Wang, Z., Magnon, G. C., White, S. P., Greene, R. K., Vaillancourt, D. E., and Mosconi, M. W. (2015). Individuals with autism spectrum disorder show abnormalities during initial and subsequent phases of precision gripping. *J. Neurophysiol.* 113, 1989–2001. doi: 10.1152/jn.00661.2014

Zuhlke, C., Budnik, A., Gehlken, U., Dalski, A., Purmann, S., Naumann, M., et al. (2004). FMR1 premutation as a rare cause of late onset ataxia - Evidence for FXTAS in female carriers. *J. Neurol.* 251, 1418–1419. doi: 10.1007/s00415-004-0558-1

9

Molecular Systems Biology of Neurodevelopmental Disorders, Rett Syndrome as an Archetype

Victor Faundez [1], *Meghan Wynne* [1], *Amanda Crocker* [2] *and Daniel Tarquinio* [3]*

[1]*Department of Cell Biology, Emory University, Atlanta, GA, United States,* [2]*Program in Neuroscience, Middlebury College, Middlebury, VT, United States,* [3]*Rare Neurological Diseases (Private Research Institution), Atlanta, GA, United States*

***Correspondence:**
Daniel Tarquinio
daniel@rareneuro.com

Neurodevelopmental disorders represent a challenging biological and medical problem due to their genetic and phenotypic complexity. In many cases, we lack the comprehensive understanding of disease mechanisms necessary for targeted therapeutic development. One key component that could improve both mechanistic understanding and clinical trial design is reliable molecular biomarkers. Presently, no objective biological markers exist to evaluate most neurodevelopmental disorders. Here, we discuss how systems biology and "omic" approaches can address the mechanistic and biomarker limitations in these afflictions. We present heuristic principles for testing the potential of systems biology to identify mechanisms and biomarkers of disease in the example of Rett syndrome, a neurodevelopmental disorder caused by a well-defined monogenic defect in methyl-CpG-binding protein 2 (MECP2). We propose that such an approach can not only aid in monitoring clinical disease severity but also provide a measure of target engagement in clinical trials. By deepening our understanding of the "big picture" of systems biology, this approach could even help generate hypotheses for drug development programs, hopefully resulting in new treatments for these devastating conditions.

Keywords: Rett, autism, biomarker, clinical trials, genealogical proteomics, precision medicine

INTRODUCTION

Rett syndrome is a devastating neurodevelopmental disorder caused by mutations in a gene responsible for both activating and repressing gene transcription: methyl CpG binding protein 2 gene (*MECP2*; Amir et al., 1999). Rett syndrome is an X linked disease that predominantly affects females (prevalence approximately 1:10,000 females; Leonard et al., 1997; Bienvenu et al., 2006; Wong and Li, 2007). Through the process of lyonization (X-chromosome inactivation), patient tissues become mosaic for *MECP2*, as both normal and mutated versions of *MECP2* are expressed. The ratio of mutant to non-mutant protein in mosaic tissue is in part responsible for determining the severity of the disorder in the individual (Amir et al., 2000). Although apparently normal in early infancy, children with Rett syndrome fail to achieve milestones in late infancy, then undergo a period of regression of language and hand use, followed by emergence of pervasive repetitive hand movements known as stereotypies. The regression period is often associated with social withdrawal, and the disorder has been classified in the past as part of the autism spectrum (Percy, 2011). However, after children with Rett syndrome emerge from the regression period, they enter a phase of stability, often with subtle developmental gains or losses, but almost never regain meaningful verbal language or hand use (Downs et al., 2010). They require constant care, often living into their 5th or 6th decade with waxing and waning periodic medical and neurological comorbidities, including epilepsy, periodic breathing disorder, disturbances of mood and behavior, pervasive growth failure, scoliosis, movement disorder, various sleep disorders, osteopenia, abnormal pubertal development, electrocardiograms with prolonged cardiac QT interval, and numerous gastrointestinal disorders (Glaze et al., 1987; FitzGerald et al., 1990; Ellaway et al., 1999; Motil et al., 2012; Tarquinio et al., 2012, 2015, 2017, 2018; Cuddapah et al., 2014; Killian et al., 2014; Jefferson et al., 2016).

Few neurodevelopmental disorders appear as amenable to targeted treatment as Rett syndrome based on preclinical evidence (Pozzo-Miller et al., 2015; Katz et al., 2016). Neurons in both individuals with Rett syndrome and mice with *Mecp2* mutations undergo normal migration but suggest developmental arrest of synaptic connections (Armstrong, 2005; Chapleau et al., 2009). No evidence of degeneration exists, and several studies have demonstrated rescue of neuropathological abnormalities in mouse models, even in adult animals (Guy et al., 2007; Robinson et al., 2012; Garg et al., 2013). Despite this evidence, human trials have failed to produce clinically meaningful change (Katz et al., 2016). On closer examination, although the preclinical evidence supporting therapeutic strategies appears strong, these disappointing trial results may stem from faulty assumptions about how these results would translate into humans. These assumptions can be divided into two broad categories: (1) mechanistic assumptions about MECP2 function; and (2) efficacy assumptions regarding how specific outcomes seen in a murine model would actually present in a human.

Molecular strategies using "omic" approaches can help to inform both the mechanisms of MeCP2 dysfunction and the pathophysiological changes we would expect to see in humans if these dysregulated mechanisms were put right. These strategies help to fill in gaps in our understanding of how dysregulated transcription of the targets of MeCP2 can result in such a protean disorder as Rett syndrome. Moreover, the findings of a comprehensive "omic" approach could result in biomarkers at various levels downstream of MeCP2. Optimally, this would result in molecular biomarkers to differentiate which populations of patients will respond best to a specific treatment, and at what developmental stage, to optimize dosing of treatment. Such biomarkers would also serve as a surrogate outcome measure of improvement in the core characteristics of disease and associated comorbidities. The omics approach accounts for the role fundamental biological components play in disease, and an omics-based biomarkers discovery program would allow for translation from basic molecular mechanisms to clinically meaningful surrogate outcome measures. A deep understanding of "omic"-based molecular phenotypes in Rett syndrome could provide a portfolio of biomarkers suitable for many drug development and clinical trial approaches.

In an effort to both improve outcome measures and develop biomarkers for Rett syndrome, the multi-center Rett syndrome Outcome Measures and Biomarker Development program[1] was established. Over the past 2 years, the program has collected data on a host of caregiver-reported, clinician-reported, and performance outcome measures in Rett syndrome subjects, and also tested a number of approaches to biomarker data collection, ranging from biometric recordings of physiological function (ECG, induction plethysmography, galvanic skin response, accelerometer and gyroscope recording of movement) to sampling tissue. This review focuses on one of the most promising approaches we have investigated, that of global interrogation of tissue protein expression.

During its inception, the principal investigators considered a number of targeted biomarkers in serum, cerebrospinal fluid (CSF), and other tissues. These included hormones such as leptin, ghrelin, and adiponectin (Blardi et al., 2009; Hara et al., 2011), and cortisol levels (Echenne et al., 1991). We also considered physiological markers such as skin temperature (Symons et al., 2015), and both eye tracking and pupillometry (Farzin et al., 2011; Rose et al., 2013). Since our initial review, other targeted markers have received attention, including immune and enzymatic markers as well as neurophysiological tests such as auditory and visual evoked potentials (Papini et al., 2014; LeBlanc et al., 2015; Hayek et al., 2017; Key et al., 2019). Ultimately, since all of these biomarkers are far downstream to the regulatory effects exerted by the MeCP2 protein, we opted to focus on a minimally biased global approach to measure the effects of dysregulation due to loss of function in *MECP2*.

We have collected skin biopsies and whole blood on approximately two dozen families (often as trios with parents and affected child) and banked these tissues for testing of "omic" biomarkers. We are also currently in the process of evaluating the results of multi-tissue omics in the *Mecp2* null male mouse to evaluate the degree to which translational assumptions from the animal model to the human hold true. The focus on male mice, as a first step, stems from the fact that most published research in Rett mouse models has been carried out in males. This approach has been embraced in an effort to minimize experimental noise introduced by brain X chromosome mosaicism in female Rett models (Braunschweig et al., 2004; Chahrour and Zoghbi, 2007; Renthal et al., 2018). However, it is clear that studies in the male model of MeCP2 loss of function must be validated in female mice to rigorously validate the potential of these biomarkers for translation into the human disease.

WHAT IS THE SYSTEMS BIOLOGY AND MULTI-"OMIC" APPROACH, AND WHY IS IT RELEVANT TO NEURODEVELOPMENTAL DISORDERS?

Neurodevelopmental disorders are profoundly complex. The hypothesis that they can be understood based on reducing them to their component parts is attractive, but not likely to be true. No disorders illustrate this case more clearly than the autism spectrum disorders, now recognized collectively as a common neurodevelopmental disability (Xu et al., 2018). Complex behavioral disorders involving multiple components of an intricate network warrant a complex explanation. Thus,

[1] https://reverserett.org/research/consortia/outcome-measures-and-biomarkers-development/

the prospect that autism can be reduced to understanding the molecular biology of a single gene and protein product, so called "naïve reductionism," is untenable (Bloom, 2001; Strange, 2005). The list of autism "risk" genes, currently over 1,000, grows each year, and, due to the multi-dimensional nature of the disorder, one would be led to believe that no unifying "cause" of autism could exist (Ayhan and Konopka, 2019)[2].

Although a unifying explanation for such a complex disorder may seem far-fetched, examples of monogenetic disorders associated with autism, such as Rett syndrome, do exist. In these monogenetic disorders, perturbation of a single gene producing a single protein product causes complex neurodevelopmental disorders with a host of systemic comorbidities and striking heterogeneity. Because a deep understanding of these examples could prove seminal for this common disease, researchers have designed monogenic knockout animal models of these rare diseases and sought to understand neurodevelopmental disorders like autism from the base up (Sztainberg and Zoghbi, 2016). In the case of specific examples of syndromic autism, the explanation for how a single gene mutation can result in such a complex neurodevelopmental disorder often lies in the complex function of the protein product of the mutated gene; in Rett syndrome, MeCP2 regulates the transcription of a host of genes yet to be identified, which may number over 1,000 (Horvath and Monteggia, 2017).

While models of syndromic autism created to understand non-syndromic autism spectrum disorder, such as the mouse models of Rett syndrome and Fragile X syndrome, have reasonable construct validity and face validity, predictive validity, the ability to translate improvements in the animal to improvements in the human, has been a harder target to hit. A number of pathways amenable to human translation have been identified, and clinical trials have examined the effects of intervention in these pathways downstream of the dysfunctional protein. In these clinical trials, we expected that restoration of systems dysregulated by the causative gene would result in meaningful clinical improvement in humans. However, to date, results of these approaches have been disappointing in terms of clinical outcome measures.

A Brief History of Clinical Investigations and Therapeutic Trials in Rett Syndrome

Historically, Rett syndrome was the first pervasive developmental disorder with an identified monogenetic cause (Neul and Zoghbi, 2004). Much can be understood about neurodevelopmental disorders in general by deepening our understanding of this prototypical disorder. To understand why the omics approach can be a useful addition to the drug development process for neurodevelopmental disorders, it helps to understand the approach to molecular investigation and clinical trials. As an illustrative example, we will discuss the history of these issues in Rett syndrome.

The Rett Pathological Phenotype

The search for viable therapeutic targets in Rett syndrome began with neuropathology. The brain of Rett syndrome patients is globally abnormal, with brain weight in all age groups reduced to 60%–88% of expected weight (Jellinger et al., 1988). Structural changes include reduced volume of frontal cortex and deep nuclei; as in Parkinson disease, the substantia nigra exhibits reduced pigmentation (Jellinger, 2003). Notably, the overall appearance of the brain is normal; however, the brain is smaller, and the neuropil is denser. Neurons are both smaller and more tightly packed, and dendrites are shorter with less mature arborization (Armstrong, 1997). Overall, the neuropathology indicates developmental arrest rather than degeneration of synaptic connections (Kaufmann et al., 2005). Because Rett syndrome was historically considered as a progressive disease, with passage to a "late motor degeneration," researchers expected to find evidence of degeneration. The fact that the pathology is not consistent with the clinical decline originally attributed to patients with the disorder has led to a rethinking of the degenerative aspect of Rett syndrome (Bauman et al., 1995). Now most experts consider the normal neuronal migration, involvement of multiple neurotransmitter systems, and immature dendrites as suggestive of developmental arrest rather than neurodegeneration, and the period of arrest correlates with development in the third trimester or during early infancy (Armstrong, 2002). Together, these findings of stable developmental arrest hold promise for the premise of establishing a disease-modifying treatment.

Unraveling *MECP2* Dysfunction and Cellular Phenotype

Experimental models of Rett syndrome have helped to elucidate the neuropathological phenotype seen in humans. In murine models with mutations in *Mecp2*, both in cases of deficient or absent protein, early development is normal, after which synapses fail to mature and synaptic reorganization is deficient (Boggio et al., 2010). Recently, the structure of *MECP2* was examined and the contribution of mutations to its structural destabilization elucidated, yet the molecular mechanisms linking abnormal MeCP2 function and Rett syndrome remain largely unclear (Spiga et al., 2019). There is a wide gap of molecular knowledge between the genotype and the phenotype, which we refer to here as the mesoscale gap, encompassing how cells, tissues and organs behave in the presence of a *MECP2* mutation. A number of general explanations have been proposed to explain the mesoscale gap., Evidence supports the notions that calcium-dependent activation is abnormal in response to synaptic stimulation, and that the loss of MeCP2's epigenetic function disrupts synaptic reorganization (Chen et al., 2003). The concept of "synaptopathy" has been related to many of the clinical features present in Rett syndrome patients. Indeed, long-term potentiation is normal in early life in Mecp2 deficient mice; however, when they become symptomatic, long-term potentiation becomes abnormal, consistent with the clinical regression of language and hand use seen in patients (Weng et al., 2011). Along with decreased Mecp2 levels, the post-synaptic

[2]https://www.sfari.org/resource/sfari-gene/

protein PSD-95 is decreased, and both excitatory and inhibitory signaling are abnormal (Chao et al., 2007).

The protein MeCP2 is primarily an epigenetic protein, responsible for both repression and induction of gene transcription, as well as regulation of chromatin organization (Lyst and Bird, 2015). While MeCP2 is primarily expressed in brain tissue, the protein can be found expressed in all tissues (Kaddoum et al., 2013). When MeCP2 is either absent or functions abnormally, this results in immature neurons. Several mechanisms for this have been proposed including: over-transcription of certain genes (expected when a transcription repressor is decreased), abnormal gene repression, increased transcriptional noise, and downstream effects on other processes (Kerr and Ravine, 2003). Human point mutations have been reproduced in animals, and the degree of affinity of MeCP2 for methylated DNA correlates with severity of the mutation type for missense mutations. Although MeCP2 protein is still produced in missense mutations, an R106W mutation (which results in a severe human phenotype) decreases the affinity of MeCP2 for methylated DNA by 100-fold, whereas T158M (resulting in a less severe phenotype) only reduces binding moderately (Kudo et al., 2001). The least severe human phenotype associated with an R133C mutation in MECP2 displays similar DNA binding to that of the wild-type protein (Ballestar et al., 2000).

Both *MECP2* gain of function and loss of function cause severe neurodevelopmental disorders in humans. Although many phenotypic similarities to *MECP2* loss of function exist (intellectual disability, poor or absent speech, repetitive behaviors, seizures), individuals with *MECP2* duplication syndrome exhibit prominent anxiety, atypical social interaction, and recurrent infections (Ramocki et al., 2009; Van Esch, 2011). Based on animal studies, *MECP2* dosing has been correlated with both morphologic changes and dendritic spine density of neurons (Larimore et al., 2009). When rat embryonic hippocampal neurons are cultured with reduced levels of normal *MECP2*, shorter dendrites with normal axon length result, whereas mutant *MECP2* results in both shorter axons and dendrites. However, as one might hypothesize, overexpression by 2-fold of *MECP2* yields both longer axons and dendrites. In postnatal hippocampal slice cultures from the rat, decreased *MECP2* results in decreased spine density, while overexpression has no effect on spine density (Chapleau et al., 2009).

The excitatory-inhibitory balance is abnormal in Rett syndrome models, reflecting changes in multiple neurotransmitter systems (Shahbazian et al., 2002). In patients with Rett syndrome, CSF dopamine metabolites are reduced to 19% and serotonin metabolites to 23% of normal levels. This effect is more pronounced with severe mutations (Samaco et al., 2009). GABAergic neurons in the cortex express 50% more MeCP2 than other cortical neurons. When *MECP2* is knocked out in GABAergic cells, the human respiratory, compulsive, motor, and social phenotypes associated with Rett syndrome are recapitulated. In particular, repetitive behaviors that mimic human stereotypies are present (Chao et al., 2010). In astrocytes, dendritic and synaptic abnormalities have been associated with excessive glutamate secretion, but the clearance rate may be a culprit as well, as has been suggested by cultured knockout astrocytes with elevated glutamate clearance; this results in decreased down-regulation of excitatory amino acid transporters and excessive glutamate synthetase production (Okabe et al., 2012). Abnormal GABA release may explain prevalent seizures (Medrihan et al., 2008) while the motor and cardiorespiratory features seen in both humans and mouse models may be due to abnormal excitatory neurotransmitter release (Kron et al., 2012). When MeCP2 is selectively decreased in GABA-releasing neurons, the model exhibits repetitive behaviors, again similar to the human stereotypies, suggesting these may be due to abnormal GABAergic function (Chao et al., 2010).

The brainstem in Rett syndrome exhibits multiple abnormalities. One of these is abnormal serotonin transporter binding in the dorsal motor nucleus of the vagus, which may result in abnormal autonomic control and subsequent gastrointestinal and cardiac dysfunction (Paterson et al., 2005). In the hippocampus, synaptic connections are dysfunctional, and this could be associated with the deficits in socialization and motor apraxia in humans with Rett syndrome (Moretti et al., 2006). The hypothalamic-pituitary-adrenal axis also demonstrates abnormalities, including enhanced corticotropin-releasing hormone expression, and this could contribute to the anxiety which is prevalent in Rett syndrome (McGill et al., 2006). Brain-derived neurotrophic factor (BDNF) levels are lower than expected in the nucleus tractus solitarius, which may correlate with abnormal neuronal gating and cardiorespiratory abnormalities in Rett syndrome (Kline et al., 2010). Tyrosine hydroxylase expressing neurons are fewer in both the medulla and locus coeruleus, resulting in low levels of norepinephrine (Taneja et al., 2009). In human autopsy studies, patients with Rett syndrome have age-related changes in the glutamatergic system and NMDA receptors; at a younger age, NMDA receptor levels are increased, whereas, at an older age, NMDA receptor levels are decreased. These findings have been reproduced in *Mecp2* knockout mice (Blue et al., 2011) and may be explained by the potential regulation by MeCP2 of splicing of the NMDA subunit NR1 (Young et al., 2005). In support of this hypothesis, deletion of the NMDA receptor subunit NR2A prevents progressive visual loss in Mecp2 deficient mice (a feature not seen in humans with the disease, however; Durand et al., 2012). Collectively, these findings suggest two alternative models which remain unresolved. First, all these phenotypes are due to common MeCP2 gene targets that generate different phenotypic outcomes in different cell types or different brain regions. Alternatively, MeCP2 regulates gene expression in a cell and tissue-specific manner. These alternative hypotheses can be resolved by the identification of genes whose expression is regulated by MeCP2.

If MeCP2 Regulates Gene Transcription, What Are Its Targets?

Remarkably, despite 20 years since the discovery that *MECP2* loss of function mutations cause Rett syndrome, only a handful of putative target genes have been identified, and both the degree to which MeCP2 regulates these and the direction of dysregulation remain unclear (Amir et al., 1999; Na et al., 2013). This is despite the clear picture of dysfunction present in multiple neurotransmitter systems. Techniques such as chromatin immunoprecipitation (ChIP) combined with RNA sequencing and/or quantitative proteomics, as we will discuss below, could solve this issue entirely. In fact, recent efforts pairing experimental design with mathematical modeling are heading in this direction (Cholewa-Waclaw et al., 2019).

Although one would expect mutations in a protein responsible for DNA methylation to result in derepression of genes, this is simply not the case—instead, modest increases and decreases in gene transcription are seen in tissues (Chahrour et al., 2008; Ben-Shachar et al., 2009). There are 1,200 neuronally expressed genes sensitive to MECP2 genetic defects, as demonstrated in mouse brain or human iPSC-derived neurons (Chahrour and Zoghbi, 2007; Chahrour et al., 2008; Tanaka et al., 2014). Few of these genes have been comprehensively analyzed.

Among the few examples, regulation of BDNF by Mecp2 is both important and paradoxical. The Mecp2 protein exhibits a repressive effect on the *Bdnf* promotor (Wade, 2004). One would predict that derepression of *Bdnf* in the *Mecp2* deficient animal would result in overexpression of the BDNF protein. However, in the knockout *Mecp2* mouse model BDNF levels are low (Sun and Wu, 2006). No satisfying explanation for this phenomenon exists, although researchers have hypothesized that either reduced synaptic activity on a global level or a feedback mechanism involving over-transcription of other repressors could decrease BDNF levels. If BDNF is overexpressed in the *Mecp2* knockout mouse, this results in partial rescue of the phenotype (Chang et al., 2006; Wang et al., 2006). One study found that Mecp2 regulates the squalene epoxidase gene in mice; this gene is critical for cholesterol metabolism, and the evidence from a large suppressor screen study in the mouse model is compelling for this association. These data were supported by a study of *MECP2* in cultured human fibroblasts (Buchovecky et al., 2013b; Segatto et al., 2014).

One strategy to sort out the targets of MeCP2 regulation involves biotin tagging in female mice expressing loss-of-function mutations that cause disease in humans (Johnson et al., 2017). Using this method, the authors identified a distinct difference in gene expression between wild type cells in these animals and cells harboring a disease-causing mutation. Furthermore, they identified differences in transcript expression between the mutations in fold-changes of the transcriptome. Unfortunately, this approach does not address the problem that decreased levels of MeCP2 could independently alter gene transcription, nor does it account for the poor correlation between transcriptome and proteome found in a number of studies (Gygi et al., 1999; Chen et al., 2002; Pascal et al., 2008; Ghazalpour et al., 2011; Yeung, 2011; Horvath and Monteggia, 2017). In terms of the general classes of genes found to be upregulated or downregulated, one study found that long genes are upregulated and another found the opposite to be true (Gabel et al., 2015; Johnson et al., 2017).

TARGETED THERAPEUTICS—A ROLE FOR "OMICS"?

Despite a paucity of mechanistic arrows to connect the dots between disease phenotypes and abnormal neurotransmitters and growth factors, a number of clinical trials have been undertaken to attempt to restore abnormalities in these systems. These clinical trials were conceived to attempt to rectify the downstream dysfunction identified in both human tissues and in animal models. We have published a detailed account of these studies, so will only briefly discuss them here (Katz et al., 2016). No current strategy for treating the underlying cause of Rett syndrome exists, i.e., restoring *MECP2* function. However, ten specific dysregulated systems have been identified which are amenable to currently available therapeutics. The burden of the disorder is so high that a number of clinical trials have been undertaken with varying degrees of preclinical evidence to support them. Each has held promise, and over half were conducted with a blinded, placebo-controlled design. Although all studies reported some positive or statistically significant results, and in many cases both physicians and caregivers believed the drugs were beneficial, none have led to the adoption of a clinically meaningful treatment beyond standard supportive care. In our detailed review of these studies, we discuss the possible reasons for what amounts to failed clinical trials. In some cases, the effect, if present, was trivial. In others, the effect appeared clear in specific individuals, but the overall effect on the group was negligible. In still other cases, the improvements described by physicians and caregivers were not adequately captured in the study outcome measures. The result in all cases was that the study results were difficult to interpret.

Clinical trials are both time consuming and expensive. In rare diseases, this point is driven home by the small potential participant pool, and the fatigue induced by asking the same families to participate in trial after trial. Moreover, recent proposed studies have included both more potent drugs, such as the dissociative anesthetic Ketamine, and more risky approaches, such as injectable drugs like Copaxone and Insulin-like Growth Factor-1. Most recently, treatment strategies have turned to gene therapy, approaches in which the wild type *MECP2* gene is added to neurons using a viral vector. However, uncertainty surrounds the gene therapy clinical trial planned for 2019, since *MECP2* dosing is critical and cannot be regulated by such an approach. The strategies behind "omics" have the potential to address all of these issues: first, by providing the earliest possible indication of cellular response, or target engagement; second, by monitoring response to the treatment, both for dosing and toxicity measurements; third, as a predictive biomarker to determine response of individual subjects; and fourth, as a surrogate biomarker for clinical response. Moreover, "omic" biomarkers could provide a window into monitoring in the clinic that would prove invaluable for anticipatory guidance and targeting resources like therapy services.

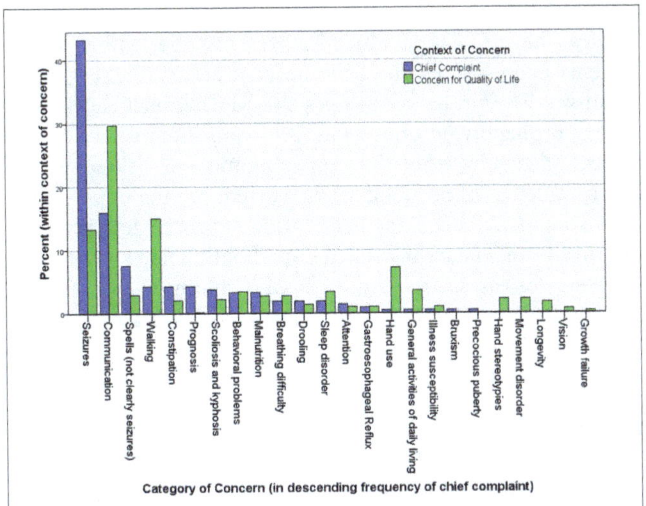

FIGURE 1 | The chief complaints (221) and other "concerns" (586) in 113 Rett syndrome patients seen in the author's (DT) clinic over a period of 2 years. Caregivers are asked to name their primary reason for the visit at the beginning of the interview. After discussing this and all related medical issues, they are asked to name the top three concerns they would address if they could. They are asked to name problems that are major contributors to morbidity that they would address if a "cure" were available, without considering available treatments. Unexpectedly, when posed this question at the end of a visit, caregivers often raise concerns for which a treatment actually exists, but that they failed to raise during the discussion of medical care.

One critical problem with therapeutic trials of drugs is that their efficacy evaluation mostly rests in clinical assessments. In Rett syndrome, the list of clinical concerns is long and complex, so summarizing these in the form of an outcome measure has proven difficult (**Figure 1**). Rett syndrome is heterogeneous on a number of levels; although four core criteria unite the group (loss of hand use and verbal language, hand stereotypies, and abnormal gait), the concerns of caregivers vary widely, and the factors contributing to disease burden are a moving target, often waxing and waning spontaneously.

A host of outcome measures and biomarkers have been used in clinical trials to try to capture this assortment of signs and symptoms (**Table 1**). Because none warrant the moniker "gold standard," most trials have chosen an assortment of outcomes, rarely using the same metric more than once, all of which have amounted to exploratory measurements. We posit that systems biology and the use of comprehensive "omics" tools to identify biomarkers hold promise for not only detecting appropriate changes in functional gene product with treatment but also potentially providing a window to measure dosing of a vector-based treatment approach. The fundamental principle is that a complex system can be understood better by considering it in its entirety, including dimensions such as time, space, and context, rather than through naïve reductionism.

The process of global, unbiased querying of systems downstream of the genetic code, involving techniques referred to as "omics" or "multi-omics," has opened the door to a vast amount of information about function, protein and genetic interactions, gene product expression, metabolite and lipid content, and complex feedback processes that integrate these molecules into pathways and in time and space. This approach has been called a "new era in *systems biology*." We define systems biology as the study of "biological systems by systematically perturbing them (biologically, genetically, or chemically); monitoring the gene, protein, and informational pathway responses; integrating these data; and ultimately, formulating mathematical models that describe the structure of the system and its response to individual perturbations" (Ideker et al., 2001; Hood et al., 2004; Weston and Hood, 2004; Hillmer, 2015). Systems biology has the potential to connect the dots between dysregulation of a single protein and a complex phenotype like Rett syndrome (Hood et al., 2004; Weston and Hood, 2004; Haas et al., 2017). The components of the "omics" are described briefly below. Taken together each can be compared to the "phenome," or the sum of traits exhibited by an organism and its component parts.

Genomics

Studies the genome, which constitutes the complete genetic material of an organism. It contains the basal information for building organisms and their cells in their whole diversity. The ability to sequence the genome once held the promise of explaining all phenotypic characteristics of human disease. However, the sequence information in the genome is static and phenotypic outcomes in human disease emerge from interactions between the genome and environment.

Epigenomics

Analyzes the modification of the structure of chromatin and modifications to DNA (such as methylation), which are referred to as the epigenome. The characterization of these modifications is the field of epigenomics. The epigenome is influenced by the environmental history of an organism, thus modifying gene expression and phenotypic outcomes. A number of known monogenic causes of autism and other neurodevelopmental disorders, including Rett syndrome, Fragile X syndrome, Angelman syndrome, and Prader-Willi syndrome, are caused by genes responsible for epigenetic modifications (Egger et al., 2004). As such, to understand the dysfunction wrought by mutations in these genes, we need to look downstream into gene expression.

Transcriptomics

Measures the transcriptome, the set of all RNAs expressed by a cell, group of cells, tissue, or organ. The transcriptome provides information about when and where genes are activated or inactivated, therefore offering a proxy for the "functional" state of a cell, tissue, or organ. The entire transcriptome can be assessed using RNA-seq, which can yield information about the presence and expression levels of an RNA, as well as splice variants, gene fusion, mutations and modifications to RNAs occurring after their transcription such as editing (Wang et al., 2009; Spies and Ciaudo, 2015).

TABLE 1 | Fifty-one outcome measures and biomarkers used in 25 clinical trials of Rett syndrome.

Category	Type	Metric
Outcome measure	Scale (Clinician)	Clinical Rett syndrome stage*
		Bayley scales of infant development
		Peabody Developmental Motor Scales
		Gesell developmental observation
		Mullen scales of early learning
		Motor behavioral assessment*
		Rett syndrome: SSI*
		Portage guide for early education (Gross/fine motor development, cognition, socialization)
		Hand Apraxia Scale
		Clinical Severity Score*
		Clinical global impression of severity and improvement
		Kerr Severity Scale*
		Aberrant behavior checklist
	Scale (Caregiver)	Vineland Adaptive Behavior Scales
		Patient well-being index
		Short-form 36
		Rett syndrome behavioral questionnaire*
		Anxiety, depression, and mood scale
		Visual analog scale of caregiver concerns
		Pediatric QOL (caregiver proxy)
		Screen for social interaction
	Clinical exam	Stereotypies
		Ambulation
		Bruxism
		Breathing dysregulation
		Social interaction
		Alertness
		Mobility and tone
		Behavior
		"Autonomic" function (breathing dysrhythmia, drooling)
		Visual attention
		Timed gait testing
	Caregiver diary	Percent reduction in seizures
		Seizure frequency
		Sleep patterns
		Overall improvement by parental report
Biomarker	Blood	Routine laboratory testing (complete blood count, serum chemistry)
		Brain-derived neurotrophic factor level
		Metabolic measures of oxidative stress
	Cerebrospinal fluid	Biogenic amines
		Brain-derived neurotrophic factor level
	Neurophysiology	Qualitative EEG features
		Quantitative EEG (frontal alpha asymmetry)
		EEG spike frequency
	Polygraphy	Induction plethysmography
		Polysomnography sleep efficiency
		Apnea index
		Respiratory disturbance index
	General physiology	Peripheral oxygen saturation
		Somatic growth
		Head circumference

*Adapted from Katz et al. (2016). *Indicates Rett syndrome specific scale.*

Proteomics

Studies the proteome which, represents the entire set of proteins expressed by the genome of a cell, tissue, organ, or organism. The proteome bridges the gap between the genetic code and phenotypic expression. Proteomic complexity cannot be predicted fully from the transcriptome (see below), and is not completely understood using current technology (Harper and Bennett, 2016). Nonetheless, this approach has provided improved understanding of the pathophysiology of cancer, infectious diseases, pre-term birth, and common diseases such as hypertension (Romero et al., 2006; Casado-Vela et al., 2011; Waterer, 2012; Tebani et al., 2016; Jean Beltran et al., 2017; Arnett and Claas, 2018).

Cistromics

The cistrome is the collection of all cis-acting targets associated to a particular trans-acting factor, such as MeCP2, at a genome-wide scale (Liu et al., 2011). Among the cistromic strategies, a powerful approach particularly relevant to *MEPC2* biology is ChIP. This technique is a hybrid of the previously mentioned strategies and permits identification of genome-wide DNA or RNA binding sites for transcription factors and other proteins. Sites are identified by immunoprecipitation of a desired protein with DNA or RNA binding capacity, followed by sequencing of the coprecipitated nucleic acid. This approach enables the identification of the putative binding sites of transcription factors, sites of epigenetic modifications in DNA and chromatin (ENCODE Project Consortium et al., 2007; ENCODE Project Consortium, 2011).

Metabolomics, Lipidomics, and Ionomics

The interaction of products of the genetic code results in an assortment of measurable phenotypic characteristics, and these have been organized into the above categories, including metabolites, lipid components, and elemental components.

We argue that the use of each one of these omic approaches, alone or in combination, is uniquely poised to identify statistically prioritized mechanisms of disease and molecular biomarkers in neurodevelopmental disorders (Mullin et al., 2013). In the next section, we discuss Rett syndrome as a prime candidate to test the power of molecular systems biology and omics approaches in the discovery of mechanisms of disease and molecular biomarkers.

GENOTYPE-PHENOTYPE ASSOCIATIONS IN RETT SYNDROME: AN INCOMPLETE STORY

Hundreds of specific *MECP2* mutations exist and the phenotypic variability of these is striking. Greater than 99% of these mutations are caused by mutations in the paternal germline, which are spontaneous; only the vast minority are inherited from mothers, who are carriers. A database cataloging both pathogenic and nonpathogenic mutations lists over 200 pathogenic mutations in *MECP2*, including eight common point mutations (four missense mutations and four nonsense mutations), and many 3′ truncations and deletions of entire exons. Together, these are found in more than 80% of individuals with Rett syndrome (Percy, 2011). In addition to the approximately 200 causative mutations, many mutations in *MECP2* have never been linked to neurodevelopmental disease (Krishnaraj et al., 2017). A minority have been associated with particularly mild cases, for example, the "preserved-speech" variant of Rett syndrome (Zappella, 1992; De Bona et al., 2000). Still others have been associated with altogether different syndromes. The A140V point mutation is the best example of this and causes PPM-X syndrome, consisting of psychosis, pyramidal signs, and macro-orchidism (Klauck et al., 2002). Although predominantly seen in males, an adolescent onset syndrome involving the A140V point mutation was described in a female with parkinsonian features and cognitive regression in adolescence (Venkateswaran et al., 2014). Although they demonstrate profoundly different human phenotypes, the mouse models that have been created with these specific human point mutations all exhibit the same neuropathological features, including abnormal neuropil density, and decreased dendritic complexity (Chapleau et al., 2009; Jentarra et al., 2010).

Considering the common mutations associated with the classic phenotype of the disorder, substantial clinical overlap exists, such that statistically significant differences in human phenotype among the mutations can only be found in large data sets between the absolute extremes of the genotypic severity scale (Cuddapah et al., 2014). In fact, it is not difficult to find an individual with the "mildest" mutation, R133C, who is phenotypically more severe than an individual with the most severe mutation, R168X. When specific components of the disease, such as seizure severity and breathing dysregulation are considered, although trends of severity can be found with respect to genotype, these are subtle, non-significant associations (Tarquinio et al., 2017, 2018).

Much of the clinical heterogeneity, even with identical point mutations, owes to the role of *MECP2* itself. The MeCP2 protein serves diverse functions that include modulation of DNA methylation, acetylation at lysine residues, interacting with RNA to influence splicing, and direct activation and repression of gene transcription. Because Rett syndrome is considered an X-linked dominant disease, lyonization (random silencing of one of the X-chromosomes in each cell early in embryonic development) has been invoked to explain this variability (Amir et al., 2000). Some individuals with very mild disease, and rare asymptomatic carriers have been identified and shown to have markedly skewed X-chromosome inactivation. Because testing can only be done easily on blood or buccal tissue, these tests only comment on peripheral silencing of the mutant gene. This is presumed to represent (to some unknown degree) X-chromosome inactivation in the brain (Huppke et al., 2006; Hardwick et al., 2007). Monozygotic twins are unusual but several pairs exist, and phenotypes are often different; this may be due to skewed X-chromosome inactivation (Ishii et al., 2001). However, X-chromosome inactivation does not explain most of the variability present in Rett syndrome (Bao et al., 2008), and may, in fact, be misleading (Takahashi et al., 2008). Other possible variables include clonal expansion of the mutant X-chromosome, but this is almost impossible to test clinically. The best example of these processes is the Calico cat, in whom patches of different hair color on every cat are the result of random distribution of X-chromosomes from the maternal and paternal cell lines during dermatogenesis. Because neurogenesis would exhibit similar clonal expansion, the distribution of mutant *MECP2* will randomly differ in various brain regions. This will occur even in Rett syndrome twins, even those with skewed X-chromosome inactivation. Although the distribution of mutant *MECP2* cannot be tested on neuronal tissue *in vivo* without invasive testing (Gibson et al., 2005), recent technological advances have made it possible to do so in select tissues (Renthal et al., 2018).

WHY IS RETT SYNDROME AN IDEAL NEURODEVELOPMENTAL DISORDER TO TESTS SYSTEMS BIOLOGY TO IDENTIFY BIOMARKERS?

Our quest for molecular biomarkers in Rett syndrome begins with the fundamental problem that there are no objective biological markers for diagnosing or evaluating any of the forms of autism spectrum disorder (Uddin et al., 2017). This fact is rooted in part on the complexity of the disease, with the majority of cases being polygenic, and the phenomenological diagnosis, which is defined by observational clinical features rather than standardized biochemical or molecular measurements (Bailey et al., 1996; Risch et al., 1999). Although no molecular biomarkers have been tied to *MECP2* dysfunction, Rett syndrome is one of the few monogenic forms of autism spectrum disorder (Katz et al., 2012; Leonard et al., 2017).

Criteria for an Ideal Disorder to Test Molecular Biomarkers

Defining molecular biomarkers for autism spectrum disorder, or any neurodevelopmental disorder, could be best materialized by considering the following heuristic criteria:

1. Disorder definition should ideally be founded on unequivocal genetic diagnosis, as is the case with Rett syndrome, or any other monogenic neurodevelopmental disorder. Rett syndrome is caused by mutations in methyl-CpG-binding protein 2 (MECP2) in >95% of patients meeting consensus clinical diagnostic criteria (Neul et al., 2010, 2014; Cuddapah et al., 2014).
2. If the disorder is well-defined genetically, then the gene affected should ideally have loss- and gain-of-function mutations in humans with a certain degree of phenotypic overlap. MECP2 mutations are ideal in this regard, as Rett syndrome is the result of loss-of-function mutations in MECP2, while duplication of the MECP2 gene causes a distinctive syndrome, the MECP2 duplication syndrome, that shares autism symptoms with Rett (OMIM: 300005[3]; Ramocki et al., 2009; Lombardi et al., 2015; Leonard et al., 2017).

[3]https://www.omim.org/entry/300005?search=mecp2&highlight=mecp2

3. High phenotypic penetrance of the mutation and consistency should exist in the clinical phenotype. Rett syndrome manifests mostly with autism and intellectual disability symptoms (Percy, 2011). This is in contrast with other neurodevelopmental disorders that can present themselves as multiple psychopathologies, even though the genetic defects are well defined, as is the case with copy number variations (Girirajan et al., 2011; Rutkowski et al., 2017).
4. There should be some knowledge about mechanisms of disease at any biological complexity level. Mechanisms of disease exist in a pathogenesis continuum along increasing levels of biological complexity. This continuum spans from the mechanisms most proximal to the mutation, such as is the role of *MECP2* as a transcriptional regulator, to mesoscale processes affected by the mutation, like cell and tissue mechanisms, to macroscale phenotypes at the level of circuit or anatomical brain dysfunction.
5. Animal and cellular models of disease should genetically and phenotypically reproduce disease features (Katz et al., 2012). These animal models are essential because they offer unlimited experimental access to all tissues, developmental stages, and levels of biological complexity along a pathogenesis continuum.
6. Cell and tissue analysis should not be constrained to neurons and brain tissue, even if the most salient pathology and clinical features point to the brain. This assertion is founded on the observation that most brain genes are expressed in diverse tissues (Uhlén et al., 2015). We would like to emphasize that in addition to searching for common mechanisms of disease shared among tissues, the advantage of conceptualizing disease as a systemic/multiorgan disorder is the immediate translational implication that biomarkers of disease could be explored in accessible tissues. For example, we could sample biomarkers in patient tissues, such as muscle, or fluids more accessible than the brain. Take for example genes involved in lipid and cholesterol metabolism, whose expression is controlled by MECP2 in brain cortex and liver (Buchovecky et al., 2013a; Kyle et al., 2016). The concept that organ-specific diseases express molecular phenotypes in multiple tissues other than the affected organ has been tested comprehensively in mouse models of organ-specific pathologies (Kozawa et al., 2018).

Rett syndrome fulfills some of these criteria for the search of biomarkers. However, we still know little about mesoscale cell and tissue mechanisms disrupted by MECP2 genetic defects (Katz et al., 2012). Despite this, we have a plethora of information about the most mutation-proximal mechanisms of MECP2 loss-of-function as a transcriptional regulator and the circuit consequences of MECP2 mutations (Na et al., 2013). The most proximal mechanisms to the mutation stem from the molecular function of MECP2 as a transcriptional regulator/repressor capable of inducing up- or down-regulation of gene transcription (Lyst and Bird, 2015; Cholewa-Waclaw et al., 2018). Nearly 1,200 neuronally expressed genes are sensitive to MECP2 genetic defects, as demonstrated in mouse brain or human iPSC-derived neurons (Chahrour and Zoghbi, 2007; Chahrour et al., 2008; Tanaka et al., 2014). These transcripts are involved in processes including neuronal differentiation, neuronal morphology and size, and function of excitatory and inhibitory synapses (Smrt et al., 2007; Chahrour et al., 2008; Na et al., 2012; Qiu et al., 2012; Yang et al., 2012). These facts about the diversity of MECP2 transcriptional targets raise key questions related to the identification of Rett syndrome molecular biomarkers: First, do gene expression products sensitive to MECP2 expression converge on discrete pathways that can be scrutinized? If there exists a molecular pathogenesis, is it shared among different cell types, regions, and developmental stages of the brain? Finally, are MEPC2 molecular mechanisms associated with MECP2-deficiency in the brain shared by non-neuronal tissues? These critical questions should inform where, when, and how we search for molecular biomarkers of disease. However, the answers to these questions still await resolution.

We favor cellular, tissue, and organ mesoscale gene and protein expression analyses of proteins or RNAs to identify potential biomarkers in animal cells and tissues as a first step. These findings can then be translated to human samples. Expression analyses allow facile exploration of biomarkers while considering the challenges and questions just described. Results from cell to organ mesoscale searches can be scaled down to be interpreted and tested in the context of mechanistic hypotheses closer to the role of MECP2 in transcriptional regulation. Conversely, the disruption of these biomarkers can be assessed in macroscale mechanisms of disease to assess their contribution to circuit dysfunction or anatomical phenotypes. The most comprehensive approach to identify mesoscale mechanisms of disease and potential biomarkers is the genome-wide interrogation of gene expression. As described above, expression can be measured at the level of coding and non-coding regulatory RNAs, as well as the proteins, transcriptomes and proteomes, respectively. Transcriptomes sample expression across the whole genome of a cell, tissue, organ, or biological fluid. The proteome coverage is at a half of all encoded proteins in humans, which are estimated to be around 20,000 (International Human Genome Sequencing Consortium, 2004; Beck et al., 2011; ENCODE Project Consortium, 2011; Nagaraj et al., 2011; Wilhelm et al., 2014). Proteomes and transcriptomes have the added advantage of being hereditable molecular phenotypes, allowing their use in family trait studies (Wu et al., 2013; Parts et al., 2014; Wright et al., 2014; Huang et al., 2015). In the case of cellular proteomes, we have demonstrated they follow genealogical relationships among subjects within a pedigree and segregate those with the disease from their non-diseased/unaffected family members (Gokhale et al., 2018; Zlatic et al., 2018). This strategy can be carried further with the pairing of classical twin studies, a number of which have been published in Rett families, and the novel techniques discussed here (van Dongen et al., 2012). The proteome has the distinctive advantage of being the executor of phenotypic programs in cells and tissues. Thus, it has the highest probability of identifying biomarkers of disease and disease mechanisms not yet recognized.

Expression levels between proteomes and transcriptomes partially correlate in normal tissues and cells

(Maier et al., 2009; Ghazalpour et al., 2011; Vogel and Marcotte, 2012). This is in part due to interplay between the coding transcriptome and the non-coding transcriptome that modulates the extent of protein expression. The partial correlation between coding transcriptome and proteome is likely to be disrupted in Rett syndrome. Defects in MECP2 alter the expression of regulatory non-coding RNA that in turn influences translation of defined mRNAs (Klein et al., 2007; Im et al., 2010; Cheng et al., 2014; Tsujimura et al., 2015). Surprisingly, even though we have catalogs of genes whose RNA expression is regulated by MECP2, we have limited understanding at a global scale of how MECP2-dependent transcriptome modifications translate into protein expression profiles in MECP2 deficient cells and tissues. Only one recent study compares the transcriptome and proteome of symptomatic Mecp2 null male mice, yet the authors report global expression correlations (Pacheco et al., 2017). In general, other proteome studies in Rett syndrome are limited in number, rely on outdated technology, and are of small sample size (Matarazzo and Ronnett, 2004; Cortelazzo et al., 2013, 2014, 2017).

The present status of "omic" technologies and the power of bioinformatic tools to distill information out of complex datasets calls for their use in renewed studies on monogenic and polygenic forms of neurodevelopmental disorders, in particular, Rett syndrome. Importantly, proteomes and transcriptomes could catalyze the discovery of cell-to-organ mesoscale disease mechanisms and biomarkers in Rett syndrome. This discovery potential stems from the capacity of these technologies to comprehensively and unbiasedly sample molecular phenotypes, irrespective of how distal a molecular phenotype is from its genetic defect.

THE RELEVANCE OF DEEPER UNDERSTANDING OF MeCP2 FUNCTION

Caregivers of individuals with Rett syndrome recognize the degree of dysfunction on many levels. Although the diagnostic criteria consist of four components, the concerns raised by caregivers evoke a more complete picture of both the neurological and systemic implications of the disorder (**Figure 1**). One can envision a monitoring biomarker that could be used to gauge dysfunction in specific pathways downstream of MeCP2. This could be used to titrate drugs used commonly in Rett syndrome at present, but currently introduced in a trial-and-error fashion. Caregivers cite their concern about prognosis, and, although rare, sudden death does occur in Rett syndrome. A prognostic biomarker could help identify individuals who are at risk, and more careful monitoring could be prescribed, whereas those at low risk could be safely reassured. We hope that this suite of omics biomarkers will some day be useful in clinical trials as a tool to determine target engagement or even a reasonably likely surrogate endpoint. Although we face a long road before such an approach may be validated, the cost of *not* pursuing this course is high. Families are already burdened by the clinical trials they are being asked to participate in at present, in terms of time, emotional, and financial costs. We owe it to them to provide metrics of improvement in measures that we can have confidence are reliable markers of improvement, and could lead to clinically meaningful change.

Hope for the Future

While our understanding of how mutations in *MECP2* cause the Rett syndrome phenotype remains incomplete, one important question has, in part, been answered. Researchers seeking to determine if a path to a clinically meaningful treatment is possible asked whether or not mature animals with defective Mecp2 could benefit from administration of the normal protein? Administering the protein and transferring it to the nucleus of neurons is technically difficult, but one elegant experiment engineered *Mecp2* null animals with a transgene. This allowed *Mecp2* to only be expressed in post-mitotic neurons. Because these animals were essentially identical to wild type animals, they concluded that *Mecp2* in postmitotic neurons could possibly rescue the phenotype in null animals. Subsequently, a genetic "switch" to silence Mecp2 in mice was engineered that could be activated after the mouse phenotype was evident. Once these mice were symptomatic, their native *Mecp2* was reactivated, and this restored a majority of function in the animals. Although this cannot be currently executed in humans, these experiments serve as proof of principle that both systemic and neurological defects, both phenotypic and those in synaptic plasticity, could be potentially reversed in mature animals if normal Mecp2 were present in the cell nuclei (Guy et al., 2007). In these and subsequent experiments, function is restored more robustly when Mecp2 is reactivated earlier in life, but rescue of the phenotype even occurs in adult mice (Robinson et al., 2012).

Although this review focuses on Rett syndrome, a number of studies of animal models of diseases including Down syndrome, neurofibromatosis type 1, tuberous sclerosis, Rubinstein–Taybi syndrome, fragile X syndrome and Angelman syndrome all suggest that neurodevelopmental deficits could be reversed, even in adult mice (Gadalla et al., 2011). We are hopeful that resolving the mesoscale gap and illustrating how cells, tissues and organs behave in the presence of a *MECP2* mutation using omics can provide a path to clinically meaningful change for these children over the next decade. Studies involving gene therapy are currently in various stages of development, both in Rett syndrome and other disorders, and these could result in profound clinical improvement over the next decade. Understanding the entire picture of how *MECP2* mutation results in the clinical phenotype of Rett syndrome through omics will allow us to design and test molecular biomarkers for response to these gene therapy strategies, and may allow the development of personalized medicine strategies to aid in the successful completion of clinical trials involving gene therapy.

AUTHOR CONTRIBUTIONS

DT and VF participated in study conceptualization, conduct of review, data collection, manuscript preparation, and approved the final manuscript as submitted. MW and AC participated in manuscript preparation, and approved the final manuscript as submitted.

FUNDING

VF is supported by grants from the Rett Syndrome Research Trust and NIH 1R56MH111459. DT is supported by grants from the Rett Syndrome Research Trust. MW is supported by the NIH Training Grant T32 GM08605. AC is supported by an Institutional Development Award (IDeA) from the National Institute of General Medicine of the National Institutes of Health under grant number P20GM103449.

ACKNOWLEDGMENTS

We thank the Rett Syndrome Research Trust for their generous support, and are deeply indebted to the families who have contributed their time to an improved understanding of neurodevelopmental disorders.

REFERENCES

Amir, R. E., Van den Veyver, I. B., Schultz, R., Malicki, D. M., Tran, C. Q., Dahle, E. J., et al. (2000). Influence of mutation type and X chromosome inactivation on Rett syndrome phenotypes. *Ann. Neurol.* 47, 670–679. doi: 10.1002/1531-8249(200005)47:5<670::aid-ana20>3.3.co;2-6

Amir, R. E., Van den Veyver, I. B., Wan, M., Tran, C. Q., Francke, U., and Zoghbi, H. Y. (1999). Rett syndrome is caused by mutations in X-linked MECP2, encoding methyl-CpG-binding protein 2. *Nat. Genet.* 23, 185–188. doi: 10.1038/13810

Armstrong, D. (1997). Recent developments in neuropathology—electron microscopy—brain pathology. *Eur. Child Adolesc. Psychiatry* 6, 69–70.

Armstrong, D. D. (2002). Neuropathology of Rett syndrome. *Ment. Retard. Dev. Disabil. Res. Rev.* 8, 72–76. doi: 10.1002/mrdd.10027

Armstrong, D. D. (2005). Neuropathology of Rett syndrome. *J. Child Neurol.* 20, 747–753. doi: 10.1177/08830738050200090901

Arnett, D. K., and Claas, S. A. (2018). Omics of blood pressure and hypertension. *Circ. Res.* 122, 1409–1419. doi: 10.1161/circresaha.118.311342

Ayhan, F., and Konopka, G. (2019). Regulatory genes and pathways disrupted in autism spectrum disorders. *Prog. Neuropsychopharmacol. Biol. Psychiatry* 89, 57–64. doi: 10.1016/j.pnpbp.2018.08.017

Bailey, A., Phillips, W., and Rutter, M. (1996). Autism: towards an integration of clinical, genetic, neuropsychological, and neurobiological perspectives. *J. Child Psychol. Psychiatry* 37, 89–126. doi: 10.1111/j.1469-7610.1996.tb01381.x

Ballestar, E., Yusufzai, T. M., and Wolffe, A. P. (2000). Effects of Rett syndrome mutations of the methyl-CpG binding domain of the transcriptional repressor MeCP2 on selectivity for association with methylated DNA. *Biochemistry* 39, 7100–7106. doi: 10.1021/bi0001271

Bao, X., Shengling, J., Fuying, S., Hong, P., Meirong, L., and Wu, X.-R. (2008). X chromosome inactivation in rett syndrome and its correlations with MeCP2 mutations and phenotype. *J. Child Neurol.* 23, 22–25. doi: 10.1177/0883073807307077

Bauman, M. L., Kemper, T. L., and Arin, D. M. (1995). Pervasive neuroanatomic abnormalities of the brain in three cases of Rett's syndrome. *Neurology* 45, 1581–1586. doi: 10.1212/wnl.45.8.1581

Beck, M., Schmidt, A., Malmstroem, J., Claassen, M., Ori, A., Szymborska, A., et al. (2011). The quantitative proteome of a human cell line. *Mol. Syst. Biol.* 7:549. doi: 10.1038/msb.2011.82

Ben-Shachar, S., Chahrour, M., Thaller, C., Shaw, C. A., and Zoghbi, H. Y. (2009). Mouse models of MeCP2 disorders share gene expression changes in the cerebellum and hypothalamus. *Hum. Mol. Genet.* 18, 2431–2442. doi: 10.1093/hmg/ddp181

Bienvenu, T., Philippe, C., De Roux, N., Raynaud, M., Bonnefond, J. P., Pasquier, L., et al. (2006). The incidence of Rett syndrome in France. *Pediatr. Neurol.* 34, 372–375. doi: 10.1016/j.pediatrneurol.2005.10.013

Blardi, P., De Lalla, A., D'Ambrogio, T., Vonella, G., Ceccatelli, L., Auteri, A., et al. (2009). Long-term plasma levels of leptin and adiponectin in Rett syndrome. *Clin. Endocrinol.* 70, 706–709. doi: 10.1111/j.1365-2265.2008.03386.x

Bloom, F. E. (2001). What does it all mean to you? *J. Neurosci.* 21, 8304–8305. doi: 10.1523/JNEUROSCI.21-21-08304.2001

Blue, M. E., Kaufmann, W. E., Bressler, J., Eyring, C., O'Driscoll, C., Naidu, S., et al. (2011). Temporal and regional alterations in NMDA receptor expression in Mecp2-null mice. *Anat. Rec.* 294, 1624–1634. doi: 10.1002/ar.21380

Boggio, E. M., Lonetti, G., Pizzorusso, T., and Giustetto, M. (2010). Synaptic determinants of rett syndrome. *Front. Synaptic Neurosci.* 2:28. doi: 10.3389/fnsyn.2010.00028

Braunschweig, D., Simcox, T., Samaco, R. C., and Lasalle, J. M. (2004). X-Chromosome inactivation ratios affect wild-type MeCP2 expression within mosaic Rett syndrome and Mecp2$^{-/+}$ mouse brain. *Hum. Mol. Genet.* 13, 1275–1286. doi: 10.1093/hmg/ddh142

Buchovecky, C. M., Hill, M. G., Borkey, J. M., Kyle, S. M., and Justice, M. J. (2013a). A protocol for evaluation of Rett Syndrome symptom improvement by metabolic modulators in *Mecp2*-Mutant mice. *Curr. Protoc. Mouse Biol.* 3, 187–204. doi: 10.1002/9780470942390.mo130157

Buchovecky, C. M., Turley, S. D., Brown, H. M., Kyle, S. M., McDonald, J. G., Liu, B., et al. (2013b). A suppressor screen in Mecp2 mutant mice implicates cholesterol metabolism in Rett syndrome. *Nat. Genet.* 45, 1013–1020. doi: 10.1038/ng.2714

Casado-Vela, J., Cebrián, A., Gómez Del Pulgar, M. T., and Lacal, J. C. (2011). Approaches for the study of cancer: towards the integration of genomics, proteomics and metabolomics. *Clin. Transl. Oncol.* 13, 617–628. doi: 10.1007/s12094-011-0707-9

Chahrour, M., Jung, S. Y., Shaw, C., Zhou, X., Wong, S. T., Qin, J., et al. (2008). MeCP2, a key contributor to neurological disease, activates and represses transcription. *Science* 320, 1224–1229. doi: 10.1126/science.1153252

Chahrour, M., and Zoghbi, H. Y. (2007). The story of Rett syndrome: from clinic to neurobiology. *Neuron* 56, 422–437. doi: 10.1016/j.neuron.2007.10.001

Chang, Q., Khare, G., Dani, V., Nelson, S., and Jaenisch, R. (2006). The disease progression of Mecp2 mutant mice is affected by the level of BDNF expression. *Neuron* 49, 341–348. doi: 10.1016/j.neuron.2005.12.027

Chao, H. T., Chen, H., Samaco, R. C., Xue, M., Chahrour, M., Yoo, J., et al. (2010). Dysfunction in GABA signalling mediates autism-like stereotypies and Rett syndrome phenotypes. *Nature* 468, 263–269. doi: 10.1038/nature09582

Chao, H. T., Zoghbi, H. Y., and Rosenmund, C. (2007). MeCP2 controls excitatory synaptic strength by regulating glutamatergic synapse number. *Neuron* 56, 58–65. doi: 10.1016/j.neuron.2007.08.018

Chapleau, C. A., Calfa, G. D., Lane, M. C., Albertson, A. J., Larimore, J. L., Kudo, S., et al. (2009). Dendritic spine pathologies in hippocampal pyramidal neurons from Rett syndrome brain and after expression of Rett-associated MECP2 mutations. *Neurobiol. Dis.* 35, 219–233. doi: 10.1016/j.nbd.2009.05.001

Chen, W. G., Chang, Q., Lin, Y., Meissner, A., West, A. E., Griffith, E. C., et al. (2003). Derepression of BDNF transcription involves calcium-dependent phosphorylation of MeCP2. *Science* 302, 885–889. doi: 10.1126/science.1086446

Chen, G., Gharib, T. G., Huang, C. C., Taylor, J. M., Misek, D. E., Kardia, S. L., et al. (2002). Discordant protein and mRNA expression in lung adenocarcinomas. *Mol. Cell. Proteomics* 1, 304–313. doi: 10.1074/mcp.m200008-mcp200

Cheng, T. L., Wang, Z., Liao, Q., Zhu, Y., Zhou, W. H., Xu, W., et al. (2014). MeCP2 suppresses nuclear microRNA processing and dendritic growth by regulating the DGCR8/Drosha complex. *Dev. Cell* 28, 547–560. doi: 10.1016/j.devcel.2014.01.032

Cholewa-Waclaw, J., Shah, R., Webb, S., Chhatbar, K., Ramsahoye, B., Pusch, O., et al. (2018). Mathematical modelling reveals how MeCP2 restrains transcriptional elongation in human neurons. *bioRxiv* [Preprint].

Cholewa-Waclaw, J., Shah, R., Webb, S., Chhatbar, K., Ramsahoye, B., Pusch, O., et al. (2019). Quantitative modelling predicts the impact of DNA methylation on RNA polymerase II traffic. *bioRxiv* [Preprint]. doi: 10.1101/391904

Cortelazzo, A., De Felice, C., Guerranti, R., Signorini, C., Leoncini, S., Pecorelli, A., et al. (2014). Subclinical inflammatory status in Rett syndrome. *Mediators Inflamm.* 2014:480980. doi: 10.1155/2014/480980

Cortelazzo, A., Guerranti, R., De Felice, C., Signorini, C., Leoncini, S., Pecorelli, A., et al. (2013). A plasma proteomic approach in Rett syndrome: classical versus preserved speech variant. *Mediators Inflamm.* 2013:438653. doi: 10.1155/2013/438653

Cortelazzo, A., Pietri, T., De Felice, C., Leoncini, S., Guerranti, R., Signorini, C., et al. (2017). Proteomic analysis of the Rett syndrome experimental model mecp2Q63X mutant zebrafish. *J. Proteomics* 154, 128–133. doi: 10.1016/j.jprot.2016.12.010

Cuddapah, V. A., Pillai, R. B., Shekar, K. V., Lane, J. B., Motil, K. J., Skinner, S. A., et al. (2014). Methyl-CpG-binding protein 2 (MECP2) mutation type is associated with disease severity in Rett syndrome. *J. Med. Genet.* 51, 152–158. doi: 10.1136/jmedgenet-2013-102113

De Bona, C., Zappella, M., Hayek, G., Meloni, I., Vitelli, F., Bruttini, M., et al. (2000). Preserved speech variant is allelic of classic Rett syndrome. *Eur. J. Hum. Genet.* 8, 325–330. doi: 10.1038/sj.ejhg.5200473

Downs, J., Bebbington, A., Jacoby, P., Williams, A. M., Ghosh, S., Kaufmann, W. E., et al. (2010). Level of purposeful hand function as a marker of clinical severity in Rett syndrome. *Dev. Med. Child Neurol.* 52, 817–823. doi: 10.1111/j.1469-8749.2010.03636.x

Durand, S., Patrizi, A., Quast, K. B., Hachigian, L., Pavlyuk, R., Saxena, A., et al. (2012). NMDA receptor regulation prevents regression of visual cortical function in the absence of Mecp2. *Neuron* 76, 1078–1090. doi: 10.1016/j.neuron.2012.12.004

Echenne, B., Bressot, N., Bassir, M., Daures, J. P., and Rabinowitz, A. (1991). Cerebrospinal fluid β-endorphin and cortisol study in Rett syndrome. *J. Child Neurol.* 6, 257–262. doi: 10.1177/088307389100600310

Egger, G., Liang, G., Aparicio, A., and Jones, P. A. (2004). Epigenetics in human disease and prospects for epigenetic therapy. *Nature* 429, 457–463. doi: 10.1038/nature02625

Ellaway, C. J., Sholler, G., Leonard, H., and Christodoulou, J. (1999). Prolonged QT interval in Rett syndrome. *Arch. Dis. Child.* 80, 470–472. doi: 10.1136/adc.80.5.470

ENCODE Project Consortium. (2011). A user's guide to the encyclopedia of DNA elements (ENCODE). *PLoS Biol.* 9:e1001046. doi: 10.1371/journal.pbio.1001046

ENCODE Project Consortium, Birney, E., Stamatoyannopoulos, J. A., Dutta, A., Guigó, R., Gingeras, T. R., et al. (2007). Identification and analysis of functional elements in 1% of the human genome by the ENCODE pilot project. *Nature* 447, 799–816. doi: 10.1038/nature05874

Farzin, F., Scaggs, F., Hervey, C., Berry-Kravis, E., and Hessl, D. (2011). Reliability of eye tracking and pupillometry measures in individuals with fragile X syndrome. *J. Autism Dev. Disord.* 41, 1515–1522. doi: 10.1007/s10803-011-1176-2

FitzGerald, P. M., Jankovic, J., and Percy, A. K. (1990). Rett syndrome and associated movement disorders. *Mov. Disord.* 5, 195–202. doi: 10.1002/mds.870050303

Gabel, H. W., Kinde, B., Stroud, H., Gilbert, C. S., Harmin, D. A., Kastan, N. R., et al. (2015). Disruption of DNA-methylation-dependent long gene repression in Rett syndrome. *Nature* 522, 89–93. doi: 10.1038/nature14319

Gadalla, K. K., Bailey, M. E., and Cobb, S. R. (2011). MeCP2 and Rett syndrome: reversibility and potential avenues for therapy. *Biochem. J.* 439, 1–14. doi: 10.1042/bj20110648

Garg, S. K., Lioy, D. T., Cheval, H., McGann, J. C., Bissonnette, J. M., Murtha, M. J., et al. (2013). Systemic delivery of MeCP2 rescues behavioral and cellular deficits in female mouse models of Rett syndrome. *J. Neurosci.* 33, 13612–13620. doi: 10.1523/JNEUROSCI.1854-13.2013

Ghazalpour, A., Bennett, B., Petyuk, V. A., Orozco, L., Hagopian, R., Mungrue, I. N., et al. (2011). Comparative analysis of proteome and transcriptome variation in mouse. *PLoS Genet.* 7:e1001393. doi: 10.1371/journal.pgen.1001393

Gibson, J. H., Williamson, S. L., Arbuckle, S., and Christodoulou, J. (2005). X chromosome inactivation patterns in brain in Rett syndrome: implications for the disease phenotype. *Brain Dev.* 27, 266–270. doi: 10.1016/j.braindev.2004.07.002

Girirajan, S., Campbell, C. D., and Eichler, E. E. (2011). Human copy number variation and complex genetic disease. *Annu. Rev. Genet.* 45, 203–226. doi: 10.1146/annurev-genet-102209-163544

Glaze, D. G., Frost, J. D. Jr., Zoghbi, H. Y., and Percy, A. K. (1987). Rett's syndrome: characterization of respiratory patterns and sleep. *Ann. Neurol.* 21, 377–382. doi: 10.1002/ana.410210410

Gokhale, A., Freeman, A. A., Hartwig, C., Bassell, J. L., Zlatic, S. A., Sapp, C., et al. (2018). Systems analysis of the 22q11.2 microdeletion syndrome converges on a mitochondrial interactome necessary for synapse function and behavior. *bioRxiv* [Preprint]. doi: 10.1101/315143

Guy, J., Gan, J., Selfridge, J., Cobb, S., and Bird, A. (2007). Reversal of neurological defects in a mouse model of Rett syndrome. *Science* 315, 1143–1147. doi: 10.1126/science.1138389

Gygi, S. P., Rochon, Y., Franza, B. R., and Aebersold, R. (1999). Correlation between protein and mRNA abundance in yeast. *Mol. Cell. Biol.* 19, 1720–1730. doi: 10.1128/mcb.19.3.1720

Haas, R., Zelezniak, A., Iacovacci, J., Kamrad, S., Townsend, S., and Ralser, M. (2017). Designing and interpreting 'multi-omic' experiments that may change our understanding of biology. *Curr. Opin. Syst. Biol.* 6, 37–45. doi: 10.1016/j.coisb.2017.08.009

Hara, M., Nishi, Y., Yamashita, Y., Yoh, J., Takahashi, S., Nagamitsu, S., et al. (2011). Ghrelin levels are reduced in Rett syndrome patients with eating difficulties. *Int. J. Dev. Neurosci.* 29, 899–902. doi: 10.1016/j.ijdevneu.2011.07.003

Hardwick, S. A., Reuter, K., Williamson, S. L., Vasudevan, V., Donald, J., Slater, K., et al. (2007). Delineation of large deletions of the MECP2 gene in Rett syndrome patients, including a familial case with a male proband. *Eur. J. Hum. Genet.* 15, 1218–1229. doi: 10.1038/sj.ejhg.5201911

Harper, J. W., and Bennett, E. J. (2016). Proteome complexity and the forces that drive proteome imbalance. *Nature* 537, 328–338. doi: 10.1038/nature19947

Hayek, J., Cervellati, C., Crivellari, I., Pecorelli, A., and Valacchi, G. (2017). Lactonase activity and lipoprotein-phospholipase A2 as possible novel serum biomarkers for the differential diagnosis of autism spectrum disorders and rett syndrome: results from a pilot study. *Oxid. Med. Cell. Longev.* 2017:5694058. doi: 10.1155/2017/5694058

Hillmer, R. A. (2015). Systems biology for biologists. *PLoS Pathog.* 11:e1004786. doi: 10.1371/journal.ppat.1004786

Hood, L., Heath, J. R., Phelps, M. E., and Lin, B. (2004). Systems biology and new technologies enable predictive and preventative medicine. *Science* 306, 640–643. doi: 10.1126/science.1104635

Horvath, P. M., and Monteggia, L. M. (2017). Engineering MeCP2 to spy on its targets. *Nat. Med.* 23, 1120–1122. doi: 10.1038/nm.4425

Huang, W., Carbone, M. A., Magwire, M. M., Peiffer, J. A., Lyman, R. F., Stone, E. A., et al. (2015). Genetic basis of transcriptome diversity in Drosophila melanogaster. *Proc. Natl. Acad. Sci. U S A* 112, E6010–E6019. doi: 10.1073/pnas.1519159112

Huppke, P., Maier, E. M., Warnke, A., Brendel, C., Laccone, F., and Gärtner, J. (2006). Very mild cases of Rett syndrome with skewed X inactivation. *J. Med. Genet.* 43, 814–816. doi: 10.1136/jmg.2006.042077

Ideker, T., Galitski, T., and Hood, L. (2001). A new approach to decoding life: systems biology. *Annu. Rev. Genomics Hum. Genet.* 2, 343–372. doi: 10.1146/annurev.genom.2.1.343

Im, H. I., Hollander, J. A., Bali, P., and Kenny, P. J. (2010). MeCP2 controls BDNF expression and cocaine intake through homeostatic interactions with microRNA-212. *Nat. Neurosci.* 13, 1120–1127. doi: 10.1038/nn.2615

International Human Genome Sequencing Consortium. (2004). Finishing the euchromatic sequence of the human genome. *Nature* 431, 931–945. doi: 10.1038/nature03001

Ishii, T., Makita, Y., Ogawa, A., Amamiya, S., Yamamoto, M., Miyamoto, A., et al. (2001). The role of different X-inactivation pattern on the variable clinical phenotype with Rett syndrome. *Brain Dev.* 23, S161–S164. doi: 10.1016/s0387-7604(01)00344-8

Jean Beltran, P. M., Federspiel, J. D., Sheng, X., and Cristea, I. M. (2017). Proteomics and integrative omic approaches for understanding host-pathogen interactions and infectious diseases. *Mol. Syst. Biol.* 13:922. doi: 10.15252/msb.20167062

Jefferson, A., Leonard, H., Siafarikas, A., Woodhead, H., Fyfe, S., Ward, L. M., et al. (2016). Clinical guidelines for management of bone health in rett syndrome based on expert consensus and available evidence. *PLoS One* 11:e0146824. doi: 10.1371/journal.pone.0146824

Jellinger, K., Armstrong, D., Zoghbi, H. Y., and Percy, A. K. (1988). Neuropathology of Rett syndrome. *Acta Neuropathol.* 76, 142–158. doi: 10.1007/bf00688098

Jellinger, K. A. (2003). Rett Syndrome—an update. *J. Neural Transm.* 110, 681–701. doi: 10.1007/s00702-003-0822-z

Jentarra, G. M., Olfers, S. L., Rice, S. G., Srivastava, N., Homanics, G. E., Blue, M., et al. (2010). Abnormalities of cell packing density and dendritic complexity in the MeCP2 A140V mouse model of Rett syndrome/X-linked mental retardation. *BMC Neurosci.* 11:19. doi: 10.1186/1471-2202-11-19

Johnson, B. S., Zhao, Y. T., Fasolino, M., Lamonica, J. M., Kim, Y. J., Georgakilas, G., et al. (2017). Biotin tagging of MeCP2 in mice reveals contextual insights into the Rett syndrome transcriptome. *Nat. Med.* 23, 1203–1214. doi: 10.1038/nm.4406

Kaddoum, L., Panayotis, N., Mazarguil, H., Giglia-Mari, G., Roux, J. C., and Joly, E. (2013). Isoform-specific anti-MeCP2 antibodies confirm that expression of the e1 isoform strongly predominates in the brain. *F1000Res.* 2:204. doi: 10.12688/f1000research.2-204.v1

Katz, D. M., Berger-Sweeney, J. E., Eubanks, J. H., Justice, M. J., Neul, J. L., Pozzo-Miller, L., et al. (2012). Preclinical research in Rett syndrome: setting the foundation for translational success. *Dis. Model. Mech.* 5, 733–745. doi: 10.1242/dmm.011007

Katz, D. M., Bird, A., Coenraads, M., Gray, S. J., Menon, D. U., Philpot, B. D., et al. (2016). Rett syndrome: crossing the threshold to clinical translation. *Trends Neurosci.* 39, 100–113. doi: 10.1016/j.tins.2015.12.008

Kaufmann, W. E., Johnston, M. V., and Blue, M. E. (2005). MeCP2 expression and function during brain development: implications for Rett syndrome's pathogenesis and clinical evolution. *Brain Dev.* 27, S77–S87. doi: 10.1016/j.braindev.2004.10.008

Kerr, A. M., and Ravine, D. (2003). Review article: breaking new ground with Rett syndrome. *J. Intellect. Disabil. Res.* 47, 580–587. doi: 10.1046/j.1365-2788.2003.00506.x

Key, A. P., Jones, D., and Peters, S. (2019). Spoken word processing in Rett syndrome: evidence from event-related potentials. *Int. J. Dev. Neurosci.* 73, 26–31. doi: 10.1016/j.ijdevneu.2019.01.001

Killian, J. T., Lane, J. B., Cutter, G. R., Skinner, S. A., Kaufmann, W. E., Tarquinio, D. C., et al. (2014). Pubertal development in rett syndrome deviates from typical females. *Pediatr. Neurol.* 51, 769–775. doi: 10.1016/j.pediatrneurol.2014.08.013

Klauck, S. M., Lindsay, S., Beyer, K. S., Splitt, M., Burn, J., and Poustka, A. (2002). A mutation hot spot for nonspecific X-linked mental retardation in the MECP2 gene causes the PPM-X syndrome. *Am. J. Hum. Genet.* 70, 1034–1037. doi: 10.1086/339553

Klein, M. E., Lioy, D. T., Ma, L., Impey, S., Mandel, G., and Goodman, R. H. (2007). Homeostatic regulation of MeCP2 expression by a CREB-induced microRNA. *Nat. Neurosci.* 10, 1513–1514. doi: 10.1038/nn2010

Kline, D. D., Ogier, M., Kunze, D. L., and Katz, D. M. (2010). Exogenous brain-derived neurotrophic factor rescues synaptic dysfunction in Mecp2-null mice. *J. Neurosci.* 30, 5303–5310. doi: 10.1523/JNEUROSCI.5503-09.2010

Kozawa, S., Ueda, R., Urayama, K., Sagawa, F., Endo, S., Shiizaki, K., et al. (2018). The body-wide transcriptome landscape of disease models. *iScience* 2, 238–268. doi: 10.1016/j.isci.2018.03.014

Krishnaraj, R., Ho, G., and Christodoulou, J. (2017). RettBASE: Rett syndrome database update. *Hum. Mutat.* 38, 922–931. doi: 10.1002/humu.23263

Kron, M., Howell, C. J., Adams, I. T., Ransbottom, M., Christian, D., Ogier, M., et al. (2012). Brain activity mapping in Mecp2 mutant mice reveals functional deficits in forebrain circuits, including key nodes in the default mode network, that are reversed with ketamine treatment. *J. Neurosci.* 32, 13860–13872. doi: 10.1523/JNEUROSCI.2159-12.2012

Kudo, S., Nomura, Y., Segawa, M., Fujita, N., Nakao, M., Dragich, J., et al. (2001). Functional analyses of MeCP2 mutations associated with Rett syndrome using transient expression systems. *Brain Dev.* 23, S165–S173. doi: 10.1016/s0387-7604(01)00345-x

Kyle, S. M., Saha, P. K., Brown, H. M., Chan, L. C., and Justice, M. J. (2016). MeCP2 co-ordinates liver lipid metabolism with the NCoR1/HDAC3 corepressor complex. *Hum. Mol. Genet.* 25, 3029–3041. doi: 10.1093/hmg/ddw156

Larimore, J. L., Chapleau, C. A., Kudo, S., Theibert, A., Percy, A. K., and Pozzo-Miller, L. (2009). Bdnf overexpression in hippocampal neurons prevents dendritic atrophy caused by Rett-associated MECP2 mutations. *Neurobiol. Dis.* 34, 199–211. doi: 10.1016/j.nbd.2008.12.011

LeBlanc, J. J., Degregorio, G., Centofante, E., Vogel-Farley, V. K., Barnes, K., Kaufmann, W. E., et al. (2015). Visual evoked potentials detect cortical processing deficits in Rett syndrome. *Ann. Neurol.* 78, 775–786. doi: 10.1002/ana.24513

Leonard, H., Bower, C., and English, D. (1997). The prevalence and incidence of Rett syndrome in Australia. *Eur. Child Adolesc. Psychiatry* 6, 8–10.

Leonard, H., Cobb, S., and Downs, J. (2017). Clinical and biological progress over 50 years in Rett syndrome. *Nat. Rev. Neurol.* 13, 37–51. doi: 10.1038/nrneurol.2016.186

Liu, T., Ortiz, J. A., Taing, L., Meyer, C. A., Lee, B., Zhang, Y., et al. (2011). Cistrome: an integrative platform for transcriptional regulation studies. *Genome Biol.* 12:R83. doi: 10.1186/gb-2011-12-8-r83

Lombardi, L. M., Baker, S. A., and Zoghbi, H. Y. (2015). MECP2 disorders: from the clinic to mice and back. *J. Clin. Invest.* 125, 2914–2923. doi: 10.1172/jci78167

Lyst, M. J., and Bird, A. (2015). Rett syndrome: a complex disorder with simple roots. *Nat. Rev. Genet.* 16, 261–275. doi: 10.1038/nrg3897

Maier, T., Guell, M., and Serrano, L. (2009). Correlation of mRNA and protein in complex biological samples. *FEBS Lett.* 583, 3966–3973. doi: 10.1016/j.febslet.2009.10.036

Matarazzo, V., and Ronnett, G. V. (2004). Temporal and regional differences in the olfactory proteome as a consequence of MeCP2 deficiency. *Proc. Natl. Acad. Sci. U S A* 101, 7763–7768. doi: 10.1073/pnas.0307083101

McGill, B. E., Bundle, S. F., Yaylaoglu, M. B., Carson, J. P., Thaller, C., and Zoghbi, H. Y. (2006). Enhanced anxiety and stress-induced corticosterone release are associated with increased Crh expression in a mouse model of Rett syndrome. *Proc. Natl. Acad. Sci. U S A* 103, 18267–18272. doi: 10.1073/pnas.0608702103

Medrihan, L., Tantalaki, E., Aramuni, G., Sargsyan, V., Dudanova, I., Missler, M., et al. (2008). Early defects of GABAergic synapses in the brain stem of a MeCP2 mouse model of Rett syndrome. *J. Neurophysiol.* 99, 112–121. doi: 10.1152/jn.00826.2007

Moretti, P., Levenson, J. M., Battaglia, F., Atkinson, R., Teague, R., Antalffy, B., et al. (2006). Learning and memory and synaptic plasticity are impaired in a mouse model of Rett syndrome. *J. Neurosci.* 26, 319–327. doi: 10.1523/JNEUROSCI.2623-05.2006

Motil, K. J., Caeg, E., Barrish, J. O., Geerts, S., Lane, J. B., Percy, A. K., et al. (2012). Gastrointestinal and nutritional problems occur frequently throughout life in girls and women with Rett syndrome. *J. Pediatr. Gastroenterol. Nutr.* 55, 292–298. doi: 10.1097/mpg.0b013e31824b6159

Mullin, A. P., Gokhale, A., Moreno-De-Luca, A., Sanyal, S., Waddington, J. L., and Faundez, V. (2013). Neurodevelopmental disorders: mechanisms and boundary definitions from genomes, interactomes and proteomes. *Transl. Psychiatry* 3:e329. doi: 10.1038/tp.2013.108

Na, E. S., Nelson, E. D., Adachi, M., Autry, A. E., Mahgoub, M. A., Kavalali, E. T., et al. (2012). A mouse model for MeCP2 duplication syndrome: MeCP2 overexpression impairs learning and memory and synaptic transmission. *J. Neurosci.* 32, 3109–3117. doi: 10.1523/JNEUROSCI.6000-11.2012

Na, E. S., Nelson, E. D., Kavalali, E. T., and Monteggia, L. M. (2013). The impact of MeCP2 loss- or gain-of-function on synaptic plasticity. *Neuropsychopharmacology* 38, 212–219. doi: 10.1038/npp.2012.116

Nagaraj, N., Wisniewski, J. R., Geiger, T., Cox, J., Kircher, M., Kelso, J., et al. (2011). Deep proteome and transcriptome mapping of a human cancer cell line. *Mol. Syst. Biol.* 7:548. doi: 10.1038/msb.2011.81

Neul, J. L., Kaufmann, W. E., Glaze, D. G., Christodoulou, J., Clarke, A. J., Bahi-Buisson, N., et al. (2010). Rett syndrome: revised diagnostic criteria and nomenclature. *Ann. Neurol.* 68, 944–950. doi: 10.1002/ana.22124

Neul, J. L., Lane, J. B., Lee, H. S., Geerts, S., Barrish, J. O., Annese, F., et al. (2014). Developmental delay in Rett syndrome: data from the natural history study. *J. Neurodev. Disord.* 6:20. doi: 10.1186/1866-1955-6-20

Neul, J. L., and Zoghbi, H. Y. (2004). Rett syndrome: a prototypical neurodevelopmental disorder. *Neuroscientist* 10, 118–128. doi: 10.1177/1073858403260995

Okabe, Y., Takahashi, T., Mitsumasu, C., Kosai, K., Tanaka, E., and Matsuishi, T. (2012). Alterations of gene expression and glutamate clearance in astrocytes derived from an MeCP2-null mouse model of Rett syndrome. *PLoS One* 7:e35354. doi: 10.1371/journal.pone.0035354

Pacheco, N. L., Heaven, M. R., Holt, L. M., Crossman, D. K., Boggio, K. J., Shaffer, S. A., et al. (2017). RNA sequencing and proteomics approaches reveal novel deficits in the cortex of Mecp2-deficient mice, a model for Rett syndrome. *Mol. Autism* 8:56. doi: 10.1186/s13229-017-0174-4

Papini, A. M., Nuti, F., Real-Fernandez, F., Rossi, G., Tiberi, C., Sabatino, G., et al. (2014). Immune dysfunction in Rett syndrome patients revealed by high levels of serum anti-N(Glc) IgM antibody fraction. *J. Immunol. Res.* 2014:260973. doi: 10.1155/2014/260973

Parts, L., Liu, Y. C., Tekkedil, M. M., Steinmetz, L. M., Caudy, A. A., Fraser, A. G., et al. (2014). Heritability and genetic basis of protein level variation in an outbred population. *Genome Res.* 24, 1363–1370. doi: 10.1101/gr.170506.113

Pascal, L. E., True, L. D., Campbell, D. S., Deutsch, E. W., Risk, M., Coleman, I. M., et al. (2008). Correlation of mRNA and protein levels: cell type-specific gene expression of cluster designation antigens in the prostate. *BMC Genomics* 9:246. doi: 10.1186/1471-2164-9-246

Paterson, D. S., Thompson, E. G., Belliveau, R. A., Antalffy, B. A., Trachtenberg, F. L., Armstrong, D. D., et al. (2005). Serotonin transporter abnormality in the dorsal motor nucleus of the vagus in Rett syndrome: potential implications for clinical autonomic dysfunction. *J. Neuropathol. Exp. Neurol.* 64, 1018–1027. doi: 10.1097/01.jnen.0000187054.59018.f2

Percy, A. K. (2011). Rett syndrome: exploring the autism link. *Arch. Neurol.* 68, 985–989. doi: 10.1001/archneurol.2011.149

Pozzo-Miller, L., Pati, S., and Percy, A. K. (2015). rett syndrome: reaching for clinical trials. *Neurotherapeutics* 12, 631–640. doi: 10.1007/s13311-015-0353-y

Qiu, Z., Sylwestrak, E. L., Lieberman, D. N., Zhang, Y., Liu, X. Y., and Ghosh, A. (2012). The Rett syndrome protein MeCP2 regulates synaptic scaling. *J. Neurosci.* 32, 989–994. doi: 10.1523/JNEUROSCI.0175-11.2012

Ramocki, M. B., Peters, S. U., Tavyev, Y. J., Zhang, F., Carvalho, C. M., Schaaf, C. P., et al. (2009). Autism and other neuropsychiatric symptoms are prevalent in individuals with MeCP2 duplication syndrome. *Ann. Neurol.* 66, 771–782. doi: 10.1002/ana.21715

Renthal, W., Boxer, L. D., Hrvatin, S., Li, E., Silberfeld, A., Nagy, M. A., et al. (2018). Characterization of human mosaic Rett syndrome brain tissue by single-nucleus RNA sequencing. *Nat. Neurosci.* 21, 1670–1679. doi: 10.1038/s41593-018-0270-6

Risch, N., Spiker, D., Lotspeich, L., Nouri, N., Hinds, D., Hallmayer, J., et al. (1999). A genomic screen of autism: evidence for a multilocus etiology. *Am. J. Hum. Genet.* 65, 493–507. doi: 10.1086/302497

Robinson, L., Guy, J., McKay, L., Brockett, E., Spike, R. C., Selfridge, J., et al. (2012). Morphological and functional reversal of phenotypes in a mouse model of Rett syndrome. *Brain* 135, 2699–2710. doi: 10.1093/brain/aws096

Romero, R., Espinoza, J., Gotsch, F., Kusanovic, J. P., Friel, L. A., Erez, O., et al. (2006). The use of high-dimensional biology (genomics, transcriptomics, proteomics and metabolomics) to understand the preterm parturition syndrome. *BJOG* 113, 118–135. doi: 10.1111/j.1471-0528.2006.01150.x

Rose, S. A., Djukic, A., Jankowski, J. J., Feldman, J. F., Fishman, I., and Valicenti-McDermott, M. (2013). Rett syndrome: an eye-tracking study of attention and recognition memory. *Dev. Med. Child Neurol.* 55, 364–371. doi: 10.1111/dmcn.12085

Rutkowski, T. P., Schroeder, J. P., Gafford, G. M., Warren, S. T., Weinshenker, D., Caspary, T., et al. (2017). Unraveling the genetic architecture of copy number variants associated with schizophrenia and other neuropsychiatric disorders. *J. Neurosci. Res.* 95, 1144–1160. doi: 10.1002/jnr.23970

Samaco, R. C., Mandel-Brehm, C., Chao, H. T., Ward, C. S., Fyffe-Maricich, S. L., Ren, J., et al. (2009). Loss of MeCP2 in aminergic neurons causes cell-autonomous defects in neurotransmitter synthesis and specific behavioral abnormalities. *Proc. Natl. Acad. Sci. U S A* 106, 21966–21971. doi: 10.1073/pnas.0912257106

Segatto, M., Trapani, L., Di Tunno, I., Sticozzi, C., Valacchi, G., Hayek, J., et al. (2014). Cholesterol metabolism is altered in rett syndrome: a study on plasma and primary cultured fibroblasts derived from patients. *PLoS One* 9:e104834. doi: 10.1371/journal.pone.0104834

Shahbazian, M., Young, J., Yuva-Paylor, L., Spencer, C., Antalffy, B., Noebels, J., et al. (2002). Mice with truncated MeCP2 recapitulate many Rett syndrome features and display hyperacetylation of histone H3. *Neuron* 35, 243–254. doi: 10.1016/s0896-6273(02)00768-7

Smrt, R. D., Eaves-Egenes, J., Barkho, B. Z., Santistevan, N. J., Zhao, C., Aimone, J. B., et al. (2007). Mecp2 deficiency leads to delayed maturation and altered gene expression in hippocampal neurons. *Neurobiol. Dis.* 27, 77–89. doi: 10.1016/j.nbd.2007.04.005

Spies, D., and Ciaudo, C. (2015). Dynamics in transcriptomics: advancements in RNA-seq time course and downstream analysis. *Comput. Struct. Biotechnol. J.* 13, 469–477. doi: 10.1016/j.csbj.2015.08.004

Spiga, O., Gardini, S., Rossi, N., Cicaloni, V., Pettini, F., Niccolai, N., et al. (2019). Structural investigation of Rett-inducing MeCP2 mutations. *Genes Dis.* 6, 31–34. doi: 10.1016/j.gendis.2018.09.005

Strange, K. (2005). The end of "naive reductionism": rise of systems biology or renaissance of physiology? *Am. J. Physiol. Cell Physiol.* 288, C968–C974. doi: 10.1152/ajpcell.00598.2004

Sun, Y. E., and Wu, H. (2006). The ups and downs of BDNF in Rett syndrome. *Neuron* 49, 321–323. doi: 10.1016/j.neuron.2006.01.014

Symons, F. J., Byiers, B., Hoch, J., Dimian, A., Barney, C., Feyma, T., et al. (2015). Infrared thermal analysis and individual differences in skin temperature asymmetry in rett syndrome. *Pediatr. Neurol.* 53, 169–172. doi: 10.1016/j.pediatrneurol.2015.03.018

Sztainberg, Y., and Zoghbi, H. Y. (2016). Lessons learned from studying syndromic autism spectrum disorders. *Nat. Neurosci.* 19, 1408–1417. doi: 10.1038/nn.4420

Takahashi, S., Ohinata, J., Makita, Y., Suzuki, N., Araki, A., Sasaki, A., et al. (2008). Skewed X chromosome inactivation failed to explain the normal phenotype of a carrier female with MECP2 mutation resulting in Rett syndrome. *Clin. Genet.* 73, 257–261. doi: 10.1111/j.1399-0004.2007.00944.x

Tanaka, Y., Kim, K. Y., Zhong, M., Pan, X., Weissman, S. M., and Park, I. H. (2014). Transcriptional regulation in pluripotent stem cells by methyl CpG-binding protein 2 (MeCP2). *Hum. Mol. Genet.* 23, 1045–1055. doi: 10.1093/hmg/ddt500

Taneja, P., Ogier, M., Brooks-Harris, G., Schmid, D. A., Katz, D. M., and Nelson, S. B. (2009). Pathophysiology of locus ceruleus neurons in a mouse model of Rett syndrome. *J. Neurosci.* 29, 12187–12195. doi: 10.1523/JNEUROSCI.3156-09.2009

Tarquinio, D. C., Hou, W., Berg, A., Kaufmann, W. E., Lane, J. B., Skinner, S. A., et al. (2017). Longitudinal course of epilepsy in Rett syndrome and related disorders. *Brain* 140, 306–318. doi: 10.1093/brain/aww302

Tarquinio, D. C., Hou, W., Neul, J. L., Berkmen, G. K., Drummond, J., Aronoff, E., et al. (2018). The course of awake breathing disturbances across the lifespan in Rett syndrome. *Brain Dev.* 40, 515–529. doi: 10.1016/j.braindev.2018.03.010

Tarquinio, D. C., Hou, W., Neul, J. L., Kaufmann, W. E., Glaze, D. G., Motil, K. J., et al. (2015). The changing face of survival in rett syndrome and MECP2-related disorders. *Pediatr. Neurol.* 53, 402–411. doi: 10.1016/j.pediatrneurol.2015.06.003

Tarquinio, D. C., Motil, K. J., Hou, W., Lee, H. S., Glaze, D. G., Skinner, S. A., et al. (2012). Growth failure and outcome in Rett syndrome: specific growth references. *Neurology* 79, 1653–1661. doi: 10.1212/wnl.0b013e31826e9a70

Tebani, A., Afonso, C., Marret, S., and Bekri, S. (2016). Omics-based strategies in precision medicine: toward a paradigm shift in inborn errors of metabolism investigations. *Int. J. Mol. Sci.* 17:E1555. doi: 10.3390/ijms17091555

Tsujimura, K., Irie, K., Nakashima, H., Egashira, Y., Fukao, Y., Fujiwara, M., et al. (2015). miR-199a links MeCP2 with mTOR signaling and its dysregulation leads to rett syndrome phenotypes. *Cell Rep* 12, 1887–1901. doi: 10.1016/j.celrep.2015.08.028

Uddin, L. Q., Dajani, D. R., Voorhies, W., Bednarz, H., and Kana, R. K. (2017). Progress and roadblocks in the search for brain-based biomarkers of autism and attention-deficit/hyperactivity disorder. *Transl. Psychiatry* 7:e1218. doi: 10.1038/tp.2017.164

Uhlén, M., Fagerberg, L., Hallstrom, B. M., Lindskog, C., Oksvold, P., Mardinoglu, A., et al. (2015). Proteomics. Tissue-based map of the human proteome. *Science* 347:1260419. doi: 10.1126/science.1260419

van Dongen, J., Slagboom, P. E., Draisma, H. H., Martin, N. G., and Boomsma, D. I. (2012). The continuing value of twin studies in the omics era. *Nat. Rev. Genet.* 13, 640–653. doi: 10.1038/nrg3243

Van Esch, H. (2011). "MECP2 duplication syndrome," in *GeneReviews*, eds R. A. Pagon, T. D. Bird, C. R. Dolan, K. Stephens and M. P. Adam (Seattle, WA: University of Washington).

Venkateswaran, S., McMillan, H. J., Doja, A., and Humphreys, P. (2014). Adolescent onset cognitive regression and neuropsychiatric symptoms associated with the A140V MECP2 mutation. *Dev. Med. Child Neurol.* 56, 91–94. doi: 10.1111/dmcn.12334

Vogel, C., and Marcotte, E. M. (2012). Insights into the regulation of protein abundance from proteomic and transcriptomic analyses. *Nat. Rev. Genet.* 13, 227–232. doi: 10.1038/nrg3185

Wade, P. A. (2004). Dynamic regulation of DNA methylation coupled transcriptional repression: BDNF regulation by MeCP2. *Bioessays* 26, 217–220. doi: 10.1002/bies.20018

Wang, H., Chan, S. A., Ogier, M., Hellard, D., Wang, Q., Smith, C., et al. (2006). Dysregulation of brain-derived neurotrophic factor expression and neurosecretory function in Mecp2 null mice. *J. Neurosci.* 26, 10911–10915. doi: 10.1523/JNEUROSCI.1810-06.2006

Wang, Z., Gerstein, M., and Snyder, M. (2009). RNA-Seq: a revolutionary tool for transcriptomics. *Nat. Rev. Genet.* 10, 57–63. doi: 10.1038/nrg2484

Waterer, G. W. (2012). Community-acquired pneumonia: genomics, epigenomics, transcriptomics, proteomics, and metabolomics. *Semin. Respir. Crit. Care Med.* 33, 257–265. doi: 10.1055/s-0032-1315637

Weng, S. M., McLeod, F., Bailey, M. E., and Cobb, S. R. (2011). Synaptic plasticity deficits in an experimental model of rett syndrome: long-term potentiation saturation and its pharmacological reversal. *Neuroscience* 180, 314–321. doi: 10.1016/j.neuroscience.2011.01.061

Weston, A. D., and Hood, L. (2004). Systems biology, proteomics and the future of health care: toward predictive, preventative and personalized medicine. *J. Proteome Res.* 3, 179–196. doi: 10.1021/pr0499693

Wilhelm, M., Schlegl, J., Hahne, H., Gholami, A. M., Lieberenz, M., Savitski, M. M., et al. (2014). Mass-spectrometry-based draft of the human proteome. *Nature* 509, 582–587. doi: 10.1038/nature13319

Wong, V. C., and Li, S. Y. (2007). Rett syndrome: prevalence among Chinese and a comparison of MECP2 mutations of classic Rett syndrome with other neurodevelopmental disorders. *J. Child Neurol.* 22, 1397–1400. doi: 10.1177/0883073807307091

Wright, F. A., Sullivan, P. F., Brooks, A. I., Zou, F., Sun, W., Xia, K., et al. (2014). Heritability and genomics of gene expression in peripheral blood. *Nat. Genet.* 46, 430–437. doi: 10.1038/ng.2951

Wu, L., Candille, S. I., Choi, Y., Xie, D., Jiang, L., Li-Pook-Than, J., et al. (2013). Variation and genetic control of protein abundance in humans. *Nature* 499, 79–82. doi: 10.1038/nature12223

Xu, G., Strathearn, L., Liu, B., and Bao, W. (2018). Prevalence of autism spectrum disorder among US children and adolescents, 2014–2016. *JAMA* 319, 81–82. doi: 10.1001/jama.2017.17812

Yang, T., Ramocki, M., Neul, J. L., Lu, W., Roberts, L., Knight, M., et al. (2012). Overexpression of methyl-CpG binding protein 2 impairs TH1 responses. *Sci. Transl. Med.* 4:163ra158. doi: 10.1126/scitranslmed.3004430

Yeung, E. S. (2011). Genome-wide correlation between mRNA and protein in a single cell. *Angew. Chem. Int. Ed. Engl.* 50, 583–585. doi: 10.1002/anie.201005969

Young, J. I., Hong, E. P., Castle, J. C., Crespo-Barreto, J., Bowman, A. B., Rose, M. F., et al. (2005). Regulation of RNA splicing by the methylation-dependent transcriptional repressor methyl-CpG binding protein 2. *Proc. Natl. Acad. Sci. U S A* 102, 17551–17558. doi: 10.1073/pnas.0507856102

Zappella, M. (1992). The Rett girls with preserved speech. *Brain Dev.* 14, 98–101. doi: 10.1016/s0387-7604(12)80094-5

Zlatic, S. A., Vrailas-Mortimer, A., Gokhale, A., Carey, L. J., Scott, E., Burch, R., et al. (2018). Rare disease mechanisms identified by genealogical proteomics of copper homeostasis mutant pedigrees. *Cell Syst.* 6, 368.e6–380.e6. doi: 10.1016/j.cels.2018.01.008

10

Peripheral Amyloid Precursor Protein Derivative Expression in Fragile X Syndrome

*Richard D. McLane[1], Lauren M. Schmitt[2], Ernest V. Pedapati[1,3,4], Rebecca C. Shaffer[2,5], Kelli C. Dominick[1,4], Paul S. Horn[3], Christina Gross[3,5] and Craig A. Erickson[1,4]**

[1] Division of Child and Adolescent Psychiatry, Cincinnati Children's Hospital Medical Center, Cincinnati, OH, United States, [2] Division of Developmental and Behavioral Pediatrics, Cincinnati Children's Hospital Medical Center, Cincinnati, OH, United States, [3] Division of Neurology, Cincinnati Children's Hospital Medical Center, Cincinnati, OH, United States, [4] Department of Psychiatry and Behavioral Neuroscience, University of Cincinnati College of Medicine, Cincinnati, OH, United States, [5] Department of Pediatrics, University of Cincinnati College of Medicine, Cincinnati, OH, United States

***Correspondence:**
Craig A. Erickson
Craig.Erickson@cchmc.org

Fragile X syndrome (FXS) is the most common inherited form of intellectual disability and is associated with increased risk for autism spectrum disorder (ASD), anxiety, ADHD, and epilepsy. While our understanding of FXS pathophysiology has improved, a lack of validated blood-based biomarkers of disease continues to impede bench-to-bedside efforts. To meet this demand, there is a growing effort to discover a reliable biomarker to inform treatment discovery and evaluate treatment target engagement. Such a marker, amyloid-beta precursor protein (APP), has shown potential dysregulation in the absence of fragile X mental retardation protein (FMRP) and may therefore be associated with FXS pathophysiology. While APP is best understood in the context of Alzheimer disease, there is a growing body of evidence suggesting the molecule and its derivatives play a broader role in regulating neuronal hyperexcitability, a well-characterized phenotype in FXS. To evaluate the viability of APP as a peripheral biological marker in FXS, we conducted an exploratory ELISA-based evaluation of plasma APP-related species involving 27 persons with FXS (mean age: 22.0 ± 11.5) and 25 age- and sex-matched persons with neurotypical development (mean age: 21.1 ± 10.7). Peripheral levels of both Aβ(1–40) and Aβ(1–42) were increased, while sAPPα was significantly decreased in persons with FXS as compared to control participants. These results suggest that dysregulated APP processing, with potential preferential β-secretase processing, may be a readily accessible marker of FXS pathophysiology.

Keywords: amyloid precursor protein, FXS, biomarker, peripheral, enzyme-linked immunosorbent assay

INTRODUCTION

Fragile X syndrome (FXS) is the most common inherited form of intellectual disability and the most common monogenic cause of autism spectrum disorder (Kosinovsky et al., 2005). FXS is an X-linked disorder affecting 1 in 4,000 males and 1 in 6,000–8,000 females, with all males and some females having significant developmental disability as well as increased risk for autism, anxiety, ADHD, and epilepsy. FXS is caused by a CGG repeat expansion in the promoter region of the fragile X mental retardation 1 gene (*FMR1*), resulting in silencing of the gene and decreased production of fragile X mental retardation protein (FMRP). FMRP is an RNA binding and carrier protein that plays a role in the transport, localization, and translational repression of at least hundreds of target mRNAs (Darnell et al., 2011; Ascano et al., 2012; Westmark, 2018). FMRP-mediated translation is necessary for regulating local protein synthesis and normal cellular processes. When FMRP is absent or expressed at low levels, dendritic spine density and abnormal spine morphology increase, leading to abnormal formation and function of synapses. As a result, neural circuitry is significantly disrupted in individuals with FXS, which is thought to account for the various neurological, behavioral, and behavioral problems associated with this intellectual disability. Although our understanding of FXS pathophysiology has improved, to date, there are still no effective targeted therapies approved in FXS. One of the obstacles preventing the development of disease-modifying treatments for FXS is a lack of useful readily accessible markers of pathophysiology. Biomarkers linked to disease mechanisms may be useful in screening participants, evaluating patient responsiveness to treatment, and identifying subgroups that may best respond to a particular treatment. In recent years, there have been efforts to identify either a single or combination of molecular markers in FXS.

Amyloid precursor protein (APP) is a transmembrane protein with a large extracellular N-terminal domain and a short cytoplasmic tail. Because APP is expressed within microglia, astrocytes, oligodendrocytes, and neurites of the brain and is primarily responsible for cell adhesion and axon pruning (Chasseigneaux and Allinquant, 2012), its regulation is critical to maintaining normal neuronal development and homeostasis (Hartmann et al., 1999; Herms et al., 2004; Guénette et al., 2006; Chasseigneaux and Allinquant, 2012). APP can be metabolized through two distinct processing pathways, the amyloidogenic and non-amyloidogenic processing pathways. In the amyloidogenic processing pathway, APP undergoes cleavage by β-secretase (BACE-1) to produce the neurotoxic amyloid peptides β-amyloid peptides 40 and 42 [Aβ(1–40) and Aβ(1–42)] (Vassar et al., 1999). These peptides are best understood in the context of Alzheimer's disease where Aβ deposition in brain has been strongly implicated in cerebral plaque formation and brain atrophy (Masters et al., 1985; Hardy and Selkoe, 2002; Persson et al., 2017). However, at lower levels, Aβ monomers are neuroprotective and have been shown to protect mature neurons against excitotoxicity (Whitson et al., 1989). β-cleavage of the soluble N-terminal domain of APP also produces secreted amyloid precursor protein β (sAPPβ) (Vassar et al., 1999). Alternatively, non-amyloidogenic, or α-secretase, processing of APP by two disintegrin and metalloproteases (ADAM-10 and ADAM-17) produces secreted amyloid precursor protein alpha (sAPPα) (Buxbaum et al., 1998; Lammich et al., 1999). Similar to Aβ, sAPPα also has neuroprotective and neurotrophic properties (Mattson et al., 1993; Smith-Swintosky et al., 1994; Luo et al., 2001; Corrigan et al., 2011; Chasseigneaux and Allinquant, 2012). However, less is known regarding altered non-amyloidogenic metabolism.

APP metabolism has been studied in the context of a variety of neurodevelopmental disorders including idiopathic autism, Angelman Syndrome, and FXS (Sokol et al., 2006; Ray et al., 2011; Erickson et al., 2014, 2016; Ray et al., 2016; Westmark et al., 2016b). Previous work has shown that FMRP directly binds and regulates *App* mRNA translation in *FMR1* KO mice (Westmark and Malter, 2007), leading to the potential investigation of APP dysregulation in FXS. In this work, genetic reduction of APP expression in *Fmr1* KO mice has been demonstrated to rescue neuronal hyperexcitability (Westmark et al., 2011b, 2016a), a well-documented neural phenotype in *Fmr1* KO mice, FXS humans, and slice physiology (Gibson et al., 2008; Choi et al., 2015; Ethridge et al., 2016, 2017; Westmark et al., 2016a; Lovelace et al., 2018). Of note, products of both amyloidogenic [Aβ(1–42)] and non-amyloidogenic (sAPPα) APP processing have been shown to enhance mGluR-dependent protein synthesis and contribute to hyperexcitability and altered synaptic plasticity in FXS (Renner et al., 2010; Westmark et al., 2011b, 2016a; Pasciuto et al., 2015). This suggests that targeting the synaptic deficits in FXS via an APP-focused approach may require pharmacotherapeutic manipulation of both amyloidogenic and non-amyloidogenic processing to restore homeostatic levels of APP metabolites (Westmark et al., 2011b, 2016a; Pasciuto et al., 2015).

Peripheral APP metabolite levels also have been reported to be altered in idiopathic ASD and FXS (Sokol et al., 2006; Bailey et al., 2008; Ray et al., 2011, 2016). For example, Ray et al. (2016) reported increased peripheral levels of sAPPα, sAPPβ, sAPP total, Aβ(1–40) and Aβ(1–42) in 18 children with FXS compared to controls. Additionally, increased levels of both sAPPα and total sAPP were found in a small sample of young ASD children with aggressive behavior compared to youth with ASD without aggressive behavior (Bailey et al., 2008). In a follow-up study, children with ASD clinically rated to have severe symptomology based on Childhood Autism Rating Scale (CARS) scores had higher levels of sAPPα than children with ASD who had mild-to-moderate rated symptomology. Additionally, authors reported reduced levels of both Aβ(1–40) and Aβ(1–42) in the more severely affected patient group (Ray et al., 2011). This suggests APP metabolite levels may track with severity of ASD symptoms, and thus may be an important marker of behavioral functioning. Furthermore, in a pilot study of individuals with ASD, our group showed that both sAPPα and sAPP total were reduced in plasma after treatment with acamprosate (Erickson et al., 2014). This suggests the potential utility of APP metabolites as pharmacodynamic markers. Together, initial findings suggest a role for APP metabolites as peripheral biomarkers in neurodevelopmental disorders, though further characterization of peripheral APP metabolites and their association with clinical features are needed in FXS.

In this study, we aimed to add to the existing understanding of peripheral APP expression in FXS by quantifying peripheral APP metabolite and processing enzyme expression in individuals with FXS compared to typically developing controls (TDC). To do so, we conducted a comprehensive evaluation of peripheral APP metabolites including sAPPα, sAPPβ, sAPP total, Aβ(1–40), and Aβ(1–42) and processing enzymes ADAM-10, ADAM-17, and BACE-1 using enzyme-linked immunosorbent assays (ELISA).

Finally, we conducted exploratory analyses looking at potential correlations between APP species and APP-associated enzymes and the clinical features of our participants.

MATERIALS AND METHODS

Participant

Plasma samples were collected from 27 individuals with FXS (15 males, 12 females) and 25 age- and sex-matched control subjects (TDC) (14 males, 11 females). Controls had no known prior diagnosis or treatment for developmental or neuropsychiatric disorders. No participant had a history of seizure disorder or current use of anticonvulsant medication, benzodiazepine, or novel potential treatment for FXS (i.e., minocycline, acamprosate, baclofen). All participants completed the Stanford-Binet Intelligence Scale, 5th Edition (SB-5) to assess intellectual functioning. SB-5 standard scores were converted to deviation scores based upon expected age-related performance to estimate intellectual ability in FXS participants for whom reducing floor effects in scores is important (Sansone et al., 2012). All participants or their legal guardians provided informed written consent or verbal assent, when appropriate. The local Institutional Review Board approved the study.

Blood Sample Collection

Blood samples were collected in 8.5 mL K_2EDTA tubes (BD Medical, 362799). Plasma samples were prepared within 1-hour post-collection. Plasma was separated from whole blood by centrifuging at 1100 × *g* for 15 min. The isolated plasma was transferred in 2 mL aliquots into several microfuge tubes and flash frozen. The samples were stored at −80°C until analysis.

Plasma Preparation

Prior to testing, the plasma samples were thawed and filtered through Corning®Costar®Spin-X®centrifuge tube filters (Corning 8163) to remove excess lipids and contaminants. Similar to previous studies (Ray et al., 2011, 2016), we found that immunodepletion of human serum albumin (HSA) improved the detection of sAPPα in plasma (data not shown). HSA was removed from plasma samples using EZAlbumin Depletion Spin Columns (BioVision, Inc., K6573). This immunosubtraction was only performed on samples used for sAPPα.

ELISA

The concentrations of sAPPα, sAPPβ, total sAPP, Aβ(1–40), Aβ(1–42), ADAM-10, ADAM-17, BACE-1, were quantified through commercially available ELISA kits from IBL America (Catalog# 27734, 27732, 27731, 27718, 27719), LifeSpan Biosciences (LS-F23768), Invitrogen Life Technologies (EHADAM17), and Biomatik (EKU02709). Samples were run according to manufacturer instructions. The assays were run over three consecutive days. On the first day, sAPPα, sAPPβ, total sAPP, Aβ(1–40), and Aβ(1–42) were prepared and allowed to incubate overnight at 4°C. The assays were completed and analyzed the following day. The third day was used to run the remaining moieties: ADAM-10, ADAM-17, and BACE-1. These assays used a biotin-streptavidin detection system that allowed for the tests to be setup and completed all within the same day. Aliquots were stored at 4°C during the 3-day period to prevent protein degradation from repeated freeze-thaw cycles. These storage conditions were tested for each moiety prior to running the experiment. In pilot experiments, no degradation of metabolites was observed up to 5 days in storage at 4°C (data not shown), confirming that these storage conditions adequately maintained sample integrity.

Ideal dilution factors were optimized for each test to allow for consistent and reproducible detection of each analyte. The dilution factors and lower limit of detection (LLOD) for each assay can be found in **Supplementary Table S1**.

Each sample was run in triplicate at the two dilutions for each analyte. The absorbance for each assay was measured using the Cytation™ 3 plate reader and Gen5™ software from BioTek Instruments, Inc. The standard curve for each assay was modeled with a 5-parameter fit, and the concentrations of the samples were calculated using this model. To limit variability, samples with a coefficient of variation exceeding 10 percent were either rerun to obtain an acceptable value or were excluded from the final analysis [sAPPα (2), ADAM-10 (Darnell et al., 2011), Aβ(1–42) (Kosinovsky et al., 2005), sAPPβ (Darnell et al., 2011), ADAM-17 (4), and BACE-1 (Ascano et al., 2012)].

Statistical Modeling

An Analysis-of-Covariance (ANCOVA) model was conducted where each amyloid was the response and diagnosis group (FXS vs. TDC) was the independent variable of interest. Covariates included sex, age, and sex*group interaction. Outliers determined by the ROUT method ($Q = 1\%$) were excluded from the analysis using GraphPad Prism version 8.01 for Windows, GraphPad Software, La Jolla, CA, United States[1] (Motulsky and Brown, 2006). Adjusted least-square means (LS means) were derived to compare group effects, or group*sex effects if the interaction term was significant. Lastly, Spearman correlation coefficients, corrected for age, were derived between the amyloid responses and FXS behavior scales for the FXS group. Consistent with prior studies (Ashwood et al., 2010; Ray et al., 2016) and the exploratory nature of this current study, correction multiple testing was not completed. Standard deviations are not available for the generalized linear models conducted here. However, pseudo-effect sizes (d*) may be derived by multiplying the resulting t-statistic (absolute value) for the LS mean differences by the square root of $(1/n_1 + 1/n_2)$, where n_1 and n_2 are the sample sizes of the two groups being compared. All statistical analyses (except for the outlier detection) were conducted using SAS®version 9.4 (SAS Institute Inc., Cary, NC, United States).

RESULTS

Patient Demographics

Results are summarized in **Table 1**. Subject groups were comprised of 27 FXS (15 males; mean age: 20.5 ± 11.6 years;

[1] www.graphpad.com

TABLE 1 | Characterization of FXS and control subjects.

Group	No.	Age	Age range	IQ	IQ range
Male					
FXS	15 (3 mosaic)	20.5 ± 11.6	5.9–40.9	44.1 ± 29.3	2.3–94.1
TDC	14	20.4 ± 11.1	5.9–43.5	101.5 ± 8.2	90.8–113.7
Female					
FXS	12	23.8 ± 11.5	8.0–42.9	65.9 ± 22.2	23.9–98.9
TDC	11	22.0 ± 10.7	8.1–39.8	99.6 ± 3.6	95.5–107.4

Age ranges and IQ scores were measured for both FXS and control subjects.

range: 5.9-40.9, 12 females; mean age: 23.8 ± 11.5 years; range: 8.0-42.9) and 25 age- and sex- matched neurotypical controls (14 males; mean age: 20.4 ± 11.1; range: 5.9-43.5, 11 females; 22.0 ± 10.7; range: 8.1-39.8). FXS participants were significantly more impacted (Deviation IQ = 54.0 ± 29.0; range: 2.3–98.9) than controls (Deviation IQ = 110.5 ± 6.5; range: 90.8–113.7) ($p < 0.001$). Females with FXS were (Deviation IQ = 66.7 ± 24.2; range 23.9–98.9) generally, but not significantly, higher functioning as compared to males with FXS (Deviation IQ = 44.1 ± 20.9; range 2.3–94.1) ($p = 0.879$). All except three males with FXS were full mutation. Two male mosaics were high functioning with deviation IQ scores greater than 90. However, these individuals were not found to impact the results observed.

APP Metabolites Are Differentially Expressed in FXS

Results are summarized in **Supplementary Table S2**. Analytes showing differential expression in the FXS group compared to TDC group are described here. sAPPα levels were significantly reduced in FXS relative to TDC ($p = 0.0003$, $d^* = 1.13$).

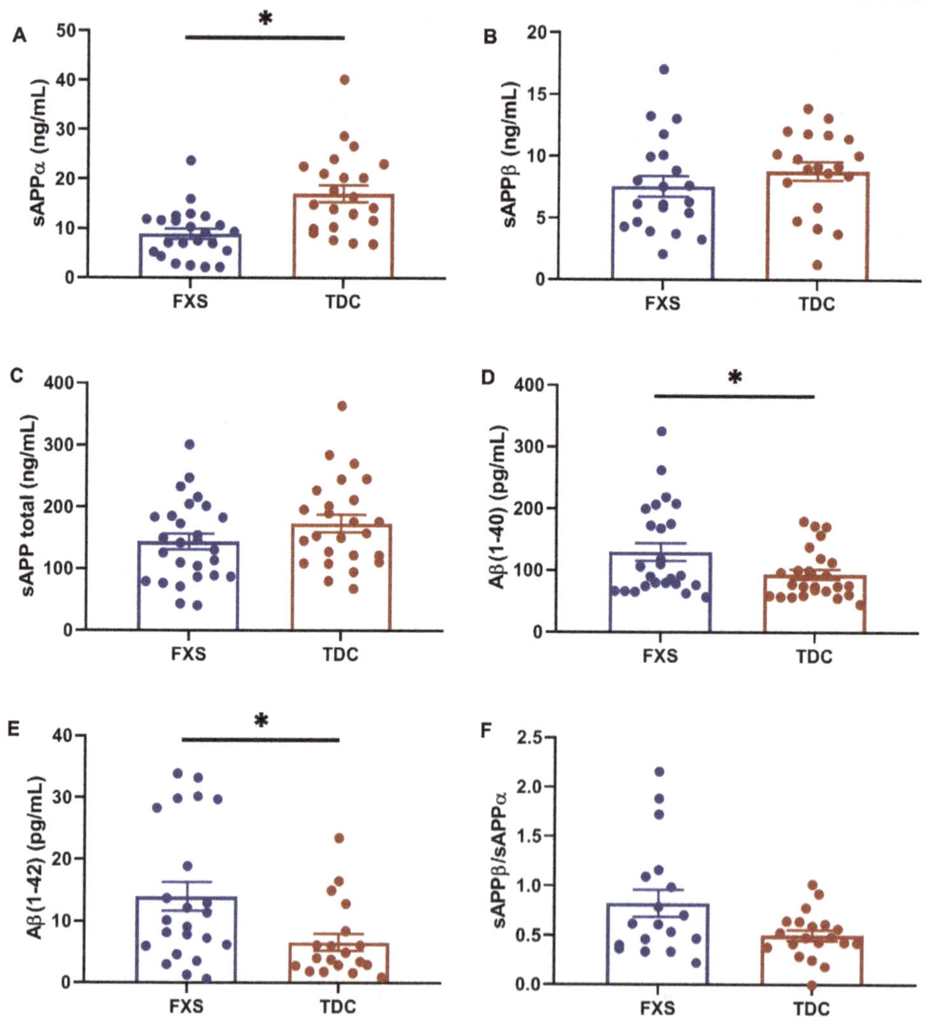

FIGURE 1 | Expression of APP metabolites in plasma from FXS and TDC subjects. Plasma levels of sAPPα, sAPPβ, sAPP total (α and β), Aβ (1–40), and Aβ (1–42) were measured using ELISA in both FXS and TDC participants. Outliers determined by the ROUT method were excluded from analysis [sAPPα (FXS = 3, TDC = 1), sAPPβ (FXS = 2, TDC = 1), Aβ(1–42) (FXS = 1, TDC = 3)]. **(A)** sAPPα was found to be significantly decreased in subjects with FXS as compared to controls ($p = 0.0003$). **(B,C)** Neither sAPPβ nor sAPP total levels were found to be significantly different between groups. **(D,E)** Both Aβ(1–40) and Aβ(1–42) were significantly increased in subjects with FXS as compared to controls ($p = 0.0169$ and 0.0098). **(F)** No significant difference was observed in the ratio of sAPPβ/sAPPα. $^*p > 0.05$.

Aβ(1–40) ($p = 0.0169$, $d^* = 0.70$) and Aβ(1–42) ($p = 0.0098$, $d^* = 0.85$) were significantly increased in FXS participants compared to TDC participants. Neither age nor sex differences contributed to these effects. Significant group differences were not observed in the expression of sAPPβ or sAPP total ($p > 0.05$). Additionally, no group difference in the ratio of sAPPβ/sAPPα were noted when evaluating for any differences in the balance of non-amyloidogenic versus amyloidogenic processing of APP (**Figure 1**). No correlations between APP metabolites were observed ($p > 0.05$, data not shown).

APP Processing Enzyme Levels Are Unaltered in FXS

Plasma levels of enzymes contributing to the amyloidogenic (BACE-1) and non-amyloidogenic (ADAM-10 and ADAM-17) were measured to see if differences in APP metabolites could be attributed to abnormal enzyme concentrations. However, no significant differences in total enzyme levels were found between groups (**Figure 2**). Additionally, no correlations were found between enzyme and metabolite concentrations using generalized mixed linear modeling with lognormal regression (**Supplementary Table S3**).

Expression of Metabolites and Enzymes Changes With Age

The effect of age was analyzed with respect to metabolite and enzyme expression (**Figure 3**). Both sAPPβ and sAPP total levels were found to significantly decrease with age in both groups ($p = 0.0074, 0.0112$). Similarly, Aβ(1–40) levels were inversely proportional to age ($p = 0.0644$) for both FXS and TDC groups. While both major metabolites of β-cleavage were found to decrease with age, BACE-1 levels appeared to increase with age ($p = 0.0548$) for each group. Neither sex nor mosaicism were found to affect the expression of any of the APP metabolites or enzymes measured.

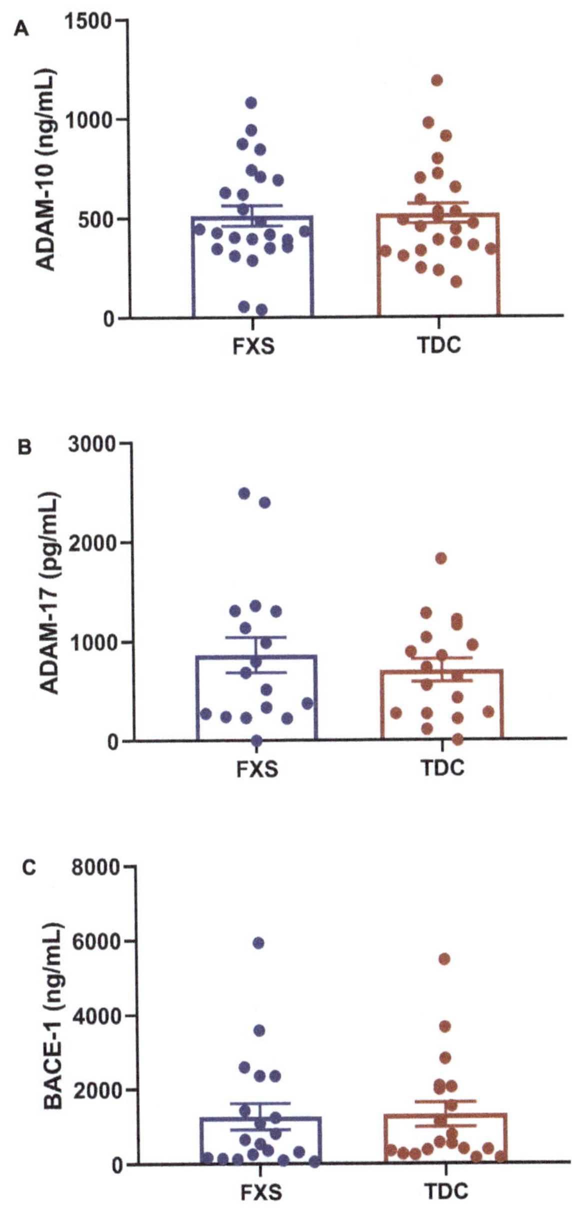

FIGURE 2 | Plasma levels of APP processing enzymes in FXS and control subjects. Plasma levels ADAM-10, ADAM-17, and BACE-1 were measured using ELISA in both FXS and TDC subjects. Outliers determined by the ROUT method were excluded from analysis [BACE-1 (FXS = 3, TDC = 1) and ADAM-17 (FXS = 3, TDC = 3)] **(A–C)** No significant differences were observed in the expression of ADAM-10, ADAM-17, and BACE-1 ($p > 0.05$).

DISCUSSION

We report a distinct molecular phenotype in our FXS participants as compared to matched controls with a significant decrease in peripheral levels of sAPPα and significant increases in peripheral levels of both Aβ(1–40) and Aβ(1–42). These results suggest potential preferential amyloidogenic, or β-secretase, processing of APP in individuals with FXS, as found in Alzheimer disease.

Similar to our findings, increased plasma concentrations of Aβ monomers have been previously reported in FXS (Westmark et al., 2011b; Ray et al., 2016). Although excess Aβ(1–40) and Aβ(1–42) are best understood in the context of Alzheimer disease, there are multiple ways that it can contribute to key phenotypes in FXS. In the brain, Aβ can significantly alter the excitability of the system both directly and indirectly. In APP overexpressing hippocampal slice neurons, Aβ has been shown to direct synaptic remodeling and depress excitatory synaptic signaling. Aβ levels also increase or decrease with respective excitation or depression of the neuronal activity and have been suggested to regulate hyperexcitability (Kamenetz et al., 2003). In the context of FXS, increased Aβ monomers may be indicative of a similar compensatory mechanism mediating neuronal hyperexcitability (Gibson et al., 2008; Choi et al., 2015; Ethridge et al., 2016, 2017; Westmark et al., 2016a; Lovelace et al., 2018). In contrast, excessive Aβ can form oligomers that, in conjunction with an extracellular scaffolding protein, can redistribute and reduce lateral mobility of $mGluR_5$ receptors, ultimately resulting in increased intracellular Ca^{2+} and neuronal excitation (Renner et al., 2010). Therefore, we speculate that excess Aβ could

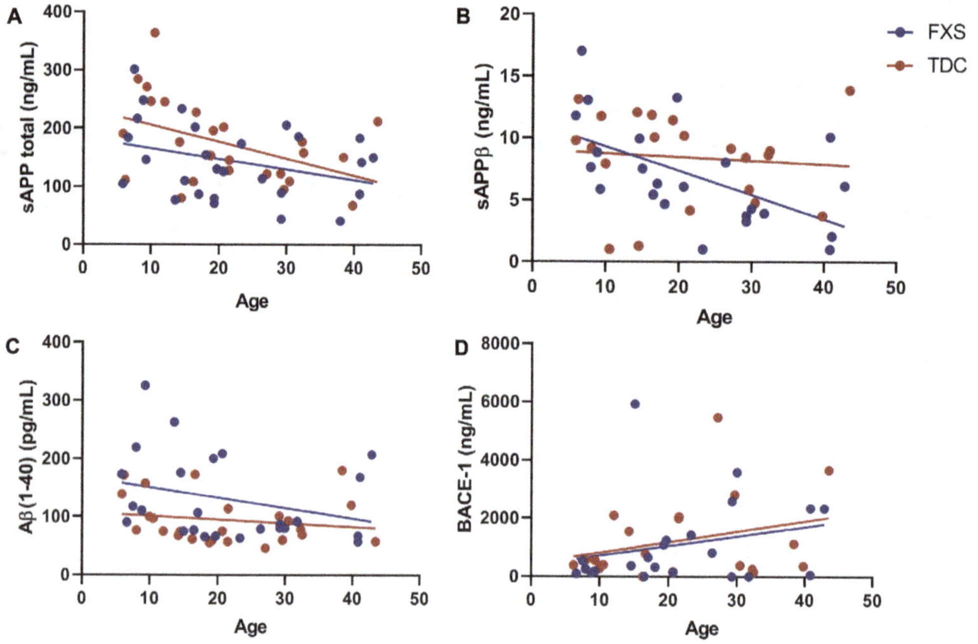

FIGURE 3 | BACE-1 activity may decrease with age. Levels of sAPP total, sAPPβ, Aβ(1–40), and BACE-1 captured by ELISA were analyzed with respect to subject age. **(A)** The expression of sAPP total decreases significantly in both FXS and TDC groups with respect to age ($p = 0.0112$). **(B)** The expression of sAPPβ decreases significantly in both FXS and TDC groups with respect to age ($p = 0.0074$). **(C)** Aβ(1–40) appears to be elevated in younger FXS patients and seems to decrease with age ($p = 0.0644$). **(D)** BACE-1 expression tended to increase with age although this trend did not reach statistical significance ($p = 0.0548$).

enhance neuronal excitability and lead to a positive feedback loop that increases hyperexcitability. Together, these findings indicate increased peripheral levels of both Aβ(1–40) and Aβ(1–42) are reflective of hyperexcitability and increased expression of APP and $mGluR_5$ in FXS. Thus, Aβ(1–40) and Aβ(1–42) each may be promising biomarkers of neural hyperexcitability in FXS.

Notably, a potential subgroup of FXS participants seem potentially represent a cluster of the highest levels of Aβ(1–42). Future studies including environmental and behavioral analyses may help to determine the cause of increased Aβ(1–42) in these individuals. For example, high fat diets have been show to promote the formation of the BACE-1/Adaptor protein-2/clathrin complex in mice, increasing the amount of intracellular BACE-1 and subsequent cleavage of APP (Maesako et al., 2015). Additionally, different behaviors, such as aggression, also correlate with levels of sAPPα in patients with ASD (Sokol et al., 2006). It could be that environmental or behavioral differences could similarly contribute to differences in peripheral metabolite expression within and between groups.

We also observed a significant reduction in peripheral sAPPα. Since both the α- and β-secretase(s) compete for APP as a substrate, the levels of their respective products also should vary inversely. With increased levels of peripheral Aβ, it is not surprising that there is a significant reduction in sAPPα. Our findings contradict previous reports by Ray et al. (2016) in which sAPPα was found to be increased in the plasma of patients with FXS. While we tested a number of plasma samples from patients with FXS from childhood to adulthood, Ray et al. (2016) only analyzed samples from children. Previous studies have shown that sAPPα is increased in juvenile *FMR1* KO brain at p21, and sAPP total is dysregulated at p21 and p30, but both return to homeostatic levels after these time points (Pasciuto et al., 2015). Restricting participant ages to children within this neurodevelopmental window may better capture potential increases in peripheral sAPPα and sAPP total.

While peripheral levels of APP metabolites were altered, we did not find any differences in the levels of their respective processing enzymes: ADAM-10, ADAM-17, and BACE-1 in FXS compared to TDC. Additionally, no correlations were found between any of the enzyme concentrations and the concentrations of their respective metabolites, importantly suggesting that total peripheral enzyme levels may not be indicative of peripheral metabolite regulation. Indeed, since ADAM-10, ADAM-17, and BACE-1 all act on numerous targets in multiple tissues, their peripheral expression may fluctuate less in response to increased APP (Barão et al., 2016; Moss and Minond, 2017; Wetzel et al., 2017). Clearance of APP metabolites from the brain and other tissues also could strongly influence peripheral metabolite levels, making the direct relationship between concentrations of enzymes and metabolites less accurate. With multiple tissue subtypes contributing to peripheral metabolite concentrations, the lack of correlation between peripheral metabolite and enzyme expression is expected. Additionally, peripheral concentrations may also not be indicative of enzymatic activity. For example, increased peripheral BACE-1 activity could result in higher turnover of sAPPβ to both Aβ peptides. This could potentially account for the differences in metabolite expression, while no differences were observed in enzyme concentration. These enzymes also could be differentially regulated during critical developmental periods not captured within our wider age range of participants. For example, in *FMR1* KO ADAM-10 expression is dysregulated in cortical neurons during a critical neurodevelopmental window in juvenile mice (Pasciuto et al., 2015). Thus, future studies are needed examine processing enzymes in a more restricted range of individuals with FXS.

Interestingly, we noted several molecular changes with age in both persons with FXS and control participants, including sAPP total, sAPPβ, Aβ(1–40), and BACE-1. Given associations were observed across both patient and control participants, this suggests that potentially developmental changes of APP metabolites and enzyme concentrations is intact in FXS. Since sAPP total is a total measure of sAPPα and sAPPβ, its significant decrease with respect to age can largely be attributed to the decrease in sAPPβ levels. Counterintuitively, while peripheral expression of both Aβ(1–40) and sAPPβ decrease with age, BACE-1 levels increase with age in both our FXS and control groups. The inverse relationship between amyloidogenic metabolites and BACE-1 reinforces that there is no clear relationship between peripheral metabolite and enzyme levels in FXS.

The results of our work should be understood within the context of the limitations of our experimental design. The greatest limitation was the overall sample size. With the significant variability of multiple metabolites with respect to age, it is possible that more subtle differences in metabolite and enzyme expression may have been captured within a narrower age range and/or a larger sample size. Correlations with clinical features such as IQ may have also been limited by sample size. Given the potential utility of APP metabolites as peripheral biomarkers in FXS, future studies including with larger participant pools need to be completed to evaluate for correlations with clinical data. Additional measures of clinical severity were not available to evaluate correlations with APP metabolites. Future work with an expanded number of subjects and deeper phenotyping will aide these efforts.

Amyloid-beta precursor protein metabolite concentrations also have a diurnal expression pattern in both cerebrospinal fluid and blood (Dobrowolska et al., 2014). Since not all blood was collected at the same time of day, relative levels of APP within participants may vary which could either prevent us from observing a small effect or lead us to observing an exaggerated effect. Additionally, blood was collected in tubes using K_2EDTA as a preservative, which has been shown to significantly reduce levels of Aβ(1–42) in plasma (Westmark et al., 2011a). Because K_2EDTA was used to collect all samples, the effect size of differences in Aβ(1–42) levels between groups may have been underestimated in this study.

We also report no differences in metabolite or enzyme expression between males, full mutation and mosaic, and females with FXS (**Supplementary Table S2**), which is somewhat unexpected. Many of the effects are subtle and may require a more sensitive platform to detect and/or larger subject cohorts to discern potentially more subtle differences. Additionally, our FXS female sample did not differ on IQ from their male counterparts, suggesting FXS males and females were similarly affected in the current study. Thus, it is possible with a more representative FXS female sample, sex differences in primary measures may emerge. Last, we are using peripheral APP metabolite and enzyme levels as a proxy to evaluate their relative expression in brain. To date, there are a very limited amount of known proteins that are expressed in parallel between brain and blood (Tajima et al., 2013). In addition to the brain, APP is also expressed in the thymus, heart, muscle, lung, kidney, adipose tissue, liver, spleen, skin, and intestine (Beer et al., 1995). Similarly, the processing enzymes are also expressed in a variety of different tissue types. Thus, blood levels of APP metabolites are most likely influenced by their expression in many organs of the body. This makes comparing peripheral APP levels to levels observed in the brain much more difficult and introduces a level of uncertainty to the measures.

CONCLUSION

In conclusion, we determined a distinct molecular pattern of APP metabolite expression with increased Aβ(1–40) and Aβ(1–42) and decreased sAPPα. While we suggest that there is increased β-secretase activity in FXS, more work needs to be completed to determine the exact mechanisms leading to increased peripheral Aβ. Still our findings provide new evidence of the promising potential of APP metabolite expression as a blood-based biomarker in FXS. Ultimately, our work highlights the need for more thorough characterization of APP expression patterns with both behavioral and electrophysiological patterns in FXS, which may provide additional insight into the mechanistic roles of APP metabolites.

ETHICS STATEMENT

All subjects gave written informed consent in accordance with the Declaration of Helsinki. The protocol was approved by the Cincinnati Children's Hospital Institutional Review Board.

AUTHOR CONTRIBUTIONS

RM aided in the study design, responsible for collecting, analyzing, and interpreting the molecular data, and writing of the manuscript. LS contributed significantly to the manuscript preparation and deviation IQ analyses. EP and KD contributed significantly to the study setup and design. RS responsible for collecting and interpreting the clinical measures. PH performed all the statistical modeling and analyses. CG aided in the study design and contributed significantly to the molecular analysis and interpretation. CE significantly contributed to the study setup and design, as well as manuscript preparation. All authors contributed substantially to the study, and read and approved the final version of the manuscript.

FUNDING

This project was supported by the Cincinnati Children's Hospital Research Foundation and the Fragile X Alliance of Ohio.

ACKNOWLEDGMENTS

The authors would like to thank Sarah Fitzpatrick, Janna Guilfoyle, Nicole Friedman, and Danielle Chin for sample collection and data acquisition.

SUPPLEMENTARY MATERIAL

TABLE S1 | Dilution factors and lower limits of detection for each ELISA. Prior to analysis, all analyte concentrations were optimized per ELISA plate. All samples were run with the dilutions listed in the table.

TABLE S2 | Analytes only significantly varied with respect to group. Levels of all analytes were captured by ELISA and analyzed with respect to group. Only sAPPα, Aβ(1–40), and Aβ(1–42) were significantly different between groups. No significant Sex*Group interactions were found for any of the analytes tested ($p > 0.05$).

TABLE S3 | Metabolite concentrations did not correlate significantly with their respective processing enzymes. The relationship between levels of APP metabolites and enzymes were examined with respect to group using generalized linear models with lognormal regression. No correlates were found to be significant ($p > 0.05$).

REFERENCES

Ascano, M. Jr., Mukherjee, N., Bandaru, P., Miller, J. B., Nusbaum, J. D., Corcoran, D. L., et al. (2012). FMRP targets distinct mRNA sequence elements to regulate protein expression. *Nature* 492, 382–386. doi: 10.1038/nature11737

Ashwood, P., Nguyen, D. V., Hessl, D., Hagerman, R. J., and Tassone, F. (2010). Plasma cytokine profiles in Fragile X subjects: is there a role for cytokines in the pathogenesis? *Brain Behav. Immun.* 24, 898–902. doi: 10.1016/j.bbi.2010.01.008

Bailey, A. R., Giunta, B. N., Obregon, D., Nikolic, W. V., Tian, J., Sanberg, C. D., et al. (2008). Peripheral biomarkers in Autism: secreted amyloid precursor protein-alpha as a probable key player in early diagnosis. *Int. J. Clin. Exp. Med.* 1, 338–344.

Barão, S., Moechars, D., Lichtenthaler, S. F., and De Strooper, B. (2016). BACE1 physiological functions may limit its use as therapeutic target for Alzheimer's disease. *Trends Neurosci.* 39, 158–169. doi: 10.1016/j.tins.2016.01.003

Beer, J., Masters, C. L., and Beyreuther, K. (1995). Cells from peripheral tissues that exhibit high APP expression are characterized by their high membrane fusion activity. *Neurodegeneration* 4, 51–59. doi: 10.1006/neur.1995.0006

Buxbaum, J. D., Liu, K.-N., Luo, Y., Slack, J. L., Stocking, K. L., Peschon, J. J., et al. (1998). Evidence that tumor necrosis factor α converting enzyme is involved in regulated α-secretase cleavage of the Alzheimer amyloid protein precursor. *J. Biol. Chem.* 273, 27765–27767. doi: 10.1074/jbc.273.43.27765

Chasseigneaux, S., and Allinquant, B. (2012). Functions of Aβ, sAPPα and sAPPβ: similarities and differences. *J. Neurochem.* 120(Suppl. 1), 99–108.

Choi, C. H., Schoenfeld, B. P., Weisz, E. D., Bell, A. J., Chambers, D. B., Hinchey, J., et al. (2015). PDE-4 inhibition rescues aberrant synaptic plasticity in Drosophila and mouse models of fragile X syndrome. *J. Neurosci.* 35, 396–408. doi: 10.1523/JNEUROSCI.1356-12.2015

Corrigan, F., Pham, C. L. L., Vink, R., Blumbergs, P. C., Masters, C. L., van den Heuvel, C., et al. (2011). The neuroprotective domains of the amyloid precursor protein, in traumatic brain injury, are located in the two growth factor domains. *Brain Res.* 1378, 137–143. doi: 10.1016/j.brainres.2010.12.077

Darnell, J. C., Van Driesche, S. J., Zhang, C., Hung, K. Y., Mele, A., Fraser, C. E., et al. (2011). FMRP stalls ribosomal translocation on mRNAs linked to synaptic function and autism. *Cell* 146, 247–261. doi: 10.1016/j.cell.2011.06.013

Dobrowolska, J. A., Kasten, T., Huang, Y., Benzinger, T. L., Sigurdson, W., Ovod, V., et al. (2014). Diurnal patterns of soluble amyloid precursor protein metabolites in the human central nervous system. *PLoS One* 9:e89998. doi: 10.1371/journal.pone.0089998

Erickson, C. A., Ray, B., Maloney, B., Wink, L. K., Bowers, K., Schaefer, T. L., et al. (2014). Impact of acamprosate on plasma amyloid-beta precursor protein in youth: a pilot analysis in fragile X syndrome-associated and idiopathic autism spectrum disorder suggests a pharmacodynamic protein marker. *J. Psychiatr. Res.* 59, 220–228. doi: 10.1016/j.jpsychires.2014.07.011

Erickson, C. A., Wink, L. K., Baindu, B., Ray, B., Schaefer, T. L., Pedapati, E. V., et al. (2016). Analysis of peripheral amyloid precursor protein in angelman syndrome. *Am. J. Med. Genet. A* 170, 2334–2337. doi: 10.1002/ajmg.a.37811

Ethridge, L. E., White, S. P., Mosconi, M. W., Wang, J., Byerly, M. J., and Sweeney, J. A. (2016). Reduced habituation of auditory evoked potentials indicate cortical hyper-excitability in Fragile X Syndrome. *Transl. Psychiatry* 6:e787. doi: 10.1038/tp.2016.48

Ethridge, L. E., White, S. P., Mosconi, M. W., Wang, J., Pedapati, E. V., Erickson, C. A., et al. (2017). Neural synchronization deficits linked to cortical hyper-excitability and auditory hypersensitivity in fragile X syndrome. *Mol. Autism* 8:22. doi: 10.1186/s13229-017-0140-1

Gibson, J. R., Bartley, A. F., Hays, S. A., and Huber, K. M. (2008). Imbalance of neocortical excitation and inhibition and altered UP states reflect network hyperexcitability in the mouse model of fragile X syndrome. *J. Neurophysiol.* 100, 2615–2626. doi: 10.1152/jn.90752.2008

Guénette, S., Chang, Y., Hiesberger, T., Richardson, J. A., Eckman, C. B., Eckman, E. A., et al. (2006). Essential roles for the FE65 amyloid precursor protein-interacting proteins in brain development. *EMBO J.* 25, 420–431. doi: 10.1038/sj.emboj.7600926

Hardy, J., and Selkoe, D. J. (2002). The amyloid hypothesis of Alzheimer's disease: progress and problems on the road to therapeutics. *Science* 297, 353–356. doi: 10.1126/science.1072994

Hartmann, D., Strooper, B. D., and Saftig, P. (1999). Presenilin-1 deficiency leads to loss of Cajal–Retzius neurons and cortical dysplasia similar to human type 2 lissencephaly. *Curr. Biol.* 9, 719–727. doi: 10.1016/s0960-9822(99)80331-5

Herms, J., Anliker, B., Heber, S., Ring, S., Fuhrmann, M., Kretzschmar, H., et al. (2004). Cortical dysplasia resembling human type 2 lissencephaly in mice lacking all three APP family members. *EMBO J.* 23:4106. doi: 10.1038/sj.emboj.7600390

Kamenetz, F., Tomita, T., Hsieh, H., Seabrook, G., Borchelt, D., Iwatsubo, T., et al. (2003). APP processing and synaptic function. *Neuron* 37, 925–937. doi: 10.1016/s0896-6273(03)00124-7

Kosinovsky, B., Hermon, S., Yoran-Hegesh, R., Golomb, A., Senecky, Y., Goez, H., et al. (2005). The yield of laboratory investigations in children with infantile autism. *J. Neural Transm.* 112, 587–596. doi: 10.1007/s00702-004-0198-8

Lammich, S., Kojro, E., Postina, R., Gilbert, S., Pfeiffer, R., Jasionowski, M., et al. (1999). Constitutive and regulated α-secretase cleavage of Alzheimer's amyloid precursor protein by a disintegrin metalloprotease. *Proc. Natl. Acad. Sci. U.S.A.* 96, 3922–3927. doi: 10.1073/pnas.96.7.3922

Lovelace, J. W., Ethell, I. M., Binder, D. K., and Razak, K. A. (2018). Translation-relevant EEG phenotypes in a mouse model of Fragile X Syndrome. *Neurobiol. Dis.* 115, 39–48. doi: 10.1016/j.nbd.2018.03.012

Luo, J. J., Wallace, M. S., Hawver, D. B., Kusiak, J. W., and Wallace, W. C. (2001). Characterization of the neurotrophic interaction between nerve growth factor and secreted alpha-amyloid precursor protein. *J. Neurosci. Res.* 63, 410–420. doi: 10.1002/1097-4547(20010301)63:5<410::aid-jnr1036>3.0.co;2-b

Maesako, M., Uemura, M., Tashiro, Y., Sasaki, K., Watanabe, K., Noda, Y., et al. (2015). High fat diet enhances β-Site cleavage of amyloid precursor protein (APP) via Promoting β-site APP cleaving enzyme 1/Adaptor Protein 2/Clathrin complex formation. *PLoS One* 10:e0131199. doi: 10.1371/journal.pone.0131199

Masters, C. L., Simms, G., Weinman, N. A., Multhaup, G., McDonald, B. L., and Beyreuther, K. (1985). Amyloid plaque core protein in Alzheimer disease and Down Syndrome. *Proc. Natl. Acad. Sci. U.S.A.* 82, 4245–4249. doi: 10.1073/pnas.82.12.4245

Mattson, M. P., Cheng, B., Culwell, A. R., Esch, F. S., Lieberburg, I., and Rydel, R. E. (1993). Evidence for excitoprotective and intraneuronal calcium-regulating roles for secreted forms of the β-amyloid precursor protein. *Neuron* 10, 243–254. doi: 10.1016/0896-6273(93)90315-i

Moss, M. L., and Minond, D. (2017). Recent advances in ADAM17 research: a promising target for cancer and inflammation. *J. Mediat. Inflamm.* 2017:9673537. doi: 10.1155/2017/9673537

Motulsky, H. J., and Brown, R. E. (2006). Detecting outliers when fitting data with nonlinear regression – a new method based on robust nonlinear regression and the false discovery rate. *BMC Bioinformatics* 7:123. doi: 10.1186/1471-2105-7-123

Pasciuto, E., Ahmed, T., Wahle, T., Gardoni, F., D'Andrea, L., Pacini, L., et al. (2015). Dysregulated ADAM10-Mediated processing of APP during a critical time window leads to synaptic deficits in fragile X syndrome. *Neuron* 87, 382–398. doi: 10.1016/j.neuron.2015.06.032

Persson, K., Eldholm, R. S., Barca, M. L., Cavallin, L., Ferreira, D., Knapskog, A. B., et al. (2017). MRI-assessed atrophy subtypes in Alzheimer's disease and the cognitive reserve hypothesis. *PLoS One* 12:e0186595. doi: 10.1371/journal.pone.0186595

Ray, B., Long, J. M., Sokol, D. K., and Lahiri, D. K. (2011). Increased secreted amyloid precursor protein-alpha (sAPPalpha) in severe autism: proposal of a specific, anabolic pathway and putative biomarker. *PLoS One* 6:e20405. doi: 10.1371/journal.pone.0020405

Ray, B., Sokol, D. K., Maloney, B., and Lahiri, D. K. (2016). Finding novel distinctions between the sAPPalpha-mediated anabolic biochemical pathways in autism spectrum disorder and Fragile X Syndrome plasma and brain tissue. *Sci. Rep.* 6:26052. doi: 10.1038/srep26052

Renner, M., Lacor, P. N., Velasco, P. T., Xu, J., Contractor, A., Klein, W. L., et al. (2010). Deleterious effects of Amyloid β Oligomers acting as an extracellular scaffold for mGluR5. *Neuron* 66, 739–754. doi: 10.1016/j.neuron.2010.04.029

Sansone, S. M., Widaman, K. F., Hall, S. S., Reiss, A. L., Lightbody, A., Kaufmann, W. E., et al. (2012). Psychometric study of the aberrant behavior checklist in fragile X syndrome and implications for targeted treatment. *J. Autism Dev. Disord.* 42, 1377–1392. doi: 10.1007/s10803-011-1370-2

Smith-Swintosky, V. L., Pettigrew, L. C., Craddock, S. D., Culwell, A. R., Rydel, R. E., and Mattson, M. P. (1994). Secreted forms of β-Amyloid precursor protein protect against ischemic brain injur. *J. Neurochem.* 63, 781–784. doi: 10.1046/j.1471-4159.1994.63020781.x

Sokol, D. K., Chen, D., Farlow, M. R., Dunn, D. W., Maloney, B., Zimmer, J. A., et al. (2006). High levels of Alzheimer beta-amyloid precursor protein (APP) in children with severely autistic behavior and aggression. *J. Child Neurol.* 21, 444–449. doi: 10.1177/08830738060210062201

Tajima, Y., Ishikawa, M., Maekawa, K., Murayama, M., Senoo, Y., Nishimaki-Mogami, T., et al. (2013). Lipidomic analysis of brain tissues and plasma in a mouse model expressing mutated human amyloid precursor protein/tau for Alzheimer's disease. *Lipids Health Dis.* 12:68. doi: 10.1186/1476-511X-12-68

Vassar, R., Bennett, B. D., Babu-Khan, S., Kahn, S., Mendiaz, E. A., Denis, P., et al. (1999). β-Secretase cleavage of Alzheimer's amyloid precursor protein by the transmembrane aspartic protease BACE. *Science* 286, 735–741. doi: 10.1126/science.286.5440.735

Westmark, C. J. (2018). Fragile X and APP: a decade in review, a vision for the future. *Mol. Neurobiol.* 56, 3904–3921. doi: 10.1007/s12035-018-1344-x

Westmark, C. J., Chuang, S. C., Hays, S. A., Filon, M. J., Ray, B. C., Westmark, P. R., et al. (2016a). APP causes hyperexcitability in Fragile X Mice. *Front. Mol. Neurosci.* 9:147. doi: 10.3389/fnmol.2016.00147

Westmark, C. J., Sokol, D. K., Maloney, B., and Lahiri, D. K. (2016b). Novel roles of amyloid-beta precursor protein metabolites in fragile X syndrome and autism. *Mol. Psychiatry* 21, 1333–1341. doi: 10.1038/mp.2016.134

Westmark, C. J., Hervey, C. M., Berry-Kravis, E. M., and Malter, J. S. (2011a). Effect of anticoagulants on Amyloid β-Protein precursor and amyloid beta levels in plasma. *J. Alzheimers Dis. Parkinsonism* 1:101.

Westmark, C. J., Westmark, P. R., O'Riordan, K. J., Ray, B. C., Hervey, C. M., Salamat, M. S., et al. (2011b). Reversal of fragile X phenotypes by manipulation of AbetaPP/Abeta levels in Fmr1KO mice. *PLoS One* 6:e26549. doi: 10.1371/journal.pone.0026549

Westmark, C. J., and Malter, J. S. (2007). FMRP mediates mGluR5-dependent translation of amyloid precursor protein. *PLoS Biol.* 5:e52. doi: 10.1371/journal.pbio.0050052

Wetzel, S., Seipold, L., and Saftig, P. (2017). The metalloproteinase ADAM10: a useful therapeutic target? *Biochim. Biophys. Acta Mol. Cell Res.* 1864(11 Pt B), 2071–2081. doi: 10.1016/j.bbamcr.2017.06.005

Whitson, J. S., Selkoe, D. J., and Cotman, C. W. (1989). Amyloid beta protein enhances the survival of hippocampal neurons in vitro. *Science* 243, 1488–1490. doi: 10.1126/science.2928783

11

Continuous Theta-Burst Stimulation in Children with High-Functioning Autism Spectrum Disorder and Typically Developing Children

Ali Jannati[1,2]*, Gabrielle Block*[1,2†], *Mary A. Ryan*[1,2], *Harper L. Kaye*[1], *Fae B. Kayarian*[2], *Shahid Bashir*[3], *Lindsay M. Oberman*[4†], *Alvaro Pascual-Leone*[2,5] *and Alexander Rotenberg*[1,2]*

[1]*Neuromodulation Program and Division of Epilepsy and Clinical Neurophysiology, Department of Neurology, Boston Children's Hospital, Harvard Medical School, Boston, MA, United States,* [2]*Berenson-Allen Center for Noninvasive Brain Stimulation and Division of Cognitive Neurology, Department of Neurology, Beth Israel Deaconess Medical Center, Harvard Medical School, Boston, MA, United States,* [3]*Neuroscience Center, King Fahad Specialist Hospital Dammam, Dammam, Saudi Arabia,* [4]*Neuroplasticity and Autism Spectrum Disorder Program, Department of Psychiatry and Human Behavior, E. P. Bradley Hospital, Warren Alpert Medical School, Brown University, East Providence, RI, United States,* [5]*Institut Guttman de Neurorehabilitació, Universitat Autónoma de Barcelona, Badalona, Spain*

Correspondence:
Ali Jannati
ali.jannati@childrens.harvard.edu
Alexander Rotenberg
alexander.rotenberg@childrens.harvard.edu

Objectives: A neurophysiologic biomarker for autism spectrum disorder (ASD) is highly desirable and can improve diagnosis, monitoring, and assessment of therapeutic response among children with ASD. We investigated the utility of continuous theta-burst stimulation (cTBS) applied to the motor cortex (M1) as a biomarker for children and adolescents with high-functioning (HF) ASD compared to their age- and gender-matched typically developing (TD) controls. We also compared the developmental trajectory of long-term depression- (LTD-) like plasticity in the two groups. Finally, we explored the influence of a common brain-derived neurotrophic factor *(BDNF)* polymorphism on cTBS aftereffects in a subset of the ASD group.

Methods: Twenty-nine children and adolescents (age range 10–16) in ASD (n = 11) and TD (n = 18) groups underwent M1 cTBS. Changes in MEP amplitude at 5–60 min post-cTBS and their cumulative measures in each group were calculated. We also assessed the relationship between age and maximum cTBS-induced MEP suppression (ΔMEP_{Max}) in each group. Finally, we compared cTBS aftereffects in *BDNF* Val/Val (n = 4) and Val/Met (n = 4) ASD participants.

Results: Cumulative cTBS aftereffects were significantly more facilitatory in the ASD group than in the TD group (P_{FDR}'s < 0.03). ΔMEP_{Max} was negatively correlated with age in the ASD group (r = −0.67, P = 0.025), but not in the TD group (r = −0.12,

Abbreviations: ADHD, attention-deficit/hyperactivity disorder; AMT, active motor threshold; *BDNF*, brain-derived neurotrophic factor; cTBS, continuous theta-burst stimulation; ΔMEP, natural log-transformed, baseline-corrected amplitude of motor evoked potentials; EEG, electroencephalography; EMG, electromyography; FDR, false discovery rate; fMRI, functional magnetic resonance imaging; GABA, gamma-aminobutyric acid; HF, high-functioning; IQ, intelligence quotient; iTBS, intermittent theta-burst stimulation; LF, low-functioning; LTD, long-term depression; LTP, long-term potentiation; MEP, motor evoked potential; Met, metionine; PAS, paired associative stimulation; PCR, polymerase chain reaction; RMT, resting motor threshold; rTMS, repetitive transcranial magnetic stimulation; SICI, short-interval intracortical cortical inhibition; SNP, single-nucleotide polymorphism; TMS, transcranial magnetic stimulation; Tn, at *n* minutes post-cTBS; Val, valine; %Δ, percent change from the baseline.

$P = 0.65$). Cumulative cTBS aftereffects were not significantly different between the two *BDNF* subgroups (P-values > 0.18).

Conclusions: The results support the utility of cTBS measures of cortical plasticity as a biomarker for children and adolescents with HF-ASD and an aberrant developmental trajectory of LTD-like plasticity in ASD.

Keywords: transcranial magnetic stimulation, continuous theta-burst stimulation, plasticity, biomarker, autism spectrum disorder, BDNF

INTRODUCTION

Autism spectrum disorder (ASD) is characterized by social communication deficits and restricted, repetitive, and stereotyped behaviors and interests (American Psychiatric Association, 2013). Due to the large variability in the clinical phenotype of ASD and manifestation of symptoms over a range of ages in childhood, a clinical diagnosis of ASD can be challenging and is often not made until 3–5 years of age. For this reason, a neurophysiologic ASD biomarker is highly desirable, particularly for improving diagnostic specificity and for enabling metrics of therapeutic target-engagement and outcomes.

Aberrant synaptic plasticity in patients with ASD can be measured *in vivo* at the circuit level by transcranial magnetic stimulation (TMS; Huang et al., 2005; Hallett, 2007; Pascual-Leone et al., 2011). TMS enables focal noninvasive brain stimulation by electromagnetic induction (Barker et al., 1985; Kobayashi and Pascual-Leone, 2003; Hallett, 2007), to evoke or modulate neural activity in a given brain region or network (Valero-Cabré et al., 2017). When the recommended guidelines are followed (Rossi et al., 2009; Rossini et al., 2015), TMS is safe and well-tolerated, even in pediatric populations (Garvey and Gilbert, 2004; Rajapakse and Kirton, 2013; Hameed et al., 2017). TMS, when combined with electromyography (EMG), electroencephalography (EEG), or neuroimaging such as functional magnetic resonance imaging (fMRI) can quantify the extent of modulation of cortical reactivity induced by an intervention, providing an index of brain plasticity (Pascual-Leone et al., 2011).

Patterned repetitive TMS (rTMS) protocols in humans approximate experimental protocols that predictably induce long-term depression (LTD) and long-term potentiation (LTP) of synaptic strength in animal models (Huang et al., 2005, 2008). A form of rTMS termed continuous theta-burst stimulation (cTBS) consists of 50 Hz bursts of three TMS pulses repeated at 5 Hz for a total of 600 pulses over 40 s (Huang et al., 2005). Following cTBS of the primary motor cortex (M1), the average amplitude of motor evoked potentials (MEPs) induced by single TMS pulses is typically reduced by 25% for up to 50 min, before returning to pre-cTBS baseline (Wischnewski and Schutter, 2015). The cTBS-induced neuromodulatory effect has LTD-like characteristics (Cárdenas-Morales et al., 2011) and involves mechanisms of GABAergic and glutamatergic plasticity (Stagg et al., 2009; Trippe et al., 2009; Benali et al., 2011). Thus, cTBS aftereffects provide a neurophysiologic index of the mechanism of LTD-like cortical plasticity that is abnormal in patients with ASD (Pascual-Leone et al., 2005, 2011; Oberman et al., 2010).

Pursuant to cTBS (Oberman et al., 2012), adults with high-functioning (HF) ASD have greater and longer-lasting MEP suppression as compared to neurotypical (NT) controls, indicating an exaggerated, *hyperplastic*, response to patterned cortical stimulation. Additionally (Oberman et al., 2014), cTBS measures of plasticity among children and adolescents with HF-ASD demonstrate a positive linear relationship between age and the extent of cTBS-induced modulation. These findings reveal an age-related increase in LTD-like plasticity in childhood and adolescence.

We now extend the scope of previous cTBS studies in 10–16 years old children with high-functioning ASD addressing two questions: (1) are cTBS aftereffects different between ASD and typically developing (TD) groups? (i.e., is the cTBS biomarker adequate to distinguish children and adolescents with HF-ASD from age-matched TD controls?); and (2) does the developmental trajectory of cortical plasticity, as measured by cTBS aftereffects, differ between the two groups? (i.e., is there cortical dysmaturity in children with HF-ASD associated with delayed or aberrant maturation of LTD-like plasticity as measured by cTBS?). We also conduct pilot analysis on a subset of the ASD group, to test whether cTBS measures of plasticity were affected by a common single-nucleotide polymorphism (SNP) in the brain-derived neurotrophic factor (*BDNF*) gene, Val66Met, which has influences on rTMS measures of cortical plasticity in healthy subjects (Cheeran et al., 2008; Antal et al., 2010; Lee et al., 2013; Chang et al., 2014; Di Lazzaro et al., 2015; Fried et al., 2017; Jannati et al., 2017; Jannati et al., 2019).

MATERIALS AND METHODS

Participants

Twenty-nine individuals participated in this study, which was approved by the local Institutional Review Board in accordance with the Declaration of Helsinki. All participants or their parents/legal guardians provided written informed consent/assent prior to enrollment and received age-appropriate monetary compensation in the form of a gift card upon completion. No participants endorsed TMS-specific contraindications (Rossi et al., 2009), and neurological examination was unremarkable for all participants enrolled. The two study populations were as follows: (1) high-functioning children with idiopathic ASD (n = 11; *ASD group*); and

(2) neurotypical age- and gender-matched controls (n = 18; *TD group*). The TD group were originally recruited as part of a separate and unrelated study, and not for the purpose of comparing cTBS responses between TD and ASD children. Participants were recruited through local community advertisements, and local autism associations and clinics. All participants in the ASD group carried a prior clinical diagnosis made by a psychiatrist or clinical psychologist, met diagnostic criteria for ASD as defined by the *Diagnostic and Statistical Manual of Mental Disorders*, 5th edition (DSM-5©; American Psychiatric Association, 2013), and underwent independent neuropsychological assessment *via* the Autism Diagnostic Observation Schedule (ADOS; mean score = 10.82; SD = 3.28). Participants in the ASD group underwent a comprehensive neurological exam by a board-certified pediatric neurologist (Alexander Rotenberg, study M.D.) to confirm the absence of impaired gross or fine motor function. Participants in the TD group had no neurological or psychological disorder. Lastly, all participants were screened following published recommendations endorsed by the International Federation of Clinical Neurophysiology (see **Table 1** for detailed demographic information).

Neuropsychological Testing

The ADOS (Lord et al., 2000), and the Abbreviated Battery of Stanford–Binet IV intelligence scale (Thorndike et al., 1986) were completed for the ASD group. IQ scores were obtained prior to enrollment only for children with ASD to ensure patients with intellectual disability or low-functioning ASD were excluded from enrollment. IQ testing was not performed for TD children, with the assumption that the IQ of TD children falls within the normal limits of the general pediatric population.

We limited the enrollment of our ASD participants to HF children for two reasons: (1) lack of established feasibility of TMS/cTBS procedures in children with LF ASD; and (2) to reduce the heterogeneity of our pool of children with ASD, which are by nature, a heterogeneous population. As such, the findings reported in this study may be specific only to children and adolescents with HF-ASD.

Genetic Testing

Saliva samples from participants in the ASD group (n = 8) were used to assess *BDNF* Val66Met SNP. The remaining three participants in the ASD group did not provide consent for DNA sampling and were thus not included in this subset.

Aliquot (700 μl) extraction of genomic DNA was performed on saliva samples collected using the Oragene Discover OGR-250 Kit (DNA Genotek Inc., Ottawa, ON, Canada). DNA was extracted from samples using standard methodology and the prepIT•L2P reagent (DNA Genotek Inc, 2015). The following quality control metrics were performed on each sample: PicoGreen fluorometry for double-stranded DNA quantification, Nanodrop spectrophotometry as an estimate of sample purity using A260/A280 ratios and agarose gel electrophoresis for visualization of DNA integrity.

The rs6265 SNP of the *BDNF* gene was analyzed using a TaqMan single-tube genotyping assay, which uses polymerase chain reaction (PCR) amplification and a pair of fluorescent dye detectors that target the SNP. One fluorescent dye is attached to the detector that is a perfect match to the first allele and a different fluorescent dye is attached to the detector that is a perfect match to the second allele. During PCR, the polymerase releases the fluorescent probe into solution where it is detected using endpoint analysis in an Applied Biosystems Inc. (Foster City, CA, USA) 7900HT Real-Time instrument. Primers and probes were also obtained through Applied Biosystems.

Because DNA samples were not available for the TD group, and a difference in rs6265 SNP prevalence in the ASD and TD groups could give rise to a difference in cTBS responses exhibited by the two groups, we estimated the probability that two hypothetical ASD and TD groups with sample sizes of 11 and 18, respectively, would have significantly different *BDNF* Met−:Met+ ratios. The minor allele frequency of the rs6265 SNP in the admixed American population in The 1000 Genomes Project Consortium et al. (2015) is approximately 0.153, which translates to 71.79%, 25.88%, and 2.33% for the prevalence of *BDNF* Val/Val, Val/Met, and Met/Met genotypes, respectively. Based on a 0.718:0.282 prevalence ratio of Met−:Met+ genotypes, we then conducted separate Monte Carlo simulations (Rubinstein and Kroese, 2016), each with 10,000 iterations, to estimate the probability that either 1, 2, . . ., or 11 subjects in the ASD group, and either 1, 2, . . ., or 18 subjects in the TD group would have a *BDNF* Met− genotype. We then conducted separate Fisher's exact tests for all possible combinations of numbers of *BDNF* Met− subjects in the two groups and identified the scenarios in which the Met−:Met+ ratio would be significantly different between the two groups. For each of those scenarios, we then calculated the joint probability of the two relevant events in the two groups. Finally, we summated the probabilities of all those mutually exclusive scenarios to obtain an estimate of the overall probability that two groups of 11 and 18 subjects randomly sampled from the admixed American population would be significantly different from one another in *BDNF* Met−:Met+ ratio.

Transcranial Magnetic Stimulation

Participants were seated in a comfortable reclining chair with the right arm and hand in a natural pronated position. They were instructed to keep their right hand as still and relaxed as possible throughout the experiment. They were also monitored for drowsiness and were asked to keep their eyes open during the TMS application.

All TMS procedures followed the recommended guidelines endorsed by the International Federation of Clinical Neurophysiology (Rossi et al., 2009; Rossini et al., 2015). Single TMS pulses and cTBS were applied to the left M1 at 120% of individual resting motor threshold (RMT) and 80% of active motor threshold (AMT), respectively, as biphasic pulses with an anteroposterior–posteroanterior (AP-PA) induced current direction in the brain. All stimulation was delivered using a hand-held figure-of-eight coil (outer diameter: 70 mm) attached to a Magstim Rapid² Plus[1] (Magstim Company Limited, Whitland, UK) stimulator.

TABLE 1 | Demographics, neuropsychological measures, and medications for individual participants.

Group	Participant No.	Age	IQ	*BDNF*	Neuroactive medication	Comorbidities	ADOS score
ASD (n = 11)		M = 13.09 (SD = 1.97)	M = 103.55 (SD = 12.43)	4 Val/Val; 4 Val/Met	10 Yes; 1 None	9 Yes; 2 None	M = 10.82 (SD = 3.28)
	AS1	10–15	106	Val/Val	Dexmethylphenidate; Sertraline	ADHD; Anxiety	11
	AS2	10–15	82	Val/Val	None	None	13
	AS3	10–15	100	Val/Met	Flouxetine	Depression	15
	AS4	10–15	100	Val/Met	Adderall	ADHD; Asthma	7
	AS5	10–15	121	Val/Val	Clonidine; Melatonin; Sertraline	Anxiety; Depression; Asthma	10
	AS6	10–15	100	Val/Met	Dexmethylphenidate; Melatonin; Fluoxetine	Anxiety; Depression	9
	AS7	10–15	100	Val/Met	Clonidine; Methylphenidate	ADHD	10
	AS8	15–20	124	Val/Val	Melatonin; Methylphenidate	ADHD; PTSD; Asthma	16
	AS9	10–15	91	-	Melatonin	None	14
	AS10	10–15	100	-	Flouxetine; Thyroid tablets	Depression; Hypothyroidism	7
	AS11	10–15	115	-	Dexmethylphenidate	ADHD	7
TD (n = 18)		M = 13.44 (SD = 1.85)			0 Yes; 18 None	0 Yes; 18 None	-
	TD1	10–15			None	None	N/A
	TD2	15–20			None	None	N/A
	TD3	10–15			None	None	N/A
	TD4	10–15			None	None	N/A
	TD5	10–15			None	None	N/A
	TD6	10–15			None	None	N/A
	TD7	15–20			None	None	N/A
	TD8	10–15			None	None	N/A
	TD9	10–15			None	None	N/A
	TD10	15–20			None	None	N/A
	TD11	10–15			None	None	N/A
	TD12	10–15			None	None	N/A
	TD13	10–15			None	None	N/A
	TD14	10–15			None	None	N/A
	TD15	10–15			None	None	N/A
	TD16	10–15			None	None	N/A
	TD17	10–15			None	None	N/A
	TD18	15–20			None	None	N/A

Group averages are presented as means and standard deviations (in parentheses). IQ scores were estimated using the Abbreviated Battery of Stanford-Binet IV intelligence scale. IQ, BDNF, and handedness data were not available for the TD group. Age range (instead of individual age) and no individual gender information are provided to avoid the possibility of publishing personally identifiable data. Three participants in the ASD group did not complete BDNF genotyping. ADHD; attention-deficit/hyperactivity disorder; ADOS, Autism Diagnostic Observation Schedule; ASD, autism spectrum disorder; BDNF, brain- derived neurotrophic factor; Met, metionine; PTSD, posttraumatic stress disorder; TD, typically developing; Val, Valine.

The coil was held tangentially to the participant's head surface, with the handle pointing occipitally and positioned at 45° relative to the mid-sagittal axis of the participant's head. The optimal spot for the maximal TMS-induced motor responses of the right first dorsal interosseous (FDI) muscle ("motor hotspot") was localized. A Polaris infrared-optical tracking system (Northern Digital Inc., Waterloo, ON, Canada) and a frameless stereotactic neuronavigation system (Brainsight, Rogue Research Inc., Montreal, QC, Canada) with a brain MRI template were used to ensure consistent targeting throughout the experiment. Each participant's head was registered to the MRI template using defined cranial landmarks to ensure the coil position and orientation was consistent with the MRI template (Ruohonen and Karhu, 2010).

Surface EMG electrodes were placed over the FDI belly (negative) and the first interphalangeal joint of the second finger (positive). The ground electrode was placed over the ipsilateral ulnar styloid process. The TMS system delivered triggered pulses that synchronized the TMS and EMG systems.

At the start of each TMS session the FDI motor hotspot was located per patient and individual RMT, defined as the lowest stimulation intensity necessary to elicit an MEP of $\geq$50 μV in at least five of 10 pulses from the relaxed right FDI, was obtained. To assess pre-cTBS cortico-motor reactivity, three blocks of 30 single TMS pulses in the ASD group, and two blocks of 20 single TMS pulses in the TD group, were applied to M1 with a 5–10-min inter-block interval, at a random 4–6-s inter-pulse interval, as done in previous studies (Pechmann et al., 2012; Gomes-Osman and Field-Fote, 2015; Davila-Pérez et al., 2018).

The different number of single TMS pulses administered at baseline (90 vs. 40) and in each post-cTBS block (30 vs. 20) in the two groups was due to site-specific approval of the experimental protocol utilized at each research site. This difference was unlikely, however, to give rise to differing baseline MEP amplitude estimates between the two groups, as recent studies have found applying at least 20 single TMS pulses yields a reliable estimate of MEP amplitude at a given time point (Chang et al., 2016; Goldsworthy et al., 2016). In each block, individual MEPs >2.5 SD from the mean were excluded. The mean ($\pm$SD) number of MEPs in total excluded from all blocks in each subject was 4.63 ($\pm$ 1.6) and 2.22 ($\pm$1.4) in the ASD and TD groups, respectively. This means that even in occasional post-cTBS blocks in the ASD group in which one (or, rarely, two) MEPs were excluded, there were 19 (or, rarely, 18) pulses remaining in each block, which has been shown to yield estimates of MEP amplitude with excellent internal consistency (Chang et al., 2016). To ensure hand relaxation was maintained throughout the experiment, real-time EMG was monitored to ensure the pre-TMS EMG activity did not exceed ~100 μV, which is the amplitude typically considered to be discernible activity from background EMG (Stinear and Byblow, 2002; Sartori et al., 2013; Benussi et al., 2018). Participants were also monitored for drowsiness and were asked to keep their eyes open for the duration of the stimulation session.

Baseline MEP amplitude was calculated as the average of the peak-to-peak amplitude of MEPs in the three blocks. AMT was then assessed as the lowest intensity that elicited MEPs $\geq$200 μV in at least five of 10 pulses with the FDI slightly contracted. Live EMG was monitored during the AMT assessment to ensure consistent contraction between ~100–200 μV. After a 5-min break, during which participants were instructed to maintain hand relaxation to control the effects of voluntary hand movements on cTBS responses (Iezzi et al., 2008), cTBS was applied as 200 bursts of three pulses at 50 Hz, repeated at 200-ms intervals for 40 s (for a total of 600 pulses). Cortico-motor reactivity was reassessed at 5, 10, 20, 30, 40, 50, and 60 min post-cTBS (*T5–T60*).

Statistical Analyses

Study data were collected and managed using Research Electronic Data Capture (REDCap) electronic data capture tools hosted at Beth Israel Deaconess Medical Center (Harris et al., 2009, 2019). MATLAB R2016b (The MathWorks, Natick, MA, USA) and Stata 13.1 (StataCorp., College Station, TX, USA) were used for data analyses and simulations. G*Power 3.1.9 (Faul et al., 2007) was used for power and sample-size calculations.

Data from each TMS visit included: (a) RMT and AMT, expressed as percentage of maximum stimulator output (MSO); (b) baseline MEP amplitude, calculated as the average of baseline MEP amplitude in three blocks of 30 single TMS pulses; and (c) percent change in the average amplitude of 30 MEPs at T5–T60 relative to baseline (%Δ) for each participant.

The Shapiro–Wilk found significant deviations in MEP amplitudes from the normal distribution. Thus, we first baseline-corrected each post-cTBS amplitude by dividing it by the average baseline MEP amplitude in that individual participant. We then natural log-transformed the baseline-corrected MEP amplitudes at each post-cTBS time point (ΔMEP, Nielsen, 1996a,b; Pasqualetti and Ferreri, 2011) and averaged them over participants separately for each group. The following measures were also calculated: maximum suppression of MEPs during 60 min post-cTBS (ΔMEP_{Max}) and the *signed* area-under-the-curve (AUC) of ΔMEPs over T5–T10, T5–T20,. . ., and T5–T60 intervals. To calculate the ΔMEP_{Max} for each participant, we chose the post-cTBS block (T5–T60) in which the ΔMEP showed the maximum suppression relative to the baseline MEP amplitude. Cumulative AUCs of the ΔMEPs enable numerical integration of cTBS-induced changes in MEP amplitude over successively larger intervals following cTBS. Such measures are more robust to the large inter-and intra-individual variability of MEP amplitudes typically observed at individual time points post-cTBS (López-Alonso et al., 2014; Vernet et al., 2014; Vallence et al., 2015; Hordacre et al., 2017; Jannati et al., 2017, 2019) and can be advantageous in studies with smaller sample sizes.

Grand-average values for all cTBS measures were calculated separately for each time point in each group and were compared between the two groups using independent-samples *t*-tests. Similar analyses were conducted for the two small *BDNF* subgroups ($n = 4$ per subgroup) of the ASD group. We conducted a sample-size analysis based on the preliminary results from the *BDNF* subgroups in order to estimate the number of participants per *BDNF* subgroup required to detect a significant difference between the cumulative AUC measures of cTBS aftereffects over each interval. Comparisons of proportions were conducted using Fisher's exact test. Pearson product-moment correlation coefficient was used to assess the relationship between ΔMEP_{Max} and age in each group. All analyses were two-tailed, and α and β levels were set to 0.05 and 0.80, respectively. False discovery rate (FDR; Benjamini and Yekutieli, 2001) was used to adjust the *P*-values for multiple testing.

To obtain a rough estimate on the extent to which our small sample sizes—combined with the interindividual variability of MEP changes in response to cTBS—resulted in reduced power, we conducted a *post hoc* power calculation for the whole sample over each post-cTBS interval (but see Hoenig and Heisey, 2001 for the limited usefulness of this approach) and a pre-hoc sample-size calculation for the analyses comparing cTBS responses in the two *BDNF* subgroups of the ASD group.

To control for the number of pre- and post-cTBS MEPs in the two groups, we selected a subset of data from the ASD group such that both the number of baseline MEPs and the number of MEPs in each post-cTBS block included in the analysis would be equal in the two groups. Out of the 90 baseline MEPs, we selected the last 40 MEPs before cTBS to calculate the baseline MEP amplitude for each subject in the ASD group. We also selected the 20 MEPs out of 30 MEPs in each post-cTBS block that centered around the time point of interest (10, 20,. . ., and 60 min post-cTBS), and then log-transformed the baseline-corrected MEPs and recalculated the cumulative AUC measures of cTBS aftereffects for the ASD group. To account for the occasional MEP amplitudes excluded from each block in the TD group that was >2.5 SD, we continued to exclude any MEP that had been excluded from each block in the original, larger ASD dataset. Finally, we compared those cumulative measures of cTBS aftereffects with the corresponding measures in the TD group, as described above.

Even though our post-cTBS MEP measures are already baseline-corrected, it is still possible that a difference in the absolute baseline MEP amplitude between the two groups contributes to a difference in cTBS aftereffects. Because, as reported below, we found a significant difference in baseline MEP amplitude between the two groups, we set out to create the largest ASD and TD subgroups that would have comparable baseline MEP amplitude, and then compared the cTBS aftereffects between those subgroups.

Because several subjects in the ASD group had comorbid attention-deficit/hyperactivity disorder (ADHD; **Table 1**), and in pediatric ADHD there is impaired GABA-mediated plasticity as measured by paired-pulse TMS (Dutra et al., 2016; Gilbert et al., 2019), we repeated the calculation of cumulative AUC measures of cTBS aftereffects and their comparison between the ASD and TD groups after excluding the five ASD subjects with a documented clinical diagnosis of ADHD.

Side-Effect Monitoring

Immediately following the TMS session, a side-effects questionnaire was completed by the experimenter. Participants were asked to report whether they experienced any of the following side effects: headache, neck pain, scalp pain or irritation, difficulty hearing, thinking or concentrating, change in mood, or to report any other change or side effect they experienced. The experimenter also noted whether the participant experienced a syncopal event or seizure. If the participant reported any side effects following the stimulation, the severity and duration were documented.

RESULTS

The ASD and TD groups were comparable in age and sex ratio (P-values > 0.61). Demographics, neuropsychological measures, and medications for individual participants are presented in **Table 1**.

cTBS Is Safe and Tolerable in Children

All participants tolerated cTBS and single-pulse stimulation without any serious adverse event. One participant reported mild scalp irritation (on the forehead underneath the headband holding the subject tracker of the neuronavigation system), which was resolved quickly without medication. No other adverse events were reported.

cTBS Measures of Plasticity Differentiate Between ASD and TD Children

The difference in cumulative AUC measures of cTBS aftereffects between the two groups was significant over all the intervals (P_{FDR}'s < 0.03), indicating greater *facilitatory* response to cTBS in the ASD group relative to the TD group. Post-cTBS data from one participant in the ASD group were not obtained beyond T10 due to technical difficulties. Grand-average ΔMEPs at individual post-cTBS time points in the two groups are presented in **Figure 1A**. Cumulative AUCs of the ΔMEPs and their 95% confidence intervals (CI) over T5–T10, T5–T20,. . ., and T5–T60 intervals for the two groups are presented in **Figure 1B**.

The baseline MEP amplitude (mean $\pm$ SD) in the ASD group, 0.37 mV $\pm$ 0.27, was significantly smaller than in the TD group, 1.19 mV $\pm$ 0.41, $t_{(27)} = 5.96$, $P < 0.001$. The largest ASD and TD subgroups that would have a comparable baseline MEP amplitude consist of only five participants per subgroup. The baseline MEP amplitude [mean $\pm$ (SD)] in the two resulting subgroups with $n = 5$ are comparable: 0.62 mV ($\pm$0.17) in the ASD subgroup and 0.72 mV ($\pm$0.17) in the TD subgroup, $t_{(8)} = 0.91$, $P = 0.39$. There is no significant difference in cumulative AUC ΔMEP measures between the two subgroups over any of the post-cTBS intervals (P-values > 0.58).

The effect sizes based on the difference in cumulative AUC measure of cTBS aftereffects between the ASD and TD groups over T5–T10, T5–T20,. . ., and T5–T60 intervals are 0.85, 0.84, 0.79, 0.70, 0.65, and 0.65, respectively. Assuming two-tailed, independent-samples t-tests with $\alpha = 0.05$, the *post hoc* power to detect a significant difference between the two groups are estimated as 57.2%, 56.2%, 51.2%, 42.2%, 37.4%, and 37.4%, respectively.

The Monte Carlo simulations find in a group of 11 subjects, the estimated probability that either 1, 2,. . ., or 11 subjects would have a *BDNF* Met—genotype is < 0.0001, 0.0002, 0.003, 0.012, 0.043, 0.115, 0.198, 0.266, 0.218, 0.113, and 0.027, respectively. In a group of 18 subjects, the estimated probability that either

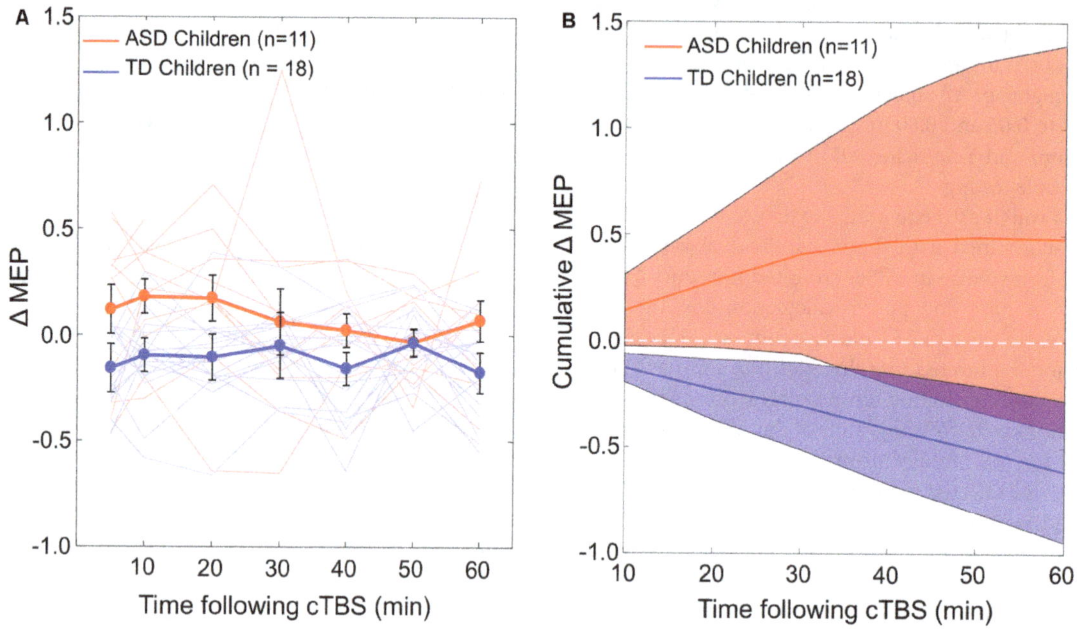

FIGURE 1 | (A) Individual and grand-average change from baseline in MEP amplitude recorded from the right FDI muscle at 5–60 min following cTBS of the left motor cortex in ASD and TD groups. Error bars represent standard error of the mean. **(B)** Cumulative AUCs of the ΔMEPs and their 95% CI over T5–T10, T5–T20, . . ., and T5–T60 intervals for the two groups (the end time-point of each interval is labeled on the abscissa). The cumulative AUC measures were significantly more positive in the ASD group than in the TD group over all the T5–T10 to T5–T60 intervals (P_{FDR}'s < 0.03). ASD, autism spectrum disorder; AUC, area-under-the-curve; CI, confidence interval; cTBS, continuous theta-burst stimulation; ΔMEP, natural log-transformed, baseline-corrected amplitude of motor evoked potentials; FDI, first dorsal interosseous; FDR, false discovery rate; MEP, motor evoked potential; TD, typically developing; *Tm–Tn*, over *m* to *n* minutes following cTBS.

1, 2,. . ., or 18 subjects would have a *BDNF* Met—genotype is <0.0001 (for 1-5 such subjects), 0.001, 0.003, 0.010, 0.031, 0.064, 0.120, 0.177, 0.208, 0.185, 0.127, 0.062, 0.019, and 0.002, respectively. After summating the probability of all scenarios in which a two-tailed Fisher's exact test would find a significant difference in *BDNF* Met−:Met+ ratio between the ASD and TD groups, we obtain an overall probability of 0.0426.

After equalizing the number of pre- and post-cTBS MEPs in the two groups, the cumulative AUC measures of cTBS aftereffects do not change substantially compared to the measures obtained with the complete ASD dataset. The mean (±SD) cumulative AUC of ΔMEP over T5-T10, T5-T20,. . ., and T5-T60 intervals in this subset of data from the ASD group is 0.085 (±0.24), 0.18 (±0.45), 0.22 (±0.67), 0.24 (±0.80), 0.20 (± 0.92), and 0.14 (±1.06), respectively. These measures remain significantly more facilitatory in the ASD group than in the TD group over all the intervals from T5-T10 to T5-T50 (P_{FDR}'s < 0.047), but not over T5-T60 (P_{FDR} = 0.053).

After excluding the five subjects in the ASD group who had comorbid ADHD, the cumulative AUC measures of cTBS aftereffects remain significantly more facilitatory in the ASD group compared to the TD group over all intervals (P_{FDR}'s < 0.001).

cTBS Aftereffects Have a Developmental Trajectory in Children with ASD

ΔMEP_{Max} is correlated with age in the ASD group (r = -0.67, P = 0.025), but not in the TD group (r = -0.12, P = 0.65). The relationship between age and the maximum cTBS-induced suppression of MEPs (ΔMEP_{Max}) during the first 60 min post-cTBS in the two groups are illustrated in **Figure 2**.

BDNF and cTBS Measures of Plasticity in ASD

The difference in cumulative AUC measures of cTBS aftereffects between the two *BDNF* subgroups (Val/Val and Val/Met) of the ASD group is not statistically significant (P-values > 0.08). Grand-average ΔMEPs at individual post-cTBS time points in the two *BDNF* subgroups are presented in **Figure 3A**. Cumulative AUCs of the ΔMEPs and their 95% CI over T0–T10, T0–T20, . . ., and T0–T60 intervals for the two *BDNF* subgroups are presented in **Figure 3B**.

Based on the results from eight participants with available *BDNF* data, the effect size based on the difference in cumulative AUC measure of cTBS aftereffects over each interval ranges from 0.78 to 0.87. Assuming a 1:1 ratio between the two subgroups, the sample size in each *BDNF* subgroup required to detect those effect sizes with 80% power ranges from 27 to 22, respectively.

DISCUSSION

We find, considering the caveats and confounders discussed below, the responses to M1 cTBS can differentiate between 10-16 years old children with HF-ASD and their age-, gender, and IQ-matched TD children. This is due to more-facilitatory

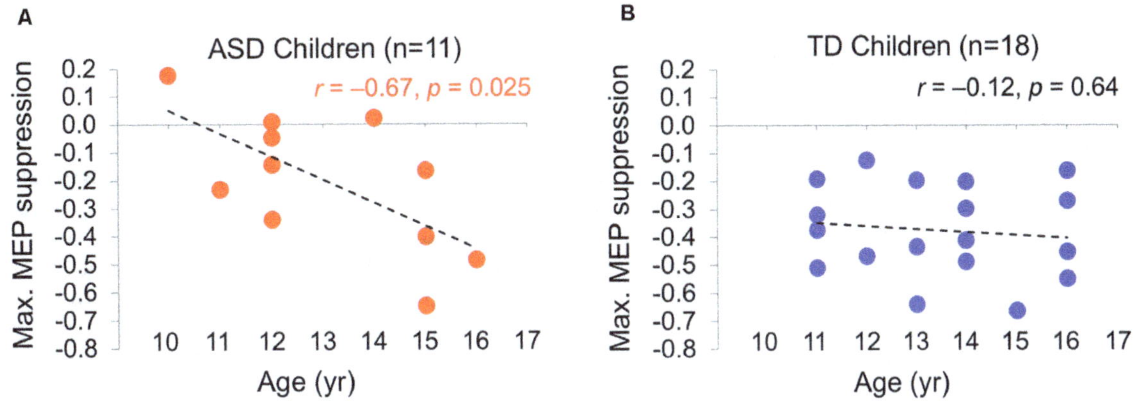

FIGURE 2 | The relationship between the maximum cTBS-induced suppression in the natural log-transformed, baseline-corrected MEP amplitude (Max. MEP suppression) and age in ASD **(A)** and TD **(B)** groups. Max. MEP suppression was negatively correlated with age in the ASD group ($r = -0.67$, $P = 0.025$), but not in the TD group ($r = -0.12$, $P = 0.65$). Dashed lines represent the slopes of the linear regression fit. ASD, autism spectrum disorder; cTBS, continuous theta-burst stimulation; MEP, motor evoked potential; TD, typically developing.

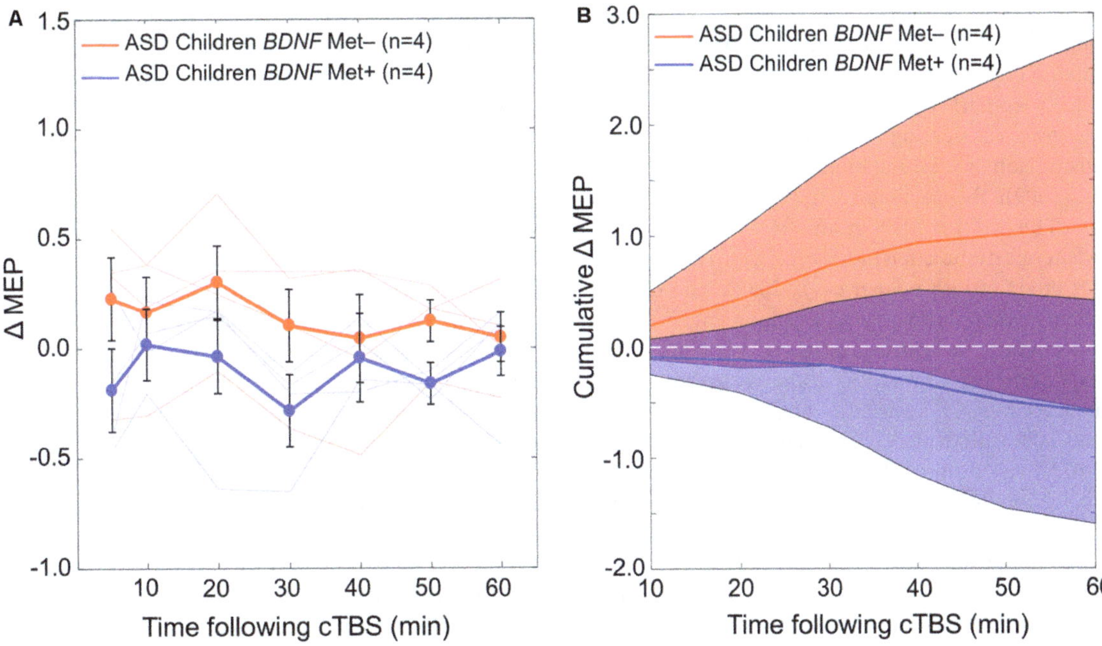

FIGURE 3 | (A) Changes in individual and grand-average MEPs recorded from the right FDI muscle at 5–60 min following cTBS of the left primary motor cortex in *BDNF* Met– (Val/Val) and Met+ (Val/Met) subgroups of participants with ASD. Error bars represent standard error of the mean. **(B)** Cumulative AUCs of the ΔMEPs and their 95% CI over T5–T10, T5–T20, ..., and T5–T60 intervals for the two *BDNF* subgroups (the end time-point of each interval is labeled on the abscissa). The cumulative AUC measures were not significantly different between the two *BDNF* subgroups over any of the intervals (*P*-values > 0.18). ASD, autism spectrum disorder; AUC, area-under-the-curve; *BDNF*, brain-derived neurotrophic factor; CI, confidence interval; cTBS, continuous theta-burst stimulation; ΔMEP, natural log-transformed, baseline-corrected amplitude of motor evoked potentials; FDI, first dorsal interosseous; FDR, false discovery rate; MEP, motor evoked potential; Met, methionine; TD, typically developing; *Tm–Tn*, over *m* to *n* minutes following cTBS; Val, valine.

cTBS aftereffects in MEPs in the ASD group relative to the TD group. We argue this difference is not likely to be due to potential confounds such as differences in the number of pre- and post-cTBS MEPs, *BDNF* Val66Met SNP, ADHD comorbidity, or neuroactive medications between the two groups. Moreover, we report an age-related increase in the maximum cTBS-induced suppression of MEPs in the ASD group, but not in the TD group, suggesting a dysmaturity in LTD-like plasticity in children with ASD. These results indicate the importance of further investigations of the utility of M1 cTBS as a potential physiologic biomarker for children and adolescents with HF-ASD.

TMS Safety and Tolerability in Children

All participants tolerated the stimulation, and only one participant reported a minor scalp irritation that resolved quickly without medication. The present study adds to the growing literature documenting the safety and tolerability of rTMS in children and in individuals with ASD (Garvey and Gilbert, 2004; Frye et al., 2008; Croarkin et al., 2011; Oberman et al., 2012, 2014, 2016; Wu et al., 2012; Rajapakse and Kirton, 2013; Hong et al., 2015; Pedapati et al., 2015; Hameed et al., 2017).

cTBS as a Biomarker for Children and Adolescents With ASD

We find that the pattern of cTBS aftereffects during the first 60 min post-cTBS successfully differentiates between the ASD and TD groups. Namely, the ASD group shows significantly more facilitatory responses to cTBS than the TD group throughout the assessed post-cTBS interval (**Figure 1**). Notably, this pattern of results is not driven by one or two particular post-cTBS time points, which can be prone to the large inter- and intra-individual variability in cTBS responses observed in adults (López-Alonso et al., 2014; Vernet et al., 2014; Vallence et al., 2015; Hordacre et al., 2017; Jannati et al., 2017, 2019).

The finding that the ASD group exhibits a distinct pattern of cTBS from their TD counterparts indicates the potential utility of M1 cTBS as a biomarker for children and adolescents with HF-ASD. Moreover, considering the involvement of GABAergic synaptic transmission in cTBS aftereffects (Stagg et al., 2009; Trippe et al., 2009), the facilitatory (rather than inhibitory) responses to cTBS in the ASD group further supports the notion of GABAergic dysfunction in ASD (LeBlanc and Fagiolini, 2011; Ben-Ari et al., 2012; Coghlan et al., 2012). The effect of GABAergic transmission during typical development shifts from excitatory to inhibitory through sequential activation of chloride (Cl^-) cotransporters NKCC1 and KCC2 and *via* age-dependent reduction of intracellular Cl^- concentration (Yamada et al., 2004; Ben-Ari et al., 2007). Rodent ASD models indicate a delayed shift of GABA activity from excitatory to inhibitory, which can be restored behaviorally and electrophysiologically by *in utero* administration of the NKCC1 inhibitor bumetanide (Tyzio et al., 2014). Similarly, bumetanide treatment may mitigate core ASD symptoms in children and adolescents (Lemonnier et al., 2017). We thus suggest that cTBS measures of M1 plasticity in ASD can be used to assess baseline cortico-motor reactivity, probe-target engagement, and monitor therapeutic response to experimental pharmacotherapy (e.g., bumetanide; Lemonnier et al., 2017) and, potentially, future rTMS treatments for ASD (Cole et al., 2019). Moreover, differential cTBS responses within the pediatric ASD population can form the physiologic basis for a clinical endophenotype that improves classification and understanding of the pathophysiology of ASD.

The more-facilitatory response to cTBS in the ASD group relative to the TD group is consistent with the results of previous studies that have found impaired LTP-like changes in MEPs in individuals with ASD by paired associative stimulation (PAS; Jung et al., 2013) and iTBS (Oberman et al., 2012; Pedapati et al., 2016). Given that cTBS also likely engages GABAergic mechanisms, our results are also consistent with related findings that employ other TMS-derived biomarkers. For instance, $GABA_A$ergic activity, as measured by short-interval intracortical cortical inhibition (SICI), was associated with a delay in language acquisition in adults with ASD (Enticott et al., 2013).

Present and Anticipated Confounders

Although the post-cTBS measures reported in the present study are already adjusted for baseline MEP amplitude at the individual level, it is possible that a difference in the baseline MEP amplitude at the group level contributes to the observed differences in cTBS aftereffects between ASD and TD groups. The finding that the baseline MEP amplitude is significantly smaller in the ASD group than in the TD group can be either due to chance because of the small sample sizes or because of a real difference in input-output characteristics of MEPs in the two groups (Goetz et al., 2014). Because the largest ASD and TD subgroups with a comparable baseline MEP amplitude consist of only five participants, the present sample does not allow for a robust assessment of the effect of group-level baseline MEP amplitude on cTBS aftereffects in the two groups. Larger samples in future studies aimed at comparing rTMS responses between ASD and control populations can address this limitation by ensuring comparable baseline MEP amplitudes at the group level between the two groups.

Our analysis controlling for the number of baseline and post-cTBS MEPs shows that the differences in cumulative measures of cTBS aftereffects, at least from T5–T10 to T5–T50, are not due to differences in the number of baseline MEPs (90 vs. 40) or the number of MEPs in each post-cTBS block (30 vs. 20) between the ASD and TD groups.

One issue that needs to be considered in comparing cTBS responses between the ASD and TD groups is the potential effects of neuroactive medications on cTBS responses. It is plausible that at least some of those medications influence the pattern of cTBS aftereffects in ASD participants and thus the difference between the two groups. There is, however, considerable variability in the type of those medications received by our ASD participants, which makes it unlikely that all or a majority of them have a similar effect on the plasticity mechanisms indexed by cTBS aftereffects. To maintain the external validity of the findings of studies aimed at developing biomarkers or therapeutics for the ASD population, it is necessary to include patients who are under treatment by neuroactive medications prescribed for common comorbidities such as depression, anxiety, and ADHD.

Another issue in comparing cTBS responses between the ASD and TD groups is the possibility that there is a significant difference in *BDNF* Met−:Met+ ratio between the two groups. Such difference can give rise to an observed difference in cTBS responses between the two groups that are not necessarily associated with an ASD diagnosis but with the composition of *BDNF* genotypes in the two groups. Our simulations, however, do not find such a possibility to be very likely in the present study. We find, assuming random sampling from the admixed American population, there is a ~4.3% chance that two groups of 11 and 18 subjects are significantly different from one another in the *BDNF* Met−:Met+ ratio.

Potential confound due to psychiatric comorbidities in the ASD group is another factor that can mediate the difference in cTBS responses between the two groups. One common comorbidity in ASD is ADHD (Craig et al., 2015), in which abnormal GABA-mediated plasticity measured by paired-pulse TMS has been observed (Dutra et al., 2016; Gilbert et al., 2019). After excluding five subjects in the ASD group with documented ADHD comorbidity, we still find significantly greater cumulative facilitatory aftereffects of cTBS in the ASD-without-ADHD subgroup than in the TD group across all post-cTBS intervals. These results show that the observed differences between the whole ASD group and the TD group cannot not be due to the effects of ADHD comorbidity on cTBS responses. In general, nonetheless, in studies comparing plasticity responses of ASD and control populations, the potential effects of common psychiatric comorbidities such as depression, anxiety, and ADHD on TMS measures of plasticity, should be considered.

Interestingly, the overall pattern of cTBS responses in the ASD group in the present study is not necessarily what one would expect based on previous results. Namely, a previous cTBS study from our group (Oberman et al., 2014) found only one-third of children and adolescents with ASD showed facilitatory responses to cTBS. This difference in results can be due to several factors:

(1) The large inter-individual variability in response to cTBS among healthy adults is now well-established (Hamada et al., 2013; Goldsworthy et al., 2014; López-Alonso et al., 2014; Nettekoven et al., 2015; Vallence et al., 2015; Hordacre et al., 2017; Jannati et al., 2017). A similar degree of variability in cTBS responses in TD children and among clinical pediatric populations such as children with ASD is reasonable to expect. By mere virtue of random sampling from a large spectrum of responses, such variability can give rise to seemingly inconsistent results in small sample sizes that may not capture the entire gamut of cTBS responses in healthy and clinical populations. In fact, our *post hoc* power calculation for the whole sample indicates that the present study is underpowered, especially beyond the T5–T20 interval. Larger sample sizes would perhaps have resulted in more-robust differences, and/or over longer intervals, between the two groups. We thus anticipate that this power analysis will enable the design of future studies with larger sample sizes that are required to confirm and extend the present results.

(2) The difference in the proportion of participants with *BDNF* Val/Met genotype, which has been shown to influence cTBS and other rTMS measures of neuroplasticity (Cheeran et al., 2008; Antal et al., 2010; Lee et al., 2013; Chang et al., 2014; Di Lazzaro et al., 2015; Fried et al., 2017; Jannati et al., 2017, 2019) may have contributed to the different results.

(3) Differences in other demographic, neuropsychological, and genetic factors as well as neuroactive medications received by the participants in the ASD group could have given rise to the different patterns of cTBS response in the two studies.

These potential confounds underscore the need for replication of present findings in future cTBS studies with large samples of children and adolescents with ASD in order to overcome, or control for, some of these factors. Another important reason for replicating the present findings is to assess the test-retest reliability of M1 cTBS aftereffects in both HF-ASD and TD children. This is underscored by the recent findings in healthy adults that indicate low-to-moderate reliability of most cTBS aftereffects (Jannati et al., 2019).

Regarding potential selection and outcome biases in recruiting the participants in the TD group, it should be noted that because the TD subjects were recruited as part of an unrelated study—and not for the purpose of comparing their cTBS responses with those of ASD children—such biases did not play a role in recruiting the TD subjects.

Developmental Trajectory of cTBS Responses in ASD

Consistent with the previously reported age-related increase in the duration of cTBS-induced modulation in children and adolescents with ASD (Oberman et al., 2014), we find an age-related increase in the maximum cTBS-induced suppression of MEP during 60 min post-cTBS in the ASD group, but not in the TD group. Namely, older participants with ASD tend to exhibit greater cTBS-induced LTD-like plasticity than younger participants with ASD, whereas there is no such developmental trajectory in the TD group (at least in the age range of 11–16). Caution should be exercised in interpreting these correlations, however, because of the short dynamic range of age in the two groups. Assuming these results are confirmed in larger studies in the future and over wider age ranges, they suggest a dysmaturity in LTD-like plasticity as measured by cTBS in children with ASD, perhaps arising from a dysfunction in the shift of GABAergic activity from excitatory to inhibitory. Since $GABA_A$-receptor activity is involved in generating the cTBS aftereffects, such dysfunction would cause the ASD participants to achieve greater inhibitory cTBS responses as they grow older. In contrast, because the GABAergic shift presumably occurs earlier in TD children, they may achieve greater cTBS-induced inhibition at a younger age and then plateau at older ages. These results hint at the utility of cTBS measures of plasticity as longitudinal tools for monitoring the development of cortical plasticity and/or gradual response to potential treatments among children and adolescents with ASD. Because the slope of such developmental trajectory is likely to vary across individuals with ASD, a substantial number of subjects at any given age may be necessary to obtain robust "growth curves" for cortical plasticity in pediatric ASD populations.

BDNF Polymorphism and cTBS Aftereffects in ASD

The role of *BDNF* Val66Met SNP in influencing rTMS plasticity measures in adults has been investigated in several studies (Cheeran et al., 2008; Antal et al., 2010; Lee et al., 2013; Chang et al., 2014; Di Lazzaro et al., 2015; Fried et al., 2017; Jannati et al., 2017, 2019). *BDNF* Met carrier status is known to be associated with impaired N-Methyl-D-aspartate-(NMDA)-dependent LTD (Woo et al., 2005), aberrant GABAergic synaptic transmission (Abidin et al., 2008), reduced cTBS-induced inhibition of MEPs (Chung et al., 2016), and, in some cases, paradoxical cTBS-induced facilitation of MEPs (Gentner et al., 2008; Goldsworthy et al., 2012; Hellriegel et al., 2012; Brownjohn et al., 2014; Jannati et al., 2017, 2019). In contrast with these results, the *BDNF* Met+ children with ASD in the present study exhibit a numerically more-*inhibitory* response than the *BDNF* Met− children at all individual post-cTBS time points, even though the difference between two subgroups is not statistically significant. Because of the small sample sizes, it is difficult to infer whether the seemingly opposite effect of *BDNF* Met carrier status on cTBS response in children with ASD compared to adults is due to: (1) sampling error arising from small sample sizes; or (2) a dysfunction in GABAergic shift that causes the *BDNF* SNP to have an opposite influence on cTBS aftereffects in children with ASD compared to healthy individuals.

CONCLUSION

Considering the discussed limitations and potential confounders, cTBS-derived metrics may enable practical and safe physiologic biomarkers in pediatric ASD. Given that such measures can be applied repeatedly to individuals, our data also point to prospects for probing developmentally regulated features of cortical plasticity in ASD and perhaps other neurodevelopmental disorders. Because of its high tolerability by patients with ASD, cTBS offers an opportunity to study the mechanisms and alterations of neural plasticity in the ASD population. These proof-of-principle findings in the motor cortex can be followed in future studies through extra motor stimulation in TMS-EEG or similar protocols.

ETHICS STATEMENT

This study was approved by the Institutional Review Boards at Boston Children's Hospital and King Saud University, where the research took place, in accordance with the Declaration of Helsinki. All participants provided written informed consent/assent prior to enrollment and received monetary compensation upon completion.

AUTHOR CONTRIBUTIONS

AJ, LO, AP-L, and AR conceived and designed the study. AJ, GB, MR, HK, FK, SB, and LO collected the data. AJ analyzed the data and drafted the manuscript. AJ, AP-L, and AR interpreted the data. All authors revised the manuscript, approved the final version, and agreed to be accountable for the content of the work.

FUNDING

This study was primarily funded by the National Institutes of Health (NIH R01 MH100186). AJ was further supported by postdoctoral fellowships from the Natural Sciences and Engineering Research Council of Canada (NSERC 454617) and the Canadian Institutes of Health Research (CIHR 41791). LO was further supported by the Simons Foundation Autism Research Initiative (SFARI) and the Nancy Lurie Marks Family Foundation. AP-L was further supported by the Sidney R. Baer Jr. Foundation, the NIH (R01 HD069776, R01 NS073601, R21 MH099196, R21 NS085491, R21 HD07616), the Football Players Health Study at Harvard University, and Harvard Catalyst | The Harvard Clinical and Translational Science Center (NCRR and the NCATS NIH, UL1 RR025758). AR was further supported by the NIH (R01 NS088583), The Boston Children's Hospital Translational Research Program, Autism Speaks, Massachusetts Life Sciences, The Assimon Family, Brainsway, CRE Medical, Eisai, Neuroelectrics, Roche, Sage Therapeutics, and Takeda Medical. The content is solely the responsibility of the authors and does not necessarily represent the official views of Harvard Catalyst, Harvard University and its affiliated academic health care centers, the National Institutes of Health, or any of the other listed granting agencies.

ACKNOWLEDGMENTS

We thank the Neurodevelopmental and Behavioral Core at Boston Children's Hospital for conducting the Autism Diagnostic Observation Schedule (ADOS), and Ann Connor and Joanna Macone (Beth Israel Deaconess Medical Center) for assistance with regulatory oversight and compliance.

REFERENCES

Abidin, I., Eysel, U. T., Lessmann, V., and Mittmann, T. (2008). Impaired GABAergic inhibition in the visual cortex of brain-derived neurotrophic factor heterozygous knockout mice: GABA release is impaired in visual cortex of BDNF heterozygous KO mice. *J. Physiol.* 586, 1885–1901. doi: 10.1113/jphysiol.2007.148627

American Psychiatric Association. (2013). *Diagnostic and Statistical Manual of Mental Disorders (DSM-5®).* Arlington: American Psychiatric Publishing.

Antal, A., Chaieb, L., Moliadze, V., Monte-Silva, K., Poreisz, C., Thirugnanasambandam, N., et al. (2010). Brain-derived neurotrophic factor (BDNF) gene polymorphisms shape cortical plasticity in humans. *Brain Stimul.* 3, 230–237. doi: 10.1016/j.brs.2009.12.003

Barker, A. T., Jalinous, R., and Freeston, I. L. (1985). Non-invasive magnetic stimulation of human motor cortex. *Lancet* 325, 1106–1107. doi: 10.1016/s0140-6736(85)92413-4

Benali, A., Trippe, J., Weiler, E., Mix, A., Petrasch-Parwez, E., Girzalsky, W., et al. (2011). Theta-burst transcranial magnetic stimulation alters cortical inhibition. *J. Neurosci.* 31, 1193–1203. doi: 10.1523/JNEUROSCI.1379-10.2011

Ben-Ari, Y., Gaiarsa, J.-L., Tyzio, R., and Khazipov, R. (2007). GABA: a pioneer transmitter that excites immature neurons and generates primitive oscillations. *Physiol. Rev.* 87, 1215–1284. doi: 10.1152/physrev.00017.2006

Ben-Ari, Y., Khalilov, I., Kahle, K. T., and Cherubini, E. (2012). The GABA excitatory/inhibitory shift in brain maturation and neurological disorders. *Neuroscientist* 18, 467–486. doi: 10.1177/1073858412438697

Benjamini, Y., and Yekutieli, D. (2001). The control of the false discovery rate in multiple testing under dependency. *Ann. Stat.* 29, 1165–1188.

Benussi, A., Dell'Era, V., Cantoni, V., Ferrari, C., Caratozzolo, S., Rozzini, L., et al. (2018). Discrimination of atypical parkinsonisms with transcranial magnetic stimulation. *Brain Stimul.* 11, 366–373. doi: 10.1016/j.brs.2017.11.013

Brownjohn, P. W., Reynolds, J. N. J., Matheson, N., Fox, J., and Shemmell, J. B. H. (2014). The effects of individualized theta burst stimulation on the excitability of the human motor system. *Brain Stimul.* 7, 260–268. doi: 10.1016/j.brs.2013.12.007

Cárdenas-Morales, L., Grön, G., and Kammer, T. (2011). Exploring the after-effects of theta burst magnetic stimulation on the human motor cortex: a functional imaging study. *Hum. Brain Mapp.* 32, 1948–1960. doi: 10.1002/hbm.21160

Chang, W. H., Bang, O. Y., Shin, Y.-I., Lee, A., Pascual-Leone, A., and Kim, Y.-H. (2014). BDNF polymorphism and differential rTMS effects on motor recovery of stroke patients. *Brain Stimul.* 7, 553–558. doi: 10.1016/j.brs.2014.03.008

Chang, W. H., Fried, P. J., Saxena, S., Jannati, A., Gomes-Osman, J., Kim, Y.-H., et al. (2016). Optimal number of pulses as outcome measures of neuronavigated transcranial magnetic stimulation. *Clin. Neurophysiol.* 127, 2892–2897. doi: 10.1016/j.clinph.2016.04.001

Cheeran, B. J., Talelli, P., Mori, F., Koch, G., Suppa, A., Edwards, M., et al. (2008). A common polymorphism in the brain-derived neurotrophic factor gene (*BDNF*) modulates human cortical plasticity and the response to rTMS. *J. Physiol.* 586, 5717–5725. doi: 10.1113/jphysiol.2008.159905

Chung, S. W., Hill, A. T., Rogasch, N. C., Hoy, K. E., and Fitzgerald, P. B. (2016). Use of theta-burst stimulation in changing excitability of motor cortex: a systematic review and meta-analysis. *Neurosci. Biobehav. Rev.* 63, 43–64. doi: 10.1016/j.neubiorev.2016.01.008

Coghlan, S., Horder, J., Inkster, B., Mendez, M. A., Murphy, D. G., and Nutt, D. J. (2012). GABA system dysfunction in autism and related disorders: from synapse to symptoms. *Neurosci. Biobehav. Rev.* 36, 2044–2055. doi: 10.1016/j.neubiorev.2012.07.005

Cole, E. J., Enticott, P. G., Oberman, L. M., Gwynette, M. F., Casanova, M. F., Jackson, S. L. J., et al. (2019). The potential of repetitive transcranial magnetic stimulation for autism spectrum disorder: a consensus statement. *Biol. Psychiatry* 85, e21–e22. doi: 10.1016/j.biopsych.2018.06.003

Craig, F., Lamanna, A. L., Margari, F., Matera, E., Simone, M., and Margari, L. (2015). Overlap between autism spectrum disorders and attention deficit hyperactivity disorder: searching for distinctive/common clinical features. *Autism Res.* 8, 328–337. doi: 10.1002/aur.1449

Croarkin, P. E., Wall, C. A., and Lee, J. (2011). Applications of transcranial magnetic stimulation (TMS) in child and adolescent psychiatry. *Int. Rev. Psychiatry* 23, 445–453. doi: 10.3109/09540261.2011.623688

Davila-Pérez, P., Jannati, A., Fried, P. J., Cudeiro Mazaira, J., and Pascual-Leone, A. (2018). The effects of waveform and current direction on the efficacy and test-retest reliability of transcranial magnetic stimulation. *Neuroscience* 393, 97–109. doi: 10.1016/j.neuroscience.2018.09.044

Di Lazzaro, V., Pellegrino, G., Di Pino, G., Corbetto, M., Ranieri, F., Brunelli, N., et al. (2015). Val66Met BDNF gene polymorphism influences human motor cortex plasticity in acute stroke. *Brain Stimul.* 8, 92–96. doi: 10.1016/j.brs.2014.08.006

DNA Genotek Inc. (2015). *Laboratory Protocol for Manual Purification of DNA from 0.5 mL of Sample.* Available online at: http://www.dnagenotek.com/US/pdf/PD-PR-006.pdf. Accessed February 01, 2016.

Dutra, T., Baltar, A., and Monte-Silva, K. (2016). Motor cortex excitability in attention-deficit hyperactivity disorder (ADHD): a systematic review and meta-analysis. *Res. Dev. Disabil.* 56, 1–9. doi: 10.1016/j.ridd.2016.01.022

Enticott, P. G., Kennedy, H. A., Rinehart, N. J., Tonge, B. J., Bradshaw, J. L., and Fitzgerald, P. B. (2013). GABAergic activity in autism spectrum disorders: an investigation of cortical inhibition *via* transcranial magnetic stimulation. *Neuropharmacology* 68, 202–209. doi: 10.1016/j.neuropharm.2012.06.017

Faul, F., Erdfelder, E., Lang, A.-G., and Buchner, A. (2007). G*Power 3: a flexible statistical power analysis program for the social, behavioral, and biomedical sciences. *Behav. Res. Methods* 39, 175–191. doi: 10.3758/bf03193146

Fried, P. J., Jannati, A., Davila-Pérez, P., and Pascual-Leone, A. (2017). Reproducibility of single-pulse, paired-pulse, and intermittent theta-burst TMS measures in healthy aging, type-2 diabetes, and Alzheimer's disease. *Front. Aging Neurosci.* 9:263. doi: 10.3389/fnagi.2017.00263

Frye, R. E., Rotenberg, A., Ousley, M., and Pascual-Leone, A. (2008). Transcranial magnetic stimulation in child neurology: current and future directions. *J. Child Neurol.* 23, 79–96. doi: 10.1177/0883073807307972

Garvey, M. A., and Gilbert, D. L. (2004). Transcranial magnetic stimulation in children. *Eur. J. Paediatr. Neurol.* 8, 7–19. doi: 10.1016/j.ejpn.2003.11.002

Gentner, R., Wankerl, K., Reinsberger, C., Zeller, D., and Classen, J. (2008). Depression of human corticospinal excitability induced by magnetic theta-burst stimulation: evidence of rapid polarity-reversing metaplasticity. *Cereb. Cortex* 18, 2046–2053. doi: 10.1093/cercor/bhm239

Gilbert, D. L., Huddleston, D. A., Wu, S. W., Pedapati, E. V., Horn, P. S., Hirabayashi, K., et al. (2019). Motor cortex inhibition and modulation in children with ADHD. *Neurology* 93, e599–e610. doi: 10.1212/WNL.0000000000007899

Goetz, S. M., Luber, B., Lisanby, S. H., and Peterchev, A. V. (2014). A novel model incorporating two variability sources for describing motor evoked potentials. *Brain Stimul.* 7, 541–552. doi: 10.1016/j.brs.2014.03.002

Goldsworthy, M. R., Hordacre, B., and Ridding, M. C. (2016). Minimum number of trials required for within- and between-session reliability of TMS measures of corticospinal excitability. *Neuroscience* 320, 205–209. doi: 10.1016/j.neuroscience.2016.02.012

Goldsworthy, M. R., Müller-Dahlhaus, F., Ridding, M. C., and Ziemann, U. (2014). Inter-subject variability of ltd-like plasticity in human motor cortex: a matter of preceding motor activation. *Brain Stimul.* 7, 864–870. doi: 10.1016/j.brs.2014.08.004

Goldsworthy, M. R., Pitcher, J. B., and Ridding, M. C. (2012). The application of spaced theta burst protocols induces long-lasting neuroplastic changes in the human motor cortex. *Eur. J. Neurosci.* 35, 125–134. doi: 10.1111/j.1460-9568.2011.07924.x

Gomes-Osman, J., and Field-Fote, E. C. (2015). Improvements in hand function in adults with chronic tetraplegia following a multiday 10-Hz repetitive transcranial magnetic stimulation intervention combined with repetitive task practice:. *J. Neurol. Phys. Ther.* 39, 23–30. doi: 10.1097/npt.0000000000000062

Hallett, M. (2007). Transcranial magnetic stimulation: a primer. *Neuron* 55, 187–199. doi: 10.1016/j.neuron.2007.06.026

Hamada, M., Murase, N., Hasan, A., Balaratnam, M., and Rothwell, J. C. (2013). The role of interneuron networks in driving human motor cortical plasticity. *Cereb. Cortex* 23, 1593–1605. doi: 10.1093/cercor/bhs147

Hameed, M. Q., Dhamne, S. C., Gersner, R., Kaye, H. L., Oberman, L. M., Pascual-Leone, A., et al. (2017). Transcranial magnetic and direct current stimulation in children. *Curr. Neurol. Neurosci. Rep.* 17:11. doi: 10.1007/s11910-017-0719-0

Harris, P. A., Taylor, R., Minor, B. L., Elliott, V., Fernandez, M., O'Neal, L., et al. (2019). The REDCap consortium: building an international community of software platform partners. *J. Biomed. Inform.* 95:103208. doi: 10.1016/j.jbi.2019.103208

Harris, P. A., Taylor, R., Thielke, R., Payne, J., Gonzalez, N., and Conde, J. G. (2009). Research electronic data capture (REDCap)—a metadata-driven methodology and workflow process for providing translational research informatics support. *J. Biomed. Inform.* 42, 377–381. doi: 10.1016/j.jbi.2008.08.010

Hellriegel, H., Schulz, E. M., Siebner, H. R., Deuschl, G., and Raethjen, J. H. (2012). Continuous theta-burst stimulation of the primary motor cortex in essential tremor. *Clin. Neurophysiol.* 123, 1010–1015. doi: 10.1016/j.clinph.2011.08.033

Hoenig, J. M., and Heisey, D. M. (2001). The abuse of power: the pervasive fallacy of power calculations for data analysis. *Am. Stat.* 55, 19–24. doi: 10.1198/000313001300339897

Hong, Y. H., Wu, S. W., Pedapati, E. V., Horn, P. S., Huddleston, D. A., Laue, C. S., et al. (2015). Safety and tolerability of theta burst stimulation vs. single and paired pulse transcranial magnetic stimulation: a comparative study of 165 pediatric subjects. *Front. Hum. Neurosci.* 9:29. doi: 10.3389/fnhum.2015.00029

Hordacre, B., Goldsworthy, M. R., Vallence, A.-M., Darvishi, S., Moezzi, B., Hamada, M., et al. (2017). Variability in neural excitability and plasticity induction in the human cortex: a brain stimulation study. *Brain Stimul.* 10, 588–595. doi: 10.1016/j.brs.2016.12.001

Huang, Y.-Z., Edwards, M. J., Rounis, E., Bhatia, K. P., and Rothwell, J. C. (2005). Theta burst stimulation of the human motor cortex. *Neuron* 45, 201–206. doi: 10.1016/j.neuron.2004.12.033

Huang, Y.-Z., Rothwell, J. C., Edwards, M. J., and Chen, R.-S. (2008). Effect of physiological activity on an NMDA-dependent form of cortical plasticity in human. *Cereb. Cortex* 18, 563–570. doi: 10.1093/cercor/bhm087

Iezzi, E., Conte, A., Suppa, A., Agostino, R., Dinapoli, L., Scontrini, A., et al. (2008). Phasic voluntary movements reverse the aftereffects of subsequent theta-burst stimulation in humans. *J. Neurophysiol.* 100, 2070–2076. doi: 10.1152/jn.90521.2008

Jannati, A., Block, G., Oberman, L. M., Rotenberg, A., and Pascual-Leone, A. (2017). Interindividual variability in response to continuous theta-burst stimulation in healthy adults. *Clin. Neurophysiol.* 128, 2268–2278. doi: 10.1016/j.clinph.2017.08.023

Jannati, A., Fried, P. J., Block, G., Oberman, L. M., Rotenberg, A., and Pascual-Leone, A. (2019). Test-retest reliability of the effects of continuous theta-burst stimulation. *Front. Neurosci.* 13:447. doi: 10.3389/fnins.2019.00447

Jung, N. H., Janzarik, W. G., Delvendahl, I., Münchau, A., Biscaldi, M., Mainberger, F., et al. (2013). Impaired induction of long-term potentiation-like plasticity in patients with high-functioning autism and Asperger syndrome: long-term Potentiation-like Plasticity in ASD. *Dev. Med. Child Neurol.* 55, 83–89. doi: 10.1111/dmcn.12012

Kobayashi, M., and Pascual-Leone, A. (2003). Transcranial magnetic stimulation in neurology. *Lancet Neurol.* 2, 145–156. doi: 10.1016/s1474-4422(03)00321-1

LeBlanc, J. J., and Fagiolini, M. (2011). Autism: a "critical period" disorder? *Neural Plast.* 2011:921680. doi: 10.1155/2011/921680

Lee, M., Kim, S. E., Kim, W. S., Lee, J., Yoo, H. K., Park, K.-D., et al. (2013). Interaction of motor training and intermittent theta burst stimulation in modulating motor cortical plasticity: influence of BDNF Val66Met polymorphism. *PLoS One* 8:e57690. doi: 10.1371/journal.pone.0057690

Lemonnier, E., Villeneuve, N., Sonie, S., Serret, S., Rosier, A., Roue, M., et al. (2017). Effects of bumetanide on neurobehavioral function in children and adolescents with autism spectrum disorders. *Transl. Psychiatry* 7:e1056. doi: 10.1038/tp.2017.10

López-Alonso, V., Cheeran, B., Río-Rodríguez, D., and Fernández-del-Olmo, M. (2014). Inter-individual variability in response to non-invasive brain stimulation paradigms. *Brain Stimul.* 7, 372–380. doi: 10.1016/j.brs.2014.02.004

Lord, C., Risi, S., Lambrecht, L., Cook, E. H. Jr., Leventhal, B. L., DiLavore, P. C., et al. (2000). The autism diagnostic observation schedule—generic: a standard measure of social and communication deficits associated with the spectrum of autism. *J. Autism Dev. Disord.* 30, 205–223. doi: 10.1023/A:1005592401947

Nettekoven, C., Volz, L. J., Leimbach, M., Pool, E.-M., Rehme, A. K., Eickhoff, S. B., et al. (2015). Inter-individual variability in cortical excitability and motor network connectivity following multiple blocks of rTMS. *NeuroImage* 118, 209–218. doi: 10.1016/j.neuroimage.2015.06.004

Nielsen, J. F. (1996a). Improvement of amplitude variability of motor evoked potentials in multiple sclerosis patients and in healthy subjects. *Electroencephalogr. Clin. Neurophysiol.* 101, 404–411. doi: 10.1016/0924-980x(96)96541-8

Nielsen, J. F. (1996b). Logarithmic distribution of amplitudes of compound muscle action potentials evoked by transcranial magnetic stimulation. *J. Clin. Neurophysiol.* 13, 423–434. doi: 10.1097/00004691-199609000-00005

Oberman, L. M., Eldaief, M., Fecteau, S., Ifert-Miller, F., Tormos, J. M., and Pascual-Leone, A. (2012). Abnormal modulation of corticospinal excitability in adults with Asperger's syndrome. *Eur. J. Neurosci.* 36, 2782–2788. doi: 10.1111/j.1460-9568.2012.08172.x

Oberman, L. M., Ifert-Miller, F., Najib, U., Bashir, S., Gonzalez-Heydrich, J., Picker, J., et al. (2016). Abnormal mechanisms of plasticity and metaplasticity in autism spectrum disorders and fragile X syndrome. *J. Child Adolesc. Psychopharmacol.* 26, 617–624. doi: 10.1089/cap.2015.0166

Oberman, L. M., Ifert-Miller, F., Najib, U., Bashir, S., Woollacott, I., Gonzalez-Heydrich, J., et al. (2010). Transcranial magnetic stimulation provides means to assess cortical plasticity and excitability in humans with fragile X syndrome and autism spectrum disorder. *Front. Synaptic Neurosci.* 2:26. doi: 10.3389/fnsyn.2010.00026

Oberman, L. M., Pascual-Leone, A., and Rotenberg, A. (2014). Modulation of corticospinal excitability by transcranial magnetic stimulation in children and adolescents with autism spectrum disorder. *Front. Hum. Neurosci.* 8:627. doi: 10.3389/fnhum.2014.00627

Pascual-Leone, A., Amedi, A., Fregni, F., and Merabet, L. B. (2005). The plastic human brain cortex. *Annu. Rev. Neurosci.* 28, 377–401. doi: 10.1146/annurev.neuro.27.070203.144216

Pascual-Leone, A., Freitas, C., Oberman, L., Horvath, J. C., Halko, M., Eldaief, M., et al. (2011). Characterizing brain cortical plasticity and network dynamics across the age-span in health and disease with TMS-EEG and TMS-fMRI. *Brain Topogr.* 24, 302–315. doi: 10.1007/s10548-011-0196-8

Pasqualetti, P., and Ferreri, F. (2011). W14.4 Amplitude values of motor evoked potentials: statistical properties and neurophysiological implications. *Clin. Neurophysiol.* 122, S44–S45. doi: 10.1016/s1388-2457(11)60148-x

Pechmann, A., Delvendahl, I., Bergmann, T. O., Ritter, C., Hartwigsen, G., Gleich, B., et al. (2012). The number of full-sine cycles per pulse influences the efficacy of multicycle transcranial magnetic stimulation. *Brain Stimul.* 5, 148–154. doi: 10.1016/j.brs.2011.02.006

Pedapati, E. V., Gilbert, D. L., Erickson, C. A., Horn, P. S., Shaffer, R. C., Wink, L. K., et al. (2016). Abnormal cortical plasticity in youth with autism spectrum disorder: a transcranial magnetic stimulation case-control pilot study. *J. Child Adolesc. Psychopharmacol.* 26, 625–631. doi: 10.1089/cap.2015.0183

Pedapati, E. V., Gilbert, D. L., Horn, P. S., Huddleston, D. A., Laue, C. S., Shahana, N., et al. (2015). Effect of 30 Hz theta burst transcranial magnetic stimulation on the primary motor cortex in children and adolescents. *Front. Hum. Neurosci.* 9:91. doi: 10.3389/fnhum.2015.00091

Rajapakse, T., and Kirton, A. (2013). Non-invasive brain stimulation in children: applications and future directions. *Transl. Neurosci.* 4, 217–233. doi: 10.2478/s13380-013-0116-3

Rossi, S., Hallett, M., Rossini, P. M., and Pascual-Leone, A. (2009). Safety, ethical considerations, and application guidelines for the use of transcranial magnetic stimulation in clinical practice and research. *Clin. Neurophysiol.* 120, 2008–2039. doi: 10.1016/j.clinph.2009.08.016

Rossini, P. M., Burke, D., Chen, R., Cohen, L. G., Daskalakis, Z., Di Iorio, R., et al. (2015). Non-invasive electrical and magnetic stimulation of the brain, spinal cord, roots and peripheral nerves: basic principles and procedures for routine clinical and research application. An updated report from an I.F.C.N. Committee. *Clin. Neurophysiol.* 126, 1071–1107. doi: 10.1016/j.clinph.2015.02.001

Rubinstein, R. Y., and Kroese, D. P. (2016). *Simulation and the Monte Carlo Method.* New York, NY: John Wiley & Sons.

Ruohonen, J., and Karhu, J. (2010). Navigated transcranial magnetic stimulation. *Neurophysiol. Clin.* 40, 7–17. doi: 10.1016/j.neucli.2010.01.006

Sartori, L., Begliomini, C., and Castiello, U. (2013). Motor resonance in left- and right-handers: evidence for effector-independent motor representations. *Front. Hum. Neurosci.* 7:33. doi: 10.3389/fnhum.2013.00033

Stagg, C. J., Wylezinska, M., Matthews, P. M., Johansen-Berg, H., Jezzard, P., Rothwell, J. C., et al. (2009). Neurochemical effects of theta burst stimulation as assessed by magnetic resonance spectroscopy. *J. Neurophysiol.* 101, 2872–2877. doi: 10.1152/jn.91060.2008

Stinear, J. W., and Byblow, W. D. (2002). Disinhibition in the human motor cortex is enhanced by synchronous upper limb movements. *J. Physiol.* 543, 307–316. doi: 10.1113/jphysiol.2002.023986

The 1000 Genomes Project Consortium, J. O., Auton, A., Brooks, L. D., Durbin, R. M., Garrison, E. P., Kang, H. M., et al. (2015). A global reference for human genetic variation. *Nature* 526, 68–74. doi: 10.1038/nature15393

Thorndike, R. L., Hagen, E. P., and Sattler, J. M. (1986). *Stanford-Binet Intelligence Scale.* Itasca, IL: Riverside Publishing Company.

Trippe, J., Mix, A., Aydin-Abidin, S., Funke, K., and Benali, A. (2009). Theta burst and conventional low-frequency rTMS differentially affect GABAergic neurotransmission in the rat cortex. *Exp. Brain Res.* 199, 411–421. doi: 10.1007/s00221-009-1961-8

Tyzio, R., Nardou, R., Ferrari, D. C., Tsintsadze, T., Shahrokhi, A., Eftekhari, S., et al. (2014). Oxytocin-mediated GABA inhibition during delivery attenuates autism pathogenesis in rodent offspring. *Science* 343, 675–679. doi: 10.1126/science.1247190

Valero-Cabré, A., Amengual, J. L., Stengel, C., Pascual-Leone, A., and Coubard, O. A. (2017). Transcranial magnetic stimulation in basic and clinical neuroscience: a comprehensive review of fundamental principles and novel insights. *Neurosci. Biobehav. Rev.* 83, 381–404. doi: 10.1016/j.neubiorev.2017.10.006

Vallence, A.-M., Goldsworthy, M. R., Hodyl, N. A., Semmler, J. G., Pitcher, J. B., and Ridding, M. C. (2015). Inter- and intra-subject variability of motor cortex plasticity following continuous theta-burst stimulation. *Neuroscience* 304, 266–278. doi: 10.1016/j.neuroscience.2015.07.043

Vernet, M., Bashir, S., Yoo, W.-K., Oberman, L. M., Mizrahi, I., Ifert-Miller, F., et al. (2014). Reproducibility of the effects of theta burst stimulation on motor cortical plasticity in healthy participants. *Clin. Neurophysiol.* 125, 320–326. doi: 10.1016/j.clinph.2013.07.004

Wischnewski, M., and Schutter, D. J. L. G. (2015). Efficacy and time course of theta burst stimulation in healthy humans. *Brain Stimul.* 8, 685–692. doi: 10.1016/j.brs.2015.03.004

Woo, N. H., Teng, H. K., Siao, C.-J., Chiaruttini, C., Pang, P. T., Milner, T. A., et al. (2005). Activation of p75NTR by proBDNF facilitates hippocampal long-term depression. *Nat. Neurosci.* 8, 1069–1077. doi: 10.1038/nn1510

Wu, S. W., Shahana, N., Huddleston, D. A., Lewis, A. N., and Gilbert, D. L. (2012). Safety and tolerability of theta-burst transcranial magnetic stimulation in children. *Dev. Med. Child Neurol.* 54, 636–639. doi: 10.1111/j.1469-8749.2012.04300.x

Yamada, J., Okabe, A., Toyoda, H., Kilb, W., Luhmann, H. J., and Fukuda, A. (2004). Cl- uptake promoting depolarizing GABA actions in immature rat neocortical neurones is mediated by NKCC1. *J. Physiol.* 557, 829–841. doi: 10.1113/jphysiol.2004.062471

12

A MEG Study of Acute Arbaclofen (STX-209) Administration

Timothy P. L. Roberts[1], Luke Bloy[1], Lisa Blaskey[1,2], Emily Kuschner[1,2], Leah Gaetz[1,2], Ayesha Anwar[1,2], Matt Ku[1], Marissa Dipiero[1], Amanda Bennett[3] and J. Christopher Edgar[1]*

[1]Lurie Family Foundations MEG Imaging Center, Department of Radiology, The Children's Hospital of Philadelphia, Philadelphia, PA, United States, [2]Center for Autism Research, Department of Pediatrics, The Children's Hospital of Philadelphia, Philadelphia, PA, United States, [3]Department of Pediatrics, The Children's Hospital of Philadelphia, Philadelphia, PA, United States

***Correspondence:**
Timothy P. L. Roberts
robertstim@email.chop.edu

Several electrophysiological parameters, including the auditory evoked response component M50/M100 latencies and the phase synchrony of transient and steady-state gamma-band oscillations have been implicated as atypical (to various extents) in autism spectrum disorder (ASD). Furthermore, some hypotheses suggest that an underlying neurobiological mechanism for these observations might be atypical local circuit function indexed by atypical levels of inhibitory neurotransmitter, GABA. This study was a randomized, placebo-controlled, double-blind, escalating-dose, acute investigation conducted in 25 14–18 year-old adolescents with ASD. The study assessed the sensitivity of magnetoencephalography (MEG) and MEGAPRESS "GABA" magnetic resonance spectroscopy (MRS) to monitor dose-dependent acute effects, as well as seeking to define properties of the pre-drug "baseline" electrophysiological and GABA signatures that might predict responsiveness to the GABA-B agonist, arbaclofen (STX-209). Overall, GABA levels and gamma-band oscillatory activity showed no acute changes at either low (15 mg) or high (30 mg) dose. Evoked M50 response latency measures tended to shorten (normalize), but there was heterogeneity across the group in M50 latency response, with only a subset of participants (n = 6) showing significant M50 latency shortening, and only at the 15 mg dose. Findings thus suggest that MEG M50 latency measures show acute effects of arbaclofen administration in select individuals, perhaps reflecting effective target engagement. Whether these subjects have a greater trend towards clinical benefit remains to be established. Finally, findings also provide preliminary support for the use of objective electrophysiological measures upon which to base inclusion for optimal enrichment of populations to be included in full-scale clinical trials of arbaclofen.

Keywords: ASD, MEG (magnetoencephalography), arbaclofen, GABA, biomarker

INTRODUCTION

Although the drug arbaclofen (STX-209) is a promising candidate for pharmaceutical therapy for use in autism spectrum disorder (ASD; Veenstra-VanderWeele et al., 2017) and fragile X syndrome (Berry-Kravis et al., 2012, 2017; Henderson et al., 2012; Qin et al., 2015), unsuccessful clinical trial outcomes challenge the excitation/inhibition imbalance hypothesis of ASD (Rubenstein and Merzenich, 2003), that helped motivate the development of arbaclofen. Specifically, arbaclofen, a GABA-B agonist, was expected to restore a balance to putative excitatory-inhibitory neural circuit abnormalities in ASD and thus improve ASD symptoms. A failed clinical trial, however, is not infrequent, and in the present study we adopt the hypothesis that the phenotypic heterogeneity of ASD arises from heterogeneity in the underlying neurobiological basis. Given between-individual differences in the neurobiology of ASD, broad inclusion criteria in clinical trials, as commonly employed, would diminish the ability to resolve positive change if the drug was only effective only in a subset of participants.

To begin exploring the above, it is of interest to demonstrate, in an acute setting, whether a participant who is a potential candidate for inclusion in a clinical trial manifests evidence in support of pharmaceutical target engagement *via* a single "test" dose administration. This, however, requires an acute readout. With respect to changes in symptoms associated with a disorder, an acute readout is unlikely to be a behavioral measure (e.g., in ASD, changes in repetitive behaviors) as behavioral and symptom changes in ASD likely occur over an extended period of time (weeks to months). If achievable, however, an acute exam (or series of exams) might also provide a rational approach towards optimal dosing, without waiting weeks for behavioral changes. Furthermore, if only a subset of potential participants did exhibit an acute drug-related response, examination of this subgroup might identify candidates distinguished by demographic or other baseline characteristics.

The following report describes a single-center, randomized, placebo-controlled, double-blind, acute "biomarker" study of the pharmaceutical arbaclofen (STX-209) in 25 adolescent males with a diagnosis of ASD. The study examined the possibility that a brief and passive magnetoencephalography (MEG) electrophysiological study consisting of a pure tone auditory exam as well as a 40 Hz auditory steady-state response (ASSR) exam would demonstrate STX-209 associated changes to superior temporal gyrus auditory encoding processes in an acute ~1 h setting. Several candidate measures were assessed including the latency of a response to pure tones (M50 response, being the earliest component measurable of the auditory evoked response, although likely analogous to later components such as the M100) and the phase coherence of 40 Hz oscillatory activity, as an index of cortical circuit function. Both of these electrophysiological measures were selected to be examined in left and right primary/secondary auditory cortex given previous studies showing abnormalities in these responses in ASD and given that these auditory responses are thought to depend, in part, on the integrity of inhibitory-interneuron and pyramidal cell cortical circuits (Gandal et al., 2010; Roberts et al., 2010; Port et al., 2014; Rojas and Wilson, 2014; Edgar et al., 2015a,b). Finally, it was also hypothesized that edited magnetic resonance spectroscopy (MRS) acquired pre- and post-administration of STX-209 would reveal changes in the levels of the inhibitory neurotransmitter GABA.

MATERIALS AND METHODS

This study was approved by the local Institutional Review Board and all participants' families gave written informed consent. When competent to do so, the adolescent participants gave verbal assent to participate.

Twenty-five adolescent males with a diagnosis of ASD were enrolled. Two subjects were excluded from analyses due to an incorrect consenting procedure. One subject withdrew from participation during the study. One other subject was screened out at neuropsychological assessment. Three participants were left-handed and one was ambidextrous.

This study was conducted "double blind." That is, drug and placebo were identically packaged (by the supplying source) and handled by the institutional investigational drug service (IDS). For the three visits, dose was administered in two oral pills (drug was 15 mg/pill, so DD, DP, PP, where D = 15 mg drug and P = placebo). The IDS devised a randomization structure that was not released to the investigators until after data was acquired and analyzed. The only constraint on randomization was imposed by the FDA that, while placebo could occur 1st, 2nd or 3rd in the series, 30 mg should never precede 15 mg. As such there were three randomization options: P,15,30 or 15,P,30 or 15,30,P. Since subjects received two identical-appearing pills on each occasion they were blinded. Since the randomization scheme was not made known to the investigators until after the data analysis was complete, they too were blinded.

Participant demographics are shown in **Table 1** and the study design depicted in **Figure 1**. At the first visit, a full neuropsychological evaluation was conducted including Autism Diagnostic Observation-2 (ADOS-2; Lord et al., 2012), Social Responsiveness Scale 2 (SRS-2; Constantino and Gruber, 2012), Social Communication Questionnaire (SCQ; Rutter et al., 2003) for diagnostic confirmation and the Wechsler Abbreviated Scale of Intelligence-II (Wechsler, 2011) and the Clinical Evaluation of Language Fundamentals—Fifth Edition (CELF-5) for characterization of cognitive (full scale intelligence quotient, FSIQ) and language abilities (core language standard score).

On three subsequent visits, at weekly intervals, participants underwent a protocol of baseline MEG followed immediately by MRI/MRS. Participants then received either placebo or arbaclofen at 15 mg or 30 mg dose (in each case, two identical-appearing oral tablets). After approximately 1 h, MRS was repeated, followed by a MEG protocol identical to the baseline MEG exam. The entire imaging-drug-imaging process lasted approximately 3 h. Since the half-life of arbaclofen is reported as 4–5 h (Berry-Kravis et al., 2017), residual effects are considered unlikely after a 1-week interval.

TABLE 1 | Demographics.

	Age	ADOS-calibrated severity score	SRS T-score	SCQ Total score	FSIQ Standard score	CELF-5 Standard score
Sample Mean ± SD (*N* = 21)	15.8 ± 0.8 years	7.6 ± 2.1	70.1 ± 12.2	19.8 ± 7.8	75.2 ± 19.1	61.9 ± 18.2

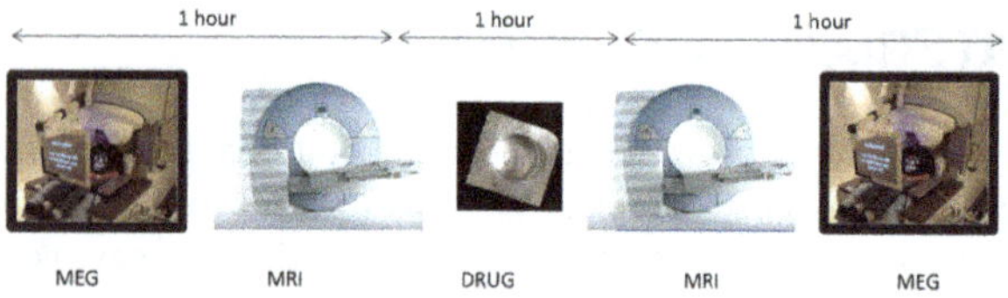

FIGURE 1 | On three subsequent visits, at weekly intervals, participants underwent a protocol of baseline magnetoencephalography (MEG) followed immediately by MRI/magnetic resonance spectroscopy (MRS). Participants then received either placebo or arbaclofen at 15 mg or 30 mg dose. After approximately 1 h, MRS was repeated, followed by a MEG protocol identical to the baseline MEG exam. The entire imaging-drug-imaging process lasted approximately 3 h.

Paradigms and Stimuli

Two auditory exams were administered. The first auditory exam ("M50 Exam") consisted of simple sinusoidal tones of 500 Hz frequency and 300 ms duration played binaurally at 45 dB Sensation Level (SL) corresponding to a pleasant conversational level (note SL loudness presents an equivalent sensory sensation, after determining individual hearing thresholds). Stimuli were presented through piezoelectric transducers and ear tip inserts (ER3A, Etymotic, IL, USA), with the inter-stimulus-interval (ISI) randomly varying between 600 and 2,000 ms, and with 520 trials collected over approximately 14 min. The second auditory exam ("40 Hz ASSR Exam") consisted of a 500 Hz stimulus modulated at 40 Hz, with the modulation depth 100%. Stimuli of 1 s duration were presented with a 4 s offset-to-onset ISI (± 2 s), with 100 trials collected over approximately 17 min.

MRI/MRS

MRI/MRS was performed on a 3T Siemens Verio MR scanner. A 3D isotropic T1-weighted structural MRI (sMRI) was acquired for the purposes of MEG source modeling. A single voxel edited MRS MEGAPRESS sequence was also administered (Mescher et al., 1998), with a voxel of 4 × 3 × 2 cm placed in the left superior temporal gyrus, and with TR/TE = 1,500/80 ms. To minimize the impact of coedited macromolecules (widely acknowledged in the conventional MEGAPRESS sequence), a modification was implemented in which the "off" pulse was delivered at 1.5 ppm frequency (symmetric about 1.7 ppm with the traditional "on" pulse at 1.9 ppm). This achieves a level of macromolecule suppression, while only extending the echo time moderately from 68 ms to 80 ms (Edden et al., 2012).

MEG Recording and Analysis

MEG data were obtained in a magnetically shielded room using a 275-channel whole-cortex CTF magnetometer (CTF MEG, Coquitlam, BC, Canada). At the start of the session, three head-position indicator coils were attached to the scalp to provide continuous specification of the position and orientation of the MEG sensors relative to the head (Roberts et al., 2010). To minimize fatigue and encourage an awake state, subjects viewed a silent movie projected on to a screen positioned at a comfortable viewing distance. To aid in the identification of eye-blink activity, the electro-oculogram (EOG, bipolar oblique, upper right and lower left sites) was collected. To later co-register MEG and sMRI data, three anatomical landmarks (nasion and right and left preauricular points) as well as an additional 200+ points on the scalp and face were digitized for each participant using a probe position identification system (Polhemus, Colchester, VT, USA). MEG data were recorded at a sample rate of 1,200 Hz per channel using 3rd order synthetic gradiometer noise reduction and DC offset correction.

For both auditory exams, to coregister MEG and sMRI data, an affine transformation matrix that involved rotation and translation between the MEG and sMRI coordinate systems was obtained *via* a least-square match of the probe position identification points to the surface of the scalp and face. For both auditory exams, to correct for eye blinks, a typical eye blink was manually identified in the raw data (including EOG) for each participant. The pattern search function in BESA Research 6.1 (BESA GmbH, Germany) scanned the raw data to identify other blinks and computed an eye-blink average. An eye blink was modeled by its first component topography from principal component analysis (PCA), typically accounting for more than 99% of the variance in the eye-blink average. Scanning the eye blink corrected raw data, epochs with artifacts other than blinks were rejected by amplitude and gradient criteria (amplitude >300 fT, gradients >25 fT/cm).

For the pure auditory exam, non-contaminated epochs were averaged (−100 ms to 500 ms) and a 1 Hz (24 dB/octave, zero-phase) to 40 Hz (48 dB/octave, zero-phase) band-pass filter applied. Using all 275 channels of MEG data, determination of the latency of M50 sources in the left and right STG was accomplished by applying a standard source model to transform each individual's raw MEG surface activity into brain space (MEG data co-registered to each subject's T1-weighted 3D MRI) using a model with multiple sources (Scherg and Picton, 1991; Scherg and Ebersole, 1993; Scherg and Berg, 1996). In particular, the standard source model applied to each subject was constructed by including left and right STG dipole sources (placed at left and right Heschl's gyrus) and the eye-blink source vector derived for each participant (Lins et al., 1993; Berg and Scherg, 1994). This source model served as a source montage for the raw MEG (Scherg and Picton, 1991; Scherg and Ebersole, 1993). As such, the MEG sensor data was transformed from channel space into brain source space where the visualized waveforms were the modeled source activities. To obtain left and right M50 latency measures, for each participant, left and right dipoles were oriented at the maximum M50 response. Thus, estimates of left and right M50 activity were obtained using an individualized anatomical constraint, with an orientation of the M50 dipoles optimized for each participant. Left and right M50 (50–125 ms) peaks were defined from the source waveforms, given appropriate magnetic field topography (ensuring the consistent orientation of neuronal current dipoles), and the latency at the left and right peak recorded.

For the ASSR exam, after artifact rejection, a band-pass filter (Butterworth) was applied with a center frequency of 40 Hz and a 20 Hz width (a band-pass filter is superior to using separate low- and high-pass filters for extracting MEG activity in narrow frequency bands) with 100% of the activity passed at 40 Hz and 50% amplitude cut offs at 30 Hz and 50 Hz. For modeling the 40 Hz steady-state response, data −500 to 1,000 ms post-stimulus were selected, with a 300 ms starting point as the amplitude-modulated 40 Hz steady-state response does not fully develop until after 250–300 ms (Ross et al., 2002). In particular, left and right STG 40 Hz steady-state dipole orientations were obtained from the 300–1,000 ms ASSR interval. Once the source model was created, the calculation of single-trial phase for the left and right STG sources used procedures outlined in Hoechstetter et al. (2004), where for each participant the derived source model was applied to the raw unfiltered data. The transformation from the time domain to the time-frequency domain used the complex demodulation technique (wavelet transformation) procedures (Papp and Ktonas, 1977) implemented in BESA 6.0, using frequencies between 4 and 60 Hz in steps of 2 Hz. Forty hertz steady-state Phase-locking (PL) was examined. PL measures were extracted from the single-trial complex time-frequency matrix. In particular, a measure of PL referred to as intertrial coherence (ITC) was computed. ITC is a normalized measure with ITC = 1 reflecting no trial-to-trial phase variability and ITC = 0 reflecting maximal phase variability across trials. For each participant, a single left and right ITC value was obtained as the average ITC within a 300–1,000 ms and 38–42 Hz interval.

Statistics

For each dependent variable (left and right M50 latency, left and right 40 Hz ASSR ITC, and GABA/Cr), and separate for each dose, a linear mixed model (LMM) examined fixed effects of pre/post-drug, hemisphere and age, along with their interactions, and with subject as a random effect. Additionally, for each parameter, a "baseline" pre-drug/placebo standard deviation (SD) was computed from the three baseline recordings. A population SD was then estimated as the average of this baseline SD across all subjects. This was then used to recast post- vs. pre-drug (or placebo) changes in each measure as a Z-score (where a Z-score of 1 corresponds to a change in the measure of equal magnitude to the population SD). Expressing the drug/placebo-related changes in each measure as a Z-score provided ready comparative visualization of changes in measures that otherwise have very different units. Positive Z-scores represented positive changes in the measure, and negative Z-scores indicated negative changes. As an example, for M50 latency, a Z-score of "−1" is equivalent to a latency shortening of magnitude 1 population SD (approximately 5 ms). Changes were considered noteworthy when the $|Z|$ score exceeded 2.57 (corresponding to a <1% probability of the change being by chance).

RESULTS

For placebo and for the 30 mg dose, there was no significant effect of pre- to post- placebo/drug administration on M50 latency (see **Table 2**). However, for the 15 mg dose, there was a significant shortening effect on M50 latency (pre: 94 ms ± 4 ms vs. post: 88 ms ± 4 ms, $p < 0.01$). *Post hoc t*-tests revealed an effect for the right hemisphere M50 response (pre: 97 ms ± 4 ms vs. post: 88 ms ± 4 ms, $p = 0.012$). The left hemisphere showed no significant pre- to post-difference (pre: 92 ms ± 4 ms vs. post: 87 ms ± 4 ms, $p = 0.2$). For the 40 ASSR ITC and for GABA/Cr MRS, there were no significant group effects at any dose or placebo (see **Table 2**).

Figure 2A shows an example of the M50 magnetic field topography, modeled as the anatomic source(s) shown in **Figure 2B** at the peak M50 deflection (**Figure 2C**, blue dashed line). **Figure 2C** shows an example of STX-209-related shortening of the M50 peak latency in a single individual pre- and post-15 mg STX209, along with a representative example (**Figure 2D**) from a non-responding participant at the same dose.

Examination of the pre- to post-changes in each target parameter (bilateral M50 latency, bilateral 40 Hz ASSR ITC, and left-hemispheric GABA/Cr) revealed that the target parameters showed little change in most individuals, with occasional statistical anomalies—~1 per measure as might be expected by chance. **Figure 3** shows each individual's data at each dose, expressed as a color-coded Z-score.

Although most parameters showed little change as a function of STX-209 or placebo (with typically only one Z-outlier and with no systematic directional bias), the 15 mg dose appeared to have a conspicuous effect on the M50 latency. As shown in **Figure 3**, M50 latency Z-score graphs (circled), several participants had high negative M50 latency Z-scores at 15 mg. Furthermore, the direction of the effect (latency shortening) was the same for all participants showing an effect (i.e., there were no participants with a significant latency elongation). This observation [several Z-outliers and a directional bias (suggesting an effect not due to random chance)] motivated consideration of M50 latency as the most sensitive measurement of an acute dose-dependent effect. To this end, a subgroup of participants were defined as "M50 Responders" if their latency shortening exceeded a Z-threshold of −2.57 (equivalent to the 99% percentile). Analyses comparing six "M50 Responders" and 15 "M50 non-Responders" showed the expected finding of the "M50 Responders" having greater pre- to post- 15 mg dose M50 shortening than the "M50 non-Responders" with an interaction term of $F_{(1,57)} = 16.02$, $p < 0.001$) (see **Table 3**). Of note, however, 40 Hz ASSR ITC also differed between "M50 Responders" and "M50 non-Responders" (interaction term: $F_{(1,57)} = 5.496$, $p = 0.023$). There was no "M50 Responders" vs. "M50 non-Responders" group difference for GABA (interaction term: $F_{(1,25)} = 0.061$,

TABLE 2 | Group effects of Arbaclofen administration on MEG/MRS measures.

Placebo	**Pre-administration**	**Post-administration**	**Statistics/*p*-value**
M50 latency	93 ms ± 4 ms	93 ms ± 4 ms	$F_{(1,54.2)} = 0.006, p = 0.941$
Steady state phase locking (ITC)	0.24 ± 0.11	0.34 ± 0.12	$F_{(1,58.1)} = 0.369, p = 0.55$
GABA/Cr	0.151 ± 0.017	0.153 ± 0.015	$F_{(1,27)} = 0.004, t = -0.065, p = 0.95$
15 mg dose	Pre-administration	Post-administration	*p*-value
M50 latency	**94 ms ± 4 ms**	**88 ms ± 4 ms**	$\mathbf{F_{(1,56.0)} = 7.48, p = 0.008}$
Steady state phase locking (ITC)	0.28 ± 0.03	0.28 ± 0.03	$F_{(1,55.0)} = 0.089, p = 0.77$
GABA/Cr	0.153 ± 0.017	0.155 ± 0.019	$F_{(1,27)} = 0.004, t = -0.060, p = 0.95$
30 mg dose	Pre-administration	Post-administration	*p*-value
M50 latency	92 ms ± 4 ms	92 ms ± 4 ms	$F_{(1,51.5)} = 0.021, p = 0.89$
Steady state phase locking (ITC)	0.28 ± 0.03	0.28 ± 0.03	$F_{(1,49.7)} = 0.138, p = 0.71$
GABA/Cr	0.149 ± 0.014	0.163 ± 0.015	$F_{(1,30)} = 0.526, t = -0.726, p = 0.47$

Bold face values achieve statistical significance as indicated in the far right column.

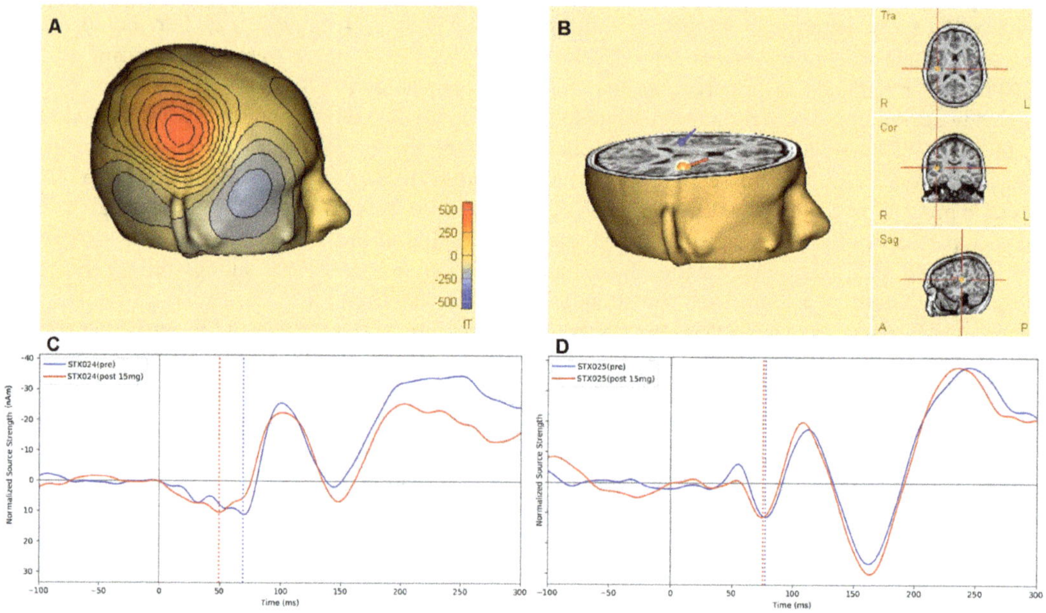

FIGURE 2 | **(A)** An example of the M50 scalp magnetic field topography (over the right hemisphere) modeled by the anatomic source depicted in **(B)** and corresponding to the M50 peak deflection (dashed line at 71 ms post-stimulus) of the pre-dose source activity waveform (blue) of **(C)**, which shows the STX-209 related shortening (arrow) of the M50 latency in the modeled source waveform for a single individual pre- (blue) vs. post (red) 15 mg STX209 administration. **(D)** A corresponding example of auditory evoked waveforms from a non-responding individual pre and post a similar dose. Dotted black line marks the stimulus onset, while dotted blue (and red) lines mark the M50 response pre and post 15 mg STX209 administration. Note, by convention and for ready comparison to the ERP literature, in which negativities are shown as positive excursions from baseline and positivities are shown below the x-axis, we show the M50 response as negatively-signed and the later M100 response as positively-signed.

$p = 0.806$). "M50 Responders" and "M50 non-Responders" also did not differ on any target parameter for either placebo or the 30 mg dose.

Examination of the baseline parameters of the six "M50 Responders" compared to the 15 "M50 non-Responders" revealed significant baseline prolongation of M50 latency ("M50 Responders" 112 ms ± 8 ms vs. "M50 non-Responders": 87 ms ± 5 ms, $p < 0.05$). A significant interaction between hemisphere and response status ($p = 0.05$), prompted evaluation of group baseline M50 latency differences in each hemisphere. Whereas right-hemisphere group differences were significant ("M50 Responders": 120 ms ± 8 ms vs. "M50 non-Responders": 87 ms ± 5 ms, $p = 0.004$), only a trend level group finding was observed in the left hemisphere ("M50 Responders": 104 ms ± 8 ms vs. "M50 non-Responders": 87 ms ± 5 ms, $p = 0.09$). Baseline 40 Hz ASSR ITC values did not differ between groups ("M50 Responders": 0.157 ± −0.014 vs. "M50 non-Responders": 0.153 ± −0.026, $p = 0.62$). Baseline GABA levels also did not differ between groups ("M50 Responders": 0.159 ± −0.022 vs. "M50 non-Responders": 0.140 ± −0.034, $p = 0.65$).

Examination of "M50 Responders" and "M50 non-Responders" group differences on demographic measures (two-sample *t*-test) showed no group difference in age, ADOS-CSS, SRS, SCQ, full-scale IQ, or CELF-5 core language index (**Table 4**).

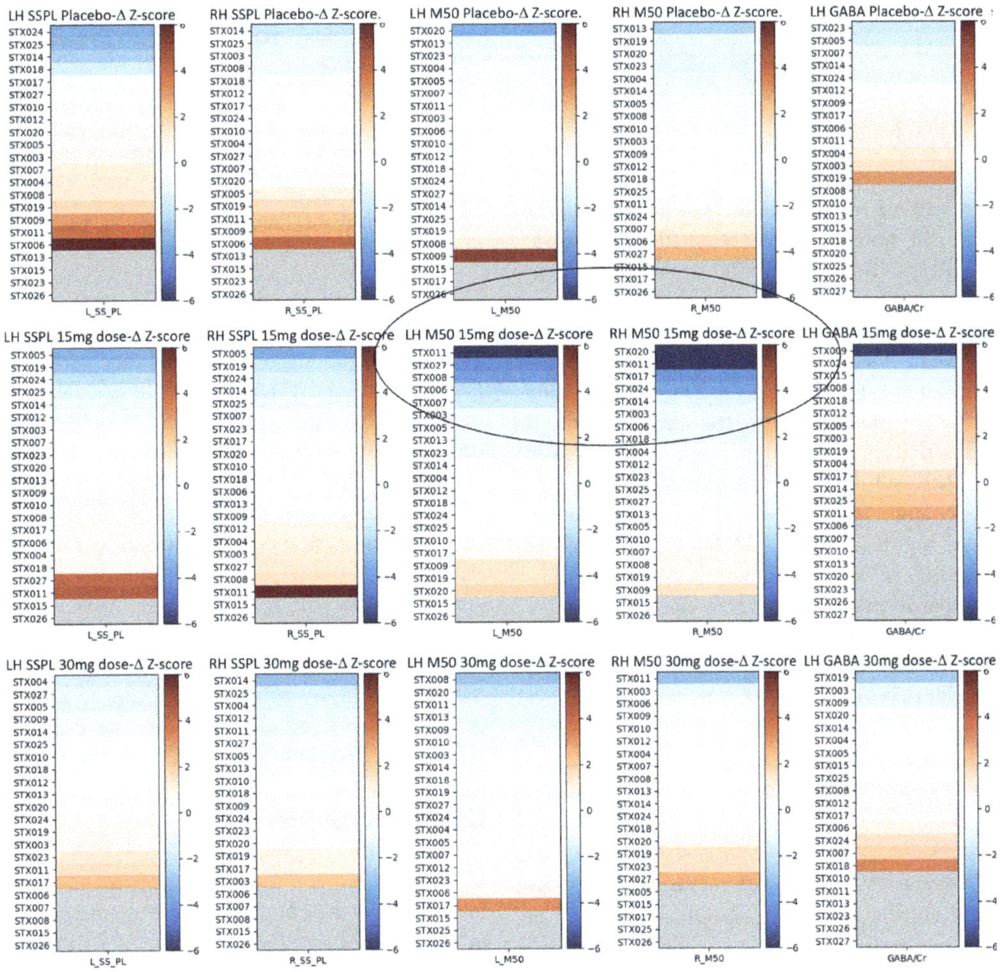

FIGURE 3 | *Z*-score graphs for the imaging target variables for all participants and all measures. Interval changes post- vs. pre-administration of drug/placebo are represented in terms of *Z*-scores, where a $Z = 1$ for any measure equals a change equivalent to the population average SD of that measure across the three pre-drug/placebo baseline scans. Circled are the participants with high negative M50 latency *Z*-scores at 15 mg. The selection of responders vs. non-responders was based on a $|Z| > 2.57$ (equivalent to the 99th percentile). In each plot, subjects are identified by their subject ID (STX###) and ranked in order of their post vs. pre-effect size for each measure as a *Z*-score based on the SD derived from the three baseline scans for each measure averaged across all subjects. Hemisphere is noted as LH vs. RH. SSPL, steady state phase locking; M50, M50 latency. Increasing dependent variable values are depicted in red, and decreases in blue, with the strength of the color indicating the magnitude of the change.

TABLE 3 | Changes in target parameters with 15 mg dose, separated according to "M50 Responsiveness".

M50 latency (ms)	Pre-administration	Post-administration	*p*-value
non-Responder	87 ms ± 4 ms	86 ms ± 4 ms	$F_{(1,57)} = 0.143, p = 0.71$
Responder	**112 ms ± 7 ms**	**92 ms ± 7 ms**	$\mathbf{F_{(1,57)} = 25.315, p < 0.001}$
Steady state phase locking (ITC)			
non-Responder	0.286 ± 0.035	0.264 ± 30.035	$F_{(1,57)} = 1.063, p = 0.307$
Responder	**0.253 ± 0.054**	**0.325 ± 0.054**	$\mathbf{F_{(1,57)} = 4.524, p = 0.038}$
GABA			
Non-Responder	0.159 ± 0.022	0.156 ± 0.023	$F_{(1,25)} = 0.007, p = 0.934$
Responder	0.140 ± 0.034	0.152 ± 0.036	$F_{(1,25)} = 0.058, p = 0.812$

Bold face values achieve statistical significance as indicated in the far right column.

DISCUSSION

Although the sample size is too small to draw strong conclusions, analyses suggested an effect of STX-209 on brain activity in only a subset of the adolescents, and only at a specific dose. In particular, 6 out of 21 adolescents (~30%) showed a significant shortening of M50 latency in response to 15 mg of arbaclofen. No other pre- to post-treatment effects were observed for any

TABLE 4 | Characteristics of "M50 Responders".

	Age (years)	ADOS-CSS	SRS	SCQ	Full Scale IQ	CELF-5
"M50 Responders"	16.2 ± 0.6	7.4 ± 2.6	73 ± 11	23 ± 11	72 ± 18	56 ± 12
"M50 non-Responders"	15.7 ± 0.9	7.3 ± 2.3	67 ± 13	19 ± 6	77 ± 20	64 ± 20
p-value (*t*-test)	0.20	0.96	0.33	0.37	0.58	0.26

other brain measure (40 Hz ASSR or GABA) or any other dose (placebo or 30 mg). Of note, however, when the group was divided into "M50 Responders" and "M50 non-Responders," according to their drug-related changes in M50 latency, significant STX-209 pre- to post-treatment changes were also observed for the 40 Hz ASSR ITC, with significantly higher PL *after* administration of 15 mg of STX-209. Upregulation of 40 Hz ASSR PL is consistent with the theorized mode of action of arbaclofen in a model of pyramidal interneuron network gamma (PING; Whittington et al., 2000; Jensen et al., 2014). Finally, no change in GABA level was identified at placebo, 15 mg or 30 mg dose, and GABA levels did not differ between "M50 Responders" and "M50 non-Responders." The absence of acute response in the MRS parameter "GABA/Cr," although counterintuitive, may, in fact, reflect the insensitivity of this measure to GABA compartmentalization or activity (on an acute timescale). While tonic GABA decrements have been reported in some cortices in ASD, it is not necessarily expected that such regionally-coarse GABA estimates (24cc) would be responsive to acute changes related to pharmaceuticals like arbaclofen.

Present findings thus suggest superior temporal gyrus M50 latency as a sensitive probe of arbaclofen activity in a subset of individuals and at a specific dose. When comparing "M50 Responder" and "M50 non-Responder," the "M50 Responder" participants were found to have significantly longer M50 latencies at baseline (pre-drug) than the "M50 non-Responder" participants. Although this suggests that a pre-existing prolonged M50 latency may be a predictor of response to STX-209, it is important to note that some of the responsive individuals would not have been distinguished based on their baseline M50 latency alone given significant overlap between the two groups. As such, relying only on baseline M50 latency assessment and not a "test drug dose" to identify potential responders for a STX-209 clinical trial would diminish sensitivity. It is also of note that there were no baseline differences in any other MEG or MRS variable, or group differences on any of the clinical assessments of ASD severity, or cognitive or language ability. The findings highlight the utility of MEG as a modality providing exquisite temporal resolution as well as sufficient source modeling to reject surface artifact and distinguish hemispheric sources. Of note, pharmacodynamic studies using electroencephalography (EEG) either spontaneous or with stimulation as evoked potentials have been proposed for drug effect monitoring, predicting response and dose optimization for many disorders and phenomena including seizure disorders, mood disorders as well as analgesia and anesthesia—for a review, see Bewernitz and Derendorf (2012). There has, however, been less extensive work in neurodevelopmental disorders.

That the drug response in M50 latency (and also 40 Hz ASSR ITC in the subgroup of "M50 Responders") occurred only at the 15 mg dose may suggest the need for optimal dose assessments, perhaps achieved *via* the acute dose-escalating paradigm used in this study. As the 15 mg M50 latency effect was not always observed bilaterally, this also indicates the need to examine left and right auditory activity separately. The basis for a hemisphere-specific effect in some individuals remains to be elucidated.

Two major study limitations are of note. First, although suggesting the biological activity of the drug, there is no guarantee that M50 latency responsiveness predicts a good clinical outcome in an extended clinical trial. Second, and conversely, absence of M50 latency responsiveness in a short monitoring (1 h) acute single-dose administration does not predict absence of clinical response; a single dose may be insufficient drug and a 1 h observation period may be too short.

CONCLUSION

MEG measures of auditory sensory processing appear responsive to a particular dose of the GABA-B agonist, STX-209 (arbaclofen) in a subset of adolescents with ASD. It is possible that this responsiveness indicates an observable marker of differential drug biological activity in some individuals vs. others. This phenomenon could potentially be exploited as an inclusion criterion for clinical trial recruitment enrichment. Furthermore, the dose-specificity of this responsiveness could provide a mechanism for rapid determination of biologically-optimal dose. There were no observed differentiating responses in basal GABA level, estimated by MRS, either indicating the insensitivity of the MRS method or the lack of bulk GABA concentration changes associated with single-dose arbaclofen administration. Findings should be treated with caution given the small sample of responders, but indicate the possibility of observing heterogeneous responses to arbaclofen across an ASD population (possibly diminishing statistical power in a clinical trial designed to assess drug efficacy), as well as offering a tantalizing potential approach to biologically-based stratification for clinical trial enrichment and, ultimately, patient management.

ETHICS STATEMENT

The studies involving human participants were reviewed and approved by Children's Hospital of Philadelphia IRB. Written informed consent to participate in this study was provided by the participants' legal guardian/next of kin.

AUTHOR CONTRIBUTIONS

TR, JE, LBla, AB and EK contributed to the conception and design of the study. AA and LG managed recruitment, regulatory reporting and compliance. AB was study physician. AB conducted clinical assessment. LBla and EK conducted neuropsychological assessments. MK and MD acquired the data. TR, LBlo, MK and MD performed the data analysis. TR, JE and LBlo performed the statistical analysis. TR wrote the first draft of the manuscript. JE, LBla and EK wrote sections of the manuscript. All authors contributed to manuscript revision, read and approved the submitted version.

FUNDING

This study was supported by a grant to TR from the Simons Foundation/Clinical Research Associates. Support was also provided by the Neuroimaging/Neurocircuitry core of the CHOP/Penn IDDRC (National Institutes of Health; NIH U54-HD086984 and R01-DC008871).

ACKNOWLEDGMENTS

TR gratefully acknowledges the Oberkircher Family for the Oberkircher Family Chair in Pediatric Radiology at CHOP. We are grateful to Siemens Medical Solutions, Erlangen, Germany for use of the WIP529 edited MRS sequence. We thank Dr. Paul Wang for insightful comments and discussions.

REFERENCES

Berg, P., and Scherg, M. (1994). A multiple source approach to the correction of eye artifacts. *Electroencephalogr. Clin. Neurophysiol.* 90, 229–241. doi: 10.1016/0013-4694(94)90094-9

Berry-Kravis, E., Hagerman, R., Visootsak, J., Budimirovic, D., Kaufmann, W. E., Cherubini, M., et al. (2017). Arbaclofen in fragile X syndrome: results of phase 3 trials. *J. Neurodev. Disord.* 9:3. doi: 10.1186/s11689-016-9181-6

Berry-Kravis, E. M., Hessl, D., Rathmell, B., Zarevics, P., Cherubini, M., Walton-Bowen, K., et al. (2012). Effects of STX209 (arbaclofen) on neurobehavioral function in children and adults with fragile X syndrome: a randomized, controlled, phase 2 trial. *Sci. Transl. Med.* 4:152ra127. doi: 10.1126/scitranslmed.3004214

Bewernitz, M., and Derendorf, H. (2012). Electroencephalogram-based pharmacodynamic measures: a review. *Int. J. Clin. Pharmacol. Ther.* 50, 162–184. doi: 10.5414/cp201484

Constantino, J. N., and Gruber, C. P. (2012). *Social Responsiveness Scale.* 2nd Edn. Los Angeles, CA: Western Psychological Services.

Edden, R. A., Puts, N. A., and Barker, P. B. (2012). Macromolecule-suppressed GABA-edited magnetic resonance spectroscopy at 3T. *Magn. Reson. Med.* 68, 657–661. doi: 10.1002/mrm.24391

Edgar, J. C., Fisk Iv, C. L., Berman, J. I., Chudnovskaya, D., Liu, S., Pandey, J., et al. (2015a). Auditory encoding abnormalities in children with autism spectrum disorder suggest delayed development of auditory cortex. *Mol. Autism* 6:69. doi: 10.1186/s13229-015-0065-5

Edgar, J. C., Khan, S. Y., Blaskey, L., Chow, V. Y., Rey, M., Gaetz, W., et al. (2015b). Neuromagnetic oscillations predict evoked-response latency delays and core language deficits in autism spectrum disorders. *J. Autism Dev. Disord.* 45, 395–405. doi: 10.1007/s10803-013-1904-x

Gandal, M. J., Edgar, J. C., Ehrlichman, R. S., Mehta, M., Roberts, T. P., and Siegel, S. J. (2010). Validating γ oscillations and delayed auditory responses as translational biomarkers of autism. *Biol. Psychiatry* 68, 1100–1106. doi: 10.1016/j.biopsych.2010.09.031

Henderson, C., Wijetunge, L., Kinoshita, M. N., Shumway, M., Hammond, R. S., Postma, F. R., et al. (2012). Reversal of disease-related pathologies in the fragile X mouse model by selective activation of GABAB receptors with arbaclofen. *Sci. Transl. Med.* 4:152ra128. doi: 10.1126/scitranslmed.3004218

Hoechstetter, K., Bornfleth, H., Weckesser, D., Ille, N., Berg, P., and Scherg, M. (2004). BESA source coherence: a new method to study cortical oscillatory coupling. *Brain Topogr.* 16, 233–238. doi: 10.1023/b:brat.0000032857.55223.5d

Jensen, O., Spaak, E., and Zumer, J. M. (2014). "Human brain oscillations: from physiological mechanisms to analysis and cognition," in *Magnetoencephalography From Signals to Dynamic Cortical Networks*, eds S. Supek, and C. J. Aine (Berlin Heidelberg: Springer-Verlag), 359–403.

Lins, O. G., Picton, T. W., Berg, P., and Scherg, M. (1993). Ocular artifacts in EEG and event-related potentials. I: scalp topography. *Brain Topogr.* 6, 51–63. doi: 10.1007/bf01234127

Lord, C., DiLavore, P. C., and Gotham, K. (2012). *Autism Diagnostic Observation Schedule.* 2nd Edn. Torrance, CA: Western Psychological Services.

Mescher, M., Merkle, H., Kirsch, J., Garwood, M., and Gruetter, R. (1998). Simultaneous *in vivo* spectral editing and water suppression. *NMR Biomed.* 11, 266–272. doi: 10.1002/(sici)1099-1492(199810)11:6<266::aid-nbm530>3.3.co;2-a

Papp, N., and Ktonas, P. (1977). Critical evaluation of complex demodulation techniques for the quantification of bioelectrical activity. *Biomed. Sci. Instrum.* 13, 135–145.

Port, R. G., Gandal, M. J., Roberts, T. P., Siegel, S. J., and Carlson, G. C. (2014). Convergence of circuit dysfunction in ASD: a common bridge between diverse genetic and environmental risk factors and common clinical electrophysiology. *Front. Cell. Neurosci.* 8:414. doi: 10.3389/fncel.2014.00414

Qin, M., Huang, T., Kader, M., Krych, L., Xia, Z., Burlin, T., et al. (2015). R-baclofen reverses a social behavior deficit and elevated protein synthesis in a mouse model of Fragile X syndrome. *Int. J. Neuropsychopharmacol.* 18:pyv034. doi: 10.1093/ijnp/pyv034

Roberts, T. P., Khan, S. Y., Rey, M., Monroe, J. F., Cannon, K., Blaskey, L., et al. (2010). MEG detection of delayed auditory evoked responses in autism spectrum disorders: towards an imaging biomarker for autism. *Autism Res.* 3, 8–18. doi: 10.1002/aur.111

Rojas, D. C., and Wilson, L. B. (2014). γ-band abnormalities as markers of autism spectrum disorders. *Biomark. Med.* 8, 353–368. doi: 10.2217/bmm.14.15

Ross, B., Picton, T. W., and Pantev, C. (2002). Temporal integration in the human auditory cortex as represented by the development of the steady-state magnetic field. *Hear. Res.* 165, 68–84. doi: 10.1016/s0378-5955(02)00285-x

Rubenstein, J. L., and Merzenich, M. M. (2003). Model of autism: increased ratio of excitation/inhibition in key neural systems. *Genes Brain Behav.* 2, 255–267. doi: 10.1034/j.1601-183x.2003.00037.x

Rutter, M., Bailey, A., and Lloyd, C. (2003). *SCQ: Social Communication Questionnaire.* Los Angeles, CA: Western Psychological Services.

Scherg, M., and Berg, P. (1996). New concepts of brain source imaging and localization. *Electroencephalogr. Clin. Neurophysiol. Suppl.* 46, 127–137.

Scherg, M., and Ebersole, J. S. (1993). Models of brain sources. *Brain Topogr.* 5, 419–423. doi: 10.1007/bf01128700

Scherg, M., and Picton, T. W. (1991). Separation and identification of event-related potential components by brain electric source analysis. *Electroencephalogr. Clin. Neurophysiol. Suppl.* 42, 24–37.

Veenstra-VanderWeele, J., Cook, E. H., King, B. H., Zarevics, P., Cherubini, M., Walton-Bowen, K., et al. (2017). Arbaclofen in children and adolescents with autism spectrum disorder: a randomized, controlled, phase 2 trial. *Neuropsychopharmacology* 42, 1390–1398. doi: 10.1038/npp.2016.237

Wechsler, D. (2011). *Wechsler Abbreviated Scale of Intelligence.* 2nd Edn. San Antonio, TX: Pearson.

Whittington, M. A., Traub, R. D., Kopell, N., Ermentrout, B., and Buhl, E. H. (2000). Inhibition-based rhythms: experimental and mathematical observations on network dynamics. *Int. J. Psychophysiol.* 38, 315–336. doi: 10.1016/s0167-8760(00)00173-2

13

Investigating Potential Biomarkers in Autism Spectrum Disorder

Carolyn Bridgemohan[1,2], David M. Cochran[3,4], Yamini J. Howe[2,5], Katherine Pawlowski[1], Andrew W. Zimmerman[3,4], George M. Anderson[6], Roula Choueiri[3,4], Laura Sices[7,8], Karen J. Miller[9,10], Monica Ultmann[9,10], Jessica Helt[5], Peter W. Forbes[1], Laura Farfel[7,9,11], Stephanie J. Brewster[1], Jean A. Frazier[3,4,12†] and Ann M. Neumeyer[2,5†] on behalf of the Autism Consortium Biomarkers Study Clinicians*

[1] Boston Children's Hospital, Boston, MA, United States, [2] Harvard Medical School, Boston, MA, United States, [3] University of Massachusetts Memorial Medical Center, Worcester, MA, United States, [4] University of Massachusetts Medical School, Worcester, MA, United States, [5] Lurie Center for Autism, Massachusetts General Hospital for Children, Lexington, MA, United States, [6] Child Study Center, Yale University School of Medicine, New Haven, CT, United States, [7] Boston University Medical Center, Boston, MA, United States, [8] Boston University School of Medicine, Boston, MA, United States, [9] Center for Children with Special Needs, Floating Children's Hospital at Tufts Medical Center, Boston, MA, United States, [10] Tufts University School of Medicine, Boston, MA, United States, [11] Autism Consortium at Harvard Medical School, Boston, MA, United States, [12] Eunice Kennedy Shriver Center, University of Massachusetts Medical School, Worcester, MA, United States

***Correspondence:**
Carolyn Bridgemohan
Carolyn.bridgemohan@childrens.harvard.edu

† These authors have contributed equally to this work

Background: Early identification and treatment of individuals with autism spectrum disorder (ASD) improves outcomes, but specific evidence needed to individualize treatment recommendations is lacking. Biomarkers that could be routinely measured within the clinical setting could potentially transform clinical care for patients with ASD. This demonstration project employed collection of biomarker data during regular autism specialty clinical visits and explored the relationship of biomarkers with clinical ASD symptoms.

Methods: Eighty-three children with ASD, aged 5–10 years, completed a multi-site feasibility study integrating the collection of biochemical (blood serotonin, urine melatonin sulfate excretion) and clinical (head circumference, dysmorphology exam, digit ratio, cognitive and behavioral function) biomarkers during routine ASD clinic visits. Parents completed a demographic survey and the Aberrant Behavior Checklist-Community. Cognitive function was determined by record review. Data analysis utilized Wilcoxon two-sample tests and Spearman correlations.

Results: Participants were 82% male, 63% White, 19% Hispanic, with a broad range of functioning. Group means indicated hyperserotonemia. In a single regression analysis adjusting for race and median household income, higher income was associated with higher levels of blood serotonin and urine melatonin sulfate excretion levels ($p = 0.004$ and $p = 0.04$, respectively). Melatonin correlated negatively with age ($p = 0.048$) and reported neurologic problems ($p = 0.02$). Dysmorphic status correlated with higher reported stereotyped behavior ($p = 0.02$) and inappropriate speech ($p = 0.04$).

Conclusion: This demonstration project employed collection of multiple biomarkers, allowed for examination of associations between biochemical and clinical measures, and identified several findings that suggest direction for future studies. This clinical research model has promise for integrative biomarker research in individuals with complex, heterogeneous neurodevelopmental disorders such as ASD.

Keywords: autism, ASD, biomarkers, serotonin, melatonin, dysmorphology, clinical research

INTRODUCTION

Autism spectrum disorder (ASD) is a highly heritable, heterogeneous neurodevelopmental disorder characterized by impaired social interaction and communication as well as restricted, repetitive behavior presenting in early childhood (American Psychiatric Association and DSM-5 Task Force, 2013). There is no curative treatment for ASD, but early intensive behavioral treatment can significantly improve long-term developmental outcomes (Lord and Mcgee, 2001; Estes et al., 2015; Reichow et al., 2018). However, specific measures needed to individualize treatment recommendations are lacking. Biomarkers could potentially identify clinically meaningful subgroups within highly heterogeneous populations and thus allow for more precise, individualized medical care by identifying risk, confirming diagnosis or guiding response to treatments (National Research Council, 2011; Veenstra-VanderWeele and Blakely, 2012; Insel, 2014; Interagency Autism CoordinatingCommittee [IACC], 2014; Ruggeri et al., 2014; De Los Reyes and Aldao, 2015; Varcin and Nelson, 2016). Recent authors have advocated for simultaneous measurement of multiple biomarkers to inform the understanding of the numerous systems and complex interactions that are likely to be involved in heterogeneous conditions (Hammock et al., 2012; Schendel et al., 2012; Ruggeri et al., 2014).

An extensive body of research is emerging on potential biomarkers in ASD including genetic, biochemical, proteomic, metabolomic, immune and redox markers as well as neuroimaging, electrophysiologic, physical and behavioral characteristics (Wang et al., 2011; Frustaci et al., 2012; Tordjman et al., 2013; Gabriele et al., 2014; Ruggeri et al., 2014; Varcin and Nelson, 2016).

Biochemical markers include neurotransmitters, hormones and markers of immune function and inflammation. Studies have consistently shown higher mean levels of platelet serotonin in individuals with ASD compared to controls (Schain and Freedman, 1961; Anderson et al., 1987; Cook and Leventhal, 1996; Mulder et al., 2004; Hammock et al., 2012; Gabriele et al., 2014; Pagan et al., 2014). Prior studies have also shown lower plasma levels of the pineal hormone melatonin and overnight urinary excretion of its major metabolite, melatonin sulfate, in individuals with ASD (Tordjman et al., 2005; Pagan et al., 2014). These biochemical markers can also vary with race, age, and gender (McBride et al., 1998; Duffy et al., 2011; Hammock et al., 2012). For example, elevations in platelet serotonin are particularly notable in prepubertal children with ASD (McBride et al., 1998).

A small number of studies have examined relationships between the chosen biomarkers and clinical characteristics in children with ASD. Elevated platelet serotonin levels have been associated in ASD with poorer speech development (Hranilovic et al., 2007), impaired social communication and play skills (Mulder et al., 2010), disruptive behavior (Kuperman et al., 1987), self-injury (Kolevzon et al., 2010), and higher autism severity (Abdulamir et al., 2018). Reduced urinary melatonin was associated with impaired social communication and play skills in ASD (Tordjman et al., 2012), and with higher serotonin levels (Mulder et al., 2010). Physical features such as macrocephaly, lower 2D:4D ratio and dysmorphic features are more common in individuals with ASD compared to controls and may correlate with symptom severity including lower IQ, language deficits and comorbid seizures (Courchesne et al., 1999, 2011; Manning et al., 2001; Miles et al., 2005; Sacco et al., 2007; Schaefer and Mendelsohn, 2008; Miller et al., 2010; Honekopp, 2012). Given the high rates of co-occurring conditions such as GI problems, sleep problems and seizures in ASD, studies examining the relationships of these conditions to biomarkers of interest could further inform understanding of subpopulations within the autism spectrum (Aldinger et al., 2015; Kohane, 2015).

Recently, studies have examined correlations between biomarkers or assessed more than one biomarker simultaneously (Sacco et al., 2010; Hammock et al., 2012; Schendel et al., 2012; Pagan et al., 2014; Ruggeri et al., 2014). For example, Hammock and colleagues found that oxytocin and serotonin were inversely related in individuals with ASD (Hammock et al., 2012). Pagan and colleagues examined associations of biomarkers with autism severity and clinical symptoms (e.g., melatonin with sleep disruption) and found that combined analysis of serotonin, *N*-acetylserotonin and melatonin levels in individuals differentiated individuals with autism from controls with 80% sensitivity and 85% specificity (Pagan et al., 2014). Sacco and colleagues collected information on a number of clinical traits in a study population and identified clusters of phenotypes (Sacco et al., 2010). The SEED study, a large national epidemiologic study of individuals with ASD and controls, is gathering data on multiple biomarkers and clinical characteristics (Schendel et al., 2012).

These types of studies can help elucidate potential etiologic pathways, distinguish cases from controls and identify subgroups of patients who may be phenotypically similar. One limitation of prior research, however, has been small sample sizes and participation bias. Identification of biomarkers that could be measured within the clinical setting would target large numbers of participants and potentially transform clinical care for patients with ASD (Hammock et al., 2012). Relatively few biomarkers, however, have been studied systematically in children with ASD, and the cost and feasibility of biomarker measurement varies. For example, neurophysiological biomarkers such as EEG require specialized equipment and staff training and cannot be easily completed during a regular follow-up clinic visit (Varcin and Nelson, 2016).

The clinical setting remains a relatively untapped resource for investigation of neurodevelopmental disorders including ASD for several reasons, among them differing priorities between clinical care and research, practical challenges including limited research infrastructure and cultural and attitudinal barriers in many clinical settings. Additionally, the specific core features of ASD such as sensory sensitivity and behavioral rigidity present barriers for individuals to participate in research.

To address these challenges, we conducted a multi-site demonstration project that evaluated the feasibility of integrating collection of biomarker and clinical data during ASD specialty clinic visits (Sices et al., 2017). Our primary hypotheses related to feasibility of the research model and we found that individuals with a range of developmental and behavioral functioning were able to participate and that the study activities did not interfere with clinical care. As part of the study, we collected multiple biomarkers on each participant to maximize the information collected in conjunction with a scheduled clinical visit (as opposed to a separate research visit). Our approach to assessment of correlations between biomarkers was exploratory. The chosen biomarkers, platelet serotonin and urinary melatonin sulfate, head circumference, dysmorphic status, and ratio of second and fourth digits (2D:4D), had prior evidence of association with ASD and could be measured with relative ease, efficiency and economy across multiple sites (Honekopp, 2012; Schendel et al., 2012; Teatero and Netley, 2013; Ruggeri et al., 2014; Mackus et al., 2017; Paynter et al., 2018).

This paper describes the range for platelet serotonin, urinary melatonin sulfate, head circumference, dysmorphic status and 2D:4D ratio in our clinical study population. In addition, this paper explores potential relationships among individual biomarkers, demographic features including sex, socioeconomic status (SES), and clinical features including cognitive level, behavioral function and co-morbid medical symptoms.

MATERIALS AND METHODS

Participants

We recruited participants from five academic medical centers in Massachusetts that specialize in ASD assessment and treatment. Recruitment and classification procedures have been described previously (Sices et al., 2017). This study was approved by the Institutional Review Board at the lead site (Boston Children's Hospital).

Children between 5 and 10 years old with a prior clinical diagnosis of ASD and scheduled for a regular clinic follow-up visit between April 2014–May 2015 at one of the five research sites were eligible to participate in the study. ASD diagnoses were verified by the children's clinicians, all of whom were pediatric specialists with expertise in the diagnosis and treatment of ASD (developmental behavioral pediatricians, pediatric neurologists, nurse practitioners, and child psychiatrists). Participants' ages were limited to between 5 and 10 years to improve stability of the ASD diagnosis and to increase the likelihood of pre-pubertal status, as some biomarkers vary with puberty.

Only one child per family was enrolled in the study. Exclusion criteria included having a non-English speaking caregiver or taking medication that could affect serotonin or melatonin metabolism within 2–6 weeks of the study visit (**Supplementary Table 1**). There were no exclusions for epilepsy, language impairment, level of intellectual functioning, or known genetic syndrome. Prior to conducting study activities, written informed consent was obtained from the participant's legal guardian and informed assent was elicited from children age 7 years and older, who were able.

Data/Sample Collection Measures

Parents/guardians completed a demographic and medical history form including birth history, medications, co-morbid medical symptoms, and family medical history. Parents/guardians also completed the Aberrant Behavior Checklist-Community (ABC-C), a 58-item behavioral functioning measure for children and adults with developmental disabilities that includes five subscales: irritability and agitation; lethargy and social withdrawal; stereotypic behavior; hyperactivity and non-compliance; and inappropriate speech (Aman et al., 1985). Scoring was completed using the method validated for children with ASD (Kaat et al., 2014).

Research staff reviewed medical records for each participant to identify results of the most recent cognitive testing (developmental or IQ test results). To allow for comparison amongst the various developmental and intellectual assessment measures documented across all participants, only non-verbal cognitive scores (Bayley cognitive score or non-verbal IQ) were analyzed. Study data were collected and managed using REDCap (Research Electronic Data Capture), a secure, web-based application for electronic data capture hosted at the lead site.

We estimated household income based on participant zip code as a proxy for SES. We assigned the median income reported in the 2012 U.S. Census for each participant's zip code. Zip code regions were assigned to a quintile based on the national breakdown of income distribution (Geronimus and Bound, 1998; U.S. Department of Commerce, 2013).

As a part of each participant's clinic visit, clinicians or their clinical staff obtained measurements of head circumference, height and weight. Clinicians then recorded results of a standardized dysmorphology examination (Miles et al., 2008; Sices et al., 2017). Photocopies of each participant's hands were obtained by study staff following the clinic visit to provide 2D:4D ratios using established methodology (Manning et al., 1998). Photocopies that were not clear or did not demonstrate clear markings of the digits were omitted from analysis.

A 3 mL EDTA-anticoagulated whole blood sample was obtained from each participant for platelet count and serotonin analysis. Automated platelet count measurements were performed locally at each respective study site within

24 h of collection. Aliquots of whole blood were stored at −80°C until shipment on dry ice to the Anderson research laboratory at Yale University for platelet (whole blood) serotonin measurement, using previously published methodology (Anderson et al., 1987; Epperson et al., 2001). Overnight urine sample was collected for melatonin sulfate and creatinine analyses either from a first morning void, or an overnight diaper, thus representing nighttime production of melatonin for all samples. Urine samples were similarly stored at −80°C until shipment on dry ice to the Anderson laboratory. Melatonin sulfate-like immunoreactivity was measured by ELISA kit provided by IBL International (Toronto, ON, Canada) and creatinine levels were determined by HPLC using UV absorbance detection (240 nm) following 10-fold dilution (Hausen et al., 1981).

Statistical Analysis and Considerations

Wilcoxon two-sample tests were used throughout to test for differences between groups of participants with and without a given characteristic. Spearman correlations were computed to estimate correlation between two continuous variables. Income was analyzed as a continuous variable. Race was challenging to analyze due to the small number of participants endorsing some racial categories, the number of participants selecting more than one category and the number selecting only the 'Other' category, which was not further specified. Linear regression models were used to test for effects of race and median household income on the two primary biomarker outcomes (platelet serotonin and urinary melatonin sulfate). A p-value ≤ 0.05 was used as a cut-off for statistical significance. All tests were two-sided. Due to the exploratory nature of the study, no adjustments were made for multiple comparisons (Rothman, 1990).

RESULTS

A total of 88 participants were enrolled in the study; five were subsequently excluded from data analysis resulting in an analyzable sample of 83. Of the five excluded individuals, two did not provide at least one sample for biochemical measurement (blood for platelet serotonin or urine for melatonin sulfate excretion), two were discovered to be taking medications not disclosed at time of enrollment [fluoxetine ($n = 1$) and melatonin ($n = 1$)], and one voluntarily withdrew from the study.

Group Descriptive Statistics

Demographics

Participant demographics are summarized in **Table 1**. The mean age of participants was 7.4 ± 1.6 years and 82% were male. Participants identified race and ethnicity by checking as many categories as applied. Overall, 63% endorsed White only, 7% Black only, 5% Asian only, 13% endorsed more than one racial category and 14% endorsed an "Other" category that was not further specified. Nineteen percent endorsed Hispanic ethnicity. Mean average income (estimated from zip code of residence) was $57,700 (SD 19,800), with a range from $26,944 to $121,693 across all participants (**Table 1**).

TABLE 1 | Demographics and characteristics of study participants.

Sex	***n* (%)**
Female	15 (18%)
Male	68 (82%)
Race*	***n* (%)**
Single Race	72 (87%)
American Indian/Alaskan Native	0 (0%)
Asian	4 (5%)
Black/African American	6 (7%)
Other	10 (12%)
White/Caucasian	52 (63%)
Multiple Races	11 (13%)
Black and American Indian/Alaskan	1 (1%)
Black and White	5 (6%)
White and American Indian/Alaskan	1 (1%)
White and Asian	1 (1%)
White and Black and American Indian/Alaskan	1 (1%)
White and Other	2 (2%)
Ethnicity	**n (%)**
Hispanic	16 (19%)
Non-Hispanic	66 (80%)
Unknown	1 (1%)
Age	**Mean (SD)**
Age at diagnosis (years)	3.2 (1.6)
Age at visit (years)	7.4 (1.6)
Income^	**Mean (SD), Median**
Income of participant's zip code	$57.7K ($19.8K), $55.6
Cognitive Function	**N, Mean (SD)**
Non-verbal cognitive score	50, 88 (19)
***ABC-C*# Checklist Subscale Score (n = 81)**	**Mean (SD)**
Irritability	13.5 (9.9)
Withdrawal	11.2 (7.8)
Stereotypy	5.5 (4.6)
Hyperactivity	15.3 (8.8)
Inappropriate Speech	4.7 (3.4)
Genetic Testing	**N (%)**
Had Genetic Testing Reported	58 (70%)
Known Genetic Syndrome	1 (%)
Variant of Unknown Significance	7 (%)

**Participants could endorse any applicable race; all responses tallied. #Aberrant Behavior Checklist – Community. ^Based on U.S. Census data from the 2012 Census.*

Developmental Function

ABC-C score distributions for the study group were comparable with recently published norms for children with ASD and represented a range of behavioral function (Kaat et al., 2014). Cognitive test results were available for 65 participants (78%). Mean age at cognitive testing was 5.4 years (SD = 2.2 years). Mean time elapsed from date of cognitive testing to date of biomarker sample collection was 2.3 years (SD = 1.8 years). Reported non-verbal standard scores ranged from 43 to 121 (mean = 88, SD = 19) with 14% having a non-verbal cognitive score below 70. Genetic testing results were reported for 58 patients. Of those, 1 had a genetic syndrome and 7 had a variant of unknown significance (**Table 1**).

Biomarkers

Discussion of study activity completion rates and feasibility has been previously described (Sices et al., 2017). Mean values and standard deviations as well as completion/collection rates for each of the biomarkers are shown in **Table 2**.

Biochemical Markers

The serotonin and urinary melatonin sulfate excretion measures were non-normally distributed (Shapiro–Wilk tests, all p-values < 0.001). Mean levels for platelet serotonin in our participant group were elevated from previously published norms (McBride et al., 1998) consistent with the presence of hyperserotonemia. Urinary melatonin sulfate excretion rates in our ASD participant group, however, were not lower than prior reported rates in control populations (Tordjman et al., 2005) (**Table 2**).

Age was negatively correlated with melatonin sulfate excretion ($r = -0.26$, $p = 0.048$). We did not find an age association for serotonin. Contrary to previously published results, we did not identify a negative correlation between platelet serotonin and melatonin sulfate excretion levels ($r = -0.008$, $p = 0.95$). In addition, there were no correlations between platelet serotonin and melatonin sulfate excretion levels and sex, ethnicity, non-verbal cognitive level, or ABC-C subscale scores (**Table 3**).

Due to the limited numbers of participants endorsing certain race categories we were not able to conduct comparative analyses. We examined platelet serotonin level and melatonin excretion rate by household income. The bivariate correlation of platelet serotonin and median household income was positive but did not reach statistical significance ($r = 0.20$, $p = 0.09$). In a single linear regression model testing for the effects both of race and of median household income on platelet serotonin, however, race and income were each independently associated with platelet serotonin. Household income was significantly associated with higher platelet serotonin levels in this regression with mean platelet serotonin increasing an estimated 9.8 points per $10K increase in household income ($p = 0.004$).

Melatonin sulfate and median household income were positively correlated ($r = 0.25$, $p = 0.03$) in bivariate analysis. In the linear regression model, higher median household income was associated with higher melatonin sulfate excretion levels with an estimated increase of 13.8 ng/mg creatinine per $10K increase in household income ($p = 0.04$).

TABLE 2 | Biomarker completion rates and group mean values.

Measure	*N* (%) completing measure	Mean (SD) or *N* (%) dysmorphic
Serotonin (ng/mL)	73 (88%)	236 (92)
Platelet serotonin (ng/billion platelets)	71 (86%)	822 (407)
Urinary melatonin sulfate (ng/mg creatinine)	71 (86%)	131 (78)
Head circumference (z-score)	72 (87%)	0.77 (1.19)
2D:4D right hand	63 (76%)	0.96 (0.04)
2D:4D left hand	35 (42%)	0.96 (0.04)
Dysmorphology exam	75 (90%)	6 (8%)

Physical Markers

2D:4D values were consistent with prior reports showing ratios for ASD participants below published norms (Manning et al., 2001). Head circumference values had a mean z-score 0.77 with range from −1.72 to 3.60. Twelve of the 72 participants (17%) with head circumference measurements were macrocephalic (z-score > 2SD). Dysmorphology examination was performed on 75 participants: 6 (8%) were identified as dysmorphic. Additionally, 42 of these participants (55%) had an abnormal finding in one or more body regions with the most frequently identified regions being the ear (20%), hair pattern (18%) and philtrum (16%). Dysmorphic status did not correlate with report of abnormal genetic test results. Only 3 of the 6 dysmorphic participants had cognitive testing results, scores ranged from 70 to 100 (**Table 2**).

Co-occuring Conditions

Participants had high rates of caregiver reported co-occuring medical and psychiatric conditions including: 52% with gastrointestinal (GI) conditions, 40% with sleep problems, 41% with psychiatric conditions (including 25% with ADHD and 5% with anxiety disorder), 31% with history of regression in developmental skills, and 20% with neurologic conditions (including 7% with seizures) (**Table 4**).

TABLE 3 | Biochemical markers by demographic characteristics.

Patient characteristics	Platelet serotonin (ng/billion platelets) *n*, mean (SD)	*p*-Value	Urinary melatonin sulfate excretion (ng/mg creatinine) *n*, mean (SD)	*p*-Value
Sex		0.10		0.20
Male	59, 852.5 (427.4)		58, 125.6 (77.9)	
Female	12, 671.0 (245.6)		13, 152.6 (76.1)	
Ethnicity		0.50		0.44
Hispanic	15, 732.9 (235.0)		14, 121.1 (72.2)	
Other	56, 845.6 (440.3)		56, 134.3 (79.6)	
Non-verbal IQ		0.28		0.29
Below 70	7, 1042.5 (657.2)		2, 144.0 (2.8)	
70 or above	38, 800.3 (401.4)		40, 131.5 (79.0)	

TABLE 4 | Caregiver-reported comorbid conditions.

Condition	*N* (%)
Neurodevelopmental/neurologic problems	
Premature birth	11 (13%)
History of regression	26 (31%)
Neurologic conditions	17 (20%)
Seizures	6 (7%)
Headaches	2 (2%)
Sleep problems	
Any sleep problem	33 (40%)
Difficulty going to bed	15 (18%)
Difficulty falling asleep	19 (23%)
Unusually tired/sleepy during the day	13 (16%)
Difficulty waking up	13 (16%)
Very long or frequent naps	6 (7%)
Frequent or prolonged awakenings at night	17 (20%)
Sleepwalking or frequent nightmares	5 (6%)
No regular bed time and wake time	13 (16%)
Gastrointestinal problems	
Any GI condition	43 (52%)
Constipation	35 (42%)
Diarrhea	15 (18%)
Gastro-esophageal reflux disease (GERD)	10 (12%)
Psychiatric and behavioral conditions	
Any psychiatric disorder	34 (41%)
Anxiety disorder	4 (5%)
OCD	1 (1%)
ADHD	21 (25%)
Disruptive behavior disorder	6 (7%)
Depressive disorder	1 (1%)
Mood disorder	1 (1%)
Self-injurious	3 (4%)
Pica	2 (2%)
Enuresis or encopresis	2 (2%)

Totals do not add up to 100% as some participants reported more than one condition in each category. No caregivers reported schizophrenia or psychosis.

Correlations of Biochemical Measures With Participant Characteristics

Biochemical Measures, Physical Characteristics, and Behavioral Functioning

Platelet serotonin levels and melatonin sulfate excretion were not significantly correlated with head circumference z-score, 2D:4D ratio, or dysmorphology status. There were also no associations among the physical measures (head circumference, 2D:4D, and dysmorphology status). Patients with dysmorphic status scored significantly higher than other patients on two of the ABC subscales [stereotypic behaviors: 10.0 (*SD*: 4.0) vs. 5.1 (*SD*: 4.5), $p = 0.019$; inappropriate speech 7.0 (*SD*: 2.9) vs. 4.5 (*SD*: 3.5), $p = 0.043$].

Biochemical Markers and Co-occurring Conditions

We examined correlations between both urinary melatonin sulfate excretion and platelet serotonin with co-occurring conditions including GI and neurologic problems, seizures, and sleep conditions reported by caregivers (**Table 5**). Patients with neurologic conditions ($n = 15$) had lower melatonin sulfate excretion than patients without these conditions [respectively: mean (SD): 91.4 (42.5) vs. 145.7 (81.3), $p = 0.02$]. There was no difference in mean age of participants with and without neurologic conditions ($p = 0.69$). No association was found between melatonin sulfate excretion and reported sleep problems (**Table 5**). We identified a trend toward an association between higher platelet serotonin levels and reported GI conditions (medians: 778 vs. 702, $p = 0.08$) Three participants had platelet serotonin values above 2000 ng/billion platelets (one was > 2 SD and the other two were > 3 SD above the mean); all three participants endorsed GI symptoms.

DISCUSSION

In this pilot demonstration feasibility project, collection of multiple biomarkers during a regularly scheduled ASD specialty clinical visit allowed for the examination of associations between biochemical and clinical measures, and identified several findings that suggest direction for future studies. While our findings for individual biochemical and clinical biomarkers should not be viewed as definitive, we found associations between platelet serotonin and melatonin sulfate excretion with patient demographic and clinical characteristics that illustrate the potential of this approach to generate important information about multiple biomarkers and functional domains within a single heterogeneous clinical patient population.

Consistent with prior research, we identified elevated platelet serotonin levels in our sample, with means and ranges similar to previously published data for children with ASD (McBride et al., 1998; Mulder et al., 2004; Hammock et al., 2012). In contrast to previous studies, urinary melatonin sulfate excretion rates in our ASD participant group were not lower than prior reported rates in control populations (Tordjman et al., 2005). However, the limited available data on a similar age range and using a similar analytical methodology limit comparison of the melatonin sulfate results to prior reports. The overall racial distribution and the high proportion of participants endorsing more than one race precluded analysis of biomarker levels by race. Unexpectedly, however, we found that higher income, independent of race, was associated with higher platelet serotonin and higher melatonin sulfate excretion. The reasons for this are likely complex, as income estimated by zip code was used as a proxy for SES and may reflect multiple social and environmental factors including diet. Lower melatonin sulfate excretion was associated with increasing age during childhood in our sample as has been previously reported (Tordjman et al., 2005). In contrast, we did not find an age-based variation in platelet serotonin whereas prior studies found that serotonin levels correlate negatively with age in children with ASD (McBride et al., 1998; Hammock et al., 2012). This may be explained by the narrow age range of our study. A more recent study did not find an age-based difference in serotonin when comparing individuals with ASD who were below 16 years with those at or above 16 years (Pagan et al., 2014). Additionally, although a prior

TABLE 5 | Mean and standard deviation (SD) for biochemical markers in patients with co-morbid medical conditions, and comparisons between participants endorsing and not endorsing these conditions.

Co-morbid conditions	Platelet serotonin (ng/billion platelets)		Urinary melatonin sulfate (ng/mg creatinine)	
	n, Mean (SD)	*p*-Value	*n*, Mean (SD)	*p*-Value
Gastrointestinal problem*		0.08		0.55
Yes	34, 934.3 (521.5)		36, 137.6 (86.4)	
No	37, 718.4 (222.5)		34, 120.9 (67.7)	
Neurologic problem*		0.85		0.02**
Yes	14, 858.8 (568.8)		15, 91.4 (42.5)	
No	52, 805.9 (372.5)		53, 145.7 (81.3)	
Seizures*		0.85		0.12
Yes	5, 1068.2 (955.3)		4, 81.0 (46.7)	
No	57, 798.8 (359.4)		60, 141.0 (78.5)	
Any sleep problem		0.16		0.27
Yes	27, 761.4 (395.0)		29, 111.4 (61.0)	
No	44, 858.9 (414.0)		42, 143.7 (85.7)	

*Participants endorsing "not sure" for Gastrointestinal ($N = 1$) or Neurologic problem ($N = 6$), or "suspected" or "not sure" for Seizures ($N = 10$) excluded from analysis.
**Significant at $p < 0.05$.

study showed a negative correlation between platelet serotonin and urinary melatonin (Mulder et al., 2010), the Pagan study did not find this correlation in a multi-aged (children and adults) sample of 230 patients with ASD (Pagan et al., 2014). Further studies with detailed sociodemographic variables will be needed to clarify these findings.

Frequencies of dysmorphic physical features in the study sample were similar to prior published findings for children with ASD. Dysmorphology examination identified six participants (8%) as dysmorphic using the scoring algorithm described by Miles et al. (2008). This compares to a rate of 12% reported as dysmorphic by Miles for a population of patients with autistic disorder. Of note, we did not preferentially select patients from settings that would typically have higher levels of dysmorphic features such as genetic specialty clinics. Although we did not have sufficient power to examine the relationship of dysmorphic status and cognitive functioning, dysmorphic status was correlated with higher ratings on the ABC stereotypy and inappropriate speech domains, suggesting higher symptom severity. This is consistent with prior studies documenting that patients with "syndromic autism" have more severe phenotypes (Miles et al., 2005; Schaefer and Mendelsohn, 2008).

Caregiver reported frequencies of comorbid medical and psychiatric conditions including developmental regression, sleep problems, ADHD, GI symptoms, and seizures were similar to those reported in other ASD cohorts (Richdale, 1999; Goldberg et al., 2003; Lord et al., 2004; Polimeni et al., 2005; Leyfer et al., 2006; Ibrahim et al., 2009; Buie et al., 2010; Murray, 2010; Aldinger et al., 2015). Study participants had lower levels of anxiety (5%) than previously reported (Filipek et al., 2000; Myers and Johnson, 2007; Volkmar et al., 2014), most likely explained by the study exclusion criteria that restricted participants on medications known to influence serotonin levels.

Serotonin [5-hydroxytryptamine (5-HT)] and melatonin are important in neurogenesis, synaptogenesis, mood, sleep, and GI function (Gabriele et al., 2014). Gastrointestinal symptoms were reported by 51% of participants, consistent with prior studies showing rates of GI symptoms ranging from 9 to 91% in children with ASD (Molloy and Manning-Courtney, 2003; Valicenti-McDermott et al., 2006; Ibrahim et al., 2009; Buie et al., 2010). A recent meta-analysis reported an odds ratio of 4.42 for GI problems in children with ASD (McElhanon et al., 2014). We did not identify significant associations between GI symptoms and platelet serotonin or melatonin sulfate excretion. However, we did observe a trend-level association between higher platelet serotonin and reported GI symptoms. In addition, three participants who were outliers with very high platelet serotonin (above 2000 ng/billion platelets) all reported GI symptoms. This is consistent with a recent study examining whole blood serotonin levels and co-occurring GI symptoms in 82 children age 6–15 years with ASD that identified a moderate positive correlation ($r = 0.23$, $p = 0.048$) between GI symptom score and serotonin levels in Caucasian participants (Marler et al., 2016). In addition, specific serotonin-related gene variants in individuals with ASD may contribute to gastrointestinal disturbance (Abdelrahman et al., 2014). Future studies examining serotonin levels in patients with ASD and co-occurring GI problems appear warranted.

Melatonin sulfate excretion was negatively associated with reported neurologic problems ($p = 0.02$), with much of the association due to lower levels in participants reporting diagnosed or suspected seizures. The rate of seizures (7%) was lower than that reported for other populations of children and adolescents with ASD. However, the age range of our study participants was between the two peak onset periods for seizures in ASD, early childhood and adolescence (Filipek et al., 2000; Myers and Johnson, 2007). An analysis of medical conditions in the AGRE and Simons Simplex Cohort (SSC) found similar rates of seizures (12.2 and 5.3% respectively) in two cohorts with mean age 9.2 and 9.0 years (Aldinger et al., 2015). Prior studies document lower melatonin secretion in individuals with refractory epilepsy compared to controls, and elevated melatonin levels following seizures; importantly, these studies did not examine associations with ASD (Bazil et al., 2000; Yalyn et al., 2006; Paprocka et al., 2010). Future studies examining urinary melatonin sulfate excretion levels in individuals with ASD and epilepsy would be of interest.

Variants in melatonin pathway genes have been associated with sleep onset delay (Veatch et al., 2015) and melatonin administration has been associated with improvements in sleep in children with ASD (Doyen et al., 2011; Guenole et al., 2011; Rossignol and Frye, 2011; Malow et al., 2012). Lower melatonin sulfate excretion levels were associated with reported insomnia in a population of 145 children and adults with ASD (Pagan et al., 2014). However, despite a high rate of reported sleep problems in our cohort (40%), there was no association found with melatonin sulfate excretion rates. This might be due to exclusion from study participation of individuals who were currently taking melatonin. Our rates of reported sleep problems were similar to those in unrestricted ASD populations (Sikora et al., 2012) but lower than those reported in the AGRE cohort (55.5%) and SSC (72.5%) (Aldinger et al., 2015).

Our study had several limitations. As this was a pilot demonstration study evaluating the feasibility of collecting data during specialty clinical visits, we did not have a control group. However, our primary intent was to examine whether and how individual biomarkers were inter-related within this clinical ASD population. Recruitment was solely from subspecialty tertiary care clinics. Our sample, however, was representative of the general population of individuals with ASD with regard to biomarker values and symptom severity. In addition, we view the direct integration of the research study within clinical visits as a strength that demonstrates the feasibility of the model.

The average income of our participants, as estimated by their home zip codes, is above the national average, and none of our participants were in the lowest national income quintile. However, the income ranges for participants are in line with the region surrounding all five clinical sites (U.S. Department of Commerce, 2013). We note that 11% of our participants endorsed more than one race. Given changing national demographics, it will become ever more important to consider how to best categorize and analyze data with respect to race and ethnicity.

We relied on expert clinician determination of ASD diagnosis, and parent report of behavioral function and comorbid medical and psychiatric symptoms. Cognitive data were historical, utilized a variety of measures, and were not concurrent with biomarker collection. In addition, availability of cognitive evaluation data, age at evaluation, and timing relative to this study varied across subjects (Sices et al., 2017).

Diet can affect both platelet serotonin and melatonin levels; however, dietary histories were not obtained. We also did not evaluate complete Tanner Staging or blood work to assess pubertal stage. Exclusion of individuals taking medications/supplements that could influence serotonin or melatonin levels likely reduced participation from some individuals with disruptive behavior, anxiety, and sleep problems.

The sample size, in combination with missing data for some variables, limited our power to identify smaller correlations. In the future, the use of clinical registries across multiple sites would facilitate systematic and consistent collection of data and tracking of outcomes for larger samples. Due to the exploratory nature of our study we did not correct for multiple comparisons, which increased the risk of Type I errors. Power was also impacted by the heterogeneity of the population sample. Future studies may need to look at subgroups of patients with particular symptom presentations or enriched samples to improve the ability to identify relationships.

This study examined potential correlations among biomarkers gathered during or in association with ASD specialty clinic visits. We found interesting potential correlations between biochemical markers, SES, and neurologic and GI symptoms that may be further explored in future studies. This translational research model has promise for defining subgroups of patients based on biomarker profiles and can help guide future studies on the use of biomarkers for individualized prognosis and treatment planning in individuals with complex, heterogeneous neurodevelopmental disorders such as ASD.

MEMBERS OF THE AUTISM CONSORTIUM BIOMARKERS STUDY CLINICIANS GROUP

Boston University Medical Center: Marilyn Augustyn, Stephanie Blenner, Lynn Hironaka, Jennifer Radesky, Arathi Reddy, Jayna Schumacher, Laura Sices, Robert Keder Boston Children's Hospital: Carolyn Bridgemohan, Elizabeth Harstad, April Levin, Leonard Rappaport, Alison Schonwald, Sarah Spence, Laura Weissman Center for Children With Special Needs, Floating Children's Hospital at Tufts Medical Center: A. Stacie Colwell, Carmina Erdei, Eric Goepfert, Karen J. Miller, Christina Sakai, Monica Ultmann, L. Erik Von Hahn Lurie Center for Autism, Massachusetts General Hospital for Children: Jessica Helt, Yamini J. Howe, Ann M. Neumeyer, Christine Stine University of Massachusetts Memorial Medical Center: Roula Choueiri, David M. Cochran, Jean A. Frazier, Andrew W. Zimmerman.

ETHICS STATEMENT

This study was approved by the Institutional Review Board at the lead site (Boston Children's Hospital): Assurance Identification No. FWA00002071 IRB Registration No. IRB00000352.

AUTHOR CONTRIBUTIONS

CB conceived of the study, participated in the design and coordination, analysis and interpretation of results and drafted the manuscript. DC, YH, LS, AZ, RC, SB, JF, and AN participated in the study design, coordination, analysis and interpretation of results and helped draft the manuscript. KM, MU, KP, LF, and JH participated in the coordination, analysis and interpretation of results and helped draft the manuscript. PF completed the statistical analysis, interpreted the results and helped draft the manuscript. GA participated in the design of the study, performance of biochemical measurements, interpretation of results and helped draft the manuscript. All authors read and approved the final manuscript.

FUNDING

This work was supported by grants from the Simons Foundation Autism Research Initiative (SFARI) award # 290933 to The Autism Consortium and award # 412328 to CB.

This work was conducted with support from The Harvard Catalyst Clinical and Translational Science Center (National Center for Research Resources and the National Center for Advancing Translational Sciences, National Institutes of Health Award UL1 TR001102) (NCATS grant #8UL1TR000170) and financial contributions from Harvard University and its affiliated academic healthcare centers.

ACKNOWLEDGMENTS

Simons Foundation Autism Research Initiative (SFARI); The Autism Consortium, Dierdre Phillips Executive Director; Leonard Rappaport, Sarah Spence, Marilyn Augustyn, and Mustafa Sahin for their contributions to the concept and development of the study, and for their subsequent guidance and support including critical review of the manuscript draft; Walter Kaufmann for his contribution to the concept and development of the project; William Barbaresi and the Boston Children's Hospital DMC Writer's Group for critical review of manuscript drafts; the Boston Children's Hospital Translational Neuroscience Center; and all of the families who participated in this project.

REFERENCES

Abdelrahman, H. M., Sherief, L. M., Alghobashy, A. A., Abdel Salam, S. M., Hashim, H. M., Abdel Fattah, N. R., et al. (2014). Association of 5-HT2A receptor gene polymorphisms with gastrointestinal disorders in Egyptian children with autistic disorder. *Res. Dev. Disabil.* 36C, 485–490. doi: 10.1016/j.ridd.2014.10.023

Abdulamir, H. A., Abdul-Rasheed, O. F., and Abdulghani, E. A. (2018). Serotonin and serotonin transporter levels in autistic children. *Saudi Med. J.* 39, 487–494. doi: 10.15537/smj.2018.5.21751

Aldinger, K. A., Lane, C. J., Veenstra-VanderWeele, J., and Levitt, P. (2015). Patterns of risk for multiple co-occurring medical conditions replicate across distinct cohorts of children with autism spectrum disorder. *Autism Res.* 8, 771–781. doi: 10.1002/aur.1492

Aman, M. G., Singh, N. N., Stewart, A. W., and Field, C. J. (1985). The aberrant behavior checklist: a behavior rating scale for the assessment of treatment effects. *Am. J. Ment. Defic.* 89, 485–491.

American Psychiatric Association, and DSM-5 Task Force (2013). *Diagnostic and Statistical Manual of Mental Disorders: DSM-5*. Washington, DC: American Psychiatric Association.

Anderson, G. M., Feibel, F. C., and Cohen, D. J. (1987). Determination of serotonin in whole blood, platelet-rich plasma, platelet-poor plasma and plasma ultrafiltrate. *Life Sci.* 40, 1063–1070. doi: 10.1016/0024-3205(87)90568-6

Bazil, C. W., Short, D., Crispin, D., and Zheng, W. (2000). Patients with intractable epilepsy have low melatonin, which increases following seizures. *Neurology* 55, 1746–1748. doi: 10.1212/wnl.55.11.1746

Buie, T., Fuchs, G. J. III, Furuta, G. T., Kooros, K., Levy, J., Lewis, J. D., et al. (2010). Recommendations for evaluation and treatment of common gastrointestinal problems in children with ASDs. *Pediatrics* 125(Suppl.), S19–S29. doi: 10.1542/peds.2009-1878D

Cook, E. H., and Leventhal, B. L. (1996). The serotonin system in autism. *Curr. Opin. Pediatr.* 8, 348–354. doi: 10.1097/00008480-199608000-00008

Courchesne, E., Campbell, K., and Solso, S. (2011). Brain growth across the life span in autism: age-specific changes in anatomical pathology. *Brain Res.* 1380, 138–145. doi: 10.1016/j.brainres.2010.09.101

Courchesne, E., Muller, R. A., and Saitoh, O. (1999). Brain weight in autism: normal in the majority of cases, megalencephalic in rare cases. *Neurology* 52, 1057–1059.

De Los Reyes, A., and Aldao, A. (2015). Introduction to the special issue: toward implementing physiological measures in clinical child and adolescent assessments. *J. Clin. Child Adolesc. Psychol.* 44, 221–237. doi: 10.1080/15374416.2014.891227

Doyen, C., Mighiu, D., Kaye, K., Colineaux, C., Beaumanoir, C., Mouraeff, Y., et al. (2011). Melatonin in children with autistic spectrum disorders: recent and practical data. *Eur. Child Adolesc. Psychiatry* 20, 231–239. doi: 10.1007/s00787-011-0162-168

Duffy, J. F., Cain, S. W., Chang, A.-M., Phillips, A. J. K., Munch, M. Y., Gronfier, C., et al. (2011). Sex difference in the near-24-hour intrinsic period of the human circadian timing system. *Proc. Natl. Acad. Sci. U.S.A.* 108(Suppl.), 15602–15608. doi: 10.1073/pnas.1010666108

Epperson, N., Czarkowski, K. A., Ward-O'Brien, D., Weiss, E., Gueorguieva, R., Jatlow, P., et al. (2001). Maternal sertraline treatment and serotonin transport in breast-feeding mother-infant pairs. *Am. J. Psychiatry* 158, 1631–1637. doi: 10.1176/appi.ajp.158.10.1631

Estes, A., Munson, J., Rogers, S. J., Greenson, J., Winter, J., and Dawson, G. (2015). Long-term outcomes of early intervention in 6-year-old children with autism spectrum disorder. *J. Am. Acad. Child Adolesc. Psychiatry* 54, 580–587. doi: 10.1016/j.jaac.2015.04.005

Filipek, P. A., Accardo, P. J., Ashwal, S., Baranek, G. T., Cook, E. H. J., Dawson, G., et al. (2000). Practice parameter: screening and diagnosis of autism: report of the quality standards subcommittee of the american academy of neurology and the child neurology society. *Neurology* 55, 468–479.

Frustaci, A., Neri, M., Cesario, A., Adams, J. B., Domenici, E., Dalla Bernardina, B., et al. (2012). Oxidative stress-related biomarkers in autism: systematic review and meta-analyses. *Free Radic. Biol. Med.* 52, 2128–2141. doi: 10.1016/j.freeradbiomed.2012.03.011

Gabriele, S., Sacco, R., and Persico, A. M. (2014). Blood serotonin levels in autism spectrum disorder: a systematic review and meta-analysis. *Eur. Neuropsychopharmacol.* 24, 919–929. doi: 10.1016/j.euroneuro.2014.02.004

Geronimus, A. T., and Bound, J. (1998). Use of census-based aggregate variables to proxy for socioeconomic group: evidence from national samples. *Am. J. Epidemiol.* 148, 475–486. doi: 10.1093/oxfordjournals.aje.a009673

Goldberg, W. A., Osann, K., Filipek, P. A., Laulhere, T., Jarvis, K., Modahl, C., et al. (2003). Language and other regression: assessment and timing. *J. Autism Dev. Disord.* 33, 607–616. doi: 10.1023/b:jadd.0000005998.47370.ef

Guenole, F., Godbout, R., Nicolas, A., Franco, P., Claustrat, B., and Baleyte, J.-M. (2011). Melatonin for disordered sleep in individuals with autism spectrum disorders: systematic review and discussion. *Sleep Med. Rev.* 15, 379–387. doi: 10.1016/j.smrv.2011.02.001

Hammock, E., Veenstra-VanderWeele, J., Yan, Z., Kerr, T. M., Morris, M., Anderson, G. M., et al. (2012). Examining autism spectrum disorders by biomarkers: example from the oxytocin and serotonin systems. *J. Am. Acad. Child Adolesc. Psychiatry* 51, 712–721.e1. doi: 10.1016/j.jaac.2012.04.010

Hausen, A., Fuchs, D., and Wachter, H. (1981). Determination of creatinine in urine by high performance liquid chromatography (HPLC) (author's transl). *J. Clin. Chem. Clin. Biochem.* 19, 375–378.

Honekopp, J. (2012). Digit ratio 2D:4D in relation to autism spectrum disorders, empathizing, and systemizing: a quantitative review. *Autism Res.* 5, 221–230. doi: 10.1002/aur.1230

Hranilovic, D., Bujas-Petkovic, Z., Vragovic, R., Vuk, T., Hock, K., and Jernej, B. (2007). Hyperserotonemia in adults with autistic disorder. *J. Autism Dev. Disord.* 37, 1934–1940. doi: 10.1007/s10803-006-0324-326

Ibrahim, S. H., Voigt, R. G., Katusic, S. K., Weaver, A. L., and Barbaresi, W. J. (2009). Incidence of gastrointestinal symptoms in children with autism: a population-based study. *Pediatrics* 124, 680–686. doi: 10.1542/peds.2008-2933

Insel, T. R. (2014). The NIMH research domain criteria (RDoC) project: precision medicine for psychiatry. *Am. J. Psychiatry* 171, 395–397. doi: 10.1176/appi.ajp.2014.14020138

Interagency Autism CoordinatingCommittee [IACC] (2014). IACC Strategic Plan for Autism Spectrum Disorder Research – 2013 Update. doi: 10.1176/appi.ajp.2014.14020138

Kaat, A. J., Lecavalier, L., and Aman, M. G. (2014). Validity of the aberrant behavior checklist in children with autism spectrum disorder. *J. Autism Dev. Disord.* 44, 1103–1116. doi: 10.1007/s10803-013-1970-1970

Kohane, I. S. (2015). An autism case history to review the systematic analysis of large-scale data to refine the diagnosis and treatment of neuropsychiatric disorders. *Biol. Psychiatry* 77, 59–65. doi: 10.1016/j.biopsych.2014.05.024

Kolevzon, A., Newcorn, J. H., Kryzak, L., Chaplin, W., Watner, D., Hollander, E., et al. (2010). Relationship between whole blood serotonin and repetitive behaviors in autism. *Psychiatry Res.* 175, 274–276. doi: 10.1016/j.psychres.2009.02.008

Kuperman, S., Beeghly, J., Burns, T., and Tsai, L. (1987). Association of serotonin concentration to behavior and IQ in autistic children. *J. Autism Dev. Disord.* 17, 133–140. doi: 10.1007/bf01487265

Leyfer, O. T., Folstein, S. E., Bacalman, S., Davis, N. O., Dinh, E., Morgan, J., et al. (2006). Comorbid psychiatric disorders in children with autism: interview development and rates of disorders. *J. Autism Dev. Disord.* 36, 849–861. doi: 10.1007/s10803-006-0123-120

Lord, A. C., and Mcgee, J. P. (2001). "National academy of sciences committee on educational interventions for children with autism," in *Educating Children with Autism*, eds J. P. McGee and C. Lord (Washington, DC: National Academy Press), 211–229.

Lord, C., Shulman, C., and DiLavore, P. (2004). Regression and word loss in autistic spectrum disorders. *J. Child Psychol. Psychiatry* 45, 936–955. doi: 10.1111/j.1469-7610.2004.t01-1-00287.x

Mackus, M., de Kruijff, D., Otten, L. S., Kraneveld, A. D., Garssen, J., and Verster, J. C. (2017). The 2D: 4D digit ratio as a biomarker for autism spectrum disorder. *Autism Res. Treat.* 2017:1048302. doi: 10.1155/2017/1048302

Malow, B., Adkins, K. W., McGrew, S. G., Wang, L., Goldman, S. E., Fawkes, D., et al. (2012). Melatonin for sleep in children with autism: a controlled trial examining dose, tolerability, and outcomes. *J. Autism Dev. Disord.* 42, 1729–1737. doi: 10.1007/s10803-011-1418-1413

Manning, J. T., Baron-Cohen, S., Wheelwright, S., and Sanders, G. (2001). The 2nd to 4th digit ratio and autism. *Dev. Med. Child Neurol.* 43, 160–164. doi: 10.1111/j.1469-8749.2001.tb00181.x

Manning, J. T., Scutt, D., Wilson, J., and Lewis-Jones, D. I. (1998). The ratio of 2nd to 4th digit length: a predictor of sperm numbers and concentrations of testosterone, luteinizing hormone and oestrogen. *Hum. Reprod.* 13, 3000–3004. doi: 10.1093/humrep/13.11.3000

Marler, S., Ferguson, B. J., Lee, E. B., Peters, B., Williams, K. C., McDonnell, E., et al. (2016). Brief report: whole blood serotonin levels and gastrointestinal symptoms in autism spectrum disorder. *J. Autism Dev. Disord.* 46, 1124–1130. doi: 10.1007/s10803-015-2646-2648

McBride, P. A., Anderson, G. M., Hertzig, M. E., Snow, M. E., Thompson, S. M., Khait, V. D., et al. (1998). Effects of diagnosis, race, and puberty on platelet serotonin levels in autism and mental retardation. *J. Am. Acad. Child Adolesc. Psychiatry* 37, 767–776. doi: 10.1097/00004583-199807000-199807017

McElhanon, B. O., McCracken, C., Karpen, S., and Sharp, W. G. (2014). Gastrointestinal symptoms in autism spectrum disorder: a meta-analysis. *Pediatrics* 133, 872–883. doi: 10.1542/peds.2013-3995

Miles, J. H., Takahashi, T. N., Bagby, S., Sahota, P. K., Vaslow, D. F., Wang, C. H., et al. (2005). Essential versus complex autism: definition of fundamental prognostic subtypes. *Am. J. Med. Genet. A* 135, 171–180. doi: 10.1002/ajmg.a.30590

Miles, J. H., Takahashi, T. N., Hong, J., Munden, N., Flournoy, N., Braddock, S. R., et al. (2008). Development and validation of a measure of dysmorphology: useful for autism subgroup classification. *Am. J. Med. Genet. A* 146A, 1101–1116. doi: 10.1002/ajmg.a.32244

Miller, D. T., Adam, M. P., Aradhya, S., Biesecker, L. G., Brothman, A. R., Carter, N. P., et al. (2010). Consensus statement: chromosomal microarray is a first-tier clinical diagnostic test for individuals with developmental disabilities or congenital anomalies. *Am. J. Hum. Genet.* 86, 749–764. doi: 10.1016/j.ajhg.2010.04.006

Molloy, C. A., and Manning-Courtney, P. (2003). Prevalence of chronic gastrointestinal symptoms in children with autism and autistic spectrum disorders. *Autism* 7, 165–171. doi: 10.1177/1362361303007002004

Mulder, E. J., Anderson, G. M., Kema, I. P., de Bildt, A., van Lang, N. D. J., den Boer, J. A., et al. (2004). Platelet serotonin levels in pervasive developmental disorders and mental retardation: diagnostic group differences, within-group distribution, and behavioral correlates. *J. Am. Acad. Child Adolesc. Psychiatry* 43, 491–499. doi: 10.1097/00004583-200404000-200404016

Mulder, E. J., Anderson, G. M., Kemperman, R. F. J., Oosterloo-Duinkerken, A., Minderaa, R. B., and Kema, I. P. (2010). Urinary excretion of 5-hydroxyindoleacetic acid, serotonin and 6-sulphatoxymelatonin in normoserotonemic and hyperserotonemic autistic individuals. *Neuropsychobiology* 61, 27–32. doi: 10.1159/000258640

Murray, M. J. (2010). Attention-deficit/hyperactivity disorder in the context of autism spectrum disorders. *Curr. Psychiatry Rep.* 12, 382–388. doi: 10.1007/s11920-010-0145-143

Myers, S. M., and Johnson, C. P. (2007). Management of children with autism spectrum disorders. *Pediatrics* 120, 1162–1182. doi: 10.1542/peds.2007-2362

National Research Council (2011). *Toward Precision Medicine: Building a Knowledge Network for Biomedical Research and a New Taxonomy of Disease.* Washington, DC: The National Academies Press, doi: 10.17226/13284

Pagan, C., Delorme, R., Callebert, J., Goubran-Botros, H., Amsellem, F., Drouot, X., et al. (2014). The serotonin-N-acetylserotonin-melatonin pathway as a biomarker for autism spectrum disorders. *Transl. Psychiatry* 4:e479. doi: 10.1038/tp.2014.120

Paprocka, J., Dec, R., Jamroz, E., and Marszal, E. (2010). Melatonin and childhood refractory epilepsy–a pilot study. *Med. Sci. Monit.* 16, CR389–CR396.

Paynter, J., Sulek, R., Luskin-Saxby, S., Trembath, D., and Keen, D. (2018). Allied health professionals' knowledge and use of ASD intervention practices. *J. Autism Dev. Disord.* 48, 2335–2349. doi: 10.1007/s10803-018-3505-3501

Polimeni, M. A., Richdale, A. L., and Francis, A. J. P. (2005). A survey of sleep problems in autism, Asperger's disorder and typically developing children. *J. Intellect. Disabil. Res.* 49, 260–268. doi: 10.1111/j.1365-2788.2005.00642.x

Reichow, B., Hume, K., Barton, E. E., and Boyd, B. A. (2018). Early intensive behavioral intervention (EIBI) for young children with autism spectrum disorders (ASD). *Cochrane Database Syst. Rev.* 5:CD009260. doi: 10.1002/14651858.CD009260.pub3

Richdale, A. L. (1999). Sleep problems in autism: prevalence, cause, and intervention. *Dev. Med. Child Neurol.* 41, 60–66. doi: 10.1111/j.1469-8749.1999.tb00012.x

Rossignol, D. A., and Frye, R. E. (2011). Melatonin in autism spectrum disorders: a systematic review and meta-analysis. *Dev. Med. Child Neurol.* 53, 783–792. doi: 10.1111/j.1469-8749.2011.03980.x

Rothman, K. J. (1990). No adjustments are needed for multiple comparisons. *Epidemiology* 1, 43–46. doi: 10.1097/00001648-199001000-00010

Ruggeri, B., Sarkans, U., Schumann, G., and Persico, A. M. (2014). Biomarkers in autism spectrum disorder: the old and the new. *Psychopharmacology* 231, 1201–1216. doi: 10.1007/s00213-013-3290-3297

Sacco, R., Curatolo, P., Manzi, B., Militerni, R., Bravaccio, C., Frolli, A., et al. (2010). Principal pathogenetic components and biological endophenotypes in autism spectrum disorders. *Autism Res.* 3, 237–252. doi: 10.1002/aur.151

Sacco, R., Militerni, R., Frolli, A., Bravaccio, C., Gritti, A., Elia, M., et al. (2007). Clinical, morphological, and biochemical correlates of head circumference in autism. *Biol. Psychiatry* 62, 1038–1047. doi: 10.1016/j.biopsych.2007.04.039

Schaefer, G. B., and Mendelsohn, N. J. (2008). Clinical genetics evaluation in identifying the etiology of autism spectrum disorders. *Genet. Med.* 10, 301–305. doi: 10.1097/GIM.0b013e31816b5cc9

Schain, R. J., and Freedman, D. X. (1961). Studies on 5-hydroxyindole metabolism in autistic and other mentally retarded children. *J. Pediatr.* 58, 315–320. doi: 10.1016/s0022-3476(61)80261-8

Schendel, D. E., Diguiseppi, C., Croen, L. A., Fallin, M. D., Reed, P. L., Schieve, L. A., et al. (2012). The study to explore early development (SEED): a multisite epidemiologic study of autism by the centers for autism and developmental disabilities research and epidemiology (CADDRE) network. *J. Autism Dev. Disord.* 42, 2121–2140. doi: 10.1007/s10803-012-1461-1468

Sices, L., Pawlowski, K., Farfel, L., Phillips, D., Howe, Y., Cochran, D. M., et al. (2017). Feasibility of conducting autism biomarker research in the clinical setting. *J. Dev. Behav. Pediatr.* 38, 483–492. doi: 10.1097/DBP.0000000000000470

Sikora, D. M., Johnson, K., Clemons, T., and Katz, T. (2012). The relationship between sleep problems and daytime behavior in children of different ages with autism spectrum disorders. *Pediatrics* 130(Suppl.), S83–S90. doi: 10.1542/peds.2012-0900F

Teatero, M. L., and Netley, C. (2013). A critical review of the research on the extreme male brain theory and digit ratio (2D:4D). *J. Autism Dev. Disord.* 43, 2664–2676. doi: 10.1007/s10803-013-1819-1816

Tordjman, S., Anderson, G. M., Bellissant, E., Botbol, M., Charbuy, H., Camus, F., et al. (2012). Day and nighttime excretion of 6-sulphatoxymelatonin in adolescents and young adults with autistic disorder. *Psychoneuroendocrinology* 37, 1990–1997. doi: 10.1016/j.psyneuen.2012.04.013

Tordjman, S., Anderson, G. M., Pichard, N., Charbuy, H., and Touitou, Y. (2005). Nocturnal excretion of 6-sulphatoxymelatonin in children and adolescents with autistic disorder. *Biol. Psychiatry* 57, 134–138. doi: 10.1016/j.biopsych.2004.11.003

Tordjman, S., Najjar, I., Bellissant, E., Anderson, G. M., Barburoth, M., Cohen, D., et al. (2013). Advances in the research of melatonin in autism spectrum disorders: literature review and new perspectives. *Int. J. Mol. Sci.* 14, 20508–20542. doi: 10.3390/ijms141020508

U.S. Department of Commerce (2013). *US Census Bureau Income Current Population Survey*. Available at: http://www.census.gov/hhes/www/cpstables/032013/hhinc/toc.htm (accessed March 31, 2016)

Valicenti-McDermott, M., McVicar, K., Rapin, I., Wershil, B. K., Cohen, H., and Shinnar, S. (2006). Frequency of gastrointestinal symptoms in children with autistic spectrum disorders and association with family history of autoimmune disease. *J. Dev. Behav. Pediatr.* 27, S128–S136.

Varcin, K. J., and Nelson, C. A. III (2016). A developmental neuroscience approach to the search for biomarkers in autism spectrum disorder. *Curr. Opin. Neurol.* 29, 123–129. doi: 10.1097/WCO.0000000000000298

Veatch, O. J., Pendergast, J. S., Allen, M. J., Leu, R. M., Johnson, C. H., Elsea, S. H., et al. (2015). Genetic variation in melatonin pathway enzymes in children with autism spectrum disorder and comorbid sleep onset delay. *J. Autism Dev. Disord.* 45, 100–110. doi: 10.1007/s10803-014-2197-2194

Veenstra-VanderWeele, J., and Blakely, R. D. (2012). Networking in autism: leveraging genetic, biomarker and model system findings in the search for new treatments. *Neuropsychopharmacology* 37, 196–212. doi: 10.1038/npp.2011.185

Volkmar, F., Siegel, M., Woodbury-Smith, M., King, B., McCracken, J., and State, M. (2014). Practice parameter for the assessment and treatment of children and adolescents with autism spectrum disorder. *J. Am. Acad. Child Adolesc. Psychiatry* 53, 237–257. doi: 10.1016/j.jaac.2013.10.013

Wang, L., Angley, M. T., Gerber, J. P., and Sorich, M. J. (2011). A review of candidate urinary biomarkers for autism spectrum disorder. *Biomarkers* 16, 537–552. doi: 10.3109/1354750X.2011.598564

Yalyn, O., Arman, F., Erdogan, F., and Kula, M. (2006). A comparison of the circadian rhythms and the levels of melatonin in patients with diurnal and nocturnal complex partial seizures. *Epilepsy Behav.* 8, 542–546. doi: 10.1016/j.yebeh.2005.12.015

14

Reproducibility of Structural and Diffusion Tensor Imaging in the TACERN Multi-Center Study

Anna K. Prohl[1], Benoit Scherrer[1], Xavier Tomas-Fernandez[1], Rajna Filip-Dhima[2], Kush Kapur[2], Clemente Velasco-Annis[1], Sean Clancy[1], Erin Carmody[2], Meghan Dean[2], Molly Valle[2], Sanjay P. Prabhu[3], Jurriaan M. Peters[1,2], E. Martina Bebin[4], Darcy A. Krueger[5], Hope Northrup[6], Joyce Y. Wu[7], Mustafa Sahin[2,8], and Simon K. Warfield[1] on behalf of the TACERN Study Group*

[1] Computational Radiology Laboratory, Department of Radiology, Boston Children's Hospital, Harvard Medical School, Harvard University, Boston, MA, United States, [2] Department of Neurology, Boston Children's Hospital, Harvard Medical School, Harvard University, Boston, MA, United States, [3] Division of Neuroradiology, Department of Radiology, Boston Children's Hospital, Harvard Medical School, Harvard University, Boston, MA, United States, [4] Department of Neurology, University of Alabama at Birmingham, Birmingham, AL, United States, [5] Department of Neurology and Rehabilitation Medicine, Cincinnati Children's Hospital Medical Center, Cincinnati, OH, United States, [6] Department of Pediatrics, McGovern Medical School, University of Texas Health Science Center at Houston, Houston, TX, United States, [7] Division of Pediatric Neurology, UCLA Mattel Children's Hospital, David Geffen School of Medicine, University of California, Los Angeles, Los Angeles, CA, United States, [8] F.M. Kirby Neurobiology Center, Boston Children's Hospital, Harvard Medical School, Harvard University, Boston, MA, United States

***Correspondence:**
Simon K. Warfield
simon.warfield@childrens.harvard.edu

Background: Multi-site MRI studies are often necessary for recruiting sufficiently sized samples when studying rare conditions. However, they require pooling data from multiple scanners into a single data set, and therefore it is critical to evaluate the variability of quantitative MRI measures within and across scanners used in multi-site studies. The aim of this study was to evaluate the reproducibility of structural and diffusion weighted (DW) MRI measurements acquired on seven scanners at five medical centers as part of the Tuberous Sclerosis Complex Autism Center of Excellence Research Network (TACERN) multisite study.

Methods: The American College of Radiology (ACR) phantom was imaged monthly to measure reproducibility of signal intensity and uniformity within and across seven 3T scanners from General Electric, Philips, and Siemens vendors. One healthy adult male volunteer was imaged repeatedly on all seven scanners under the TACERN structural and DW protocol (5 b = 0 s/mm^2 and 30 b = 1000 s/mm^2) over a period of 5 years (age 22–27 years). Reproducibility of inter- and intra-scanner brain segmentation volumes and diffusion tensor imaging metrics fractional anisotropy (FA) and mean diffusivity (MD) within white matter regions was quantified with coefficient of variation.

Results: The American College of Radiology Phantom signal intensity and uniformity were similar across scanners and changed little over time, with a mean intra-scanner coefficient of variation of 3.6 and 1.8%, respectively. The mean inter- and intra-scanner coefficients of variation of brain structure volumes derived from T1-weighted (T1w) images of the human phantom were 3.3 and 1.1%, respectively. The mean inter- and intra-scanner coefficients of variation of FA in white matter regions were 4.5 and 2.5%, while the mean inter- and intra-scanner coefficients of variation of MD in white matter regions were 5.4 and 1.5%.

Conclusion: Our results suggest that volumetric and diffusion tensor imaging (DTI) measurements are highly reproducible between and within scanners and provide typical variation amplitudes that can be used as references to interpret future findings in the TACERN network.

Keywords: MRI, quality assurance, reproducibility, multicenter study, brain, ACR, phantom

INTRODUCTION

The Tuberous Sclerosis Complex Autism Center of Excellence Research Network study is a multi-center study examining neurodevelopment in infants with TSC, a rare genetic disorder associated with a high incidence (26–50%) of ASD (Jeste et al., 2008, 2014; Capal et al., 2017). One of the goals of TACERN is to acquire prospective, longitudinal structural and diffusion weighted (DW), MRI of TSC infants over the first 3 years of life, and implement advanced quantitative neuroimaging techniques to detect MRI biomarkers that predict development of ASD (Davis et al., 2017). Specifically, TACERN seeks to characterize the development of brain morphometry from structural MRI and white matter connectivity from DTI, and evaluate the relationship of these quantitative MRI measures with ASD outcome in TSC patients.

Although multi-center studies aid in recruitment of sufficiently sized samples of patients with rare conditions like TSC from diverse geographies, they also require rigorous quality control to minimize site-related bias. Multi-center, longitudinal MRI studies use multiple scanners, potentially from different vendors, and use different software to characterize deviations in quantitative MRI measures that may be associated with disease. To reliably detect disease-related changes in quantitative MRI measures, it is critical to harmonize MRI protocols across sites, adhere to strict quality control procedures, and to measure variation in MR images that may arise due to scanner-related sources of noise, and artifact (Pagani et al., 2010). Sources of variability in MR images include, but are not limited to: partial volume averaging, variations in signal intensity arising from spatially varying coil sensitivity profiles and B_1 transmit field inhomogeneity, table vibration, thermal noise in the coils and subject that create stochastic variability in the image pixels, and geometric distortion resulting from B_0 inhomogeneity, and gradient non-linearity (Morelli et al., 2011). The normal amplitude of hardware-induced variations in MR images can be detected and quantified using phantoms, and can be used to remove the effect of system variability from quantitative MRI measures of subjects (Keenan et al., 2018).

The American College of Radiology accreditation program has developed a designated MR protocol and phantom designed to facilitate scanner quality control. The ACR phantom is a short, hollow acrylic plastic cylinder of standard dimensions, filled with nickel chloride, and sodium chloride. Structures within the phantom allow for measurements of image quality, including SNR and image intensity uniformity (American College of Radiology, 2018). Previous reports indicate that frequent, repeat imaging of the ACR phantom is an effective method for monitoring and evaluating image quality, and is useful in multisite studies (Chen et al., 2004; Ihalainen et al., 2011; Davids et al., 2014).

However, the ACR phantom does not accurately reproduce all properties of *in-vivo* tissue, such as its microscopic diffusion properties. The lack of a validated phantom for DWI with FA and MD similar to those seen in humans makes the accurate assessment of DWI reproducibility across scanners challenging. The best alternative to date is to scan a living human phantom on each scanner. Repeated imaging of the same human on all study scanners has successfully characterized the normal physical and physiological variability in numerous multi-center studies (Vollmar et al., 2010; Fox et al., 2012; Zhu et al., 2012; Grech-Sollars et al., 2015; Palacios et al., 2017; Duchesne et al., 2019).

The goal of this work was to determine the reproducibility of MRI structural and diffusion data acquired on seven scanners over 5 years as part of the TACERN study. Monthly ACR phantom imaging was performed to measure variation in signal intensity and uniformity within and across scanners. A single healthy volunteer was also imaged on each scanner under the TACERN imaging protocol when possible with a goal of every six months at each site for a total of 26 scans. We analyzed all images using the same processing pipeline which included a fully automatic computation of the volume of brain structures and DTI parameters within 17 white matter regions. In order to assess the reproducibility, we calculated the coefficient of variation (CV) for ACR phantom intensity measures and the human phantom volumetric and DTI measures. Our results indicate good reproducibility of quantitative MRI measures across and within scanners and will inform future interpretation of MRI findings in the TACERN network.

Abbreviations: ACR, American College of Radiology; ASD, autism spectrum disorders; BCH, Boston Children's Hospital; CCHMC, Cincinnati Children's Hospital Medical Center; CUSP, cube and sphere; CV, coefficient of variation; DTI, diffusion tensor imaging; DWI, diffusion weighted imaging; FA, fractional anisotropy; FOV, field of view; GE, General Electric; ICC, intracranial cavity; IU, integral uniformity; MD, mean diffusivity; MRI, magnetic resonance imaging; PSTAPLE, probabilistic simultaneous truth and performance level estimation; ROI, region of interest; SD, standard deviation; SNR, signal to noise ratio; T1w, T1-weighted; T2w, T2-weighted; TACERN, Tuberous Sclerosis Complex Autism Center of Excellence Research Network; TE, echo time; TR, repetition time; TSC, tuberous sclerosis complex; UAB, University of Alabama; UCLA, University of California Los Angeles; UTH, University of Texas Houston.

MATERIALS AND METHODS

Study Design and Sample

This study was performed to measure the variability of quantitative structural and DW brain MRI measurements across multiple scanners used in the TACERN study, an ongoing, prospective, longitudinal, multi-site study investigating MRI biomarkers of ASD in infants with TSC. TACERN sites include BCH, CCHMC, UAB, UCLA, and McGovern Medical School at University of Texas Health Science Center (UTH).

Image quality was evaluated with two methods: (1) The ACR phantom was imaged monthly under the standardized ACR phantom protocol to evaluate the stability of MR signal intensity and uniformity over the study period. (2) A healthy adult male volunteer was imaged under the TACERN MRI protocol on every study scanner over a period of 5 years (age 22–27 years) to evaluate the variability of quantitative MRI measurements that will be made in the TSC cohort. The human phantom was scanned every 6 months at each site, when possible. At each bi-annual scan session, scan-rescan, or back-to-back imaging of the volunteer under identical TACERN protocols with a brief exit and re-entry of the scanner between scan sessions, was achieved when possible, given the scheduling demands of the clinical scanners used in this study. Scan-rescan is valuable because it reduces the magnitude of anatomical changes that may occur with time in the subject and narrows the sources of measurement variability to those associated with the scanner and subject repositioning (Wei et al., 2004; Velasco-Annis et al., 2018). Each human phantom scan was analyzed with the fully automated TACERN MRI analysis pipeline, that includes a whole brain labeling and volumetric analysis of cortical, subcortical, cerebellar, white matter, and ventricular brain structures. The pipeline also includes a DTI analysis, which computes the single tensor field and labels regions of white matter for tract selection (pipeline described below). Brain structure volumes and white matter DTI metrics were compared across scans acquired on the same scanner (intra-scanner) and across all scanners (inter-scanner) to evaluate the reproducibility of quantitative MRI measurements. All study procedures were approved by the Institutional Review Board at each site, and the human phantom provided written informed consent.

MRI Acquisition

MRI scans were acquired at 3T on seven scanners and five scanner models, including one GE Signa HDxt, one Philips Achieva, two Philips Ingenia, one Siemens Skyra and two Siemens TrioTim scanners with 32, 12, and 8 channel head coils. Software upgrades occurred on two of the seven scanners during the course of the study (**Table 1**). Scanner B replaced scanner A at BCH after 3.7 years of research use and scanner E replaced scanner D at CCHMC after 1.5 years of research use.

Monthly ACR Phantom scans were acquired on all study scanners under the standardized ACR phantom MRI protocol, which includes an axial T1w fast spin echo (matrix = 256 × 256, FOV = 250 mm, number of slices = 11, slice thickness = 5.0 mm, slice gap = 5.0 mm, resolution = 1.0 mm^3 × 1.0 mm^3 × 10.0 mm^3, TR = 500 ms, TE = 20 ms, and Flip angle = 90 deg) and axial T2w fast spin echo (geometry matched to ACR T1w, TR = 2000 ms, TE = 20, and 80 ms).

Human phantom scans were performed awake or in natural sleep under the TACERN consensus clinical imaging protocol that includes high resolution, routine clinical imaging sequences used for annual surveillance imaging of TSC patients, plus additional multi *b*-value DW research sequences. Imaging protocols were harmonized to the extent permitted by each platform. Acquisition parameters used on each scanner are detailed in **Table 1**. The protocol includes a 1.0 mm^3 × 1.0 mm^3 × 1.0 mm^3 sagittal T1w image, 0.4 mm^2 × 0.4 mm^2 in-plane resolution axial T2w image, 30 high angular resolution b = 1000 s/mm^2, and 6 b = 0 s/mm^2 DW images at 1.7 mm^2 × 1.7 mm^2 in-plane resolution and 2.0 mm slice thickness. One b = 0 s/mm^2 DWI was acquired with reversed phase-encoding direction for distortion compensation, covering the entire brain.

Quality Assurance

MRI data were transmitted to and evaluated at the Computational Radiology Lab at BCH. MRI metadata were reviewed for protocol compliance. Scans that did not adhere to study protocols were excluded (15 ACR, 0 human phantom). Images were reviewed by an expert rater for extent of brain coverage and artifacts resulting from a variety of sources, including but not limited to subject motion, flow, radiofrequency leak, table vibration, magnetic susceptibility, and venetian blind artifact. Artifacts were not found in ACR T1w images or human phantom T1w, T2w, or DW images.

ACR MRI Processing

All MRI processing and analyses were completed using the Computational Radiology Kit[1]. ACR phantom processing was completed using a fully automated processing pipeline. Each ACR phantom T1w image was aligned to a common reference ACR T1w image using rigid registration with mutual information metric. Regions of interest (ROI) were drawn on the common ACR T1w reference, as defined by the ACR Phantom Guide, and were used to measure SNR and IU (**Figure 1**; American College of Radiology, 2018).

A signal ROI was drawn on axial slices 6 through 10 in a uniform, high signal region of the template ACR phantom (volume = 21028 mm^3, area/slice = 400 mm^2). A background ROI was drawn on axial slices 2 through 10 (volume = 18024 mm^3, area/slice = 182 mm^2) in the background adjacent to the ACR phantom. The SNR was calculated using the mean of the signal ROI, $\bar{x}_{Signal}$, and the SD of the background ROI, $\sigma_{Background}$, as follows:

$$SNR = \frac{\bar{x}_{Signal}}{\sigma_{Background}}$$

Integral uniformity was measured in a large, circular uniform region on slice 7 of the template ACR phantom

[1] http://crl.med.harvard.edu

TABLE 1 | Clinical T1, T2, and Diffusion-weighted MR protocols for the TACERN study.

	BCH		UCLA	CCHMC		UAB	UTH
ScannerID	A	B	C	D	E	F	G
Field strength (T)	3	3	3	3	3	3	3
Manufacturer	Siemens	Siemens	Siemens	Philips	Philips	Philips	General Electric
Model	TrioTim	Skyra	TrioTim	Achieva	Ingenia	Ingenia	Signa HDxt
Software versions	syngoMRB17	syngoMRE11	syngoMRB17	3.2.1	5.1.9; 5.3.0	4.1.3; 5.1.7; and 5.3.0	HD 16
Number of head coil channels	32	32	12	32	32	32	8
T1-weighted							
Orientation	sagittal	sagittal	sagittal	sagittal	sagittal	sagittal	sagittal
Field of view (mm)	256 × 256	224 × 224	256 × 256	220 × 220	220 × 220	220 × 220	220 × 220
Matrix	256 × 256	256 × 256	256 × 256	224 × 224	224 × 224	224 × 224	256 × 256
Number of slices	176	192	176	176	176	176	172
Resolution (mm)	1.0 × 1.0 × 1.0	0.9 × 0.9 × 0.9	1.0 × 1.0 × 1.0	1.0 × 1.0 × 1.0	0.9 × 0.9 × 1.0	1.0 × 1.0 × 1.0	0.9 × 0.9 × 1.0
Repetition time (ms)	8	8	8	8	8	8	6
Echo time (ms)	4	2	4	4	4	4	3
Bandwidth (Hz/Px)	199	200	199	191	191	191	244
Inversion time (ms)	1100	1100	1100	1100	1100	1100	1100
Flip angle (deg)	7	7	7	7	7	7	7
Number of averages	1	1	1	1	1	1	1
T2-weighted							
Orientation	axial	axial	axial	axial	axial	axial	axial
Field of view (mm)	159 × 200	162 × 200	159 × 200	200 × 200	200 × 200	200 × 200	200 × 200
Matrix	408 × 512	364 × 448	408 × 512	512 × 512	512 × 512	512 × 512	512 × 512
Number of slices	76	90	76	76	76	76	76
Resolution (mm)	0.4 × 0.4 × 2.0	0.4 × 0.4 × 2.0	0.4 × 0.4 × 2.0	0.4 × 0.4 × 2.0	0.4 × 0.4 × 2.0	0.4 × 0.4 × 2.0	0.4 x 0.4 × 2.0
Repetition time (ms)	14850	10900	14850	9366	7182	10300	15000
Echo time (ms)	79	82	79	79	79	79	76
Bandwidth (Hz/Px)	208	225	208	196	200	196	244
Flip angle (deg)	90	90	90	90	90	90	90
Number of averages	2	2	2	2	2	2	2
Diffusion-weighted							
Orientation	axial	axial	axial	axial	axial	axial	axial
Field of view (mm)	220 × 220	220 × 220	220 × 220	220 × 220	220 × 220	220 × 220	220 × 220
Matrix	128 × 128	128 × 128	128 × 128	128 × 128	128 × 128	128 × 128	256 × 256
Number of slices	74	74	74	68	72	72	48
Resolution (mm)	1.7 × 1.7 × 2.0	1.7 × 1.7 × 2.0	1.7 × 1.7 × 2.0	1.7 × 1.7 × 2.0	1.7 × 1.7 × 2.0	1.7 × 1.7 × 2.0	0.9 × 0.9 × 2.0
Repetition time (ms)	6448	6800	10900	10400	11300	15000	12700
Echo time (ms)	88	94	88	64	98	78	87
Bandwidth (Hz/Px)	1395	1500	1395	2378	1144	1276	1953
Flip Angle (deg)	90	90	90	90	90	90	90
Number of averages	1	1	1	1	1	1	1
b-values (number of directions)	0 (13)	0 (13)	0 (15)	0 (3)	0 (18)	0 (24)	0 (15)
	400 (6)	400 (6)	–	–	400 (6)	–	–
	600 (6)	600 (6)	–	–	600 (6)	–	–
	800 (6)	800 (6)	–	–	800 (6)	–	–
	1000 (30)	1000 (30)	1000 (30)	1000 (30)	1000 (30)	1000 (30)	1000 (30)
	1050–1850 (20)	1050–1850 (20)	1050–1850 (20)	1050–1850 (20)	1050–1850 (20)	1050–1850 (20)	–
	2000 (6)	2000 (6)	2000 (6)	2000 (6)	2000 (6)	2000 (6)	–
	–	–	2500 (30)	2500 (30)	2500 (30)	2500 (30)	2500 (30)
	3000 (4)	3000 (4)	3000 (4)	3000 (4)	3000 (4)	3000 (4)	3000 (31)

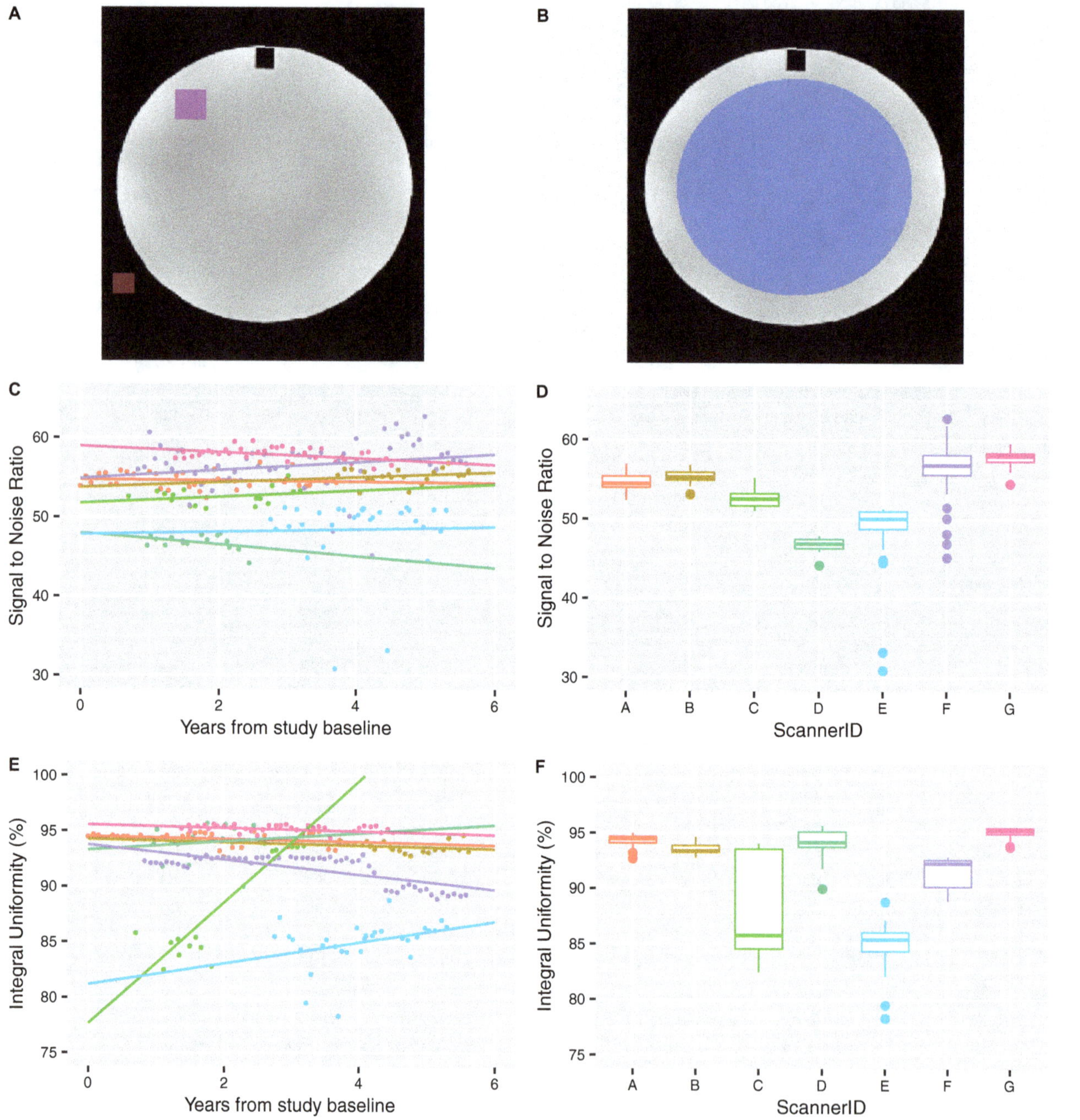

FIGURE 1 | (A) A signal ROI (purple) and a background ROI (red) are used to calculate the SNR in the ACR phantom T1w image. **(B)** A large, circular ROI (blue) overlaid on an ideally uniform region of the ACR phantom T1w image is used to measure percent IU. **(C)** Plot of SNR over time and **(D)** by scanner for ACR phantom T1w image. **(E)** Plot of percent IU over time and **(F)** by scanner for ACR phantom T1w image.

(volume = 1746687 mm^3; area = 174669 cm^2) (**Figure 1**). Voxels within the ROI were ordered from low to high intensity, and the image intensities of the 5th (low) and 95th (high) percentile voxels were identified and used to calculate IU as described in (Fu et al., 2006):

$$IU = 100 \times \left(1 - \left[\frac{high - low}{high + low}\right]\right)$$

Human Phantom Structural MRI Processing

All MRI processing and analyses were completed using the Computational Radiology Kit (see text footnote 1). Human phantom processing was completed using a fully automated processing pipeline. In the native space of each human phantom scan, the T2w image was aligned and resampled to the 1.0 mm$^3\times$ 1.0 mm^3 $\times$ 1.0 mm^3 T1w image using rigid registration with mutual information metric. The ICC was then segmented using a previously validated multispectral ICC segmentation method (Grau et al., 2004), and the ICC was masked from the T1w and T2w images.

Next, a fully automatic, multi-template MRI parcellation approach was used to parcellate the T1w image into ROI for volumetric analysis. We constructed a template library, composed of 18 T1w images of healthy controls, each with manual cortical, subcortical, white matter, cerebellar, and ventricular segmentations based on well-established MRI brain labeling protocols provided by the Center for Morphometric Analysis at Massachusetts General Hospital[2] (Caviness et al., 1996; Klein and Tourville, 2012). The 18 templates were each non-linearly aligned to each subject using dense registration between the T1w anatomical scans. The dense deformation field was then used to resample the template manual segmentations to the target subject anatomy, resulting in 18 template segmentations aligned to the target T1w image. A consensus segmentation was computed from all aligned segmentations using the PSTAPLE algorithm (Akhondi-Asl and Warfield, 2013). PSTAPLE uses both the label images and intensity profiles of the T1w templates to compute probability maps for each target structure, ultimately leading to a fully automatic consensus labeling of each brain. Finally, the volume of each label ($n = 38$) was computed. Subcortical and cortical volume measurements estimated by PSTAPLE have been shown to be more reproducible and accurate than Freesurfer and other similar algorithms (Velasco-Annis et al., 2018).

Human Phantom DW MRI Processing

The DW images were corrected for magnetic susceptibility distortion using the pair of b = 0 s/mm^2 images with opposite phase-encoding direction and FSL top-up (Andersson et al., 2003). Inter-volume motion correction was then performed by affine registration of each DW image to the average b = 0 s/mm^2 image. The DW images were aligned and up-sampled to the 1.0 mm^3 × 1.0 mm^3 × 1.0 mm^3 T2w resampled scan using affine registration and sinc interpolation, and the brain extracted on DWI using the previously computed ICC segmentation (Dyrby et al., 2014). A single tensor diffusion model was estimated using robust least squares in each brain voxel from which fractional anisotropy [$FA = 3Var(\lambda)/(\lambda^2{}_1 + \lambda^2{}_2 + \lambda^2{}_3)^{1/2}$] and mean diffusivity [$MD = (\lambda_1 + \lambda_2 + \lambda_3)/3$] were computed, where λ_i represent the eigenvalues of the diffusion tensor (Mori and Zhang, 2006).

Next, a fully automatic, multi-template approach was used to define 17 white matter ROIs in the native space of each human phantom DTI scan using a previously validated method (Suarez et al., 2012). A template library was constructed from whole brain DTI of 20 healthy controls, with each scan in its native space. The DTI were computed from 30 high angular resolution b = 1000 s/mm^2 and 5 b = 0 s/mm^2 TACERN protocol DW images.

For each template, scalar FA and color maps of the principal diffusion directions were computed from the DTI. ROI were hand drawn by an expert rater on the color map within white matter fiber bundles following previously defined and validated labeling schemes for tractography (Catani et al., 2005; Catani and Thiebaut de Schotten, 2008; Benjamin et al., 2014). To delineate the same white matter ROIs in the native space of each human phantom scan, the following procedure was performed for every template: the template scalar FA map was aligned to the target human phantom scalar FA map using affine registration with mutual information metric. The affine registration field was used to initialize a non-linear, dense registration of the template DTI to the human phantom DTI. The affine and dense deformation fields were then used to resample the template white matter ROIs to the human phantom native DTI space using nearest neighbor interpolation. Now with 20 sets of white matter ROIs (one for each template) aligned to the native space of the human phantom scan, a final, consensus set of white matter ROIs was computed using the STAPLE algorithm (Warfield et al., 2004). Lastly, mean FA and MD were computed in each ROI.

White Matter ROIs

The ROIs analyzed in this analysis were defined using previously validated labeling schemes for tractography and include left and right posterior limb of the internal capsule, anterior limb of the internal capsule, cingulum body, corpus callosum, and inferior extreme capsule, from here on referred to as uncinate fasciculus (Catani and Thiebaut de Schotten, 2008). The sagittal stratum was defined following the labeling technique for tractography of the optic radiations presented in (Benjamin et al., 2014). Three ROIs were placed along the arcuate fasciculi in each hemisphere; in the white matter (1) projecting from the inferior parietal lobule to the inferior frontal gyrus, (2) underlying the inferior parietal lobule, and (3) underlying the posterior superior temporal gyrus, following the labeling scheme presented in (Catani et al., 2005). From here on we refer to these ROIs as left and right arcuate fasciculus region 1, region 2, and region 3, respectively.

Statistical Analysis

We quantified reproducibility using the coefficient of variation (CV) of quantitative MR measurements. The inter-scanner (all scans across all scanners) and intra-scanner (all scans across a single scanner) CV were measured for SNR and IU of the ACR phantom, brain structure volume measurements derived from brain segmentation labels, and for FA and MD of white matter, measured within white matter labels. Intra-vendor (all scans across a single scanner vendor) CV was also computed. The CV of an MR measurement is defined as the ratio of the SD (σ) to the mean ($\bar{x}$) of the measurement, expressed as a percentage:

$$\text{Inter-scanner CV:} \quad CV_j = \frac{\sigma_j}{\bar{x}_j} \times 100\%$$

$$\text{Intra-scanner CV:} \quad CV_{ij} = \frac{\sigma_{ij}}{\bar{x}_{ij}} \times 100\%$$

$$\text{Intra-vendor CV:} \quad CV_k = \frac{\sigma_{kj}}{\bar{x}_{kj}} \times 100\%$$

where i indexes scanner, j indexes label, and k indexes scanner vendor.

[2] http://www.neuromorphometrics.org

A CV of value 0 would represent perfect reproducibility, while a greater value represents a larger SD relative to the mean of the sample. CV is an ideal measure of reproducibility of brain volume measurements because it is a dimensionless value relative to the size of the structure of interest. The analysis was completed using R software version 3.5.1.

RESULTS

ACR Phantom

There were 216 ACR phantom scans in total acquired on 7 of 7 TACERN scanners available for analysis (**Table 2**). Results of SNR and IU variability over the study period are presented in **Figure 1** and **Table 3**. SNR was highest on scanner G at 57 ± 1 and lowest on scanner D at 46.8 ± 0.9. SNR was most variable on scanner E, with a CV of 9.9%. Overall, SNR variability was low over the study period, with CV less than 2.1% on 5 of 7 scanners evaluated.

Average IU was highest on scanner A at 95.1% and lowest on scanner G at 85.0%. IU was most variable on scanner C, with a CV of 5.5%. Overall, IU was high for all scanners and IU variability was low, with an overall mean IU of 91.8% and a CV less than 2.4% on 6 of 7 scanners evaluated.

TABLE 3 | Variability of ACR Phantom T1-weighted signal to noise ratio and percent integral uniformity over the study period.

	Signal to noise ratio			Integral uniformity (%)		
Scanner	**Mean**	**SD**	**CV (%)**	**Mean (%)**	**SD (%)**	**CV (%)**
A	54	1	1.8	95.1	0.5	0.6
B	55.3	0.9	1.7	94.3	0.6	0.5
C	52.6	1.1	2.1	88.8	4.9	5.5
D	46.8	0.9	2.0	91.7	1.3	1.7
E	48.5	4.8	9.9	94.2	0.5	2.4
F	56.5	3.3	5.8	93.6	0.5	1.4
G	57	1	1.7	85.0	2.1	0.5

Human Phantom Volumetric Analysis

There were 26 human phantom scans acquired on 7 of 7 TACERN scanners available for analysis. Scan and re-scan following exit and re-entry to the scanner was possible on 5 of 7 scanners in 9 of 17 scan sessions (**Table 2**).

Figure 2 and **Table 4** display a summary of average inter- and intra-scanner volume CV across all labels. The average inter-scanner volume CV across all labels was 3.3%, and the average intra-scanner volume CV was 1.1% across all labels. Scanner B was the least variable scanner overall, with an average CV of 0.7% across all labels. Scanner G was the most variable scanner overall with an average CV of 1.4% across all labels. Intra-vendor CVs were also computed. The mean CV across all labels in Philips scans only was 1.7%, while the mean CV across all labels in Siemens scans was more variable, at 2.7%. There is a single GE scanner used in the study, and thus intra-vendor CV was not computed for GE.

Figure 3 and **Table 5** display the inter-scanner and mean intra-scanner mean, SD and CV of volume for each label. For purposes of concision, mean, SD, and CV for each label on each scanner are presented in **Supplementary Figure 1** and **Supplementary Table 1**. All inter-scanner label CVs were less than 5% with the exception of right temporal cortex (5.3%), left parietal cortex (5.4%), and extracerebral spinal fluid (9.9%). The least variable label volume across scanners was the cerebellar vermis, in the region of lobules 8, 9, and 10 (1.4%). Inter-scanner CV of left and right hippocampi and insular cortex were also less than 2%.

The mean intra-scanner label CV across all labels was 1.1% and within-label ranged from 0.5 to 3.0% for the ICC and extracerebral spinal fluid volumes, respectively (**Tables 4, 5**). The inter-scanner CV exceeded the mean intra-scanner CV by a factor of 2.5 on average and ranged from a factor of 1.1 in the right amygdala to a factor of 4.2 in the ICC.

Human Phantom DTI ROI Analysis

There were 24 human phantom scans acquired with DWI on 6 of 7 TACERN scanners available for analysis. DTI data were not available for scanner B. Scan and re-scan following exit and re-entry to the scanner was possible on 4 of 6 scanners in 8 of 16 scan sessions (**Table 2**).

Figure 2 and **Table 4** display a summary of inter- and intra-scanner FA and MD CV across all white matter labels. Overall, FA and MD in white matter labels were more variable within and across scanners than volume of brain segmentation labels. The average inter-scanner FA and MD CV across all labels was 4.5 and 5.4%, respectively. The average intra-scanner FA and MD CV across all labels was 2.5 and 1.5%, respectively. Scanners A and D were the least variable scanner overall, with average FA CVs of 1.9 and 1.6% and average MD CVs of 1.2 and 1.3%, respectively. Scanner E was the most variable scanner overall with an average FA CV of 3.7 % and an average MD CV of 1.8%. The mean FA CV across all labels in Philips scans slightly exceeded that of Siemens scans; with a mean Philips FA CV of 4.0% and a mean Siemens

TABLE 2 | Scan Information.

	Scanner	A	B	C	D	E	F	G	Overall
ACR	Number scans (% of total)	38 (18)	21 (10)	17 (8)	15 (7)	30 (13)	57 (26)	38 (18)	216
	Years over which scans were acquired	3.7	1.9	2.5	1.5	2.5	4.8	3.1	
Human phantom	Number scans (% of total)	4 (15)	2 (8)	2 (8)	3 (12)	4 (15)	7 (27)	4 (15)	26
	Number re-scans	2	1	0	1	2	3	0	9
	Years over which scans were acquired	0.8	0	3.0	0.9	1.4	4.5	4.7	

ACR, American College of Radiology.

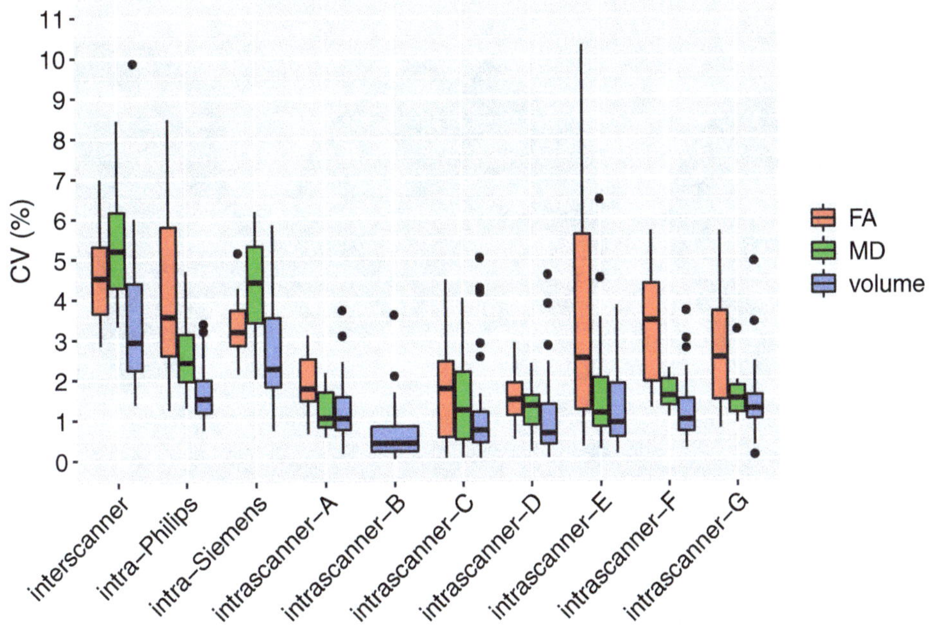

FIGURE 2 | Average inter-scanner, intra-scanner, and intra-vendor variability of all brain parcellation cortical label volumes, all white matter ROI FA, and all white matter ROI MD. Intra-GE was not computed because only one GE scanner was used in the study. DTI scans were not available from scanner B.

TABLE 4 | Average inter-scanner, intra-scanner, and intra-vendor variability of volume, FA, and MD in all labels.

	Volume		FA		MD	
	Mean CV (%)	SD CV (%)	Mean CV (%)	SD CV (%)	Mean CV (%)	SD CV (%)
Inter-scanner	3.3	1.6	4.5	1.2	5.4	1.4
Mean intra-scanner	1.1	0.2	2.5	0.9	1.5	0.2
Intra-scanner-A	1.3	0.8	1.9	0.7	1.2	0.5
Intra-scanner-B	0.7	0.7	–	–	–	–
Intra-scanner-C	1.1	1.2	1.7	1.2	1.5	1.2
Intra-scanner-D	1.0	1.0	1.6	0.7	1.3	0.5
Intra-scanner-E	1.2	1.0	3.7	3.2	1.8	1.7
Intra-scanner-F	1.2	0.8	3.3	1.4	1.7	0.4
Intra-scanner-G	1.4	0.9	2.7	1.4	1.5	0.5
Intra-vendor-Philips	1.7	0.7	4.0	2.0	2.6	0.9
Intra-vendor-Siemens	2.7	1.3	3.3	0.7	4.4	1.2

CV, coefficient of variation; FA, fractional anisotropy; MD, mean diffusivity (mm^2/s). Intra-General Electric not computed because only one General Electric scanner.

FA CV of 3.3%. In contrast, the mean MD CV across all labels in all Philips scans was lower than Siemens, with a mean Philips MD CV of 2.6%, compared to a mean Siemens MD CV of 4.4%. There is a single GE scanner used in the study, and thus intra-vendor CV was not computed for GE.

Figure 4 and **Tables 6, 7** display the mean, SD and inter and intra-scanner CV of FA and MD in all white matter labels. For purposes of concision, mean, SD, and CV of FA and MD for each label on each scanner are presented in **Supplementary Figure 1** and **Supplementary Tables 2, 3.**

Inter-scanner FA CVs were less than 5% in 12 of 17 labels evaluated and between 5 and 8% for 5 of 17 labels, including bilateral arcuate fasciculus region 3, left sagittal stratum, and right posterior limb internal capsule and uncinate fasciculus. Inter-scanner MD CVs were less than 5% in 7 of 17 labels evaluated. MD inter-scanner CV was maximal in left and right anterior limb of the internal capsule, at 8.2 and 8.1%, respectively. The least variable FA across scanners was the right arcuate fasciculus region 1 at 2.4%, while the least variable MD CV across scanners was the right arcuate fasciculus region 2.0 at 2.7%.

The FA of the corpus callosum and left and right posterior limbs of the internal capsules had the lowest average intra-scanner CV, at 1.7%, whereas the right uncinate fasciculus had the highest average intra-scanner FA CV, at 5.3%, driven by an intra-scanner CV of 10.3% on scanner E. The MD of corpus callosum had the lowest average intra-scanner CV at 1.1 %, and MD of the left and right uncinate fasciculus had the highest intra-scanner MD CV on average, at 2.5%.

The inter-scanner FA CV exceeded the mean intra-scanner FA CV by a factor of 1.9 on average and ranged from a factor of 1.0–3.0. The inter-scanner MD CV exceeded the mean intra-scanner MD CV by a factor of 3.8 on average, and ranged from a factor of 1.5–6.1.

DISCUSSION

We evaluated the reproducibility of MRI data of the ACR phantom and a traveling human phantom from seven scanners across 5 sites in a multi-site imaging study over a period of

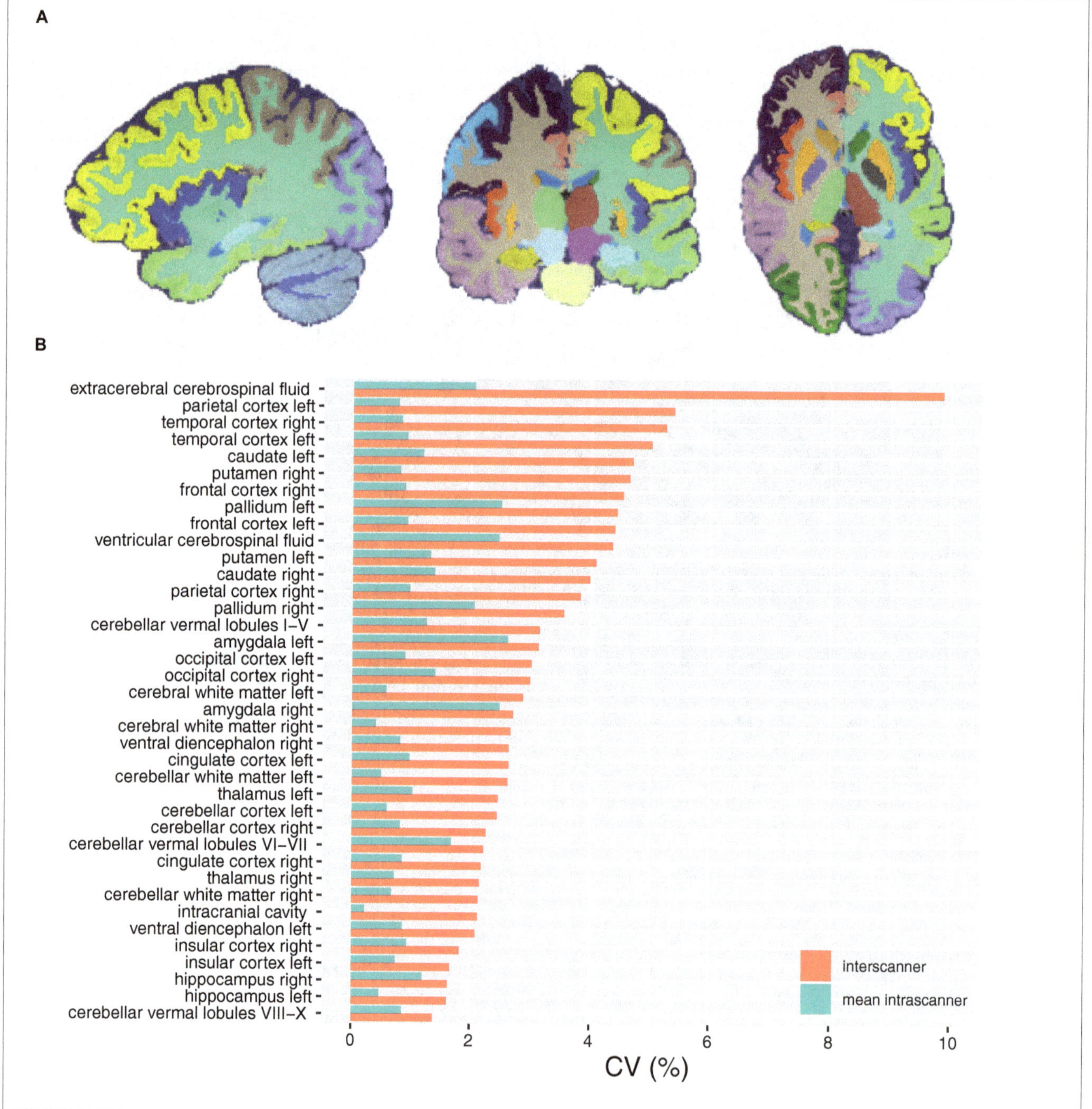

FIGURE 3 | (A) Sagittal, coronal, and axial views of a fully automatic brain parcellation result. Each color label identifies a brain structure of interest. **(B)** Inter-scanner and mean intra-scanner CV of brain parcellation label volumes.

5 years. Scanners are often subjected to system maintenance upgrades over time, and the hardware for imaging can be heterogeneous across centers. Analyzing the reproducibility of imaging measures across scanners is therefore important when combining measures from different scanners into a single dataset.

Our methods include reproducibility analyses of (1) signal intensity and uniformity using T1w images of the ACR phantom, (2) brain segmentation label volumes in a human volunteer, and (3) DTI metrics of white matter labels in a human volunteer within and across scanners used in the TACERN study. Analysis of signal intensity and uniformity demonstrate that SNR was consistent over time, with a CV of less than 2.1% in 5 of 7 scanners over time. Two scanners that underwent software upgrades demonstrated the highest SNR CV of 9.9 and 5.8%. SNR is influenced by a number of scanner-related factors, including resonance frequency, transmitter gain, scan acceleration, and coil loading (Keenan et al., 2018), any of which could vary with a

TABLE 5 | Inter and mean intra-scanner variability of brain parcellation label volumes.

Label	Measure	Mean	SD	CV (%)	Inter: intra CV ratio	Mean	SD	CV (%)	Inter: intra CV ratio
		LEFT				RIGHT			
Cerebellar cortex	inter-scanner	51274	1258	2.5	3.1	51490	1171	2.3	2.3
	Mean intra-scanner	51270	428	0.8		51501	521	1.0	
Cingulate cortex	Inter-scanner	12266	324	2.6	2.2	10869	238	2.2	2.2
	Mean intra-scanner	12338	147	1.2		10919	112	1.0	
Frontal cortex	Inter-scanner	94435	4163	4.4	3.1	96357	4384	4.6	3.3
	Mean intra-scanner	94040	1306	1.4		95936	1307	1.4	
Insular cortex	Inter-scanner	6356	106	1.7	1.9	6773	124	1.8	1.6
	Mean intra-scanner	6376	56	0.9		6804	72	1.1	
Occipital cortex	Inter-scanner	33598	1015	3.0	2.5	36392	1090	3.0	1.9
	Mean intra-scanner	33594	394	1.2		36295	584	1.6	
Parietal cortex	Inter-scanner	48671	2627	5.4	3.9	47279	1812	3.8	2.9
	Mean intra-scanner	48449	657	1.4		47204	631	1.3	
Temporal cortex	Inter-scanner	61785	3102	5.0	3.3	61533	3238	5.3	3.8
	Mean intra-scanner	61524	893	1.5		61207	853	1.4	
Cerebellar white matter	Inter-scanner	18600	487	2.6	3.3	18438	394	2.1	2.33
	Mean intra-scanner	18653	144	0.8		18491	160	0.9	
Cerebral white matter	Inter-scanner	245773	7068	2.9	3.2	249787	6668	2.7	3.9
	Mean intra-scanner	246668	2161	0.9		250626	1745	0.7	
Amygdala	Inter-scanner	1307	41	3.1	1.1	1289	35	2.7	1.1
	Mean intra-scanner	1309	35	2.7		1287	32	2.5	
Caudate	Inter-scanner	4130	195	4.7	2.9	4270	170	4.0	2.4
	Mean intra-scanner	4164	67	1.6		4305	73	1.7	
Hippocampus	Inter-scanner	4038	65	1.6	2.7	3984	65	1.6	1.2
	Mean intra-scanner	4053	25	0.6		3998	50	1.3	
Pallidum	Inter-scanner	1610	72	4.5	1.6	1666	59	3.5	1.5
	Mean intra-scanner	1622	44	2.8		1672	37	2.3	
Putamen	Inter-scanner	5432	222	4.1	2.4	5274	246	4.7	3.6
	Mean intra-scanner	5442	91	1.7		5299	68	1.3	
Thalamus	Inter-scanner	7903	194	2.5	2.1	7479	161	2.2	2.4
	Mean intra-scanner	7942	95	1.2		7517	68	0.9	
Ventral diencephalon	Inter-scanner	5592	117	2.1	2.1	5538	146	2.6	2.4
	Mean intra-scanner	5618	57	1.0		5564	58	1.1	
				BILATERAL					
Cerebellar vermal lobules I-V	Inter-scanner	4699	148	3.2	2.1				
	Mean intra-scanner	4715	70	1.5					
Cerebellar vermal lobules VI-VII	Inter-scanner	1530	34	2.2	1.2				
	Mean intra-scanner	1529	27	1.8					
Cerebellar vermal lobules VIII-X	Inter-scanner	2938	40	1.4	1.6				
	Mean intra-scanner	2935	27	0.9					
Extracerebral cerebrospinal fluid	Inter-scanner	262844	25930	9.9	3.3				
	Mean intra-scanner	267104	8091	3.0					
Intracranial cavity	Inter-scanner	1553414	33165	2.1	4.2				
	Mean intra-scanner	1560739	7326	0.5					
Ventricular cerebrospinal fluid	Inter-scanner	19614	858	4.4	1.6				
	Mean intra-scanner	19758	527	2.7					

All scans were included (n = 26).

software upgrade. Image uniformity on all scanners exceeded the ACR recommended IU of 82% or higher on 3T systems (American College of Radiology, 2018). IU was 92% on average across scanners, in line with reports of ACR IU in previous quality assurance studies (Chen et al., 2004; Davids et al., 2014). Variation in IU can be due to many factors, including but not

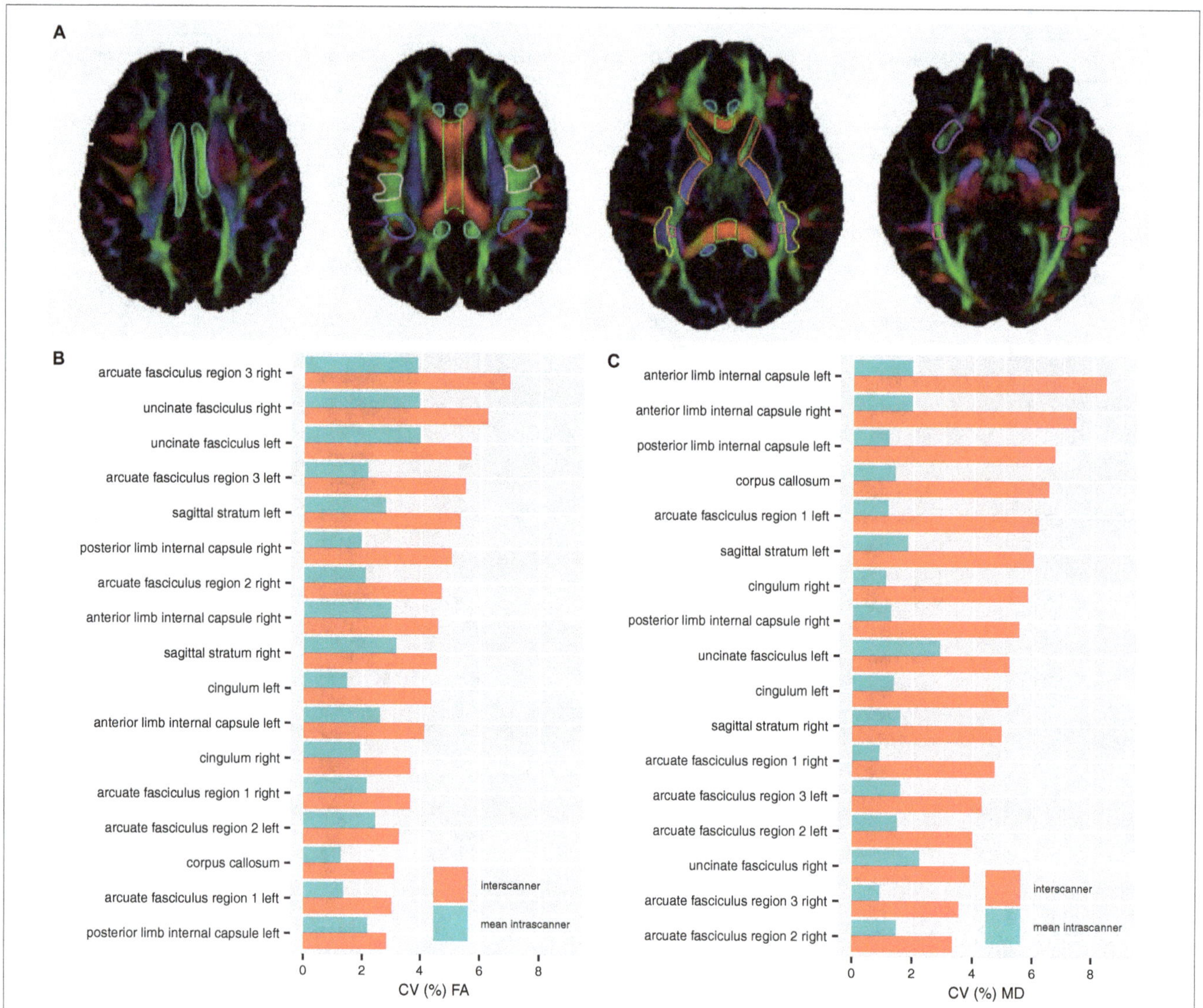

FIGURE 4 | (A) White matter ROI superimposed on a color map of the principal diffusion directions. Red color map voxels indicate left-right diffusion, green color map voxels indicate anterior-posterior diffusion, blue color map voxels indicate inferior-superior diffusion, and other colors indicate intermediate diffusion directions. Four axial slices from a single scan depict 2D slices of 3D white matter ROI, outlined in unique colors: light blue, cingulum; green, corpus callosum; white, arcuate fasciculus region 1; royal blue, arcuate fasciculus region 2; red, anterior limb of the internal capsule; orange, posterior limb of the internal capsule; yellow, arcuate fasciculus region 3; pink, sagittal stratum; and purple, uncinate fasciculus. **(B)** Inter-scanner and mean intra-scanner CV of white matter ROI FA. **(C)** Inter-scanner and mean intra-scanner CV of white matter ROI MD. Labels are ordered from bottom to top by increasing inter-scanner coefficient of variation.

limited to B_0 and B_1 non-uniformities, gradient linearity, and eddy currents (Keenan et al., 2018). Scanner C exhibited two temporally segregated clusters of IU, indicating an initial non-uniformity that was later corrected.

We found the inter-scanner variability of brain volume measurements overall was low and in line with other multisite studies of brain volume measurements. We found inter-scanner volume CV was on average 3.3%, ranged from 1.4 to 9.9%, and was less than 5% in 35 of 38 labels. Previous studies generally report average inter-scanner CV of less than 5%, depending on the brain structure analyzed (Huppertz et al., 2010; De Guio et al., 2016), and also have found a similarly high CSF inter-scanner CV of 9% (Huppertz et al., 2010). We found mean intra-scanner volume CV was on average 1.1% and ranged from 0.5 to 3.0%, similar to previous studies that report 0–3% intra-scanner CV of tissue volumes (de Boer et al., 2010; Huppertz et al., 2010; Landman et al., 2011; Maclaren et al., 2014; De Guio et al., 2016). Despite variable SNR on scanner E over the study period, scanner E volume measurements were not outlying from the rest of the data set, likely due to the robustness of the automated brain segmentation methodology.

Inter-scanner label volume CV was on average 2.5 times more variable than intra-scanner label volume CV. Higher inter-scanner compared to intra-scanner CV is expected given variation in hardware and software across scanners,

TABLE 6 | Inter and mean intra-scanner variability of FA in white matter ROIs.

Label	Measure	Mean FA	SD FA	CV (%) FA	Inter: intra CV ratio	Mean FA	SD FA	CV (%) FA	Inter: Intra CV ratio
			LEFT				**RIGHT**		
Anterior limb internal capsule	Inter-scanner	5.1	0.2	3.9	2.0	5.2	0.2	3.8	1.0
	Mean intra-scanner	5.1	0.1	2.0		5.2	0.2	3.8	
Arcuate fasciculus region 1	Inter-scanner	4.1	0.1	2.4	1.0	4.3	0.2	4.7	2.0
	Mean intra-scanner	4.1	0.1	2.4		4.3	0.1	2.3	
Arcuate fasciculus region 2	Inter-scanner	3.8	0.1	2.6	1.0	4.2	0.2	4.8	2.0
	Mean intra-scanner	3.8	0.1	2.6		4.2	0.1	2.4	
Arcuate fasciculus region 3	Inter-scanner	4.6	0.3	6.5	3.0	4.0	0.3	7.5	1.5
	Mean intra-scanner	4.6	0.1	2.2		4.0	0.2	5.0	
Cingulum	Inter-scanner	4.6	0.2	4.4	2.0	4.5	0.2	4.4	2.0
	Mean intra-scanner	4.6	0.1	2.2		4.5	0.1	2.2	
Posterior limb internal capsule	Inter-scanner	5.8	0.2	3.4	2.0	5.9	0.3	5.1	3.0
	Mean intra-scanner	5.8	0.1	1.7		5.8	0.1	1.7	
Sagittal stratum	Inter-scanner	5.0	0.3	6.0	3.0	4.6	0.2	4.4	2.0
	Mean intra-scanner	5.0	0.1	2.0		4.6	0.1	2.2	
Uncinate fasciculus	Inter-scanner	4.1	0.2	4.9	1.0	3.8	0.2	5.3	1.0
	Mean intra-scanner	4.2	0.2	4.8		3.8	0.2	5.3	
				BILATERAL					
Corpus callosum	Inter-scanner	6.1	0.2	3.3	1.9				
	Mean intra-scanner	6.0	0.1	1.7					

All scans were included (n = 24). DTI data were not available for Scanner B. FA is scaled × 10.

TABLE 7 | Inter and intra-scanner variability of MD in white matter ROIs.

Label	Measure	Mean MD	SD MD	CV (%) MD	Inter: intra CV ratio	Mean MD	SD MD	CV (%) MD	Inter: Intra CV ratio
				LEFT				**RIGHT**	
Anterior limb internal capsule	Inter-scanner	7.3	0.6	8.2	5.9	7.4	0.6	8.1	5.8
	Mean intra-scanner	7.2	0.1	1.4		7.3	0.1	1.4	
Arcuate fasciculus region 1	Inter-scanner	7.2	0.4	5.6	4.0	7.3	0.4	5.5	3.9
	Mean intra-scanner	7.2	0.1	1.4		7.3	0.1	1.4	
Arcuate fasciculus region 2	Inter-scanner	7.5	0.3	4.0	3.1	7.3	0.2	2.7	1.9
	Mean intra-scanner	7.5	0.1	1.3		7.3	0.1	1.4	
Arcuate fasciculus region 3	Inter-scanner	7.5	0.3	4.0	3.1	7.6	0.3	3.9	3.0
	Mean intra-scanner	7.5	0.1	1.3		7.6	0.1	1.3	
Cingulum	Inter-scanner	7.6	0.4	5.3	4.1	7.5	0.4	5.3	4.1
	Mean intra-scanner	7.6	0.1	1.3		7.5	0.1	1.3	
Posterior limb internal capsule	Inter-scanner	7.2	0.5	6.9	4.9	7.0	0.4	5.7	4.1
	Mean intra-scanner	7.2	0.1	1.4		7.0	0.1	1.4	
Sagittal stratum	Inter-scanner	8.3	0.5	6.0	2.5	8.1	0.4	4.9	4.1
	Mean intra-scanner	8.3	0.2	2.4		8.1	0.1	1.2	
Uncinate fasciculus	Inter-scanner	8.0	0.4	5.0	2.0	8.1	0.3	3.7	1.5
	Mean intra-scanner	8.1	0.2	2.5		8.1	0.2	2.5	
				BILATERAL					
Corpus callosum	Inter-scanner	9.0	0.6	6.7	6.1				
	Mean intra-scanner	9.0	0.1	1.1					

All scans were included (n = 24). DTI data were not available Scanner B. MD is scaled × 10,000 mm^2/s.

Members of the Tuberous Sclerosis Autism Center of Excellence Research Network (TACERN).

Member name	Affiliation	COIs/Disclosures
Simon K. Warfield, Ph.D.	Department of Radiology, Boston Children's Hospital, Boston, MA	None
Jurriaan M. Peters, MD, Ph.D.	Division of Epilepsy and Clinical Neurophysiology, Department of Neurology, Boston Children's Hospital, Boston, MA	None
Monisha Goyal, MD	Department of Neurology, University of Alabama at Birmingham, Birmingham, AL	
Deborah A. Pearson, Ph.D.	Department of Psychiatry and Behavioral Sciences, McGovern Medical School, University of Texas Health Science Center at Houston, Houston, TX	Curemark LLC–Consulting fees, Research grants and Travel Reimbursement ——————————————— *In the last year, my team has also done psych consults for Dr. Northrup's Biomarin clinical trial and Dr. Koenig's Novartis clinical trial. Thus, although I am listing myself as having received research grant funds from these projects, the funds are actually awarded to Hope and Mary Kay.* Biomarin: Research grant funds (Northrup, PI) Novartis: Research grant funds (Koenig, PI)
Marian E. Williams, Ph.D.	Keck School of Medicine of USC, University of Southern California, Los Angeles, California	None
Ellen Hanson, Ph.D.	Department of Developmental Medicine, Boston Children's Hospital, Boston, MA	None
Nicole Bing, Psy.D.	Department of Developmental and Behavioral Pediatrics, Cincinnati Children's Hospital Medical Center, Cincinnati, Ohio	
Bridget Kent, MA, CCC-SLP	Department of Developmental and Behavioral Pediatrics, Cincinnati Children's Hospital Medical Center, Cincinnati, Ohio	
Sarah O'Kelley, Ph.D.	University of Alabama at Birmingham, Birmingham, AL	
Rajna Filip-Dhima, MS	Department of Neurology, Boston Children's Hospital, Boston, MA	None
Kira Dies, ScM, CGC	Department of Neurology, Boston Children's Hospital, Boston, MA	None
Stephanie Bruns	Cincinnati Children's Hospital Medical Center, Cincinnati, OH	
Benoit Scherrer, Ph.D.	Department of Radiology, Boston Children's Hospital, Boston, MA	
Gary Cutter, Ph.D.	University of Alabama at Birmingham, Data Coordinating Center, Birmingham, AL	
Donna S. Murray, Ph.D.	Autism Speaks	None
Steven L. Roberds, Ph.D.	Tuberous Sclerosis Alliance	Research funding from Novartis

in addition to intra-scanner sources of variance including noise and subject positioning within the scanner. Within-subject biological sources of variation also contribute to inter-scanner measurement variation. Previous work has shown that time of day and level of hydration affects brain and cerebrospinal fluid volume measurements (Dieleman et al., 2017).

We found the reproducibility of DTI measurements within and across TACERN scanners is in accordance with previous studies of multisite DTI studies. Over all white matter labels, we found intra-scanner FA (2.5%) was greater than the intra-scanner MD (1.5%). Our findings are in line with past studies that generally report <3% CV FA (Heiervang et al., 2006; Zhu et al., 2012; Grech-Sollars et al., 2015; Acheson et al., 2017; Palacios et al., 2017) . Reports of MD are more variable, ranging from 0 to 7 % with most studies clustering around 2% intra-scanner CV MD (Heiervang et al., 2006; Magnotta et al., 2012; Grech-Sollars et al., 2015; Shahim et al., 2017; Nencka et al., 2018; Zhou et al., 2018).

We found an inter-scanner FA CV of 4.5%, in line with past studies of inter-scanner variability in white matter ROIs that report <5% CV for FA (Pagani et al., 2010; Vollmar et al., 2010; Grech-Sollars et al., 2015; Nencka et al., 2018). Studies of inter-scanner variability of FA within larger ROIs, such as whole brain white matter, lobar white matter, or white matter tracts generally report a CV of less than 4% (Magnotta et al., 2012; Grech-Sollars et al., 2015). For MD, we found an inter-scanner CV of 5.4%, greater than the inter-scanner FA CV. In contrast, past studies typically report an inter-scanner MD CV of <3%, lower than inter-scanner FA CV (Pagani et al., 2010; Magnotta et al., 2012; Grech-Sollars et al., 2015; Palacios et al., 2017; Nencka et al., 2018; Zhou et al., 2018). We found the average ratio of inter- to intra-scanner CV FA was approximately 2 to 1; whereas the average inter- to intra-scanner CV MD ratio was approximately 4 to 1. Thus, our data suggest that the FA is more robust to inter-scanner variations than MD.

This study is limited because scan-rescan was not possible on all study scanners due to scheduling demands of the clinical scanners utilized in the TACERN study. Thus change in subject anatomy over time is an additional source of measurement error that cannot be excluded from the intra-scanner CV metric.

CONCLUSION

Volumetric and DTI measurements acquired on TACERN study scanners are highly reproducible between and within scanners. Our findings will be useful for calculating sample sizes needed to identify group differences corresponding to pre-specified effect sizes, and for interpreting future MRI findings in the TACERN study.

ETHICS STATEMENT

All study procedures were approved by the Institutional Review Board at BCH, CCHMC, UAB, UCLA, and UTH, and the human phantom provided written informed consent.

AUTHOR CONTRIBUTIONS

AP, BS, CV-A, JP, EB, DK, HN, JW, MS, SP, and SW conceived and designed the study. All authors collected and analyzed the data. KK, AP, BS, RF-D, XT-F, JP, MS, and SW drafted a significant portion of the manuscript.

FUNDING

Research reported in this publication was supported by the National Institute of Neurological Disorders and Stroke of the National Institutes of Health (NINDS) and Eunice Kennedy Shriver National Institute of Child Health and Human Development (NICHD) under the award number U01NS082320 as well as the Intellectual and Developmental Disabilities Research Center at the Boston Children's Hospital (U54HD090255). This investigation was also supported in part by the NIH grants R01 NS079788, R01 EB019483, R44 MH086984, and by a research grant from the Boston Children's Hospital Translational Research Program. The content is solely the responsibility of the authors and does not necessarily represent the official views of the National Institutes of Health.

ACKNOWLEDGMENTS

We are sincerely indebted to the generosity of the families and patients in TSC clinics across the United States who contributed their time and effort to this study. We would also like to thank the Tuberous Sclerosis Alliance for their continued support in TSC research.

REFERENCES

Acheson, A., Wijtenburg, S. A., Rowland, L. M., Winkler, A., Mathias, C. W., Hong, L. E., et al. (2017). Reproducibility of tract-based white matter microstructural measures using the ENIGMA-DTI protocol. *Brain Behav.* 7, 1–10. doi: 10.1002/brb3.615

Akhondi-Asl, A., and Warfield, S. K. (2013). Simultaneous truth and performance level estimation through fusion of probabilistic segmentations. *IEEE Trans. Med. Imag.* 32, 1840–1852. doi: 10.1109/TMI.2013.2266258

American College of Radiology (2018). Phantom test guidance for the ACR MRI accreditation program. *Am. Coll. Radiol.* 1–28. doi: 10.2340/16501977-1025

Andersson, J. L., Skare, S., and Ashburner, J. (2003). How to correct susceptibility distortions in spin-echo echo-planar images: application to diffusion tensor imaging. *NeuroImage* 20, 870–888. doi: 10.1016/S1053-8119(03)00336-7

Benjamin, C. F., Singh, J. M., Prabhu, S. P., and Warfield, S. K. (2014). Optimization of tractography of the optic radiations. *Hum. Brain Map.* 35, 683–697. doi: 10.1002/hbm.22204

Capal, J. K., Horn, P. S., Murray, D. S., Byars, A. W., Bing, N. M., Kent, B., et al. (2017). Utility of the autism observation scale for infants in early identification of autism in tuberous sclerosis complex. *Pediatr. Neurol.* 75, 80–86. doi: 10.1016/j.pediatrneurol.2017.06.010

Catani, M., Jones, D. K., and Ffytche, D. H. (2005). Perisylvian language networks of the human brain. *Ann. Neurol.* 57, 8–16. doi: 10.1002/ana.20319

Catani, M., and Thiebaut de Schotten, M. (2008). A diffusion tensor imaging tractography atlas for virtual in vivo dissections. *Cortex* 44, 1105–1132. doi: 10.1016/j.cortex.2008.05.004

Caviness, V. S. Jr., Meyer, J., Makris, N., and Kennedy, D. N. (1996). MRI-based topographic parcellation of human neocortex: an anatomically specified method with estimate of reliability. *J. Cogn. Neurosci.* 8, 566–587. doi: 10.1162/jocn.1996.8.6.566

Chen, C. C., Wan, Y. L., Wai, Y. Y., and Liu, H. L. (2004). Quality assurance of clinical mri scanners using ACR MRI phantom: preliminary results. *J. Digit. Imag.* 17, 279–284. doi: 10.1007/s10278-004-1023-5

Davids, M., Zöllner, F. G., Ruttorf, M., Nees, F., Flor, H., Schumann, G., et al. (2014). Fully-automated quality assurance in multi-center studies using MRI phantom measurements. *Magn. Reson. Imaging* 32, 771–780. doi: 10.1016/j.mri.2014.01.017

Davis, P. E., Filip-Dhima, R., Sideridis, G., Peters, J. M., Au, K. S., Northrup, H., et al. (2017). Presentation and diagnosis of tuberous sclerosis complex in infants. *Pediatrics* 140:e20164040. doi: 10.1542/peds.2016-4040

de Boer, R., Vrooman, H. A., Ikram, M. A., Vernooij, M. W., Breteler, M. M., van der Lugt, A., et al. (2010). Accuracy and reproducibility study of automatic MRI brain tissue segmentation methods. *NeuroImage* 51, 1047–1056. doi: 10.1016/j.neuroimage.2010.03.012

De Guio, F., Jouvent, E., Biessels, G. J., Black, S. E., Brayne, C., Chen, C., et al. (2016). Reproducibility and variability of quantitative magnetic resonance imaging markers in cerebral small vessel disease. *J. Cereb. Blood Flow Metab.* 36, 1319–1337. doi: 10.1177/0271678X16647396

Dieleman, N., Koek, H. L., and Hendrikse, J. (2017). Short-term mechanisms influencing volumetric brain dynamics. *NeuroImage* 16, 507–513. doi: 10.1016/j.nicl.2017.09.002

Duchesne, S., Chouinard, I., Potvin, O., Fonov, V. S., Khademi, A., Bartha, R., et al. (2019). The canadian dementia imaging protocol: harmonizing national cohorts. *J. Magn. Reson. Imaging* 49, 456–465. doi: 10.1002/jmri.26197

Dyrby, T. B., Lundell, H., Burke, M. W., Reislev, N. L., Paulson, O. B., Ptito, M., et al. (2014). Interpolation of diffusion weighted imaging datasets. *NeuroImage* 103, 202–213. doi: 10.1016/j.neuroimage.2014.09.005

Fox, R. J., Sakaie, K., Lee, J. C., Debbins, J. P., Liu, Y., Arnold, D. L., et al. (2012). A validation study of multicenter diffusion tensor imaging: reliability of fractional anisotropy and diffusivity values. *Am. J. Neuroradiol.* 33, 695–700. doi: 10.3174/ajnr.A2844

Fu, L., Fonov, V., Pike, B., Evans, A. C., and Collins, D. L. (2006). Automated analysis of multi site MRI phantom data for the NIHPD project. *Med. Image Comput. Comput. Assist. Interv.* 9(Pt 2), 144–151. doi: 10.1007/11866763_18

Grau, V., Mewes, A. U. J., Alcañiz, M., Kikinis, R., and Warfield, S. K. (2004). Improved watershed transform for medical image segmentation using prior information. *IEEE Trans. Med. Imag.* 23, 447–458. doi: 10.1109/tmi.2004.824224

Grech-Sollars, M., Hales, P. W., Miyazaki, K., Raschke, F., Rodriguez, D., Wilson, M., et al. (2015). Multi-centre reproducibility of diffusion MRI parameters for clinical sequences in the brain. *NMR Biomed.* 28, 468–485. doi: 10.1002/nbm.3269

Heiervang, E., Behrens, T. E., Mackay, C. E., Robson, M. D., and Johansen-Berg, H. (2006). Between session reproducibility and between subject variability of diffusion mr and tractography measures. *NeuroImage* 33, 867–877. doi: 10.1016/j.neuroimage.2006.07.037

Huppertz, H. J., Kröll-Seger, J., Klöppel, S., Ganz, R. E., and Kassubek, J. (2010). Intra- and interscanner variability of automated voxel-based volumetry based on a 3D probabilistic atlas of human cerebral structures. *NeuroImage* 49, 2216–2224. doi: 10.1016/j.neuroimage.2009.10.066

Ihalainen, T. M., Lönnroth, N. T., Peltonen, J. I., Uusi-Simola, J. K., Timonen, M. H., Kuusela, L. J., et al. (2011). MRI quality assurance using the ACR phantom in a multi-unit imaging center. *Acta Oncol.* 50, 966–972. doi: 10.3109/0284186X.2011.582515

Jeste, S. S., Sahin, M., Bolton, P., Ploubidis, G. B., and Humphrey, A. (2008). Characterization of autism in young. *J. Child Neurol.* 23, 520–525.

Jeste, S. S., Wu, J. Y., Senturk, D., Varcin, K., JKo, J., McCarthy, B., et al. (2014). Early developmental trajectories associated with ASD in infants with tuberous sclerosis complex. *Neurology* 83, 160–168. doi: 10.1212/wnl.0000000000000568

Keenan, K. E., Ainslie, M., Barker, A. J., Boss, M. A., Cecil, K. M., Charles, C., et al. (2018). Quantitative magnetic resonance imaging phantoms: a review and the need for a system phantom. *Magn. Reson. Med.* 79, 48–61. doi: 10.1002/mrm.26982

Klein, A., and Tourville, J. (2012). 101 labeled brain images and a consistent human cortical labeling protocol. *Front. Neurosci.* 6:171. doi: 10.3389/fnins.2012.00171

Landman, B. A., Huang, A. J., Gifford, A., Vikram, D. S., Lim, I. A., Farrell, J. A., et al. (2011). Multi-parametric neuroimaging reproducibility: a 3-T resource study. *NeuroImage* 54, 2854–2866. doi: 10.1016/j.neuroimage.2010.11.047

Maclaren, J., Han, Z., Vos, S. B., Fischbein, N., and Bammer, R. (2014). Reliability of brain volume measurements: a test-retest dataset. *Sci. Data* 1, 1–9. doi: 10.1038/sdata.2014.37

Magnotta, V. A., Matsui, J. T., Liu, D., Johnson, H. J., Long, J. D., Bolster, B. D. Jr., et al. (2012). MultiCenter reliability of diffusion tensor imaging. *Brain Connect.* 2, 345–355. doi: 10.1089/brain.2012.0112

Morelli, J. N., Runge, V. M., Ai, F., Attenberger, U., Vu, L., Schmeets, S. H., et al. (2011). An Image-based approach to understanding the physics of MR artifacts. *RadioGraphics* 31, 849–866. doi: 10.1148/rg.313105115

Mori, S., and Zhang, J. (2006). Principles of diffusion tensor imaging and its appolications in basic neuroscience research. *Neuron* 51, 527–539. doi: 10.1016/j.neuron.2006.08.012

Nencka, A. S., Meier, T. B., Wang, Y., Muftuler, L. T., Wu, Y. C., Saykin, A. J., et al. (2018). Stability of MRI metrics in the advanced research core of the NCAA-DoD concussion assessment, research and education (CARE) consortium. *Brain Imaging Behav.* 12, 1121–1140. doi: 10.1007/s11682-017-9775-y

Pagani, E., Hirsch, J. G., Pouwels, P. J., Horsfield, M. A., Perego, E., Gass, A., et al. (2010). Intercenter differences in diffusion tensor MRI acquisition. *J Magn. Reson. Imaging* 31, 1458–1468. doi: 10.1002/jmri.22186

Palacios, E. M., Martin, A. J., Boss, M. A., Ezekiel, F., Chang, Y. S., Yuh, E. L., et al. (2017). Toward Precision and reproducibility of diffusion tensor imaging: a multicenter diffusion phantom and traveling volunteer study. *Am. J. Neuroradiol.* 38, 537–545. doi: 10.3174/ajnr.A5025

Shahim, P., Holleran, L., Kim, J. H., and Brody, D. L. (2017). Test-retest reliability of high spatial resolution diffusion tensor and diffusion kurtosis imaging. *Sci. Rep.* 7, 1–14. doi: 10.1038/s41598-017-11747-3

Suarez, R. O., Commowick, O., Prabhu, S. P., and Warfield, S. K. (2012). Automated delineation of white matter fiber tracts with a multiple region-of-interest approach. *NeuroImage* 59, 3690–3700. doi: 10.1016/j.neuroimage.2011.11.043

Velasco-Annis, C., Akhondi-Asl, A., Stamm, A., and Warfield, S. K. (2018). Reproducibility of brain MRI segmentation algorithms: empirical comparison of local MAP PSTAPLE, FREESURFER, and FSL-FIRST. *J. Neuroimaging* 28, 162–172. doi: 10.1111/jon.12483

Vollmar, C., O'Muircheartaigh, J., Barker, G. J., Symms, M. R., Thompson, P., Kumari, V., et al. (2010). Identical, but Not the same: intra-Site and inter-site reproducibility of fractional anisotropy measures on two 3.0*T scanners. NeuroImage* 51, 1384–1394. doi: 10.1016/j.neuroimage.2010.03.046

Warfield, S. K., Zou, K. H., and Wells, W. M. (2004). Simultaneous truth and performance level estimation (STAPLE). *IEEE Trans. Med. Imaging* 23, 903–921. doi: 10.1109/TMI.2004.828354

Wei, X., Guttmann, C. R., Warfield, S. K., Eliasziw, M., and Mitchell, J. R. (2004). Has your patient's multiple sclerosis lesion burden or brain atrophy actually changed? *Mult. Scler.* 10, 402–406. doi: 10.1191/1352458504ms1061oa

Zhou, X., Sakaie, K. E., Debbins, J. P., Narayanan, S., Fox, R. J., and Lowe, M. J. (2018). Scan-rescan repeatability and cross-scanner comparability of DTI metrics in healthy subjects in the SPRINT-MS multicenter trial. *Magn. Reson. Imaging* 53, 105–111. doi: 10.1016/j.mri.2018.07.011

Zhu, T., Hu, R., Qiu, X., Taylor, M., Tso, Y., Yiannoutsos, C., et al. (2012). Measurements?: a diffusion phantom and human brain study. *NeuroImage* 56, 1398–1411. doi: 10.1016/j.neuroimage.2011.02.010.Quantification

15

Auditory Processing of Speech and Tones in Children with Tuberous Sclerosis Complex

*Amanda M. O'Brien[1], Laurie Bayet[2], Katherine Riley[3], Charles A. Nelson[3,4], Mustafa Sahin[5,6] and Meera E. Modi[5,6]**

[1] Program in Speech and Hearing Bioscience and Technology, Division of Medical Sciences, Harvard University, Cambridge, MA, United States, [2] Department of Psychology, American University, Washington, DC, United States, [3] Laboratories of Cognitive Neuroscience, Division of Developmental Medicine, Boston Children's Hospital, Boston, MA, United States, [4] Harvard Graduate School of Education, Harvard University, Cambridge, MA, United States, [5] Translational Neuroscience Center, Boston Children's Hospital, Boston, MA, United States, [6] Department of Neurology, Harvard Medical School, Boston, MA, United States

Correspondence:
Meera E. Modi
meera.modi@childrens.harvard.edu

Individuals with Tuberous Sclerosis Complex (TSC) have atypical white matter integrity and neural connectivity in the brain, including language pathways. To explore functional activity associated with auditory and language processing in individuals with TSC, we used electroencephalography (EEG) to examine basic auditory correlates of detection (P1, N2, N4) and discrimination (mismatch negativity, MMN) of speech and non-speech stimuli for children with TSC and age- and sex-matched typically developing (TD) children. Children with TSC (TSC group) and without TSC (typically developing, TD group) participated in an auditory MMN paradigm containing two blocks of vowels (/a/and/u/) and two blocks of tones (800 Hz and 400 Hz). Continuous EEG data were collected. Multivariate pattern analysis (MVPA) was used to explore functional specificity of neural auditory processing. Speech-specific P1, N2, and N4 waveform components of the auditory evoked potential (AEP) were compared, and the mismatch response was calculated for both speech and tones. MVPA showed that the TD group, but not the TSC group, demonstrated above-chance pairwise decoding between speech and tones. The AEP component analysis suggested that while the TD group had an increased P1 amplitude in response to vowels compared to tones, the TSC group did not show this enhanced response to vowels. Additionally, the TD group had a greater N2 amplitude in response to vowels, but not tones, compared to the TSC group. The TSC group also demonstrated a longer N4 latency to vowels compared to tones, which was not seen in the TD group. No group differences were observed in the MMN response. In this study we identified features of the auditory response to speech sounds, but not acoustically matched tones, which differentiate children with TSC from TD children.

Keywords: Tuberous Sclerosis Complex, autism spectrum disorder, auditory evoked potential, MVPA, mismatch negativity

---

Abbreviations: AEP, auditory evoked potential; ASD, autism spectrum disorder; MVPA, multivariate pattern analysis; TSC, Tuberous Sclerosis Complex.

INTRODUCTION

Tuberous Sclerosis Complex is a genetic syndrome caused by a mutation in either the *TSC1* or *TSC2* gene. TSC is characterized by the formation of lesions on multiple organs including the brain, skin, kidneys, and lungs. Concurrent with TSC, approximately 50% of individuals are co-diagnosed with intellectual disabilities and 20–60% are co-diagnosed with ASD (Ehninger et al., 2009; Mcdonald et al., 2017), which contribute to pervasive deficits in language acquisition and development (Prather and De Vries, 2004).

Underlying these neurodevelopmental impairments, patients with TSC present with abnormalities in white matter microstructure (Peters et al., 2013), particularly within language pathways (Lewis et al., 2013). Molecular evidence suggests that the reduction in white matter in TSC is due to decreased myelination, altered axonal arborization, and synaptic formation (Tavazoie et al., 2005; Meikle et al., 2007; Choi et al., 2008; Ercan et al., 2017). While it is hypothesized that such structural differences in the brain lead to auditory and language deficits in TSC, the neural response to basic auditory and speech stimuli is not well characterized. Electroencephalography (EEG) can be used to determine if there are functional alterations in addition to structural deviations in patients with TSC. EEG is ideally suited for assessing functional activity with high temporal resolution in young and neurodevelopmentally delayed populations, as it is non-invasive and does not require active participation (Jeste et al., 2015). Further, the high temporal resolution of EEG is ideal for a time-locked exploration of early auditory processing.

In this study, we explored the neural processing of tones and speech sounds in children with TSC. The neural responses to auditory stimuli in a mismatch negativity (MMN) paradigm was compared in children with and without TSC using auditory evoked response potentials (AEP), time-resolved multivariate pattern analysis (MVPA), and MMN analysis. MVPA considers complete neural activation patterns at each individual time point, rather than focusing on one specific region and time point of interest (Cauchoix et al., 2014; Grootswagers et al., 2017; Holdgraf et al., 2017; Bayet et al., 2018). Thus, MVPA allows for the exploration of potential compensatory mechanisms of processing (i.e., unique localizations and patterns) that may be established in clinical populations due to structural aberrations. To our knowledge, this study is the first to utilize MVPA for speech sound processing in a pediatric population.

The AEP, elicited by an auditory stimulus and collected using EEG, is a traditional measure of basic auditory detection that is well conserved in typically developing populations (Picton, 2011; O'connor, 2012). Deviations from the stereotyped response, therefore, serve as an apt measure of differences in functional auditory detection and may serve as biomarkers of functional impairment in the disorder. Mismatch negativity (MMN) is a second order measure of auditory processing that represents a neural discrimination response induced by an unexpected stimulus (Naatanen et al., 2007, 2012). The MMN reflects learning and habituation while not requiring overt behavioral responses, and is thus an appropriate measure for use with clinical populations (Naatanen et al., 2012).

Early efforts suggest AEP may reflect neural disruptions in TSC. Parallel to the white matter abnormalities seen in neuroimaging in individuals with TSC and ASD, co-diagnosis is also associated with an increased latency in the N1 component of the AEP and a reduction in the MMN response to tones relative to those with TSC alone (Seri et al., 1999). The correlation between neurodevelopmental, neuroimaging and electrophysiological phenotypes in TSC empowers the use of EEG for biomarker detection. Based on the specificity of white matter abnormalities to language pathways and the prevalence of language impairment in children with TSC, we predict that MVPA and AEP analyses of the neural responses to speech and tone stimuli will reveal (1) decreased accuracy of decoding between speech and tones in the TSC population compared to typically developing children, (2) typical early sensory responses but disrupted later cognitive responses, and (3) reduced MMN response to vowel changes, but not tone changes, compared to typically developing children.

MATERIALS AND METHODS

Participants

Eleven children with a clinical diagnosis of TSC between the ages of 4 and 14, and age- and sex- matched typically developing (TD) children (mean age: 9.28) were recruited from the multidisciplinary Tuberous Sclerosis Program of the Department of Neurology at Boston Children's Hospital. Medical history for both groups including auditory deficits, visual deficits, neurological conditions and current pharmacological treatments were collected through parent questionnaire.

Nine children (mean age: 9.22; range 9.90, 4 boys) with a diagnosis of TSC were included in the study (**Table 1**). Two of the eleven recruited children with TSC were excluded due to seizure activity during the test session and excessive movement artifact. Seven participants reported a history of seizures, and five participants were being treated with seizure medication during the study. Four participants with TSC had a clinical co-diagnosis of ASD based on parent report. One participant with TSC was exposed to Spanish as a first language and English as a second language; however, because the speech sound stimuli used in this study are present in both Spanish and English, this participant

TABLE 1 | Demographic and clinical data for participants.

	Control	TSC
Age	9.24 (4.09–14.36)	9.22 (4.64–14.55)
Sex	5/9 female	5/9 female
Race	9/9 white	8/9 white
Clinical diagnosis	None	5/9 TSC 4/9 TSC + ASD
Hearing/vision	0/9 Hearing Dx 2/9 Vision Dx	0/9 Hearing Dx 3/9 Vision Dx
Language	9/9 L1: English	8/9 L1: English
Speech therapy	0/9	9/9

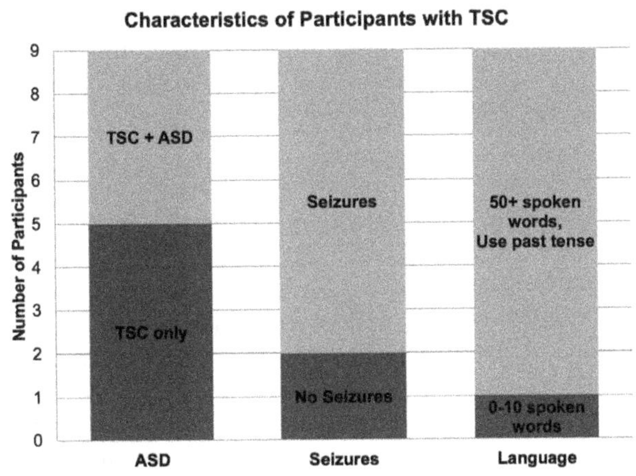

FIGURE 1 | Diagnostic, medical, and language characteristics of participants with TSC. Four of the nine participants with TSC were co-diagnosed with ASD. Seven children with TSC experienced seizures, while two children did not. Per parent report, one participant with TSC used 0–10 spoken words while the other eight children used over 50 spoken words and the past tense.

was not excluded from the study. All other participants in this group were monolingual English speakers (**Figure 1**).

Nine TD children who were age (± 6 months) and sex-matched to the TSC group (mean age: 9.28; range: 10.26; 4 males) participated in the control group. Per parent report, children in the control group had no history of neurological abnormalities or traumas, birth-related complications, developmental delays, uncorrected vision difficulties, nor immediate family history of neurodevelopmental disorders. Reports were not confirmed with medical records. One participant in the control group had simultaneous language exposure to English and German. Two participants reported English as a first language with some exposure to a second language (Italian, American Sign Language). All other participants in the control group were monolingual English speakers. No participant in either group presented with hearing abnormalities or uncorrected vision difficulties.

The Institutional Review Board at Boston Children's Hospital approved this study (P00023954). Informed written consent was obtained from the parents of each participant, and from the participants as appropriate.

Stimuli

The stimuli included two vowel sounds (/a/and/u/) and two non-speech acoustically matched tones (800 Hz and 400 Hz, respectively). A female speaker of American English recorded the vowel sounds using PRATT computer software. Each non-speech tone complement was synthesized with PRATT computer software to be within one standard deviation of the first two formants (F1, F2) of the average female formants and the corresponding recorded speech sounds (Sandoval and Utianski, 2015). Stimuli were each 300 ms in length, with a 0.05 ms on-ramp and off-ramp. Files of the tone and vowel stimuli are included as **Supplementary Material**.

Stimuli Presentation

The stimuli were presented in a within-category MMN paradigm (deviant stimuli 15%, never in succession). Participants listened to four stimuli blocks; each block contained 360 pseudo-randomly presented stimuli. Two sequential blocks contained the speech sound stimuli (i.e.,/a/then/u/) and two sequential blocks contained the non-linguistic stimuli (i.e., 800 Hz then 400 Hz). For each category (vowels or tones), each stimulus was used as both the "flip" and the "flop" variant in the MMN paradigm. For half of the participants, the speech sound stimuli blocks were played first (TSC: $n = 5$; TD: $n = 5$); for the other half of participants, the non-linguistic blocks were played first. The inter-stimulus interval was 700 ms. The stimuli intensities were equalized to be 61 dB ± 3 dB when playing through two speakers positioned bilaterally in front of the participant. The stimuli intensities were measured using a sound meter from the distance that the participants sat from the speakers. Stimuli were presented via speakers instead of earphones due to the sensory sensitivities that are often present in individuals of this demographic. The stimuli were played using E-Prime experimental software (Psychology Software Tools Incorporated, Pittsburgh, Pennsylvania).

Procedure

Participants sat in an electrically shielded and sound attenuated room. Participants passively listened to the stimuli while watching a silent video (Wall-E, Disney Pixar) on a computer monitor. An experimenter sat in the room to maintain participant engagement and ensure that participants continued to tolerate wearing the net. Breaks were provided as needed between the blocks of stimuli. The MMN procedure lasted for approximately 24 min. The stimuli were presented as a part of a battery of EEG paradigms. The entire battery was approximately 45 min long.

EEG Recording

A continuous EEG recording was collected for each participant using a 128-channel Geodesic Sensor Net (Philips Electrical Geodesics Inc., Eugene, OR). The net size was determined by the child's head circumference. EEG was recorded using Net Station Acquisition software (Philips Electrical Geodesics Inc., Eugene, OR) at a sampling rate of 1000 Hz and referenced online to the average reference. A Net Amps 300 amplifier was used to amplify the electrical signal.

Data Processing

The data were processed offline using Net Station analysis software (Philips Electrical Geodesics Inc., Eugene, OR). A bandpass filter of 0.3–30 Hz was used. The continuous recording was segmented into 600-ms epochs, including 100-ms before the onset of the stimuli as a baseline. The mean voltage during the baseline period was used for baseline correction of each epoch.

Artifact detection was automated by the Net Station program. Channels within each segment were removed if the difference between the maximum and the minimum heights of the waveform exceeded 200 μV. Segments with more than 18 eliminated channels were excluded from further analysis. The standard stimulus segments that immediately follow a deviant stimulus were also removed. If the number of good segments varied by more than five segments per condition for a given participant, segments were randomly eliminated until all conditions were within five segments of each other. Participants with fewer than 10 good segments in any given condition were excluded from further analysis ($n = 1$). The average number of good segments in an included standard condition was 212, with a range of 70–252. The average number of good segments in an included deviant condition was 47, with a range from 22 to 54.

Bad channels within the accepted segments were replaced using a spherical spline interpolation. Average waveforms for each electrode referenced to the average reference were generated for each participant, and a final baseline correction was applied. Finally, the individual trials were averaged by condition for each participant.

For MVPA, the epoch data was processed as described above (i.e., bandpass filter, segmentation, baseline correction, artifact removal); however, we did not average across the trials for each electrode. Instead, after artifact removal we re-referenced and baseline corrected the single trial data and then exported the single trial data to MATLAB to run the MVPA.

Analysis

MVPA

We utilized MVPA to explore the functional specificity of neural processing for differentiating standard speech sounds compared to standard non-speech stimuli. For each pairwise classification between the four standard stimuli, a linear classifier was trained in MATLAB on 3/4 of the trials for each participant. The other 1/4 of the trials were used to test the accuracy of classifier. We used a fourfold cross-validation with pseudo-averaging and 300 random permutations of the data (Isik et al., 2014; Grootswagers et al., 2017; Bayet et al., 2018). To prevent possible effects from the order of presentation, only trials from the second and third stimuli blocks (i.e., the two middle blocks) were used for each participant, thereby eliminating trials that are further separated by time (i.e., the first and last blocks of stimuli). The average number of included trials from a single stimuli block was 213, with a range of 70–252. Forty-eight of the electrodes were excluded from our analysis due to location on the outer rim of the electrode cap.

AEP Component Analysis

Waveforms were calculated from montages resulting from electrodes in the right frontal region. The right frontal region (electrodes 2, 3, 4, 10, 122, 123, 124) was selected as the region of interest (ROI) *a priori* to the analysis based on the implication of this region in the processing of vowel sounds and tones (Lepisto et al., 2005; Ceponiene et al., 2008; Britton et al., 2009). Further, because one of the strengths of MVPA is the identification of relevant electrode clusters during neural processing, we used the spatial resolution of the MVPA as evidence-based confirmation that the electrode clusters chosen *a priori* were indeed relevant to our paradigm. The average number of good trials included by group and condition are included in **Table 2**.

TABLE 2 | Average number of good trials per condition, by group.

Group	Vowels (standards)	Tones (standards)	Vowels (deviants)	Tones (deviants)
TSC	370 SD = 108	377 SD = 114	83 SD = 17	85 SD = 19
Control	475 SD = 42	474 SD = 40	103 SD = 7	102 SD = 7

Peak components of interest from the montage averaged waveform were selected based on their association with language processing in pediatric populations. Components of the AEP waveform mature through adolescence. The adult AEP waveform contains the following sequence of positive (P) and negative (N) inflections in response to speech and tones: P1, N1, P2, N2, N4. In contrast, children do not have noticeable N1 or P2 peaks in response to speech sounds or tones (**Figure 2**; Ceponiene et al., 2008). The P1, N2, and N4 components evident by early childhood (e.g., age 7) have been shown to reflect neural processes associated with basic auditory detection, recognition, and spectral changes in pitch and speech sound formants (Ceponiene et al., 2008). The N4 peak has been identified as particularly relevant to speech processing (Ceponiene et al., 2008). Adults and TD children demonstrate a reduced or absent N4 in response to tones, compared to a larger N4 response to speech sounds (Ceponiene et al., 2005). Data further suggest that diminished N2 and N4 peaks in response to consonant-vowel syllables are correlated with language impairment (Ceponiene et al., 2009). In light of the consistent P1, N2, and N4 in the developing pediatric AEP response, we explore these components of the auditory AEP as potential auditory biomarkers.

The waveform peaks were identified in each participant according to established pediatric time windows (Ceponiene et al., 2009): P1 (maximum positive peak between 70 and 190 ms), N2 (most negative peak between 270 and 390 ms), and N4 (most negative peak between 350 and 500 ms). The amplitudes and latencies of each peak were averaged across standard group category (i.e., responses to the standard/a/and/u/were averaged together, responses to the standard 800 Hz and 400 Hz were averaged together) by participant.

MMN

As described above, the right frontal region waveform response was also used when identifying the MMN. To confirm the presence of the MMN response, the minimum peak (between 100 and 300 ms) of the standard and deviant waveforms were compared for each condition.

To quantify the MMN, the difference waveform (response to the deviant minus response to the standard) was calculated for each stimulus between 100 and 300 ms (Lepisto et al., 2005). Difference waveforms were calculated on a per subject basis and the difference wave was used for analysis. The minimum negative peak between 100 and 300 ms was identified as the mismatch negativity amplitude. The presence of the MMN was analyzed at the population level; data was included from each participant regardless of whether an MMN was detected for an individual stimulus.

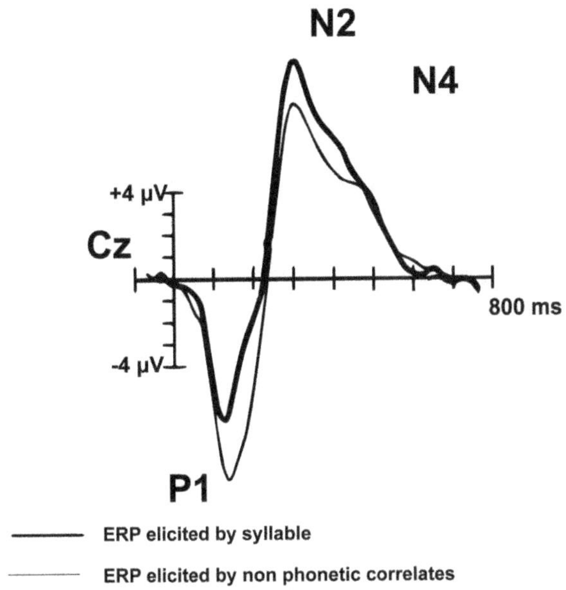

FIGURE 2 | Pediatric (n = 14) syllable (bold) and non-speech ERP grand-average waveform from Cz (adapted from Ceponiene et al., 2005). The P1, N2, and N4 peaks are evident in the pediatric auditory waveform. In contrast to the matured adult AEP waveform, the N1 and P2 peaks are not observed in children.

The literature suggests that the ASD diagnosis drives some EEG phenotypes in TSC, including the MMN response (Jeste and Nelson, 2009; Jeste et al., 2015). Acknowledging the limitations of our small sample size, we ran preliminary analyses to explore these possible trends in the MMN response of children with both TSC + ASD, compared to the MMN response of participants in the TD and TSC - ASD groups.

Statistical Analysis

MVPA

For each participant group, the accuracy of the linear classifier was determined for decoding between (1) standard tones (800 Hz vs. 400 Hz); (2) standard speech sounds (/a/vs./u/); (3) standard tones vs. standard speech; and (4) all standard stimuli (e.g.,/a/vs./u/, 800 Hz vs. 400 Hz, etc.).

Accuracy vs. chance was analyzed for both of the time windows as defined above (corrected for multiple comparisons at the FDR level) and for a cluster-level correction over time points. In the latter case, statistical significance of the classification accuracy time-series against chance was established using permutation tests (right-tail test against the chance level of 50 or 0% as appropriate, 1000 permutations) with cluster-wise correction over time-points (cluster-defining threshold p-value = 0.05, $\alpha = 0.05$) (Bayet et al., 2018; Dobs et al., 2018).

Additionally, we analyzed whether the classification accuracies (1) within and (2) between stimuli categories were above chance for each group. Average pairwise classification accuracies over two broad time windows of interest (early, 100–250 ms; late, 250–500 ms) were analyzed using Linear Mixed Effects (LME) Models to test for effects of group (TSC group/TD group) and classification type (within-domain classification, such as 400 Hz tone vs. 800 Hz tone, or cross-domain classification such as/a/vs. 800 Hz tone). A random intercept was used for each participant. Analyses of Variances (ANOVAs) were conducted to test the statistical significance of fixed effects, with follow up t-tests as appropriate.

All MVPA analyses were run in MATLAB (The MathWorks, Natick, MA).

AEP Component Analysis

To compare the amplitudes of each peak (P1, N2, N4), we completed a repeated-measures ANOVA for each peak with stimuli category (speech/tone) as within-factor and group (TSC group/TD group) as between-factor. To compare the latency of each peak (P1, N2, N4), we completed a repeated-measures ANOVA for each peak with stimuli category (speech/tone) as within-factor and group (TSC group/controls) as between factor. The AEP statistical analyses were performed with GraphPad Prism 7 for Mac OS X (GraphPad Software, Inc., La Jolla, CA). Significant main effects and interactions were followed up with unpaired t-tests between the groups. All analyses were corrected for multiple comparisons using Sidak's test of multiple comparisons. All significance levels were set at $\alpha < 0.05$. To compensate for the small sample size of our groups, *post hoc* Bayesian comparisons were conducted for the amplitude and latency of each AEP component using IBM SPSS Statistics version 25 (IBM Corp., Armonk, NY).

MMN Analysis

To confirm the presence of an MMN response in each group (TSC group/TD group), we used a t-test for both auditory conditions (speech/tone). Each t-test compared the minimum amplitude (between 100 and 300 ms) in response to the standard stimuli to that of the deviant stimuli for each group.

To compare the amplitudes of the MMN response between each group (TSC group/TD group), we used a t-test for both auditory conditions (vowels and tones). Each t-test compared the most negative amplitude of the difference waveform (deviant minus standard) between groups, for both the vowel and the tone conditions.

To explore possible trends in the MMN response driven by the ASD diagnosis, we used a one-way ANOVA to compare the three groups (TD group, TSC - ASD, TSC + ASD group) for both auditory conditions (vowels and tones). Significant effects were followed up with Dunnet's Multiple Comparisons (TD group/TSC - ASD group, TD group/TSC + ASD group). All significance levels were set at $\alpha < 0.05$. *Post hoc* Bayesian comparisons were also conducted using IBM SPSS Statistics version 25 to compensate for the small sample sizes.

The MMN statistical analyses were performed with GraphPad Prism 7 for Mac OS X (GraphPad Software, Inc., La Jolla, CA).

RESULTS

Please see **Supplementary Table S1** for the results of all statistical analyses reported below, as well as results from *post hoc* Bayesian comparisons that further supported our findings.

MVPA

There was a significant group x stimulus interaction [$F(1,32) = 6.37$, $p = 0.0168$], with more accurate decoding between stimulus class than within class in the TD group ($p = 0.0214$) but not the TSC group ($p = 0.404$) at an early time window (100–250 ms), indicating that there was significant difference in the neural response to tones vs. vowels in the TD group but not the TSC group.

The TD group had above chance decoding between speech vs. tones at early (100–250 ms; $p = 0.005$) and late (250–500 ms; $p = 0.0187$) time windows after FDR correction. A cluster analysis revealed above chance decoding between speech and tones from 110 to 449 ms for the TD group ($p < 0.05$). The TSC group did not have above chance decoding between these stimuli categories (early: $p = 0.401$; late: $p = 0.416$). A cluster analysis confirmed that decoding was not above chance in any time range for the TSC group ($p > 0.05$) (**Figure 3A**).

The MVPA revealed above chance decoding for the TD group within the speech category (/a/vs./u/) at a late time window ($p = 0.0428$) (as confirmed by the time-wise analysis finding of two significant clusters between 273–348 and 418–499 ms, $p < 0.05$), but not at an early time window ($p = 0.176$), after FDR correction (**Figure 3B**). The TSC group did not demonstrate above-chance decoding within the speech sound category at early ($p = 0.133$) or late ($p = 0.133$) time windows.

Unlike for speech, there was no above chance decoding between tones (400 Hz vs. 800 Hz) for the TD group at early ($p = 0.176$) or late ($p = 0.176$) time windows. Similarly, there was no above chance decoding between tones for the TSC group at early ($p = 0.133$) or late ($p = 0.400$) time windows (**Figure 3C**). Unexpectedly, there was above chance decoding for all stimuli within each class for the TD group at early time points ($p = 0.0428$), however, the cluster analysis at this time point was not statistically significant ($p > 0.05$). As expected, there was no above chance decoding for all stimuli within each class at late time windows ($p = 0.416$) for the TD group, or at early ($p = 0.176$) or late ($p = 0.607$) time windows for the TSC group (**Figure 3D**).

AEP Waveform Analysis

Average waveforms were generated for both the TD and the TSC groups in response to normal tones (both 400 Hz and 800 Hz together) and normal speech sounds (both/a/and/u/together), excluding the first normal stimuli after an oddball stimulus (**Figure 4A**). Averaged waveforms for each participant for both tone and speech can be seen in **Supplementary Figure S1**.

P1 Amplitude

We found a main effect of stimulus for the P1 response [$F(1,16) = 6.34$, $p = 0.0229$], with an enhanced P1 response to vowels compared to tones ($p = 0.027$) in the TD group, but not in the TSC group ($p = 0.686$). There was no effect of group [$F(1,16) = 1.71$, $p = 0.209$] or a group x stimulus interaction [$F(1,16) = 1.947$, $p = 0.182$] (**Figure 4B**). Bayesian comparisons supported these findings, as shown in **Supplementary Table S1**.

N2 Amplitude

The N2 amplitude differed significantly between groups [$F(1,16) = 6.736$, $p < 0.02$]. The TD group had significantly

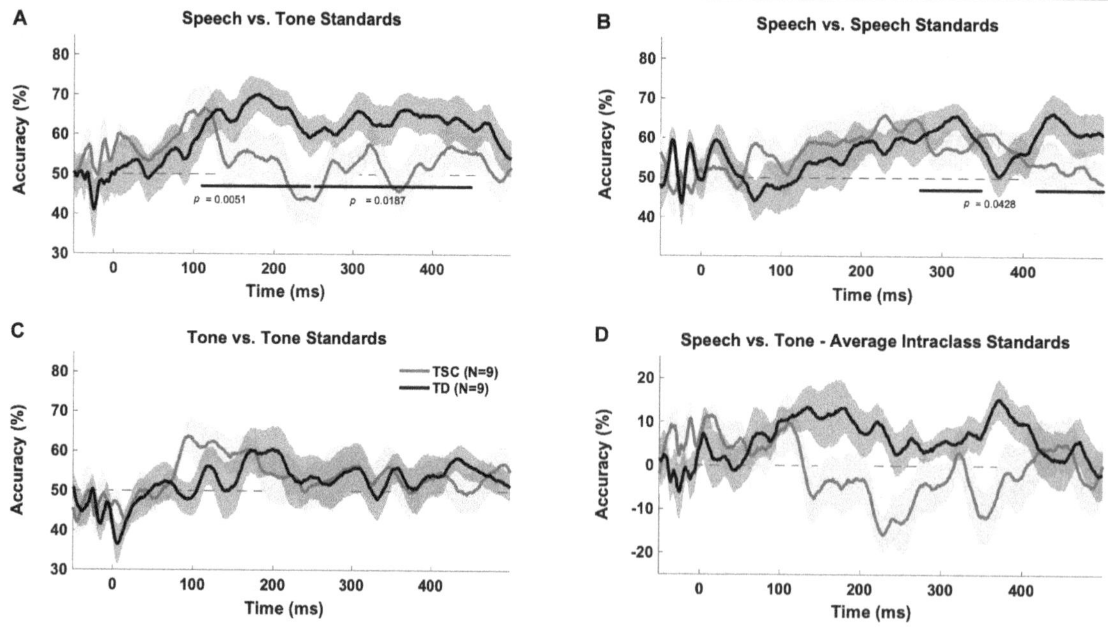

FIGURE 3 | Multivariate pattern analysis accuracy between groups. Plots represent decoding accuracy between responses to speech sounds compared to tones (/a/ + /u/vs. 800 Hz + 400 Hz) **(A)**, the standard speech sounds (/a/vs./u/) **(B)**, tones (800 vs. 400) **(C)**, and between all stimuli (/a/vs./u/vs. 800 Hz vs. 400 Hz) **(D)** for the children with TSC and typically developing children. The bold lines on the figures indicate time points of above-chance decoding in the TD group, as determined by the cluster correction method. In contrast, the TSC data did not yield significant above-chance decoding at any time point. Levels of chance were set to 50% **(A–C)** and 0% **(D)** as appropriate.

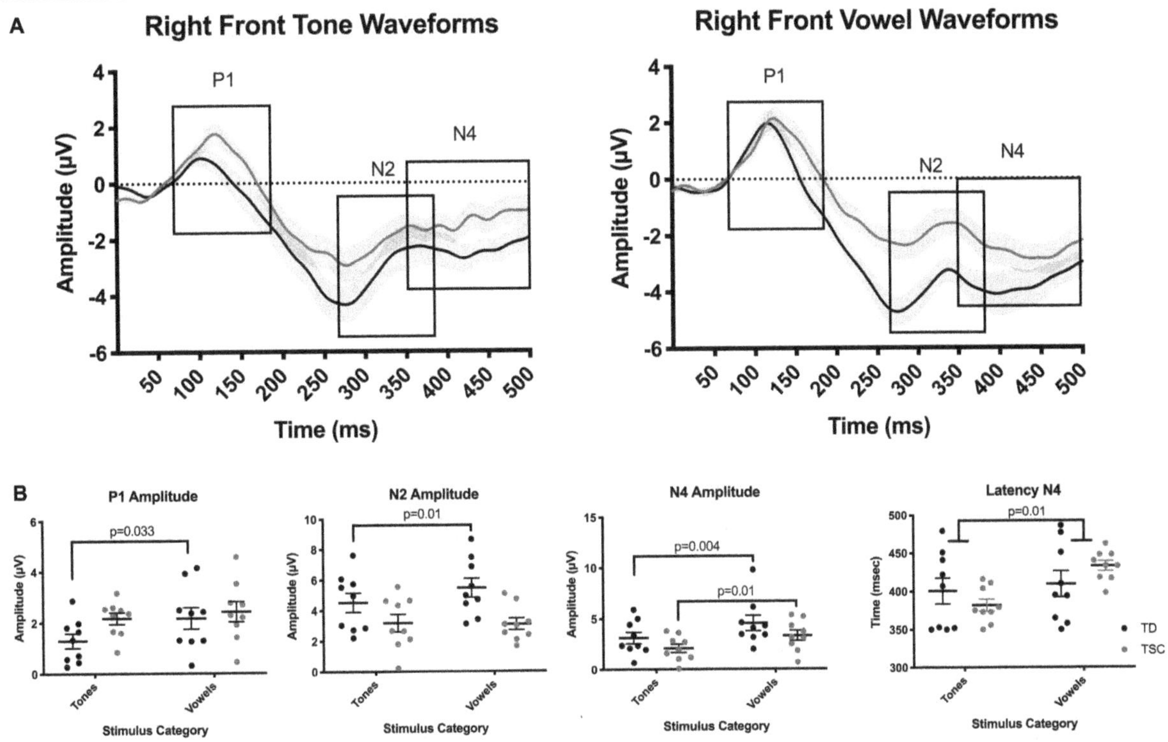

FIGURE 4 | Auditory evoked potential response to tones and vowels between groups in the right front cluster. Plots represent AEP waveform response to tones and vowels **(A)**, and absolute value in microvolts of the amplitude of each waveform component of interest (P1, N2, N4) **(B)**. There was an enhanced P1 response to vowels compared to tones in the TD group, but not in the TSC group. The TD group had significantly greater N2 amplitude in response to vowels, but not tones, compared to the TSC group. There was a greater N4 amplitude in response to vowels than tones in both the TD and TSC groups. The TSC group had significantly longer latency of the N4 in response to speech compared to tones, which was not seen in the TD group. No group or stimulus differences were observed related to the latency of P1 or N2.

greater N2 amplitude in response to vowels ($p = 0.0104$), but not to tones ($p = 0.187$), compared to the TSC group (**Figure 4B**). There was no effect of stimulus [$F(1,16) = 1.66$, $p = 0.236$] or group x stimulus interaction [$F(1,16) = 2.325$, $p = 0.147$]. Bayesian comparisons supported these findings, as shown in **Supplementary Table S1**.

N4 Amplitude

In contrast to our hypothesis, N4 amplitude did not differ by group [$F(1,16) = 2.179$, $p = 0.159$]. There was a greater N4 amplitude in response to vowels than tones [$F(1,16) = 24.35$, $p = 0.0001$] in both the TD ($p = 0.0035$) and TSC groups ($p = 0.0105$; **Figure 4B**). There was no group x stimulus interaction [$F(1,16) = 0.139$, $p = 0.715$]. Bayesian comparisons supported these findings, as shown in **Supplementary Table S1**.

P1, N2, N4 Latency

There were no significant main effects of diagnosis ($p = 0.264$) or stimuli ($p = 0.347$) for latency of the P1 component. Similarly, there were no significant main effects of diagnosis ($p = 0.190$) or stimulus ($p = 0.0802$) for the N2 peak. For the N4 latency, Levene's Test of Equal Variance determined that there was unequal variance for tones ($p = 0.006$) and vowels ($p = 0.013$). As shown by the individual data points plotted in **Figure 4B**, this difference in variance was due to the expectedly reduced, or absent, N4 response to tones but not vowels in the TD group. A non-parametric Related-Samples Wilcoxon Signed Rank Test revealed a significant effect of stimulus ($p = 0.011$), but not diagnosis ($p = 0.845$), for N4 latency (**Figure 4B**). Bayesian comparisons supported these findings, as shown in **Supplementary Table S1**.

MMN

Mismatch negativity waveform responses (indexing sound discrimination) were observed in the tone and vowel conditions for both groups. Unpaired *t*-tests revealed no significant difference between MMN amplitude between the TD and TSC groups in response to tones [$t(16) = 1.117$, $p = 0.2806$] or to vowels [$t(16) = 1.499$, $p = 0.154$] (**Figure 5**).

A one-way ANOVA exploring possible trends driven by the ASD diagnosis compared the three groups (TD, TSC − ASD, TSC + ASD) and revealed a significant difference between means of the three groups' MMN response to vowels [$F(2,15) = 4.39$, $p < 0.0174$]. *Post hoc* comparisons using the Dunnet's multiple comparisons test indicated that the mean of the TSC + ASD was significantly lower than the TD group ($p = 0.0120$), while the TSC − ASD group did not differ significantly in their MMN response from the TD group ($p > 0.999$) (**Figure 5**). There was no significant difference between the means of the three groups' MMN response to tones [$F(2,15) = 0.929$, $p = 0.416$].

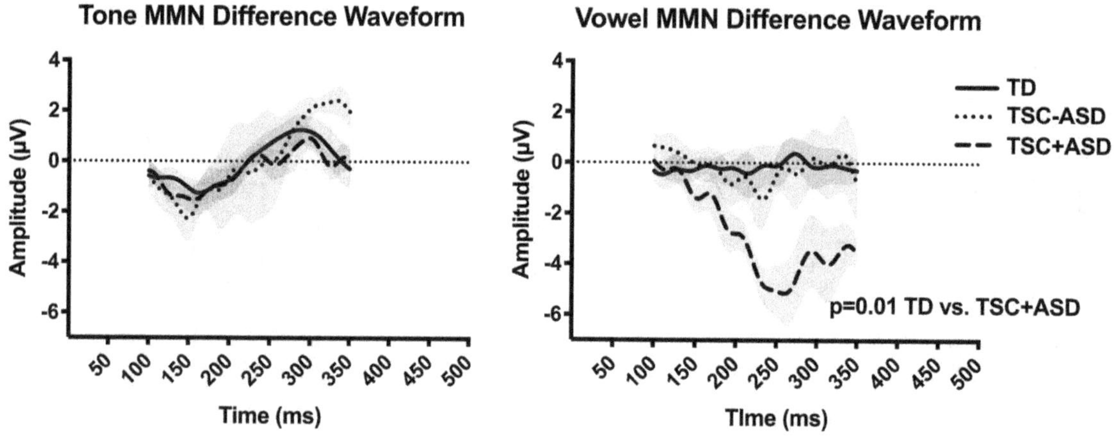

FIGURE 5 | Mismatch negativity difference waveforms (deviant response – standard response) for controls and children with TSC by ASD diagnosis. MMN difference waveforms in microvolts in response to tones and vowels by groups at the right front cluster. No group differences are observed in the MMN response to tones or vowels between typically developing children and children with TSC. When exploring MMN response by ASD diagnosis, there was a significantly enhanced MMN response to vowels, but not tones, in the TSC + ASD group compared to the TD group.

Bayesian comparisons supported these findings, as shown in **Supplementary Table S1**. Averaged difference waveforms for each participant for both tone and speech can be seen in **Supplementary Figure S2**.

DISCUSSION

Children with TSC have altered neural responses to vowels, but not tones, relative to TD children. MVPA suggests above chance decoding of speech vs. tones in the TD group but not in the TSC group. This is supported by AEP waveform analysis demonstrating an enhanced response to vowel sounds relative to tones in TD children but not in children with TSC. In the present study, TD children had an increased P1 amplitude to vowel sounds relative to tones and had a higher N2 amplitude to vowels than children with TSC. As expected, TD children had a reduced or absent N4 response to tones, compared to vowels. Children with TSC, though, did not demonstrate this absent N4 response to tones, and instead had a significantly longer latency for the N4 response than TD children. This could be due to less efficient processing, alternate processing pathways, or impaired conduction of neural signals in this population. These findings, coupled with the reduced connectivity in language related white matter tracts in this population (Lewis et al., 2013), suggest functional differences in basic speech detection for individuals with TSC.

A significant MMN response was elicited by deviant vowels and tones in both groups. We did not find a significant group difference in MMN amplitude or latency between the TD and TSC groups. In contrast to early AEP work in TSC (Seri et al., 1999), we found a preliminary trend toward an enhanced MMN response to vowels in children with TSC + ASD, as compared to the TD group and the TSC – ASD groups. This is consistent with other research that has shown an enhanced MMN in response to changes in speech pitch for children with ASD (Lepisto et al., 2005, 2008). Based on preliminary data, children with TSC + ASD, but not TSC – ASD, appear to have an enhanced attention to pitch change in speech sounds compared to TD children. This increased attention to unexpected speech sounds may contribute to downstream language processing difficulties.

Multivariate pattern analysis broadens traditional evoked potential analyses through the application of an unbiased approach to categorizing signals in both time and space. These results suggest that EEG responses from TD children show above-chance differentiation between stimulus category (speech vs. tones) in both early and late processing and within speech stimuli (/a/vs./u/) during late processing in the right frontal brain region. In contrast, EEG responses from children with TSC did not show this reliable differentiation between these stimuli categories during any time window. These outcomes potentially reflect fewer processing distinctions between speech and tones for individuals with TSC. It is also possible that children with TSC have increased heterogeneity in processing of speech and tones compared to the TD group, which may reduce the overall group-level accuracy of the linear classifier. Children with TSC contributed fewer valid trials to the analysis; although these trial numbers remain high, it is possible that the relatively lower number of valid trials could explain the lack of robust classification between auditory stimuli that was observed in this analysis. By adding MVPA as a complement to traditional methodology, we are taking full advantage of the temporal specificity that is provided from EEG in a manner that is less biased toward specific temporal windows and spatial regions in the data. It also allows for exploring cognitive variation in differentiating between stimuli, which may provide greater insight into cognition than traditional univariate analyses.

Despite the similar language abilities to the controls, as measured by a coarse language survey (**Figure 1**), we still detect basic processing differences between groups. Thus, the evoked responses to speech stimuli could represent a latent endophenotype related to language development more sensitive than overall verbal fluency. Despite the functional speech abilities of most of the participants, all individuals with TSC in our study receive speech-language therapy at school, suggesting the potential for the development of compensatory language processing strategies or language difficulties that were not fully detected by our brief parent survey. Validation of these measures as endophenotypes may provide a sensitive biomarker of language ability that could be used in clinical trials with language related outcome measures.

The apparent speech specific deficits in children with TSC are consistent with broader electrophysiological investigations into sensory processing in TSC. In the visual domain, research has demonstrated that infants with TSC do not have deficits in basic visual processing (i.e., as measured by the VEP in response to a changing checkerboard); however, adults with TSC + ASD do have deficits in socially relevant visual processing (i.e., faces) (Tye et al., 2015; Varcin et al., 2016). The current study explored basic and social processing in the auditory domain for children with TSC and found analogous outcomes: children with TSC do not have deficits in basic auditory processing (i.e., tones), however, they do have deficits in socially relevant auditory processing (i.e., speech sounds). Taken together, these outcomes suggest socially specific processing deficits in both the visual and auditory domains for individuals with TSC.

Limitations

To validate sensory evoked responses for clinical applications, it will be necessary to broaden the study population. Due to inherent challenges associated with recruiting individuals with low-incidence genetic disorders, our sample size is relatively small and spans a wide chronological age range (4–14) and developmental co-morbidity. Further, our preliminary analyses of MMN as driven by a co-diagnosis of TSC + ASD include an even smaller subgroup of participants. Cross-site investigation are currently being undertaken to recruit larger numbers of this rare population, including participants across the developmental and chronological range proposed for clinical interventions in which similar measures are being collected. The age range included in this study spans a range in which there is a maturation of the AEP response, however, age related changes of the waveform are equally reflected in both the TSC and TD populations. Characterization of the speech evoked response across these domains will contextualize its utility as a biomarker.

CONCLUSION

In this paper, we identify electrophysiological responses (P1, N2, N4) to vowel sounds, but not tones, that differentiate children with TSC from age and sex-matched controls. Processing differences suggest that children with TSC do not demonstrate the typical neural differentiation between speech compared to tones. A novel MVPA corroborates these traditional analyses with temporal specificity. The basic auditory processing deficits likely contribute to language difficulties seen in children with TSC and may serve as biomarkers of language impairment in the TSC population. Downstream effects of these basic auditory processing deficits (e.g., at the syllable, word, and sentence level) should be investigated further. Additionally, it is important to explore the responsiveness of these AEP components to behavioral and medical intervention to understand their clinical significance as biomarkers.

ETHICS STATEMENT

The Boston Children's Hospital Institutional Review Board approved this study. Informed written consent was provided by a parent or guardian of each participant. Participants provided written assent as appropriate.

AUTHOR CONTRIBUTIONS

AO'B contributed to the design of the study and analysis, contributed to the collection of the data, contributed to the data analysis and interpretation, and drafted the manuscript. LB contributed to the design of the MVPA analysis. KR contributed to the collection of the data. CN contributed to the collection of the data and revised the manuscript. MS contributed to the study design and revised the manuscript. MM conceived of the study, directed its design, coordination, analysis, and interpretation, and revised the manuscript. All authors read and approved the final version of the manuscript.

FUNDING

Funding for this study was provided by a Pfizer Neuroscience Seed Grant (2015) and by the Clinical and Translational Core of the Boston Children's Hospital IDDRC, U54HD090255.

ACKNOWLEDGMENTS

The authors would like to thank all participants and their families for their involvement in this study. The authors would also like to thank the members of the Laboratory for Cognitive Neuroscience at Boston Children's Hospital for their advice, expertise and support in the design and execution of this study.

SUPPLEMENTARY MATERIAL

FIGURE S1 | Auditory evoked potential response to tones and vowels in the right front electrode cluster. Plots represents trial averaged waveforms from each participant for each stimulus type (tones and vowels). Response to both variants of the stimulus are included in the individual average.

FIGURE S2 | Mismatch negativity difference waveforms (deviant response – standard response) for individual participants of each diagnostic group. Individual averaged waveforms were generated for both the deviant and the standard response and then subtracted for each participant to reveal the difference waveform.

TABLE S1 | Detailed presentation of statistical analyses for each of the results depicted in the figures, including both traditional and Bayesian approaches.

AUDIO S1 | 800Hz.

AUDIO S2 | 400Hz.

AUDIO S3 | /u/.

AUDIO S4 | /a/.

REFERENCES

Bayet, L., Zinszer, B., Pruitt, Z., Aslin, R. N., and Wu, R. (2018). Dynamics of neural representations when searching for exemplars and categories of human and non-human faces. *Sci. Rep.* 8:13277. doi: 10.1038/s41598-018-31526-y

Britton, B., Blumstein, S. E., Myers, E. B., and Grindrod, C. (2009). The role of spectral and durational properties on hemispheric asymmetries in vowel perception. *Neuropsychologia* 47, 1096–1106. doi: 10.1016/j.neuropsychologia.2008.12.033

Cauchoix, M., Barragan-Jason, G., Serre, T., and Barbeau, E. J. (2014). The neural dynamics of face detection in the wild revealed by MVPA. *J. Neurosci.* 34, 846–854. doi: 10.1523/JNEUROSCI.3030-13.2014

Ceponiene, R., Alku, P., Westerfield, M., Torki, M., and Townsend, J. (2005). ERPs differentiate syllable and nonphonetic sound processing in children and adults. *Psychophysiology* 42, 391–406. doi: 10.1111/j.1469-8986.2005.00305.x

Ceponiene, R., Cummings, A., Wulfeck, B., Ballantyne, A., and Townsend, J. (2009). Spectral vs. temporal auditory processing in specific language impairment: a developmental ERP study. *Brain Lang.* 110, 107–120. doi: 10.1016/j.bandl.2009.04.003

Ceponiene, R., Torki, M., Alku, P., Koyama, A., and Townsend, J. (2008). Event-related potentials reflect spectral differences in speech and non-speech stimuli in children and adults. *Clin. Neurophysiol.* 119, 1560–1577. doi: 10.1016/j.clinph.2008.03.005

Choi, Y. J., Di Nardo, A., Kramvis, I., Meikle, L., Kwiatkowski, D. J., Sahin, M., et al. (2008). Tuberous sclerosis complex proteins control axon formation. *Genes Dev.* 22, 2485–2495. doi: 10.1101/gad.1685008

Dobs, K., Isik, L., Pantazis, D., and Kanwisher, N. (2018). How face perception unfolds over time. *bioRxiv* [Preprint]. doi: 10.1101/442194

Ehninger, D., De Vries, P. J., and Silva, A. J. (2009). From mTOR to cognition: molecular and cellular mechanisms of cognitive impairments in tuberous sclerosis. *J. Intellect. Disabil. Res.* 53, 838–851. doi: 10.1111/j.1365-2788.2009.01208.x

Ercan, E., Han, J. M., Di Nardo, A., Winden, K., Han, M. J., Hoyo, L., et al. (2017). Neuronal CTGF/CCN2 negatively regulates myelination in a mouse model of tuberous sclerosis complex. *J. Exp. Med.* 214, 681–697. doi: 10.1084/jem.20160446

Grootswagers, T., Wardle, S. G., and Carlson, T. A. (2017). Decoding dynamic brain patterns from evoked responses: a tutorial on multivariate pattern analysis applied to time series neuroimaging data. *J. Cogn. Neurosci.* 29, 677–697. doi: 10.1162/jocn_a_01068

Holdgraf, C. R., Rieger, J. W., Micheli, C., Martin, S., Knight, R. T., and Theunissen, F. E. (2017). Encoding and decoding models in cognitive electrophysiology. *Front. Syst. Neurosci.* 11:61. doi: 10.3389/fnsys.2017.00061

Isik, L., Meyers, E. M., Leibo, J. Z., and Poggio, T. (2014). The dynamics of invariant object recognition in the human visual system. *J. Neurophysiol.* 111, 91–102. doi: 10.1152/jn.00394.2013

Jeste, S. S., Frohlich, J., and Loo, S. K. (2015). Electrophysiological biomarkers of diagnosis and outcome in neurodevelopmental disorders. *Curr. Opin. Neurol.* 28, 110–116. doi: 10.1097/WCO.0000000000000181

Jeste, S. S., and Nelson, C. A. III (2009). Event related potentials in the understanding of autism spectrum disorders: an analytical review. *J. Autism Dev. Disord.* 39, 495–510. doi: 10.1007/s10803-008-0652-9

Lepisto, T., Kajander, M., Vanhala, R., Alku, P., Huotilainen, M., Naatanen, R., et al. (2008). The perception of invariant speech features in children with autism. *Biol. Psychol.* 77, 25–31. doi: 10.1016/j.biopsycho.2007.08.010

Lepisto, T., Kujala, T., Vanhala, R., Alku, P., Huotilainen, M., and Naatanen, R. (2005). The discrimination of and orienting to speech and non-speech sounds in children with autism. *Brain Res.* 1066, 147–157. doi: 10.1016/j.brainres.2005.10.052

Lewis, W. W., Sahin, M., Scherrer, B., Peters, J. M., Suarez, R. O., Vogel-Farley, V. K., et al. (2013). Impaired language pathways in tuberous sclerosis complex patients with autism spectrum disorders. *Cereb. Cortex* 23, 1526–1532. doi: 10.1093/cercor/bhs135

Mcdonald, N. M., Varcin, K. J., Bhatt, R., Wu, J. Y., Sahin, M., Nelson, C. A. III, et al. (2017). Early autism symptoms in infants with tuberous sclerosis complex. *Autism Res.* 10, 1981–1990. doi: 10.1002/aur.1846

Meikle, L., Talos, D. M., Onda, H., Pollizzi, K., Rotenberg, A., Sahin, M., et al. (2007). A mouse model of tuberous sclerosis: neuronal loss of Tsc1 causes dysplastic and ectopic neurons, reduced myelination, seizure activity, and limited survival. *J. Neurosci.* 27, 5546–5558. doi: 10.1523/jneurosci.5540-06.2007

Naatanen, R., Kujala, T., Escera, C., Baldeweg, T., Kreegipuu, K., Carlson, S., et al. (2012). The mismatch negativity (MMN)–a unique window to disturbed central auditory processing in ageing and different clinical conditions. *Clin. Neurophysiol.* 123, 424–458. doi: 10.1016/j.clinph.2011.09.020

Naatanen, R., Paavilainen, P., Rinne, T., and Alho, K. (2007). The mismatch negativity (MMN) in basic research of central auditory processing: a review. *Clin. Neurophysiol.* 118, 2544–2590. doi: 10.1016/j.clinph.2007.04.026

O'connor, K. (2012). Auditory processing in autism spectrum disorder: a review. *Neurosci. Biobehav. Rev.* 36, 836–854. doi: 10.1016/j.neubiorev.2011.11.008

Peters, J. M., Taquet, M., Prohl, A. K., Scherrer, B., Van Eeghen, A. M., Prabhu, S. P., et al. (2013). Diffusion tensor imaging and related techniques in tuberous sclerosis complex: review and future directions. *Future Neurol.* 8, 583–597. doi: 10.2217/fnl.13.37

Picton, T. W. (2011). "Introduction: past, present, and potential," in *Human Auditory Evoked Potentials*, ed. T. W. Picton (San Diego, CA: Plural Publishing), 1–14.

Prather, P., and De Vries, P. J. (2004). Behavioral and cognitive aspects of tuberous sclerosis complex. *J. Child Neurol.* 19, 666–674. doi: 10.1177/08830738040190090601

Sandoval, S., and Utianski, R. (2015). Average formant trajectories. *J. Phon.* 4, 719–732. doi: 10.1044/2019_pers-sig19-2019-0002

Seri, S., Cerquiglini, A., Pisani, F., and Curatolo, P. (1999). Autism in tuberous sclerosis: evoked potential evidence for a deficit in auditory sensory processing. *Clin. Neurophysiol.* 110, 1825–1830. doi: 10.1016/s1388-2457(99)00137-6

Tavazoie, S. F., Alvarez, V. A., Ridenour, D. A., Kwiatkowski, D. J., and Sabatini, B. L. (2005). Regulation of neuronal morphology and function by the tumor suppressors Tsc1 and Tsc2. *Nat. Neurosci.* 8, 1727–1734. doi: 10.1038/nn1566

Tye, C., Farroni, T., Volein, A., Mercure, E., Tucker, L., Johnson, M. H., et al. (2015). Autism diagnosis differentiates neurophysiological responses to faces in adults with tuberous sclerosis complex. *J. Neurodev. Disord.* 7:33. doi: 10.1186/s11689-015-9129-2

Varcin, K. J., Nelson, C. A. III, Ko, J., Sahin, M., Wu, J. Y., and Jeste, S. S. (2016). Visual evoked potentials as a readout of cortical function in infants with tuberous sclerosis complex. *J. Child Neurol.* 31, 195–202. doi: 10.1177/0883073815587328

16

Auditory EEG Biomarkers in Fragile X Syndrome: Clinical Relevance

Lauren E. Ethridge[1,2], Lisa A. De Stefano[2], Lauren M. Schmitt[3,4], Nicholas E. Woodruff[2], Kara L. Brown[2], Morgan Tran[2], Jun Wang[5], Ernest V. Pedapati[4,6,7], Craig A. Erickson[4,6] and John A. Sweeney[4]*

[1] Department of Pediatrics, Section of Developmental and Behavioral Pediatrics, The University of Oklahoma Health Sciences Center, Oklahoma City, OK, United States, [2] Department of Psychology, The University of Oklahoma, Norman, OK, United States, [3] Division of Developmental and Behavioral Pediatrics, Cincinnati Children's Hospital Medical Center, Cincinnati, OH, United States, [4] Department of Psychiatry and Behavioral Neuroscience, University of Cincinnati, Cincinnati, OH, United States, [5] Department of Psychology, Zhejiang Normal University, Jinhua, China, [6] Division of Child and Adolescent Psychiatry, Cincinnati Children's Hospital Medical Center, Cincinnati, OH, United States, [7] Division of Child Neurology, Cincinnati Children's Hospital Medical Center, Cincinnati, OH, United States

Correspondence:
Lauren E. Ethridge
Lauren-Ethridge@ouhsc.edu

Sensory hypersensitivities are common and distressing features of Fragile X Syndrome (FXS). While there are many drug interventions that reduce behavioral deficits in Fmr1 mice and efforts to translate these preclinical breakthroughs into clinical trials for FXS, evidence-based clinical interventions are almost non-existent potentially due to lack of valid neural biomarkers. Local circuit function in sensory networks is dependent on the dynamic balance of activity in inhibitory/excitatory synapses. Studies are needed to examine the association of electrophysiological alterations in neural systems with sensory and other clinical features of FXS to establish their clinical relevance. Adolescents and adults with FXS (n = 38, Mean age = 25.5, std = 10.1; 13 females) and age matched typically developing controls (n = 40, Mean age = 27.7, std = 12.1; 17 females) completed auditory chirp and auditory habituation tasks while undergoing dense array electroencephalography (EEG). Amplitude, latency, and percent change (habituation) in N1 and P2 event-related potential (ERP) components were characterized for the habituation task; time-frequency calculations using Morlet wavelets characterized phase-locking and single trial power for the habituation and chirp tasks. FXS patients showed increased amplitude but some evidence for reduced habituation of the N1 ERP, and reduced phase-locking in the low and high gamma frequency range and increased low gamma power to the chirp stimulus. FXS showed increased theta power in both tasks. While the habituation finding was weaker than previously found, the remaining findings replicate our previous work in a new sample of patients with FXS. Females showed less deficit in the chirp task but not the habituation task. Abnormal increases in gamma power were related to more severe behavioral and psychiatric features as well as reductions in neurocognitive abilities. Replicating electrophysiological deficits in a new group of patients using different EEG equipment at a new data collection site with differing levels of environmental noise that were robust to data processing techniques utilizing multiple researchers, indicates a potential for scalability to multi-site clinical trials. Given the robust replicability, relevance to clinical measures, and preclinical evidence for sensitivity of these EEG measures to pharmacological intervention, the observed abnormalities may provide novel translational markers of target engagement and potentially outcome measures in large-scale studies evaluating new treatments targeting neural hyperexcitability in FXS.

Keywords: Fragile X Syndrome, EEG, chirp, habituation, gamma, sensory

INTRODUCTION

While there are many drug interventions that reduce behavioral deficits in Fmr1 mice and efforts to translate these preclinical breakthroughs into clinical trials for Fragile X Syndrome (FXS) (Tranfaglia, 2011; Wijetunge et al., 2013; Budimirovic et al., 2017; Berry-Kravis et al., 2018; Erickson et al., 2018), evidence-based clinical interventions are almost non-existent (Berry-Kravis et al., 2018). One advance that may speed progress in treatment development is the establishment of valid biomarkers of brain activity that can be used to stratify patients based on presence of abnormalities targeted by novel drugs (Erickson et al., 2018).

Auditory hypersensitivities and other sensory processing abnormalities are common in FXS as well as idiopathic autism spectrum disorder (ASD) (Takarae et al., 2007, 2014; Hagerman, 2008; Hall et al., 2009; Matsuzaki et al., 2012; Ethridge et al., 2017). Our previous electroencephalography (EEG) and event-related potential (ERP) studies demonstrated electrophysiological phenotypes that show considerable conservation across Fmr1 knock-out (KO) mice and FXS patients, indicating that they may represent promising biomarkers for FXS. However, replication in a larger independent patient population, evaluation of clinical correlates, addressing specificity, and evaluation of scalability considerations in data collection are needed to further validate these evoked EEG measures.

Our previous findings showed significantly increased non-specific gamma activity (gamma single-trial power) in FXS that was associated with a decreased ability to (1) transiently synchronize evoked gamma (the "gamma spike" during early stimulus registration), (2) to synchronize evoked gamma to a rapidly changing oscillatory "chirp" stimulus (Ethridge et al., 2017) and (3) to habituate the neural response to repeated tones (Ethridge et al., 2016). These abnormalities were associated with increased clinical measures of sensory hypersensitivity, suggesting altered gamma oscillations/neural hyper-excitability are a potential biomarker of sensory issues in FXS. Still whether this potential biomarker has clinical relevance beyond sensory issues, including links to cardinal behavioral and cognitive features, remains unknown.

Gamma band activity has established neural mechanisms, which include the local circuit glutamate/GABA interactions involving excitation onto and inhibition originating from parvalbumin positive (PV+) fast-spiking interneurons (the PING model), and mutually connected inhibitory interneurons (the ING model) (Gibson et al., 2008; Cardin et al., 2009; Tiesinga and Sejnowski, 2009). During sensory processing gamma is associated with bottom-up sensory processing of basic stimulus properties (Brosch et al., 2002). Reduced local circuit inhibition via the PING model has been proposed as a neural mechanism for sensory hypersensitivity and neural hyper-excitability in FXS (Gibson et al., 2008; Paluszkiewicz et al., 2011). Importantly, these neural phenotypes have been largely replicated in Fmr1 KO mice, including increased gamma power and abnormal synchronization at both the *in vivo* (Sinclair et al., 2017; Lovelace et al., 2018) and *in vitro* (Goswami et al., 2019) levels. Gamma power and synchronization abnormalities also show preclinical responsiveness to both genetic (Wen et al., 2018) and pharmaceutical (Sinclair et al., 2017; Lovelace et al., 2018) intervention. Together these convergent translational findings suggest altered local inhibitory networks in FXS pathophysiology can be evaluated using electrophysiology, and the findings may be predictive of clinical/behavioral pathologies relevant to drug development and testing.

The current study aimed to replicate previous EEG/ERP results in a larger sample of FXS patients from a different data collection site using different EEG equipment. The larger sample also enabled evaluation of gender differences in these phenotypes. In our previous preliminary study, clinical evaluation to establish correlation with electrophysiology was modest. In the current study, considerably more clinical data was collected to better establish the relevance of traditional electrophysiological measures with psychological and behavioral measures. We hypothesized that gamma measures would largely replicate in the new sample, be associated with both sensory and behavioral clinical measures, and be robust to reasonable levels of variability introduced by larger-scale data collection and analysis efforts. We further predicted that females with FXS would show reduced EEG/ERP abnormalities relative to males with FXS, consistent with reduced clinical/behavioral impairment in the majority of females with FXS.

MATERIALS AND METHODS

Participants

Thirty-eight adolescents and adults with full mutation FXS [Mean (M) age = 25.5, standard deviation (SD) = 10.1; age range 10–53; 13 females] and 40 age- and sex-matched typically developing controls (M age = 27.7, SD = 12.1; age range 12–57; 17 females) participated in the study (**Table 1**). Most participants completed both habituation and chirp EEG tasks, but see **Table 1** for exact demographic breakdown per

Abbreviations: Db, decibels; EEG, electroencephalography; ERP, event-related potential; FXS, Fragile X Syndrome; GLU, glutamate; Hz, Hertz; ICA, independent components analysis; IQ, intelligence quotient; ITC, inter-trial coherence; KO, knockout; Ms, milliseconds; PCA, principal components analysis; PV+, parvalbumin positive; SCQ, social communication questionnaire; SNR, signal-to-noise ratio; STP, single trial power.

TABLE 1 | Participant characteristics.

	FXS n = 38 (13 females)				**Controls n = 40 (17 females)**			
	Mean	**Std. Dev.**	**Range**		**Mean**	**Std. Dev.**	**Range**	***t* Statistic (df)**
Total sample								
Age	25.5	10.1	10 to 53	Age	27.7	12.1	12 to 57	$t(76) = 0.9, p = 0.37$
Full scale IQ	60.3	20.9	47 to 115	Full Scale IQ	103.8	10.4	85 to 124	$t(73) = 11.5, p < 0.001$
Verbal Z	−3.0	1.9	−6.5 to 0.2	Verbal Z	0.14	0.71	−1.4 to 2	$t(71) = 9.4, p < 0.001$
Non-verbal Z	−4.6	2.4	−8.6 to −0.4	Non-verbal Z	0.21	0.76	−1.1 to 1.8	$t(71) = 11.2, p < 0.001$
Deviation IQ	41.7	28.9	−10.8 to 94.1	Deviation IQ	102.7	8.4	88.9 to 120.8	$t(71) = 11.9, p < 0.001$
SCQ	14.0	7.9	1 to 29	SCQ	2.2	2.4	0 to 8	$t(63) = 8.0, p < 0.001$
	FXS n = 30 (12 females)				**Controls n = 37 (16 females)**			
	Mean	**Std. Dev.**	**Range**		**Mean**	**Std. Dev.**	**Range**	***t* Statistic (df)**
Participants completing habituation task								
Age	25.7	10.5	13 to 53	Age	26.8	11.9	12 to 45	$t(65) = 0.4, p = 0.69$
Full scale IQ	62.4	21.6	47 to 115	Full scale IQ	103.1	9.9	85 to 124	$t(62) = 10.1, p < 0.001$
Verbal Z	−2.8	1.8	−6.5 to −0.3	Verbal Z	0.1	0.6	−1.4 to 1.5	$t(60) = 8.9, p < 0.001$
Non-verbal Z	−4.6	2.6	−8.6 to −0.4	Non-verbal Z	0.2	0.8	−1.1 to 1.8	$t(60) = 10.3, p < 0.001$
Deviation IQ	43.7	30.2	−10.8 to 94.1	Deviation IQ	102.1	8.1	88.9 to 120.8	$t(60) = 11.1, p < 0.001$
SCQ	13.8	8.1	1 to 29	SCQ	2.3	2.4	0 to 8	$t(54) = 7.7, p < 0.001$
	FXS n = 36 (13 females)				**Controls n = 39 (17 females)**			
	Mean	**Std. Dev.**	**Range**		**Mean**	**Std. Dev.**	**Range**	***t* Statistic (df)**
Participants completing chirp task								
Age	25.4	10.2	10 to 53	Age	27.9	12.2	12 to 57	$t(73) = 0.9, p = 0.33$
Full scale IQ	60.7	20.4	47 to 115	Full scale IQ	104.2	10.2	85 to 124	$t(71) = 11.8, p < 0.001$
Verbal Z	−3.0	1.9	−6.5 to 0.2	Verbal Z	0.2	0.7	−1.4 to 2.0	$t(69) = 9.6, p < 0.001$
Non-verbal Z	−4.5	2.4	−8.6 to −0.4	Non-verbal Z	0.2	0.7	−1.1 to 1.8	$t(69) = 11.6, p < 0.001$
Deviation IQ	42.4	29.1	−10.8 to 94.1	Deviation IQ	102.9	8.3	88.9 to 120.8	$t(69) = 12.3, p < 0.001$
SCQ	14.0	7.9	1 to 29	SCQ	2.2	2.4	0 to 8	$t(62) = 8.2, p < 0.001$

SCQ, social and communication questionnaire.

task. Groups did not differ on proportion of each sex either overall (chi square = 0.57, p = 0.45), for the habituation task (chi square = 0.07, p = 0.79) or for the chirp task (chi square = 0.44, p = 0.51). Typically developing controls (TDC) had no known prior diagnosis or treatment for neuropsychiatric illness (reported via clinical history interview with parent or participant as appropriate). Exclusion criteria included history of seizures and current use of medications with known EEG effects, including anticonvulsant medications and benzodiazepines. Five patients were receiving atypical antipsychotics, 8 antidepressants, 8 both antipsychotics and antidepressants all on a stable dose for at least 4 weeks (see **Supplementary Table 1** for a complete list). While medication effects cannot be ruled out, removing patients based on presence of commonly prescribed psychiatric medications would produce a sample that is non-representative of the FXS population. Our previous work and other EEG studies of these drugs in psychiatric research suggest they do not have significant confounding effects on electrophysiology as measured in the current study (Mitra et al., 2015; Ahnaou et al., 2016; Clementz et al., 2016; Ethridge et al., 2016, 2017); we also did not find any significant differences between medicated and non-medicated patients on any of the EEG variables studied here.

Primary caregivers completed the following clinical assessment measures for FXS patients: The Caregiver Report Adolescent and Adult Sensory Profile (Brown et al., 2001), the Social and Communication Questionnaire (SCQ; Rutter et al., 2003), Anxiety Depression and Mood Scale (ADAMS, Esbensen et al., 2003), Aberrant Behavior Checklist-Community (ABC-C, optimized for FXS, Sansone et al., 2012). We also administered the Woodcock-Johnson III Tests of Cognitive Abilities Auditory Attention subscale (McGrew and Woodcock, 2001), the Vineland Adaptive Behavior Scales (Sparrow et al., 2005) and the computerized Test of Attentional Performance for Children (KiTAP, Knox et al., 2012). IQ was assessed for both FXS and TDC with the Stanford-Binet Intelligence Scale 5th Ed. Abbreviated IQ (Roid, 2003) using deviation scores for calculating verbal and non-verbal IQ in the lower IQ range using the technique proposed by Sansone et al. (2014). Typically developing controls completed the SCQ, ADAMS, ABC-C, and KiTAP. All participants provided written informed consent (caregiver with assent or individual consent as appropriate) prior to participation, as approved by the Cincinnati Children's Hospital Institutional Review Board.

Procedure

Habituation Task

The auditory habituation stimulus consisted of 150 stimulus trains of four 50 ms duration white noise bursts separated by 500 ms inter-stimulus intervals. Each stimulus train was separated by a 4000 ms inter-trial interval. Habituation in this task is characterized as the change in ERP amplitude for each repetition in a stimulus train compared to the ERP amplitude to the initial stimulus in a train (e.g., initial N1 to 2nd N1, 3rd N1, and 4th N1).

Chirp Task

The auditory chirp stimulus consisted of a white noise burst carrier stimulus amplitude modulated by a sinusoid linearly increasing in frequency from 0 to 100 Hz over 2000 ms (16). Chirp stimuli were presented 200 times each separated by an inter-trial interval randomly jittered between 1500 and 2000 ms. For both EEG tasks, stimuli were delivered at 65 db SPL through headphones. Participants watched a silent movie during testing to facilitate compliance with testing procedures as in prior studies (Ethridge et al., 2016, 2017).

ERP Recording

EEG was continuously recorded and digitized at 1000 Hz, filtered from 0.01 to 200 Hz, referenced to Cz, and amplified 10,000x using a 128 channel saline-based Electrical Geodesics system (EGI, Eugene, Oregon) with sensors placed approximately according to the International 10/10 system (42% of sensors in 128 channel EGI Hydrocel nets have 10–10 equivalents, while an additional 42% are within a 2 cm tolerance; Chatrian, 1985; Luu and Ferree, 2005).

EEG Analysis

Raw data were visually inspected offline. Bad sensors were interpolated (no more than 5% per subject, no more than two adjacent, 90% of participants had no sensors interpolated within the 23 channels used in the final analyses) using spherical spline interpolation implemented in BESA 6.1 (MEGIS Software, Grafelfing, Germany). Data were digitally filtered from 0.5 to 120 Hz (12 and 24 db/octave roll-off, respectively; zero-phase; 60 Hz notch). Eye movement, cardiac, and muscle movement artifacts were removed blind to participant group using independent components analysis (ICA; Infomax) implemented in EEGLAB (Delorme and Makeig, 2004) using Matlab (The Mathworks, Natick, MA, United States). Segments of data with large amounts of movement artifact were removed prior to ICA to facilitate algorithm convergence. For both tasks, data were then transformed to average reference and epoched into 3250 ms trials (−500 to 2750 ms). For ERP analyses, data were averaged across trials and baseline-corrected using the 500 ms pre-stimulus period. Any trial with post-ICA amplitude exceeding 120 μV was considered residual artifact and removed prior to averaging. ERP averages for the habituation task were then low-pass filtered at 40 Hz for ERP analyses, while chirp averages and single trial power data for both tasks were retained at a low-pass filter of 120 Hz. Number of valid trials retained after artifact correction was higher for controls compared to FXS for the habituation task (FXS M = 105.5, SD = 22.4; Control M = 119.6, SD = 20.2, $t(66)$ = 2.7, p = 0.008) and the chirp task (FXS M = 128.7, SD = 34.8; Control M = 152.9, SD = 32.7, $t(75)$ = 3.2, p = 0.002), therefore trial count was evaluated as a covariate for all analyses and retained when significant.

Analyses in our previous studies used spatial principal components analysis (PCA) on the grand average ERP in order to create component weights using all sensors (Ethridge et al., 2016, 2017). However, the use of data-driven analyses is ultimately not scalable to clinical trials, which require *a priori* thresholds and defined regions of interest that can be calculated at the individual level without waiting for availability of large group averages for patient stratification. Therefore, we selected and averaged over 23 sensors distributed across the fronto-central scalp *a priori* based on the spatial distribution most consistent with previous literature capturing auditory cortex activity (**Figure 1**; Luck, 2014) and the peak of spatial activity from our previous PCA results (Ethridge et al., 2016, 2017). All analyses were conducted on data averaged over the same 23 sensors for both tasks.

For both tasks, un-baseline-corrected epoched single-trial data were analyzed in the time-frequency domain using Morlet wavelets with 1 Hz frequency step using a linearly increasing cycle length from 1 cycle at the lowest frequency (2 Hz) to 30 cycles at the highest (120 Hz). Single-trial power (STP) and inter-trial coherence (ITC) measures obtained from this method evaluated the amplitude of response at each frequency and how stable or phase-locked responses were to the auditory stimuli across trials, respectively (Delorme and Makeig, 2004). Raw ITC values were initially corrected for trial number by subtracting the critical r value, calculated as sqrt[-1/(number of trials)*log(0.5)], for each subject based on trial count. STP and ITC values were averaged over trials for each individual and transformed into time-frequency plots down-sampled to 250 time-bins.

Single trial power was then baseline corrected using the pre-stimulus period, up to 50 ms prior to stimulus onset, to avoid windowing effects from stimulus onset-related activity. Subsequent analyses followed the same method as those done with non-baseline corrected single trial power.

Statistical Analysis

For habituation ERP analyses, the waveform components of interest were the N1 and P2 components for the initial stimulus and each repeated stimulus in the stimulus train. N1 and P2 peaks were defined as the minimum and maximum amplitudes, respectively, in a time window centered on the grand average peak amplitude $\pm$ 40 ms. Amplitude and latency were calculated for each participant average at each peak. Separate mixed effects ANOVAs were calculated for amplitude and latency of each peak with the between subjects factors group (FXS, TDC) and gender (M,F) and within subjects factor stimulus repetition (initial stimulus, repetition 1, repetition 2, repetition 3). Differences in habituation of the N1 and P2 waveforms were calculated as the group by stimulus repetition interaction, indicating a difference between groups in the change in amplitude or latency

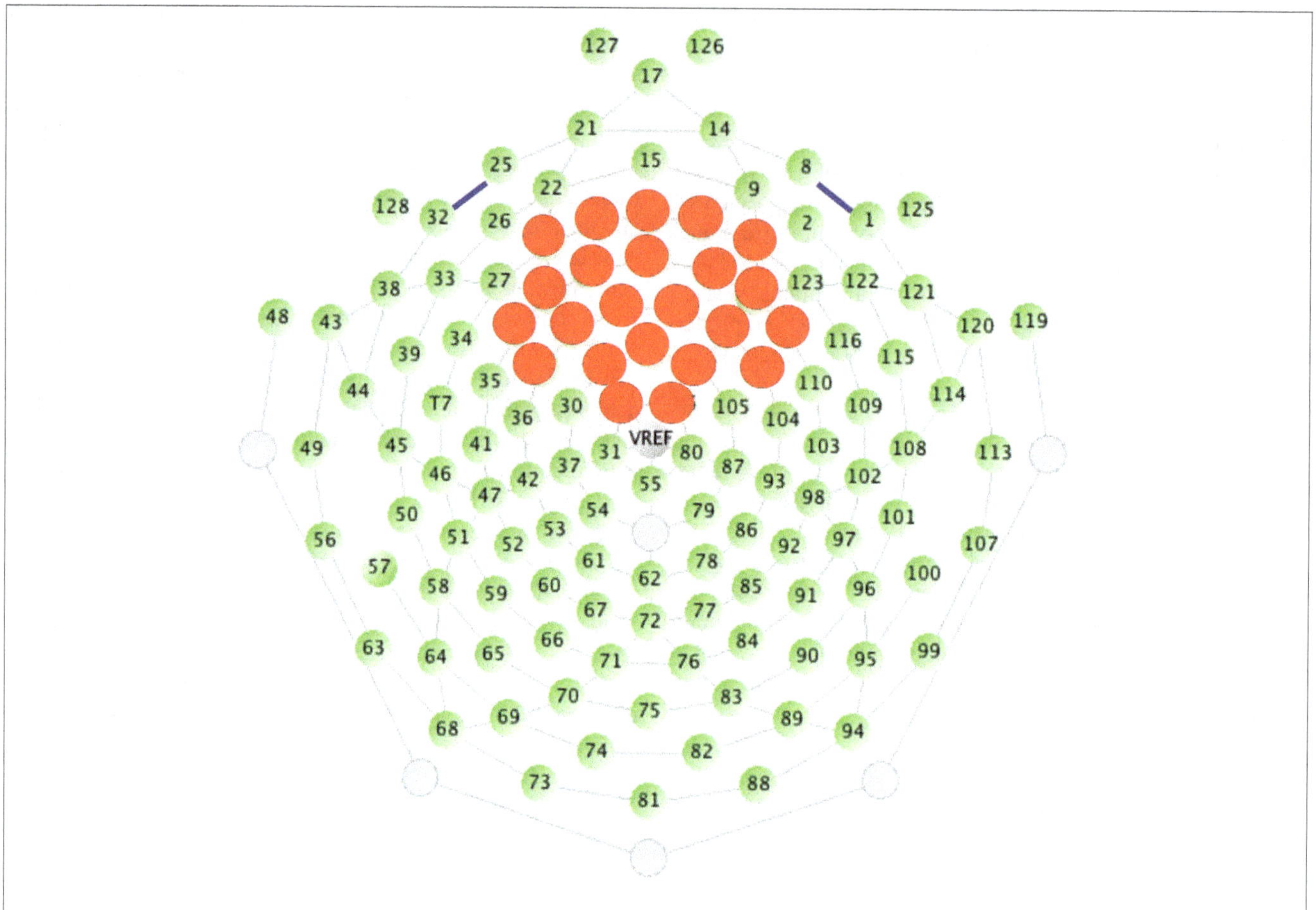

FIGURE 1 | Sensor layout for the EGI 128 channel system with selected sensors analyzed highlighted in red. Sensors were selected based on the traditional location of the N1 ERP component, originating from auditory cortices, and from previous work.

across repetitions. Habituation was also calculated as percent change in N1 amplitude across repetitions, to match with our previous work.

For single-trial EEG analyses for both tasks, point-by-point two-tailed t-tests were used to calculate group differences across the time-frequency matrix. Time-frequency clustering techniques and Monte Carlo simulations controlled for multiple comparisons (Ethridge et al., 2012, 2017). To maintain a family-wise alpha of $p < 0.01$ (corrected for multiple comparisons), a minimum of three sequential time-bins and three adjacent frequencies were required to be significant at a nominal threshold of $p < 0.05$. Data were then averaged within each cluster to produce a single value for clinical correlations as well as univariate ANOVAs with fixed factors of group and gender. For all analyses, trial number and age were evaluated as covariates and retained in the model when significant. Effect sizes are reported as partial eta squared. Means presented are estimated marginal means.

Clinical correlations were examined with all significant variables. We also examined exploratory correlations between power in all frequency bands (theta, alpha, beta, gamma) and hypothesis-driven associations between gamma STP and gamma ITC. All correlations were conducted using Spearman's rho. Clinical correlations and power band correlations were considered to be exploratory and hypothesis generating, and thus not corrected for multiple comparisons.

RESULTS

Participant Demographics

There were no significant differences between FXS and TDC in age or proportion of gender. As expected with this clinical sample, FXS had significantly lower IQ scores and significantly higher number of autism-like symptoms on the SCQ than TDC (see **Table 1** for detail).

EEG

Habituation

For N1 amplitude (**Figure 2**), there was a main effect of group, $F(1,62) = 11.833$, $p = 0.001$, ES = 0.16 indicating that FXS patients had larger N1 amplitudes ($M = -1.47$ μV, standard error (SE) = 0.13) than TDC ($M = -0.85$ μV, SE = 0.12). There was a marginal main effect of repetition $F(3,186) = 2.5$, $p = 0.05$, ES = 0.04 with a significant linear contrast $F(1,62) = 6.07$, $p = 0.02$, ES = 0.09. Pairwise comparisons to further examine this

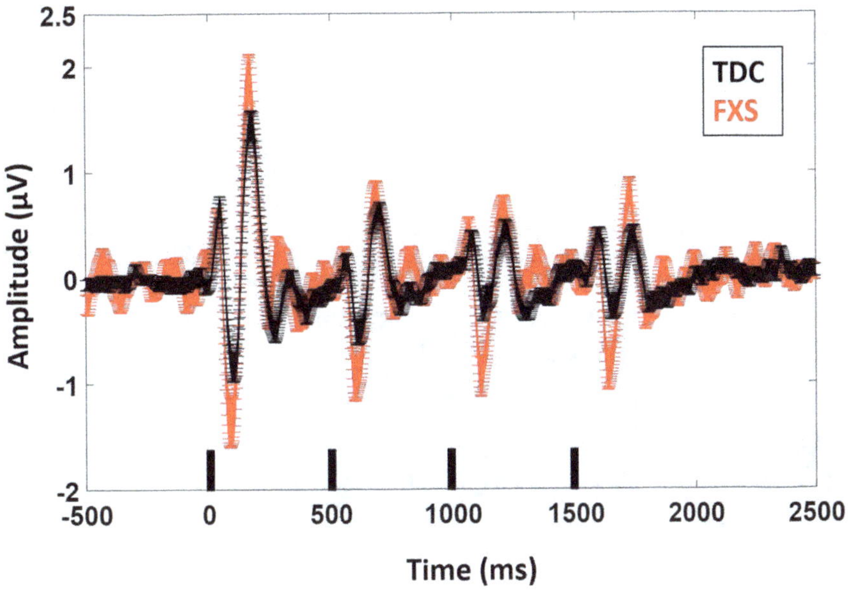

FIGURE 2 | ERP average waveforms for FXS and TDC for the habituation task. Black marks along the x-axis indicate stimulus timing for the four stimuli in each train. Error bars indicate standard error of the mean. Note the increased N1 (negative peaks) and P2 (positive peaks) amplitude in FXS relative to TDC.

combination of effects indicated that N1 amplitude significantly ($p < 0.001$ for all repetitions) decreased across repetitions relative to the initial stimulus onset, but repetitions did not differ from each other, describing the plateau effect of subsequent repetitions: (N1 initial stimulus $M = -1.60$ μV, SE = 0.13; N1 repetition 1 $M = -1.12$ μV, SE = 0.10, N1 repetition 2 $M = -0.99$ μV, SE = 0.09, N1 repetition 3 $M = -0.91$ μV, SE = 0.09). There was no group by repetition effect, $F(3,189) = 0.60$, $p = 0.61$, ES = 0.01 suggesting that while FXS had larger N1 amplitudes overall, they did not habituate differently from TDC across repetitions. A repetition by gender effect $F(3,186) = 2.67$, $p = 0.048$, ES = 0.04 suggests that females plateau more strongly than males, who continue to decrease N1 amplitude across repetitions. Age was a significant covariate in the model $F(1,62) = 7.13$, $p = 0.01$, ES = 0.10, consistent with the literature that supports effects of age on N1 amplitude (Pang and Taylor, 2000), however age did not interact significantly with repetition effects ($p = 0.21$). There was no significant effect of trial count ($p = 0.63$). Similarly to our previous findings, we also quantified N1 habituation as percent change from N1 for the initial stimulus to each subsequent stimulus, however, FXS and TDC also did not differ on this comparison, $F(2,124) = 0.61$, $p = 0.55$, ES = 0.01 across all repetitions. Estimated marginal means for this comparison did show a large difference at the final repetition (percent reduction from initial stimulus to the last repetition in the train: FXS $M = 25\%$, SE = 8%; TDC $M = 51\%$, SE = 8%), suggesting that while it was not a strong effect, FXS may have shown decreased habituation relative to TDC by the end of the stimulus train. There were no differences between groups for N1 latency. There were no significant effects of age or trial count on percent change or N1 latency (p's > 0.10).

Results were similar for P2 amplitude: there was a main effect of group, $F(1,63) = 7.5$, $p = 0.008$, ES = 0.11 indicating that FXS had larger P2 amplitudes ($M = 1.37$, SE = 0.10) than TDC ($M = 0.99$, SE = 0.09). There was a main effect of repetition, $F(3,189) = 75.35$, $p < 0.001$, ES = 0.55 indicating habituation of the P2 amplitude across repetitions (P2 initial stimulus $M = 1.95$, SE = 0.13; P2 repetition 1 $M = 0.99$, SE = 0.07, P2 repetition 2 $M = 0.94$, SE = 0.06, P2 repetition 3 $M = 0.85$, SE = 0.07). Again there were no group by repetition or gender effects, suggesting that although FXS patients had larger P2 amplitudes, they did not habituate differently. Age was not a significant covariate ($p < 0.10$). There was a main effect of group for P2 latency $F(1,62) = 5.2$, $p = 0.03$, ES = 0.08 such that FXS ($M = 173.1$ ms, SE = 2.47) had faster latencies than TDC ($M = 180.7$ ms, SE = 2.2). Age was a significant covariate $F(1,62) = 4.09$, $p = 0.04$, ES = 0.06. There were no significant effects of trial count on P2 amplitude or latency (p's > 0.05).

Point-by-point t-tests on non-baseline-corrected time-frequency plots for ITC and STP (corrected for multiple comparisons) revealed 3 time-frequency clusters with significant differences between FXS and TDC (**Figure 3**), all of which were in single trial power. Power values differences were largely consistent across the entire trial, including in the baseline, so values for each cluster were averaged across the entire trial and significant frequency range. For each of these comparisons, trial number was a significant covariate and retained in the analyses, but age was not a significant covariate. For theta (3–7 Hz) power, there was a main effect of group, $F(1,62) = 9.12$, $p = 0.004$, ES = 0.13 indicating that when correcting for number of trials, FXS ($M = 50.9$, SE = 0.44) showed higher theta power than TDC ($M = 49.1$, SE = 0.39).

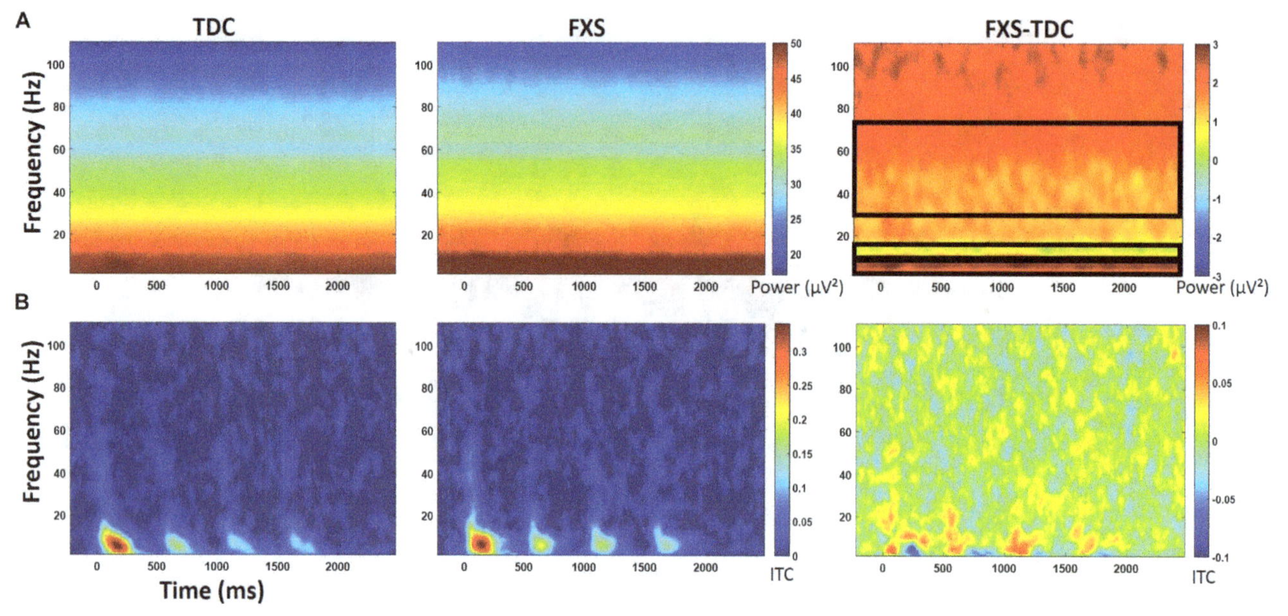

FIGURE 3 | (A) Single trial power (STP) for TDC, FXS, and difference maps (FXS minus TDC) for the habituation task. **(B)** Inter-trial coherence (ITC) for TDC, FXS, and difference maps (FXS minus TDC) for the habituation task. Black boxes in the difference maps indicate clusters with significant group differences. Warmer colors (reds, yellows) in the difference maps (right column) indicate higher phase-locking or higher power for FXS and cooler colors (blues, greens) indicate higher values for TDC.

There were no gender effects on theta power. For alpha (8–12 Hz) power, however, there was no main effect of group, but a group by gender interaction, $F(1,62) = 4.81$, $p = 0.03$, ES = 0.07. FXS females ($M = 49.2$, SE = 0.82) showed higher alpha power than TDC females ($M = 46.5$, SE = 0.75) while FXS males ($M = 48.07$, SE = 0.69) and TDC males did not differ ($M = 48.46$, SE = 0.61). For gamma (31–70 Hz) power across the entire trial, there was a marginal effect of group, $F(1,62) = 3.6$, $p = 0.06$, ES = 0.05 indicating that FXS patients ($M = 33.6$, SE = 0.42) had marginally higher gamma power than TDC ($M = 32.5$, SE = 0.38). While there was a main effect of gender, $F(1,62) = 5.63$, $p = 0.02$, ES = 0.08 (males have more power than females), there was no interaction between group and gender.

For baseline-corrected single-trial power, FXS showed increased power in the beta/low gamma range (23–33 Hz) during stimulus onset for the initial stimulus only, $F(1,63) = 10.97$, $p = 0.002$, ES = 0.15. There were no effects of age, trial count, or gender on this comparison.

Chirp

Point-by-point t-tests on time-frequency plots for ITC and STP (corrected for multiple comparisons) revealed 4 time-frequency clusters with significant differences between FXS and TDC (**Figure 4**). There was a main effect of group for alpha band (6–13 Hz) phase-locking (ITC) to the onset of the stimulus (92–308 ms post-stimulus), $F(1,70) = 7.12$, $p = 0.009$, ES = 0.09 indicating that FXS ($M = 0.14$, SE = 0.01) showed stronger phase-locking to the stimulus onset than did TDC ($M = 0.09$, SE = 0.01), consistent with habituation findings of increased ERP amplitude to auditory stimuli. Age was a significant covariate $F(1,70) = 5.55$, $p = 0.02$, ES = 0.07. There was a main effect of group for phase-locking (ITC) to the chirp stimulus (676–1066 ms post-stimulus, while the stimulus was in the low gamma oscillatory range) in the low gamma (31–57 Hz) band, $F(1,71) = 5.65$, $p = 0.02$, ES = 0.07 indicating that FXS ($M = 0.11$, SE = 0.01) were less able to lock in to the chirp oscillatory stimulus than TDC ($M = 0.15$, SE = 0.01). There was also a group by gender interaction, $F(1,71) = 5.00$, $p = 0.03$, ES = 0.07 indicating that while both males and females with FXS had lower phase-locking values, FXS females ($M = 0.13$, SE = 0.02) were more similar to both TDC females ($M = 0.14$, SE = 0.02) and TDC males ($M = 0.16$, SE = 0.02) than were FXS males ($M = 0.08$, SE = 0.02). Age was not a significant covariate ($p = 0.97$).

Gender effects were also found for ongoing (entire trial) theta power (3–7 Hz) during the chirp stimulus. First, there was a main effect of group, $F(1,70) = 8.39$, $p = 0.005$, ES = 0.11 indicating that FXS ($M = 50.68$, SE = 0.43) had higher theta (3–7 Hz) power than TDC ($M = 48.93$, SE = 0.40). There was also a group by gender interaction, $F(1,70) = 5.74$, $p = 0.02$, ES = 0.08. FXS females ($M = 51.33$, SE = 0.67) showed more theta power than TDC females ($M = 48.19$, SE = 0.58) while FXS ($M = 50.03$, SE = 0.53) and TDC ($M = 49.65$, SE = 0.52) males did not differ. For theta power, trial number was a significant covariate $F(1,70) = 7.1$, $p = 0.01$, ES = 0.09, and was retained in the analyses but age was not ($p = 0.74$).

For ongoing (entire trial) gamma (31–70 Hz) power, there was a main effect of group, $F(1,71) = 7.4$, $p = 0.008$, ES = 0.09 indicating that FXS ($M = 33.58$, SE = 0.32) showed

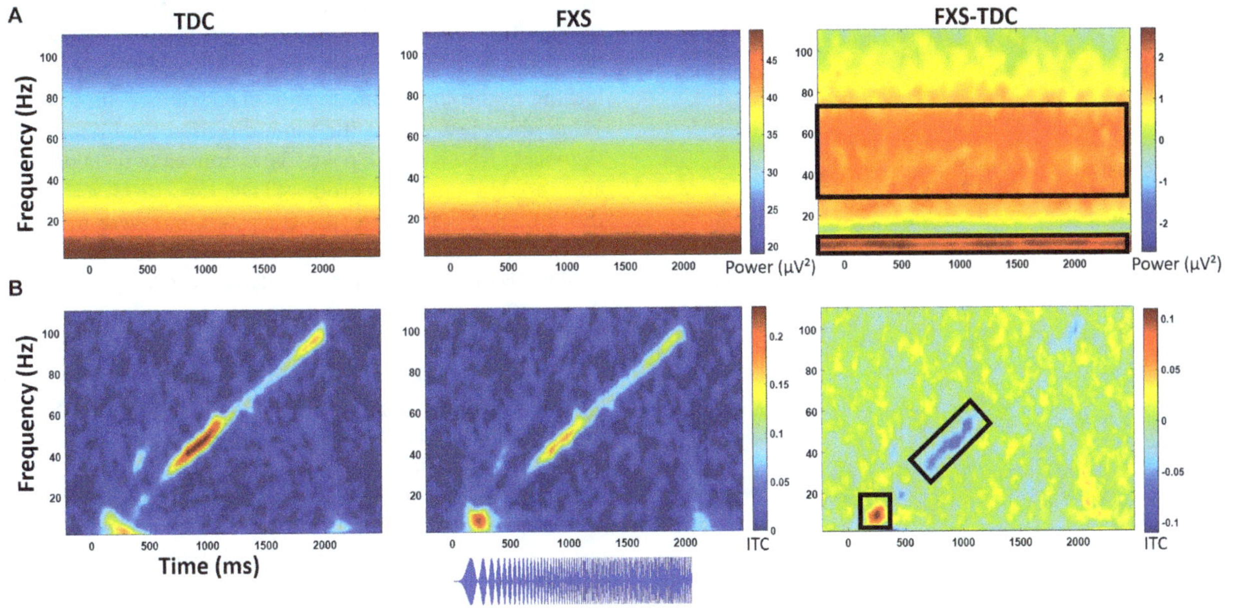

FIGURE 4 | (A) Single trial power (STP) for TDC, FXS, and difference maps (FXS minus TDC) for the chirp task. **(B)** Inter-trial coherence (ITC) for TDC, FXS, and difference maps (FXS minus TDC) for the chirp task. Black boxes in the difference maps indicate clusters with significant group differences. Warmer colors (reds, yellows) in the difference maps (right column) indicate higher phase-locking or higher power for FXS and cooler colors (blues, greens) indicate higher values for TDC. Chirp stimulus schematic is represented bottom center relative to x-axis timing.

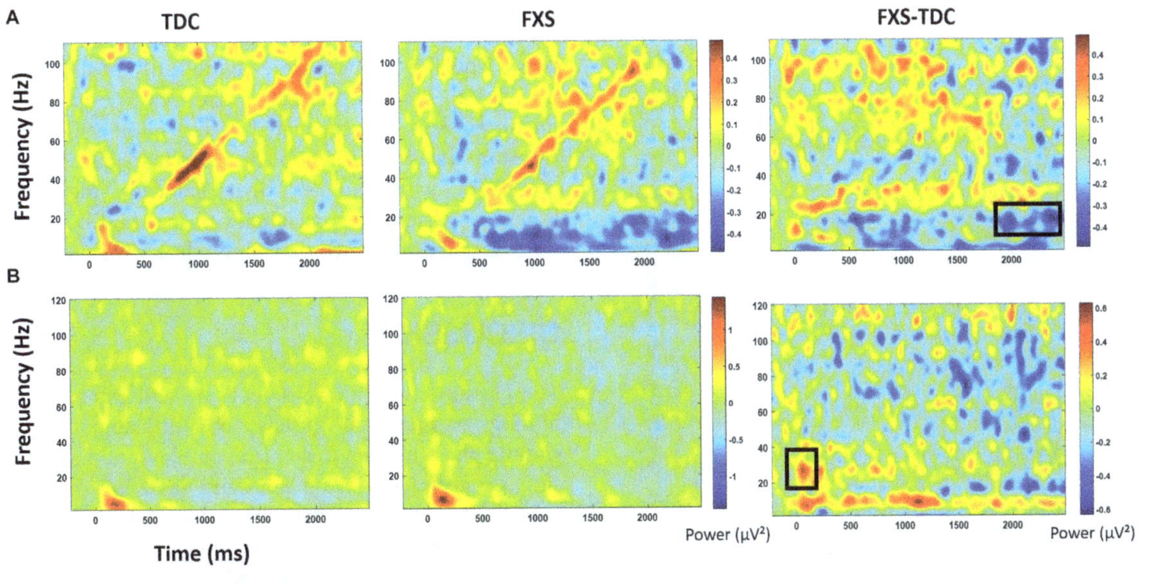

FIGURE 5 | Baseline corrected single trial power for the chirp task **(A)** and the habituation task **(B)** for TDC, FXS, and difference maps (FXS minus TDC). Black boxes in the difference maps indicate clusters with significant group differences. Warmer colors (reds, yellows) in the difference maps (right column) indicate higher power for FXS and cooler colors (blues, greens) indicate higher values for TDC.

more gamma power than TDC (M = 32.41, SE = 0.29). While there was a main effect of gender on gamma power, $F(1,71) = 6.21$, $p = 0.02$, ES = 0.08 (males have more gamma power than females in general), there was no interaction between gender and group. Age was not a significant covariate ($p = 0.07$).

For baseline-corrected single trial power (**Figure 5**), FXS showed a decrease in alpha/beta power (11–20 Hz) which became significantly different from TDC during the time period surrounding stimulus offset (~2000 to 2500 ms), $F(1,71) = 15.44$, $p < 0.001$, ES = 0.18. There were no effects of age, trial count, or gender on this group difference.

TABLE 2 | Significant clinical correlations for FXS patients.

EEG measure	SCQ total score	Deviation IQ	ABC irritability	ABC stereotopy	ABC hyperactivity	ABC inappropriate Speech	WJIII	Vineland Comm	Vineland DL	Vineland Social	Vineland Comp
Habituation											
N1 amplitude							−0.56**				
P2 amplitude											
% habituation S1–S4	0.62**								−0.48*	−0.42*	
STP theta								−0.53**	−0.45*	−0.43*	−0.49*
STP alpha								−0.43*			
STP gamma		−0.43*						−0.47*	−0.44*		−0.42*
Chirp											
ITC stimulus onset							0.47*				
ITC 40 Hz chirp	−0.53**						0.49**		0.36*	0.38*	
STP theta							0.46*				
STP gamma		−0.54**	0.37*	0.42*	0.39*	0.41*		−0.37*	−0.41*		

*Clinical variables with no significant correlations to EEG variables are not included. All correlations are Spearman's rho. All correlations represent the FXS group only. Due to the negative amplitude of the N1 ERP, negative correlations should be viewed as increased N1 amplitude correlating with increased scores on the clinical/behavioral measure. Blank = N.S. *p < 0.05, **p < 0.01.*

Gamma Power and Phase-Locking

For the chirp stimulus, increased gamma single trial power across the entire trial was correlated with decreased gamma phase-locking to the chirp stimulus for TDC (rho = −0.34, p = 0.04). While the effect was in the same direction for FXS, it was not significant (rho = −0.22, p = 0.21). Gamma and theta power were also correlated for both groups (TDC rho = 0.34, p = 0.04; FXS rho = 0.35, p = 0.03) for the chirp task but were marginal for habituation. Gamma power was also correlated with beta power (13–30 Hz) for both groups (TDC rho = 0.61, $p < 0.001$; FXS rho = 0.49, p = 0.002), but while gamma power was also correlated with alpha power in TDC (rho = 0.50, p = 0.001), it was not for FXS (rho = 0.23, p = 0.18). Measures which were captured in both tasks (single trial power for gamma and theta bands) showed good correlation across tasks for both FXS and TDC. Gamma power (TD rho = 0.71, $p < 0.001$, FXS rho = 0.76, $p < 0.001$), and theta power (TD rho = 0.67, $p < 0.001$, FXS rho = 0.71, $p < 0.001$) both showed strong correlation between chirp and habituation tasks, suggesting good fidelity and test-retest reliability not just in these measures but also in the multiple-user blinded data processing approach utilized for this study.

Exploratory Clinical Correlations

Significant correlations of electrophysiology data with clinical and behavioral measures in FXS participants are presented in **Tables 2–7**. Correlations are presented for all FXS patients first, then because gender and clinical/cognitive ability can be confounded in FXS, separated by gender. Increased gamma power and theta power were significantly related to a number of clinical ratings, including the ABC. Vineland subscale measures were also correlated with a number of spectral EEG measures across habituation and chirp tasks, primarily driven by correlations within female patients. Behavioral measures from the KiTAP were strongly correlated with spectral EEG measures, but most strongly correlated variables differed by gender.

DISCUSSION

The current study findings replicate and extend our previous findings of increased auditory N1 ERP amplitude, decreased gamma phase locking to a chirp stimulus, and increased gamma single trial power during the chirp task. We did not strongly replicate our prior finding of reduced habituation, although the general patterns seen across ERP repetitions is remarkably similar between our original study and the current. We utilized a larger sample in this study, enabling studies of effects in females who are underrepresented in the FXS research literature, and explored correlations of electrophysiological abnormalities with clinical and behavioral alterations associated with FXS. As this replication study was conducted using a new EEG system, different staff collecting and analyzing EEG data, these findings indicate both clinical scalability and clinical relevance of the electrophysiological findings.

Increased N1 ERP amplitude in FXS was replicated in this larger new sample, and we additionally found increased P2 ERP amplitude in FXS relative to TDC. In our previous work we found

TABLE 3 | Significant clinical correlations for FXS patients – males only.

EEG measure	SCQ total score	ABC social withdrawal	WJIII	Vineland DL	Vineland social	Vineland Comp
Habituation						
N1 amplitude	0.63*		−0.82**			
P2 amplitude		−0.52*				
% habituation S1–S4	0.77**			−0.69**	−0.61**	−0.48*
STP theta						
STP alpha						
STP gamma						
Chirp						
ITC stimulus onset			0.49*			
ITC 40 Hz chirp	−0.44*		0.47*			
STP theta			0.53*			
STP gamma						

*Clinical variables with no significant correlations to EEG variables are not included. All correlations are Spearman's rho. All correlations represent the FXS group only. Due to the negative amplitude of the N1 ERP, negative correlations should be viewed as increased N1 amplitude correlating with increased scores on the clinical/behavioral measure. Blank = N.S. *p < 0.05, **p < 0.01.*

TABLE 4 | Significant clinical correlations for FXS patients – females only.

EEG measure	SCQ total score	Deviation IQ	ABC irritability	ABC social avoidance	Vineland comm	Vineland DL	Vineland social	Vineland comp
Habituation								
N1 amplitude					0.71*			0.75*
P2 amplitude		−0.70*	0.74*		−0.84**	−0.73*	−0.73*	−0.75*
% habituation S1 to S4								
STP theta					−0.70*			
STP alpha								
STP gamma		−0.71*			−0.86**	−0.69*		−0.75*
Chirp								
ITC stimulus onset								
ITC 40 Hz chirp	−0.77*			−0.67*				
STP theta								
STP gamma		−0.80**						

*Clinical variables with no significant correlations to EEG variables are not included. All correlations are Spearman's rho. All correlations represent the FXS group only. Due to the negative amplitude of the N1 ERP, negative correlations should be viewed as increased N1 amplitude correlating with increased scores on the clinical/behavioral measure. Blank = N.S. *p < 0.05, **p < 0.01.*

a marginal difference in N1 ERP amplitude between groups for the response to the initial stimulus, and significant amplitude differences for repeated stimuli, although ERP waveform plots suggested potentially larger amplitudes to all four stimuli. Here with more power to detect differences between groups, we show increased N1 amplitudes to all four stimuli in the stimulus train. We additionally found increased P2 amplitudes to all four stimuli in FXS, suggesting a generally hyper-excitable response throughout stimulus processing. Although we noted a possible *post hoc* difference between groups for habituation measured as percent change from the initial stimulus (S1) to the final stimulus (S4), we did not entirely replicate previous findings of decreased habituation of the N1 response across all repetitions, suggesting that the decrement in ERP amplitudes with repeated stimulation may not be a robust observation. One possibility for the lack of replication is, in the effort to increase translation between mouse and human, the change in stimulus from a 1000 Hz tone to a white noise burst. Increased stimulation of auditory cortices may have introduced the possibility of lateral inhibition effects, which can mimic habituation by decreasing ERP amplitudes for stimuli presented in close succession (Pantev et al., 2004). Rotschafer and Razak (2013) show broadened frequency tuning curves for individual neurons in auditory cortex in fmr1 KO mice, which may make FXS particularly sensitive to lateral inhibition effects. Alternatively, inhibitory interneuron dysfunction is characteristic of FXS (Cea-Del Rio and Huntsman, 2014), which may decrease lateral inhibition in FXS (Franco et al., 2017). Future work with masking stimuli is necessary to parse these effects and provide a mechanistic explanation for the differences in habituation effects found here.

The significantly hyper-excitable response (increased N1 amplitude) to repeated stimuli may still result in an increased attention to and lack of behavioral habituation to ongoing sounds (ability to "tune out") in the environment. Indeed, for males, increased N1 amplitude was correlated with increased alertness and vigilance during Woodcock Johnson Auditory Attention

TABLE 5 | Significant behavioral correlations for FXS patients.

EEG measure	Distractor correct	Distractor errors	No distractor correct	Distract total correct	Flex correct	Go-NoGo errors
Habituation						
N1 amplitude						
P2 amplitude						
% habituation S1–S4						
STP theta						
STP alpha						
STP gamma	−0.39*			−0.39*		
Chirp						
ITC stimulus onset		0.37*				
ITC 40 Hz chirp					0.43*	
STP theta						−0.39*
STP gamma	−0.44*		−0.38*	−0.44*		

*Clinical variables with no significant correlations to EEG variables are not included. All correlations are Spearman's rho. All correlations represent the FXS group only. Due to the negative amplitude of the N1 ERP, negative correlations should be viewed as increased N1 amplitude correlating with increased scores on the clinical/behavioral measure. Blank = N.S. *p < 0.05, **p < 0.01.*

Test. Interestingly, although FXS males and females did not differ on N1 amplitudes, the clinical relevance for increased N1 amplitude shows opposite effects based on gender: for males, increased N1 amplitude was associated with decreased scores on the SCQ, indicating fewer autism-like characteristics, and increased scores on the Woodcock-Johnson Tests. Indeed, individuals with idiopathic autism commonly show *reduced* ERP amplitudes relative to TDC (Jeste and Nelson, 2009), and in this case the hyper-excitable N1 response associated hyper-vigilance may improve ability to complete cognitive tests in individuals with intellectual disability. This is the first study known to date that links neural hyper-excitability to cognitive functioning in FXS. In females, however, increased N1 and P2 amplitudes were associated with decreased scores on the Vineland Adaptive Behavior Scales. This suggests that among females with FXS, neural hyper-excitability, and in turn hyper-vigilance, may impair functional abilities more broadly. However, it remains less clear whether this a gender-effect or due to the fact that females with FXS have more modest or no intellectual disabilities. Percent habituation also showed unusual gender effects, in that males with stronger habituation showed higher SCQ scores and lower Vineland scores, while females did not show correlations between these variables and habituation, suggesting that habituation and N1 amplitude are dissociable effects and may differentially impact clinical response. However, clinical correlations are presented as exploratory analyses, and further work designed to test specific clinical hypotheses is necessary to disentangle both gender and ERP effects on clinical variables.

A new finding for the habituation task was increased theta and alpha power in FXS relative to TDC. Our previous work showed similar trends (Ethridge et al., 2016) but with increased statistical power in the current study these group differences were statistically significant. Increased theta power has been commonly found for FXS in the resting EEG literature (Sabaratnam et al., 2001; Van der Molen and Van der Molen, 2013; Wang et al., 2017) and may reflect a compensatory response to reduced alpha-range thalamic modulation of high frequency cortical oscillations (Wang et al., 2017). Both theta and alpha oscillations may reflect thalamocortical modulation, but theta modulation is typically associated with longer range integration of cortical activity measured over anterior scalp and thus may be specialized for different functions relative to alpha, which is more commonly found to couple with gamma over posterior scalp (Canolty and Knight, 2010). The group by gender interaction for alpha power is interesting, in that FXS females do not show the reduced alpha (commonly associated with thalamic modulation) power that has previously been found in resting EEG literature with FXS patients (Van der Molen and Van der Molen, 2013; Wang et al., 2017); in fact, they showed increased alpha power relative to females without FXS.

Previous EEG literature in FXS has generally been underpowered to detect gender differences. Given that males

TABLE 6 | Significant behavioral correlations for FXS patients – males only.

EEG measure	Distract total correct	Flex correct	Go-NoGo correct
Habituation			
N1 amplitude			−0.59*
P2 amplitude			
% habituation S1–S4			
STP theta			
STP alpha			
STP gamma			
Chirp			
ITC stimulus onset			
ITC 40 Hz chirp		0.52*	
STP theta			
STP gamma	−0.45*		

*Clinical variables with no significant correlations to EEG variables are not included. All correlations are Spearman's rho. All correlations represent the FXS group only. Due to the negative amplitude of the N1 ERP, negative correlations should be viewed as increased N1 amplitude correlating with increased scores on the clinical/behavioral measure. Blank = N.S. *p < 0.05, **p < 0.01.*

TABLE 7 | Significant behavioral correlations for FXS patients – females only.

EEG measure	Flex median	Flex correct
Habituation		
N1 amplitude		
P2 amplitude	0.64*	
% habituation S1 to S4		
STP theta		
STP alpha		
STP gamma		−0.63*
Chirp		
ITC stimulus onset		
ITC 40 Hz chirp		
STP theta		
STP gamma		

*EEG measures with no significant correlations to clinical variables are not included. All correlations are Spearman's rho. All correlations represent the FXS group only. Due to the negative amplitude of the N1 ERP, negative correlations should be viewed as increased N1 amplitude correlating with increased scores on the clinical/behavioral measure. Blank = N.S. *p < 0.05, **p < 0.01.*

and females both showed increased theta and gamma power and that they are correlated with each other, while alpha and gamma power are not, this finding may indicate a more complex relationship between high frequency (gamma) power abnormalities in FXS and thalamocortical modulation via alpha oscillations. This finding may be task-specific, since increased low frequency power in FXS was largely confined to the theta frequency band, where FXS females showed even more marked increases, even though both males and females with FXS showed increased gamma power. If the increased theta power does represent a compensatory effort to reduce high frequency activity as proposed previously, then this may indicate that female FXS patients may in part have higher functioning because of a more preserved ability to mobilize this response.

For the chirp task, we replicated previous findings of reduced ability to synchronize (phase-lock) high-frequency neural activity to the chirp stimulus. However, a group by gender interaction suggests that FXS females are considerably less impaired on this ability than FXS males. For both males and females, though, decreased phase locking to the chirp stimulus was associated with increased autism-like characteristics on the SCQ, similar to our previous findings (Ethridge et al., 2017). For males, cortical synchronization deficits were associated with reduced behavioral flexibility on the KiTAP, whereas the same deficits were associated with increased social problems in females. Cortical synchronization deficits were also associated with cognitive deficits on the Woodcock Johnson Auditory Attention Tests in males. Both males and females showed increased gamma power, although this finding was more robust in the chirp task, which may be due to stimulus-related effects, in that the chirp stimulus drives cortical oscillations in the gamma frequency range while the habituation task does not. For both tasks, increased gamma power was associated with decreased deviation IQ scores, suggesting a significant overall functional impairment associated with increased high-frequency neural "noise." Indeed, gamma power correlated with increased distractibility on the KiTAP test and lower adaptive behavior scores on the Vineland, the latter mostly driven by a strong relationship between gamma power and adaptive behavior scores in females. Gamma power was also associated with an increase in severity of a number of behavioral problems and psychiatric issues, including irritability, stereotyped behaviors and speech, and hyperactivity. although these correlations were not significant when separated by gender, suggesting that they may correlate most strongly to differences in symptom severity that are commonly found to be associated with gender in FXS patients. These gender differences in clinical relevance for gamma power may also reflect the gender differences seen above in the theta and alpha bands, which may suggest a different effect of low frequency modulation of gamma power between genders. Future studies with specific clinical hypotheses will be necessary to examine the relationship between gender, symptom severity and EEG abnormalities.

The significant correlation between phase-locking abnormalities and increased non-specific gamma power was only partially replicated in this study, although the direction of the effect was the same as previously found (Ethridge et al., 2017). We have characterized increased gamma power as an increase in background neural "noise," reducing overall signal-to-noise ratio (SNR) of sensory processing in auditory cortex. The overall reduction in strength for this comparison for both TD and FXS may be due to equipment differences between this study and the previous. Saline-based EEG systems like the one employed here typically have a higher impedance threshold and thus lower SNR, which although sensitive enough to capture overall group differences in gamma, may be less sensitive to capture smaller variations in gamma between individuals. Still, both gamma deficits were replicated in this sample, further highlighting deficits in neural synchronization related to local network excitation/inhibition balance supported by FXS translational rodent models and shown here to be related to core clinical deficits in FXS. In addition, the baseline-corrected single trial power findings from both tasks, of enhanced processing during the ERP at stimulus onset and then decreased or desynchronized low frequency activity during the chirp, suggest an increase in cortical "effort" accompanying processing the stimulus for FXS which may persist after stimulus offset and may indicate a potential homeostatic response to gamma processing deficits. FXS increase their gamma power relative to baseline similarly to TDC, however, the similar increase in gamma power riding on top of already significantly increased baseline power produces the group differences in un-baseline-corrected single trial gamma power and which is particularly evident during the chirp stimulus, which drives oscillatory networks at gamma frequencies. Similar findings in individuals with autism and their first degree relatives (Rojas et al., 2008; De Stefano et al., 2019) support a possible pathophysiological link in gamma power regulation across neurodevelopmental disorders.

Preclinical work in *Fmr1* knockout mice supports a mechanism for gamma abnormalities in decreased excitatory drive on fast-spiking inhibitory interneurons, resulting in increased and poorly synchronized pyramidal cell firing in the gamma range at rest and during stimulus processing

(Gibson et al., 2008). Recent work suggests that intrinsic excitability in auditory cortex appears to be largely driven by synaptic activity between layers 2/3 and layer 5, which in contrast to previous work demonstrating network synchrony deficits, show a *hyper-synchrony* (Goswami et al., 2019). This hyper-synchronous response between cortical layers in the gamma frequency band may underlie the increased overall gamma power seen when neural activity is measured at the scalp, since increased gamma oscillatory activity is necessary to produce signals measurable at distant sources. This hyper-synchrony is also consistent with previous findings of poor stimulus-related synchrony, both at the slice level (Gibson et al., 2008) and in *in vivo* reductions in gamma phase-locking in both humans (seen here) and in Fmr1 KO mice (Lovelace et al., 2018). Phase-locking is driven by a resetting of the phase of ongoing oscillations in order to process an incoming stimulus. Intrinsically hyper-synchronous, hyper-excitable networks may be difficult to disrupt and modulate in order to produce accurate phase resetting, both reducing the signal processing ability and increasing the background "noise" of off-stimulus neural firing. Interestingly, increased ability to phase-reset and phase-lock gamma oscillations to the chirp stimulus was associated with increased behavioral flexibility on the KiTAP for both males and females with FXS, suggesting that local cortical flexibility measured at the sensory level may be related to higher-order cognitive flexibility.

Translational work with Fmr1 KO mice has reported similar findings to those reported here on both the habituation (Lovelace et al., 2016) and chirp tasks (Lovelace et al., 2018). An additional important step is necessary to fully validate these measures as functional outcome measure biomarkers and translate these findings for human clinical trials: scalability. This study addresses clinical scalability in a number of ways. First, we utilized a new group of subjects from a new clinic that recruits from a geographically distinct area from our previous work. Replication of our findings in this new sample suggests that these measures are robust to differences based on recruitment area, which is particularly important for FXS clinical trials which commonly utilize multi-site data collection strategies to increase patient numbers. Second, we used a different type of EEG equipment, in this case a saline-based EGI system, as compared to our previous work which used gel-based electrodes. Although we may have observed some minor system-related differences (see discussion above on signal to noise ratio), findings appear to be largely robust to system differences as well as reduced SNR associated with the EGI nets. This finding is important as saline-based EEG systems are becoming increasingly popular due to their ease of use, comfort, speed at which they can be applied, and reduced mess, all of which are important to reducing both patient and clinician burden as well as increasing the possibility of collecting useable data from more behaviorally impaired individuals. Equipment-invariance is also important due to the significant variation in existing equipment across clinics; purchasing identical EEG systems may not be financially feasible for large multi-site studies. Third, we used a white noise carrier sound for both habituation and chirp stimuli, which differs from the 1000 Hz carrier tone used in our previous studies. The white noise carrier sound stimulates a larger area of auditory cortex and produces a more robust neural response. Because it uses a wide range of frequencies rather than just one, the white noise sound can also be directly translated to rodent models without modification for hearing thresholds. The white noise sound is also less harsh-sounding to participants, and may allow for data collection in individuals with higher levels of sensory sensitivity. Our findings appear to be robust to these practical improvements in the stimulus properties, although see the discussion above regarding the habituation findings and white noise stimuli. Finally, we collected and analyzed the current dataset using a laboratory-based approach, with multiple research assistants and multiple data analysts all contributing to data collection, preprocessing, and screening. While all researchers involved were highly trained for reliability on their respective duties, this approach stills differs considerably from our previous work, which was collected and analyzed by a single individual. The laboratory approach is more consistent with large-scale studies with multiple research teams, and indicates that our findings are robust to the increase in error variance intrinsic to procedures with more decision-makers and decision points. We also analyzed the data slightly differently in order to produce *a priori* data cut-offs that can be utilized for individual data evaluation as well as interim data analyses, rather than data-driven approaches that can only be used once the entire dataset is collected. We used pre-defined sensors rather than data-driven topographic weights based on principle components analysis. Using predefined sensors also introduces the possibility of scaling the number of sensors necessary for data collection, reducing clinical burden. Taken together with similar findings in related disorders such as autism (Orekhova et al., 2008; Van Diessen et al., 2014; De Stefano et al., 2019), the replication of our previous work using different subjects, equipment, stimuli, and laboratory-based techniques point to ERP amplitude and gamma phase-locking and power as robust, clinically scalable measures that might be useful to predict or monitor drug response in large-scale multi-site clinical trials. Strong correlations between similar measures (gamma and theta power) between tasks also suggests test-retest reliability both of the measures and the laboratory-based data analysis strategies, another important factor in clinical trial readiness. While retest reliability for ongoing gamma (McFadden et al., 2014) and theta (Tan et al., 2015) power has been previously established, these findings support retest reliability of these measures specifically for FXS, a population for which increased response variability is sometimes a concern (The additional preclinical work showing replication of deficits and responsiveness to pharmaceutical intervention in FXS mouse models (Sinclair et al., 2017; Lovelace et al., 2018) suggests these measures may provide useful candidate biomarkers for treatment response in FXS. Specifically, both gamma phase-locking and power deficits show great promise as biologically grounded and functionally robust outcome measures in future clinical trials for FXS. Given the potential link to underlying pathophysiology, these biomarkers may also be relevant for other disorders with overlapping biological pathways and/or behavioral deficits that may ultimately arise from sensory processing abnormalities.

Despite these advances, some additional questions remain. Comparative work is still necessary to assess the specificity of our findings to FXS relative to other neurodevelopmental disabilities. Second, although we did not find differences between medicated and non-medicated patients, our sample is still not large enough to address the effects of individual medications; additionally, in correlational studies medication status may be confounded with symptom severity, necessitating targeted studies with pre-post designs. Excluding medicated patients can exclude a majority of FXS patients, particularly males and those with more severe clinical presentation, significantly impacting the representativeness of our data were they to be excluded from studies. So, we chose to retain patients in this study taking psychiatric medications commonly used to treat FXS patients that are not known to have significant impact on EEG measures obtained in the present study. Further, gamma abnormalities may be due to group differences in residual movement artifact due to common reduced behavioral compliance in FXS, however, preclinical studies of this question have found enhanced gamma power in fmr1 KO mice even during movement-free periods (Lovelace et al., 2018).

Preclinical models have provided a wealth of information relevant to understanding the genetic alteration resulting in FXS and its impacts on biochemical and local circuit function, but thus far the ability to translate these results into successful human clinical trials has been lacking. One reason for this disconnect may be the lack of translational biomarkers robust to both species differences and practical differences that may hinder reproducibility. The current study provides additional support for EEG-related neurophysiological measures as biomarkers by replicating previous findings in human data and linking them to a wider array of clinical features. Work is needed to link the EEG findings to molecular and network mechanisms in preclinical work, and also continue establishing their translational robustness.

ETHICS STATEMENT

All participants provided written informed consent (caregiver with assent or individual consent as appropriate) prior to participation, as approved by the Cincinnati Children's Hospital Institutional Review Board.

AUTHOR CONTRIBUTIONS

LE aided in study design, analyzed and interpreted the data, and wrote the manuscript. LD supervised EEG data management, quality control, and preprocessing. NW, KB, and MT contributed significantly to EEG data preprocessing. LS conducted the clinical assessments and supervised EEG data collection of all participants. JW aided in manuscript preparation and data interpretation. EP supervised EEG data collection and provided extensive contribution to manuscript preparation. CE supervised clinical assessment, participant recruitment, and contributed significantly to manuscript preparation and deviation IQ analyses. JS designed the study and contributed to all aspects of the research process, most significantly in data interpretation and manuscript preparation. All authors contributed substantially to the study, and read and approved the final version of the manuscript.

FUNDING

This study was supported by NIMH/NICHD grant U54 HD082008-01 (Huber and JS). The sponsor had no further role in the research plan development, analysis, or reporting of results.

ACKNOWLEDGMENTS

The authors would like to thank Michael Hong, Lindsey Mooney, Janna, Guilfoyle, and Nicole Friedman for aid in data collection and clinical variable calculations.

REFERENCES

Ahnaou, A., Biermans, R., and Drinkenburg, W. H. (2016). Modulation of mGlu2 receptors, but not PDE10A inhibition normalizes pharmacologically-induced deviance in auditory evoked potentials and oscillations in conscious rats. *PLoS One* 11:e0147365. doi: 10.1371/journal.pone.0147365

Berry-Kravis, E. M., Lindemann, L., Jonch, A. E., Apostol, G., Bear, M. F., Carpenter, R. L., et al. (2018). Drug development for neurodevelopmental disorders: lessons learned from fragile X syndrome. *Nat. Rev. Drug. Discov.* 17, 280–299. doi: 10.1038/nrd.2017.221

Brosch, M., Budinger, E., and Scheich, H. (2002). Stimulus-related gamma oscillations in primate auditory cortex. *J. Neurophysiol.* 87, 2715–2725. doi: 10.1152/jn.2002.87.6.2715

Brown, C., Tollefson, N., Dunn, W., Cromwell, R., and Filion, D. (2001). The adult sensory profile: measuring patterns of sensory processing. *Am. J. Occup. Ther.* 55, 75–82. doi: 10.5014/ajot.55.1.75

Budimirovic, D. B., Berry-Kravis, E., Erickson, C. A., Hall, S. S., Hessl, D., Reiss, A. L., et al. (2017). Updated report on tools to measure outcomes of clinical trials in fragile X syndrome. *J. Neurodev. Disord.* 9:14. doi: 10.1186/s11689-017-9193-x

Canolty, R. T., and Knight, R. T. (2010). The functional role of cross-frequency coupling. *Trends. Cogn. Sci.* 14, 506–515. doi: 10.1016/j.tics.2010.09.001

Cardin, J. A., Carlen, M., Meletis, K., Knoblich, U., Zhang, F., Deisseroth, K., et al. (2009). Driving fast-spiking cells induces gamma rhythm and controls sensory responses. *Nature* 459, 663–667. doi: 10.1038/nature08002

Cea-Del Rio, C. A., and Huntsman, M. M. (2014). The contribution of inhibitory interneurons to circuit dysfunction in Fragile X Syndrome. *Front. Cell Neurosci.* 8:245. doi: 10.3389/fncel.2014.00245

Chatrian, G. E. (1985). Ten percent electrode system for topographic studies of spontaneous and evoked EEG activity. *Am. J. EEG Technol.* 25, 83–92. doi: 10.1080/00029238.1985.11080163

Clementz, B. A., Sweeney, J. A., Hamm, J. P., Ivleva, E. I., Ethridge, L. E., Pearlson, G. D., et al. (2016). Identification of distinct psychosis biotypes using brain-based biomarkers. *Am. J. Psychiatry* 173, 373–384. doi: 10.1176/appi.ajp.2015.14091200

De Stefano, L. A., Schmitt, L. M., White, S. P., Mosconi, M. W., Sweeney, J. A., and Ethridge, L. E. (2019). Developmental effects on auditory neural oscillatory synchronization abnormalities in autism spectrum disorder. *Front. Integr. Neurosci.* 13:34. doi: 10.3389/fnint.2019.00034

Cea-Del Rio, C. A., and Huntsman, M. M. (2014). The contribution of inhibitory interneurons to circuit dysfunction in Fragile X Syndrome. *Front. Cell Neurosci.* 8:245. doi: 10.3389/fncel.2014.00245

Chatrian, G. E. (1985). Ten percent electrode system for topographic studies of spontaneous and evoked EEG activity. *Am. J. EEG Technol.* 25, 83–92. doi: 10.1080/00029238.1985.11080163

Clementz, B. A., Sweeney, J. A., Hamm, J. P., Ivleva, E. I., Ethridge, L. E., Pearlson, G. D., et al. (2016). Identification of distinct psychosis biotypes using brain-based biomarkers. *Am. J. Psychiatry* 173, 373–384. doi: 10.1176/appi.ajp.2015.14091200

De Stefano, L. A., Schmitt, L. M., White, S. P., Mosconi, M. W., Sweeney, J. A., and Ethridge, L. E. (2019). Developmental effects on auditory neural oscillatory synchronization abnormalities in autism spectrum disorder. *Front. Integr. Neurosci.* 13:34. doi: 10.3389/fnint.2019.00034

Delorme, A., and Makeig, S. (2004). EEGLAB: an open source toolbox for analysis of single-trial EEG dynamics including independent component analysis. *J. Neurosci. Methods* 134, 9–21. doi: 10.1016/j.jneumeth.2003.10.009

Erickson, C. A., Kaufmann, W. E., Budimirovic, D. B., Lachiewicz, A., Haas-Givler, B., Miller, R. M., et al. (2018). Best practices in fragile x syndrome treatment development. *Brain Sci.* 8:E224. doi: 10.3390/brainsci8120224

Esbensen, A. J., Rojahn, J., Aman, M. G., and Ruedrich, S. (2003). Reliability and validity of an assessment instrument for anxiety, depression, and mood among individuals with mental retardation. *J. Autism Dev. Disord.* 33, 617–629. doi: 10.1023/b:jadd.0000005999.27178.55

Ethridge, L. E., Hamm, J. P., Shapiro, J. R., Summerfelt, A. T., Keedy, S. K., Stevens, M. C., et al. (2012). Neural activations during auditory oddball processing discriminating schizophrenia and psychotic bipolar disorder. *Biol. Psychiatry* 72, 766–774. doi: 10.1016/j.biopsych.2012.03.034

Ethridge, L. E., White, S. P., Mosconi, M. W., Wang, J., Byerly, M. J., and Sweeney, J. A. (2016). Reduced habituation of auditory evoked potentials indicate cortical hyper-excitability in fragile X syndrome. *Transl. Psychiatry* 6:e787. doi: 10.1038/tp.2016.48

Ethridge, L. E., White, S. P., Mosconi, M. W., Wang, J., Pedapati, E. V., Erickson, C. A., et al. (2017). Neural synchronization deficits linked to cortical hyper-excitability and auditory hypersensitivity in fragile X syndrome. *Mol. Autism* 8:22. doi: 10.1186/s13229-017-0140-141

Franco, L. M., Okray, Z., Linneweber, G. A., Hassan, B. A., and Yaksi, E. (2017). Reduced lateral inhibition impairs olfactory computations and behaviors in a drosophila model of fragile x syndrome. *Curr. Biol.* 27, 1111–1123. doi: 10.1016/j.cub.2017.02.065

Gibson, J. R., Bartley, A. F., Hays, S. A., and Huber, K. M. (2008). Imbalance of neocortical excitation and inhibition and altered UP states reflect network hyperexcitability in the mouse model of fragile X syndrome. *J. Neurophysiol.* 100, 2615–2626. doi: 10.1152/jn.90752.2008

Goswami, S., Cavalier, S., Sridhar, V., Huber, K. M., and Gibson, J. R. (2019). Local cortical circuit correlates of altered EEG in the mouse model of Fragile X syndrome. *Neurobiol. Dis.* 124, 563–572. doi: 10.1016/j.nbd.2019.01.002

Hagerman, P. J. (2008). The fragile X prevalence paradox. *J. Med. Genet.* 45, 498–499. doi: 10.1136/jmg.2008.059055

Hall, S. S., Walter, E., Sherman, E., Hoeft, F., and Reiss, A. L. (2009). The neural basis of auditory temporal discrimination in girls with fragile X syndrome. *J. Neurodev. Disord.* 1, 91–99. doi: 10.1007/s11689-009-9007-x

Jeste, S. S., and Nelson, C. A. III (2009). Event related potentials in the understanding of autism spectrum disorders: an analytical review. *J. Autism Dev. Disord.* 39, 495–510. doi: 10.1007/s10803-008-0652-659

Knox, A., Schneider, A., Abucayan, F., Hervey, C., Tran, C., Hessl, D., et al. (2012). Feasibility, reliability, and clinical validity of the test of attentional performance for children (KiTAP) in fragile X syndrome (FXS). *J. Neurodev. Disord.* 4:2. doi: 10.1186/1866-1955-4-2

Lovelace, J. W., Ethell, I. M., Binder, D. K., and Razak, K. A. (2018). Translation-relevant EEG phenotypes in a mouse model of fragile X syndrome. *Neurobiol. Dis.* 115, 39–48. doi: 10.1016/j.nbd.2018.03.012

Lovelace, J. W., Wen, T. H., Reinhard, S., Hsu, M. S., Sidhu, H., Ethell, I. M., et al. (2016). Matrix metalloproteinase-9 deletion rescues auditory evoked potential habituation deficit in a mouse model of fragile X syndrome. *Neurobiol. Dis.* 89, 126–135. doi: 10.1016/j.nbd.2016.02.002

Luck, S. J. (2014). *An Introduction to the Event-Related Potential Technique.* Cambridge, MA: The MIT Press.

Luu, P., and Ferree, T. (2005). *Determination of the Hydrocel Geodesic sensor Nets' Average Electrode Positions and their 10-10 International Equivalents. Technical Document.* Eugene, OR: Electrical Geodesics, Inc.

Matsuzaki, J., Kagitani-Shimono, K., Goto, T., Sanefuji, W., Yamamoto, T., Sakai, S., et al. (2012). Differential responses of primary auditory cortex in autistic spectrum disorder with auditory hypersensitivity. *Neuroreport* 23, 113–118. doi: 10.1097/WNR.0b013e32834ebf44

McFadden, K. L., Steinmetz, S. E., Carroll, A. M., Simon, S. T., Wallace, A., and Rojas, D. C. (2014). Test-retest reliability of the 40 Hz EEG auditory steady-state response. *PLoS One* 9:e85748. doi: 10.1371/journal.pone.0085748

McGrew, K., and Woodcock, R. (2001). *Woodcock-Johnson III Technical Manual.* Itasca, IL: Riverside Publishing.

Mitra, S., Nizamie, S. H., Goyal, N., and Tikka, S. K. (2015). Evaluation of resting state gamma power as a response marker in schizophrenia. *Psychiatry Clin. Neurosci.* 69, 630–639. doi: 10.1111/pcn.12301

Orekhova, E. V., Stroganova, T. A., Prokofyev, A. O., Nygren, G., Gillberg, C., and Elam, M. (2008). Sensory gating in young children with autism: relation to age, IQ, and EEG gamma oscillations. *Neurosci. Lett.* 434, 218–223. doi: 10.1016/j.neulet.2008.01.066

Paluszkiewicz, S. M., Olmos-Serrano, J. L., Corbin, J. G., and Huntsman, M. M. (2011). Impaired inhibitory control of cortical synchronization in fragile X syndrome. *J. Neurophysiol.* 106, 2264–2272. doi: 10.1152/jn.00421.2011

Pang, E. W., and Taylor, M. J. (2000). Tracking the development of the N1 from age 3 to adulthood: an examination of speech and non-speech stimuli. *Clin. Neurophys.* 111, 388–397. doi: 10.1016/s1388-2457(99)00259-x

Pantev, C., Okamoto, H., Ross, B., Stoll, W., Ciurlia-Guy, E., Kakigi, R., et al. (2004). Lateral inhibition and habituation of the human auditory cortex. *Eur. J. Neurosci.* 19, 2337–2344. doi: 10.1111/j.0953-816x.2004.03296.x

Roid, G. H. (2003). *Stanford-Binet Intelligence Scales*, 5th Edn. Itasca, IL: Riverside Publishing.

Rojas, D. C., Maharajh, K., Teale, P., and Rogers, S. J. (2008). Reduced neural synchronization of gamma-band MEG oscillations in first-degree relatives of children with autism. *BMC Psychiatry* 8:66. doi: 10.1186/1471-244X-8-66

Rotschafer, S., and Razak, K. (2013). Altered auditory processing in a mouse model of fragile x syndrome. *Brain Res.* 1506, 12–24. doi: 10.1016/j.brainres.2013.02.038

Rutter, M., Bailey, A., and Lord, C. (2003). *Manual for the Social Communication Questionnaire.* Los Angeles, CA: Western Psychological Services.

Sabaratnam, M., Vroegop, P. G., and Gangadharan, S. K. (2001). Epilepsy and EEG findings in 18 males with fragile X syndrome. *Seizure* 10, 60–63. doi: 10.1053/seiz.2000.0492

Sansone, S. M., Schneider, A., Bickel, E., Berry-Kravis, E., Prescott, C., and Hessl, D. (2014). Improving IQ measurement in intellectual disabilities using true deviation from population norms. *J. Neurodev. Disord.* 6:16. doi: 10.1186/1866-1955-6-16

Sansone, S. M., Widaman, K. F., Hall, S. S., Reiss, A. L., Lightbody, A., Kaufmann, W. E., et al. (2012). Psychometric study of the aberrant behavior checklist in fragile X syndrome and implications for targeted treatment. *J. Autism Dev. Disord.* 42, 1377–1392. doi: 10.1007/s10803-011-1370-1372

Sinclair, D., Featherstone, R., Naschek, M., Nam, J., Du, A., Wright, S., et al. (2017). GABA-B agonist baclofen normalizes auditory-evoked neural oscillations and behavioral deficits in the Fmr1 knockout mouse model of fragile X syndrome. *eNeuro* 4:ENEURO.0380-16.2017. doi: 10.1523/ENEURO.0380-16.2017

Sparrow, S., Cicchetti, D. V., and Balla, D. A. (2005). *Vineland Adaptive Behavior Scales.* Minneapolis, MN: NCS Pearson Inc.

Takarae, Y., Luna, B., Minshew, N. J., and Sweeney, J. A. (2014). Visual motion processing and visual sensorimotor control in autism. *J. Int. Neuropsychol. Soc.* 20, 113–122. doi: 10.1017/S1355617713001203

Takarae, Y., Minshew, N. J., Luna, B., and Sweeney, J. A. (2007). Atypical involvement of frontostriatal systems during sensorimotor control in autism. *Psychiatry Res.* 156, 117–127. doi: 10.1016/j.pscychresns.2007.03.008

Tan, H. R. M., Gross, J., and Ulhaas, P. J. (2015). MEG-measured auditory steady-state oscillations show high test-retest reliabiltiy: a sensor and source-space analysis. *Neuroimage* 122, 417–426. doi: 10.1016/j.neuroimage.2015.07.055

Tiesinga, P., and Sejnowski, T. J. (2009). Cortical enlightenment: are attentional gamma oscillations driven by ING or PING? *Neuron* 63, 727–732. doi: 10.1016/j.neuron.2009.09.009

Tranfaglia, M. R. (2011). The psychiatric presentation of fragile x: evolution of the diagnosis and treatment of the psychiatric comorbidities of fragile X syndrome. *Dev. Neurosci.* 33, 337–348. doi: 10.1159/000329421

Van der Molen, M. J., and Van der Molen, M. W. (2013). Reduced alpha and exaggerated theta power during the resting-state EEG in fragile X syndrome. *Biol. Psychol.* 92, 216–219. doi: 10.1016/j.biopsycho.2012.11.013

Van Diessen, E., Senders, J., Jansen, F. E., Boersma, M., and Bruining, H. (2014). Increased power of resting-stet gamma oscillations in autism spectrum disorder detected by routine electroencephalography. *Eur. Arch. Psychiatry Clin. Neurosci.* 265, 537–540. doi: 10.1007/s00406-014-0527-3

Wang, J., Ethridge, L. E., Mosconi, M. W., White, S. P., Binder, D. K., Pedapati, E. V., et al. (2017). A resting EEG study of neocortical hyperexcitability and altered functional connectivity in fragile X syndrome. *J. Neurodev. Disord.* 9:11. doi: 10.1186/s11689-017-9191-z

Wen, T. H., Afroz, S., Reinhard, S. M., Palacios, A. R., Tapia, K., Binder, D. K., et al. (2018). Genetic reduction of matrix metalloproteinase-9 promotes formation of perineuronal nets around parvalbumin-expressing interneurons and normalizes auditory cortex responses in developing Fmr1 knock-out mice. *Cereb. Cortex* 28, 3951–3964. doi: 10.1093/cercor/bhx258

Wijetunge, L. S., Chattarji, S., Wyllie, D. J., and Kind, P. C. (2013). Fragile X syndrome: from targets to treatments. *Neuropharmacology* 68, 83–96. doi: 10.1016/j.neuropharm.2012.11.028

17

Atypical Social Attention and Emotional Face Processing in Autism Spectrum Disorder: Insights from Face Scanning and Pupillometry

Debra L. Reisinger[1], *Rebecca C. Shaffer*[1,2], *Paul S. Horn*[2,3], *Michael P. Hong*[2], *Ernest V. Pedapati*[2,4,5], *Kelli C. Dominick*[4,5] *and Craig A. Erickson*[4,5]*

[1]*Division of Developmental and Behavioral Pediatrics, Cincinnati Children's Hospital Medical Center, Cincinnati, OH, United States,* [2]*Department of Pediatrics, University of Cincinnati College of Medicine, Cincinnati, OH, United States,* [3]*Division of Neurology, Cincinnati Children's Hospital Medical Center, Cincinnati, OH, United States,* [4]*Division of Child and Adolescent Psychiatry, Cincinnati Children's Hospital Medical Center, Cincinnati, OH, United States,* [5]*Department of Psychiatry and Behavioral Neuroscience, University of Cincinnati College of Medicine, Cincinnati, OH, United States*

Correspondence:
Craig A. Erickson
craig.erickson@cchmc.org

Social attention deficits are a hallmark characteristic within autism spectrum disorder (ASD) and have been hypothesized to have cascading effects on emotion recognition. Eye-tracking methodology has emerged as a potentially reliable, feasible, and sensitive biomarker for examining core phenotypic features of ASD; however, these findings are mixed with regards to measuring treatment change in clinical trials. The present study aimed to assess the utility of an eye-tracking paradigm to discriminate between clinical groups in social attention and emotion recognition through face scanning and pupillometry. The present study also assessed the reliability of this paradigm within the ASD sample to further our understanding of the utility of eye-tracking for future clinical trials. Participants included 42 individuals with ASD, 29 developmental disability (DD) controls, and 62 typically developing (TD) controls between 3 and 25 years of age. An emotional faces eye-tracking paradigm was administered to all participants, with the ASD group completing the paradigm a second time approximately 2 months later. Participants' average proportion of looking and number of fixations to specific areas of interest (AOI) were examined along with changes in pupil reactivity while viewing different emotional faces. Results suggest atypical face-scanning through a reduced proportion of looking and the number of fixations toward the eyes in the ASD group regardless of the emotion that was presented. Further, pupillometry measures were able to detect increases in pupil dilation to happy faces in the ASD group. Lastly, test-retest reliability coefficients varied between the poor and excellent range based on the mechanism assessed, with the proportion of looking demonstrating the highest reliability coefficients. These findings build on the promise of eye-tracking as a feasible and reliable biomarker for identifying social attention and emotion recognition deficits in ASD. Detecting differences in emotion recognition explicitly through facial scanning was not as clear. Specific mechanisms within the eye-tracking paradigm may be viable options for assessing treatment-specific outcomes.

Keywords: eye tracking, autism spectrum disorder, social attention, emotional faces, pupillometry

INTRODUCTION

Autism spectrum disorder (ASD) is a neurodevelopmental disorder characterized by significant impairments in social communication, restricted interests, and the presence of repetitive and stereotyped behaviors (American Psychiatric Association, 2013). Within the research on social communication deficits in ASD, there has been specific interest in attention to faces or social stimuli across the lifespan (for review, see Guillon et al., 2014; Chita-Tegmark, 2016). Specifically, it has been hypothesized that deficits in social attention (e.g., reduced attention to social stimuli as a whole or atypical allocation of attention to social stimuli) may cause reduced social processing and a loss of relevant information necessary for the development of appropriate social functioning. Further, these deficits in social attention may also cause difficulty in the interpretation of emotional information (Pelphrey et al., 2002; Wagner et al., 2013). In light of the knowledge surrounding these deficits, there is great interest in identifying and developing feasible, valid, and reliable outcome measures to be utilized in clinical trials that are sensitive to assess the core phenotypic features of ASD. The present study examines the utility of an emotional face eye-tracking paradigm to discriminate between clinical groups in addition to evaluating the reliability of the paradigm in ASD.

To date, there have been many studies conducted examining deficits in social attention through abnormal face scanning in ASD; however, the literature is quite mixed with regards to hypothesized causes and whether these deficits are consistently present. One proposed theory suggests individuals with ASD find attention to eyes over stimulating with a heightened sensitivity to social stimuli to support an eye "aversion" hypothesis (Dalton et al., 2005; Spezio et al., 2007b). Another possibility suggests individuals with ASD experience a reduced reward value for social stimuli (Dawson et al., 2005; Chevallier et al., 2012). Specifically, the social motivation theory implies individuals with ASD may not seek out social stimuli because eye contact and faces are not intrinsically rewarding and may not be activating their cognitive reward systems appropriately. This reduced reward is hypothesized to be causing the failure to attend to faces or to develop expertise to attend to faces, resulting in abnormal attention to faces.

Regardless of the cause, a number of studies have suggested that individuals with ASD spend less time attending to the eyes of faces and more time looking at mouths, bodies, and objects in comparison to typically developing (TD) controls across the lifespan (Klin et al., 2002; Pelphrey et al., 2002; Corden et al., 2008; Riby and Hancock, 2008; Rice et al., 2012; Hanley et al., 2013; Auyeung et al., 2015). In comparison to typical development, attention to faces and social stimuli is expected to emerge during infancy and extend into adulthood, with a preferential bias toward the eyes of faces across a variety of tasks and settings (Birmingham et al., 2008). Unfortunately, a number of studies have found no significant differences in face scanning to particular facial regions between ASD and TD controls (Wagner et al., 2013; Gillespie-Smith et al., 2014; Åsberg Johnels et al., 2014; Kwon et al., 2019). These mixed findings within the ASD literature suggest a lack of consensus on social attention deficits in ASD as measured through eye-tracking paradigms; which could be accounted for by the unknown origin of these deficits, the variability of paradigms utilized, how well these paradigms measure social attention, and how sensitive they are to the core phenotypic features of ASD.

Appropriate social attention through facial scanning is also critical for accurate emotion recognition. Within the TD literature, research has demonstrated different attention patterns in relation to positive vs. negative emotions. For example, TD individuals will fixate more on the eye region of negative emotions in contrast to the mouth region of positive emotions (Eisenbarth and Alpers, 2011; Messinger et al., 2012). In addition to the identified deficits in face scanning patterns in ASD, these deficits are further complicated when adding in emotions. Specifically, deficits in the face-scanning of different simple emotions (e.g., happy, sad, fear) have been identified through abnormal-looking time and a number of fixations toward certain regions of emotional faces (Pelphrey et al., 2002; de Wit et al., 2008). Spezio et al. (2007a,b) hypothesized adults with high-functioning ASD fail to make use of the information from the eyes when interpreting facial expressions; therefore, reduced attention to the eye region of faces may have downstream effects on emotion processing in ASD. Unfortunately, the literature is mixed in supporting this theory. According to Sawyer et al. (2012), they suggest emotion recognition cannot be fully explained by impairments in facial scanning after their results demonstrated impairments during an emotional recognition task in comparison to no impairments with facial scanning of basic and complex emotions in ASD.

Aside from examining facial scanning to assess social attention and emotion recognition impairments in ASD, emotional arousal as captured through the autonomic nervous system (ANS) can also be considered. Pupil reactivity, as measured using eye-tracking pupillometry, has been identified as a reliable indicator of emotional arousal that reflects changes in the brain activity that underlie the cognitive events of emotion processing (Bradshaw, 1967; Bradley et al., 2008; Kret, 2015). Specifically, increased sympathetic activity and decreased parasympathetic activity prompt pupil dilation resulting in pupil diameter increases being mediated by both divisions of the ANS (Steinhauer et al., 2004). More recently, pupil reactivity has been used to assess the ANS in response to social stimuli and emotion recognition in ASD during screen viewing (Falck-Ytter, 2008; Sepeta et al., 2012; Nuske et al., 2014a,b). Similar to the social attention and emotion recognition literature, there are mixed findings with respect pupil reactivity in ASD. Specifically, findings have demonstrated pupil constriction while viewing other children's faces (Anderson et al., 2006), reduced pupillary responses to fearful expressions of unfamiliar people (Nuske et al., 2014a), and increased pupil dilation while viewing inverted, but not upright, emotional faces (Falck-Ytter, 2008) in young children with ASD. Conversely, some studies have demonstrated no change in pupillary responses when viewing emotional faces (Sepeta et al., 2012; Wagner et al., 2013). Combining pupillometry as a measure of emotional arousal and face scanning as a measure of social attention to emotional faces may provide a clearer picture of emotion recognition processing in ASD; however, very few studies have explored these combined mechanisms.

Social attention has notably been identified as one of the earliest hallmark impairments in ASD with the promise of being a predictive diagnostic biomarker for ASD outcomes (Jones and Klin, 2013; Elsabbagh et al., 2014; Jones et al., 2016). These findings have now pushed the field to begin assessing and identifying effective behavioral and pharmacological treatments that can improve social functioning in ASD. Unfortunately, a significant challenge currently being faced within the ASD treatment literature is identifying reliable, valid, and feasible outcome measures that are sensitive to change in measuring the core phenotypic symptoms in ASD. Until recently, most outcome measures used in ASD treatment research have relied on caregiver report or clinician-administered assessments (Bolte and Diehl, 2013). An explicit interest in the utility of biomarkers to measure treatment change in clinical trials has emerged. A promising start for eye tracking was identified by Murias et al. (2018), where they found a strong association between a social attention eye-tracking task and caregiver reports of social communication frequently utilized in ASD clinical trials. Nevertheless, the theme of variability continues with some findings suggesting eye tracking is sensitive enough to detect treatment effects (Auyeung et al., 2015; Fletcher-Watson and Hampton, 2018) and other findings identifying change through clinical measures with no treatment change detected through eye-tracking (Bradshaw et al., 2019).

The present study aims to expand the understanding of the current literature of eye-tracking as a reliable and feasible biomarker for assessing social attention and emotion recognition using a chronologically diverse ASD sample with mentally and chronologically age-matched comparison groups. The methodology utilized in the present study mimics previous work completed by Farzin et al. (2009, 2011) that demonstrated the feasibility and reliability of an emotional faces paradigm in fragile × syndrome (FXS). Given majority of their sample had a co-occurring diagnosis of ASD (Farzin et al., 2009), this paradigm may show promise within ASD as well. It is hypothesized that individuals with ASD will demonstrate reduced attention to the eye region of different emotional faces that varies across emotions in comparison to the mentally and chronologically age-matched control groups. Further, it is hypothesized that individuals with ASD will exhibit abnormal pupil reactivity to the different emotions presented (e.g., reduced reactivity to fearful faces compared to increased reactivity to happy faces). Last, we anticipate that the paradigm will exhibit good-to-excellent reliability estimates within the ASD sample.

MATERIALS AND METHODS

Participants

Participants were drawn from a larger study examining potential biomarkers in ASD at Cincinnati Children's Hospital Medical Center. The present study included 42 individuals with ASD (83.33% male), 29 age-, gender-, and IQ-matched developmental disability (DD) controls (89.65% male), and 62 age-, gender-matched TD controls (88.79% male) between 3 and 25 years of age (M = 12.33, SD = 5.80). Of the sample, 72% were White, 12% were Black, 10% were Other/Multiracial, 3% were Hispanic/Latino, 2% were Asian, and 1% were Native Hawaiian or Other Pacific Islander. The ASD group had a confirmed diagnosis of ASD through a structured clinical interview using the Diagnostic and Statistical Manual of Mental Disorders, Fifth Edition (DSM-5) ASD criteria (American Psychiatric Association, 2013), testing with the Autism Diagnostic Observation Schedule, Second Edition (ADOS-2; Lord et al., 2012), and administration of the Social Communication Questionnaire (SCQ; Rutter et al., 2003). Further, the ASD participants did not have any known syndromic or other genetic variant associated with their ASD diagnosis. The TD control participants had no reported or suspected developmental concerns, fell in the normal range (e.g., between 90 and 125) of cognitive functioning on IQ measures administered through the study, and an SCQ total score less than 15. The DD control group was matched with a subgroup of the ASD participants with an IQ less than 90. The DD control group was also administered the ADOS-2 to ensure none of the participants had undiagnosed ASD. All participants or their guardians provided written informed consent and participant assent (if feasible) for study participation, and the study was approved by the local Institutional Review Board.

Participants' cognitive functioning was measured across all three groups utilizing the Stanford-Binet Intelligence Scales, Fifth Edition (SB-5; Roid, 2003) or the Differential Ability Scales-II (DAS-II; Elliott, 2007) to obtain a Full-Scale IQ score. One DD control participant and eight ASD participants were not able to complete one of the above cognitive measures due to behavioral concerns or functioning level. This resulted in statistically significant differences between the mean Full-Scale IQ score of the ASD group and the DD control group ($F_{(2,121)}$ = 54.70, p = 0.000); however, adding in the eight lower functioning individuals would assumedly account for these differences and decrease the ASD mean Full-Scale IQ score. These participants were still included in the original sample due to their ability to complete the eye-tracking task despite their low cognitive abilities. Participants' caregivers or guardians across all groups completed the SCQ. Participants' caregivers of the ASD group completed the Aberrant Behavior Checklist (ABC; Aman et al., 1985) and the Social Responsiveness Scale (SRS; Constantino and Gruber, 2005). No significant group differences were found based on chronological age ($F_{(2,120)}$ = 2.29, p = 0.106). As expected, significant group differences emerged across groups on the SCQ consistent with the lack of ASD diagnosis in the DD and TD control groups ($F_{(2,130)}$ = 90.79, p = 0.000). See **Table 1** for participant descriptive statistics along with the caregiver rating scales for the analyzed sample.

Apparatus and Stimuli

Eye-tracking data were collected using a Tobii (Stockholm, Sweden) T120 infrared binocular eye tracker sampling at a rate of 120 Hz to record X and Y coordinates of eye position and pupil diameter along with gaze duration. The paradigm was run on an integrated 17-inch flat-panel monitor (1,280 × 1,024 pixels resolution) running Tobii Studio (Version 3.0, Tobii Technology, Sweden). Stimuli consisted of 12 colored photographs of adult human faces (equal numbers of males and females) from the NimStim Face Stimulus Set (Tottenham et al., 2002), each showing a calm, happy, or fearful facial expression (see **Figure 1**). Each emotional face was presented on the screen for 5 s. Prior to presenting the emotional faces, a scrambled version of the face image was presented for 1 s (**Figure 1A**). Similar to Farzin et al. (2009, 2011), each face and corresponding scrambled image were matched on mean luminance, and equivalence was confirmed using a photometer (Minolta, LS-100, Osaka, Japan). Face images subtended a 12.12° by 17.19° region (the size of an actual human face) when viewed from a distance of 60 cm, and were presented on a standard 50% gray background (RGB: 128, 128, 128).

Procedure

All participants were assessed as part of the larger battery during a 1 day visit. Following clinical assessments, participants were allowed a break, if needed or requested, to ensure they were at baseline levels prior to completing the paradigm. Once participants were at their normal baseline state, they were seated in a quiet room in front of the eye tracker at a distance of 60–65 cm from the eye tracker monitor. Each participant was presented with verbal instructions to "look at the screen" or a "first-then" communication tool to demonstrate that the child would first look at the screen and then receive a trivial prize. The eye tracker was calibrated for each participant at the beginning of each session using the Tobii Studio "five-point infant calibration." Successful calibration was ascertained *via* Tobii Studio's automated validation procedure. A second attempt to calibrate was conducted if the participant did not successfully calibrate. The task was discontinued if they were not successfully calibrated after two attempts. Following calibration, participants were again instructed to look at the upcoming pictures presented on the screen through verbal instruction or a "first-then" visual prior to the start of the task. Subjects

TABLE 1 | Descriptive statistics of ASD, DD, and TD variables.

Variable	ASD					DD					TD					Group differences
	n	Mean	*SD*	Min	Max	*n*	Mean	*SD*	Min	Max	*n*	Mean	*SD*	Min	Max	*p*
Age (years)	36	14.05	5.80	3.11	21.10	28	11.25	5.17	3.73	24.60	59	11.88	5.96	3.04	25.47	0.106
Full scale IQ	30	88.07	19.71	40.00	137.00	27	73.56	10.09	51.00	88.00	59	104.41	8.99	91.00	124.00	0.000[a]
SCQ	36	19.75	5.72	7.00	33.00	28	10.25	6.17	0.00	24.00	59	5.17	4.85	0.00		0.000[b]
SRS Total T-Score	24	85.54	14.25	57.00	113.00											
ABC Irritability	24	12.42	11.00	0.00	41.00											
ABC Lethargy	24	15.92	7.96	0.00	35.00											
ABC Stereotypy	24	4.96	4.22	0.00	15.00											
ABC Hyperactivity	24	17.96	12.92	0.00	40.00											
ABC Inappropriate Speech	24	5.00	4.12	0.00	12.00											

Note. Table includes data from the analyzed sample of participants; ASD, autism spectrum disorder; DD, developmental delay controls; TD, typically developing controls; SD, standard deviation; ABC, Aberrant Behavior Checklist; SRS, Social Responsiveness Scale. [a]*Group differences found on full scale IQ (TD > ASD>DD).* [b]*Group differences found on SCQ (ASD > DD > TD).*

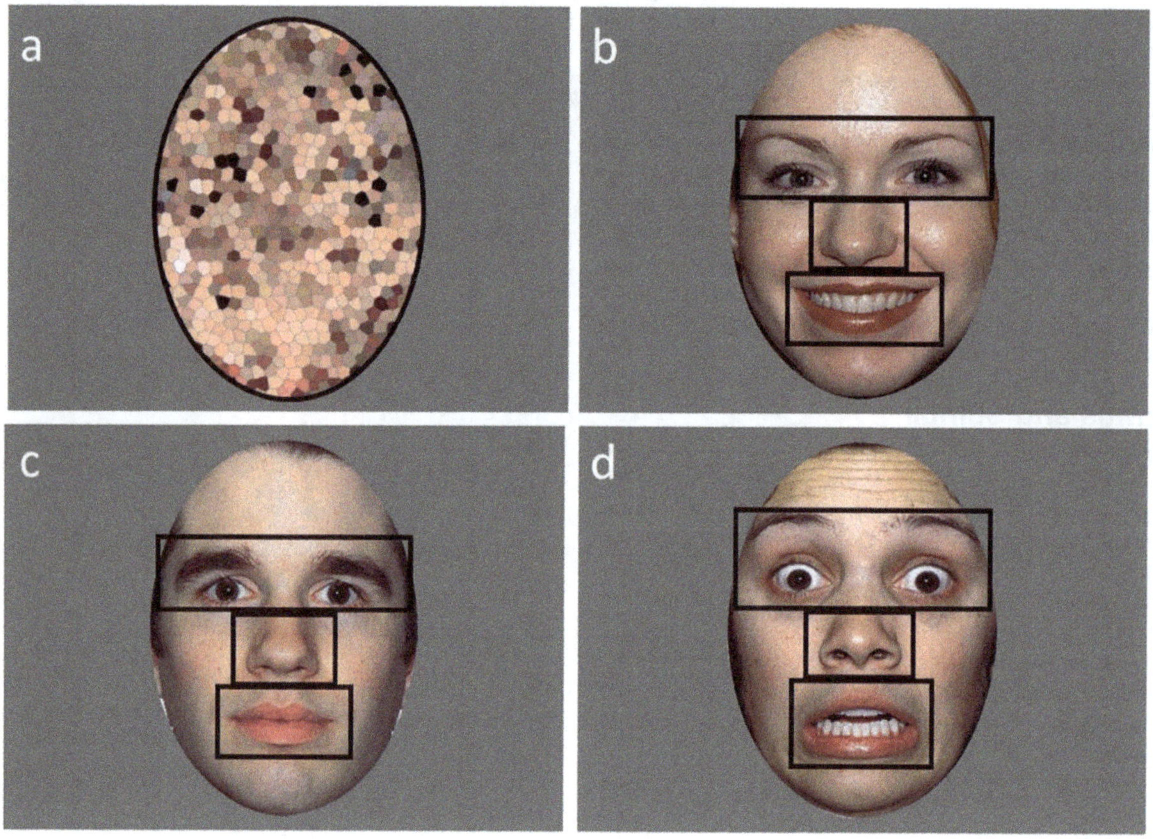

FIGURE 1 | An example of a scrambled **(A)**, happy **(B)**, calm **(C)**, and fearful **(D)** face used in the emotional faces paradigm with the areas of interests (AOI's) outlined in black.

completed one of two variations with different randomizations of the order of emotional faces. Approximately 8–12 weeks later, 19 of the participants in the ASD group returned to the lab to repeat the same battery of measures they received during the first visit. The first and second sessions were the same with respect to the order of the protocol, room set-up, and timing. Depending on which randomization order of the faces the ASD group received at their first visit, they received the other randomized order at the second visit. The second visit in the ASD group allowed us to examine the test-retest reliability of the eye-tracking measure administered. The average length of time between the first and second visits was 9.77 weeks.

Statistical Analyses

Data Extraction

Areas of interest (AOI) for the eyes (including eyebrows), nose, mouth, and other (the rest of the face minus the eyes, nose, and mouth regions) were created (**Figure 1**). A single ellipse AOI around the face was utilized for the scrambled faces. Two variables were extracted for the analyses from Tobii Studio: fixation count and proportion of looking time to each AOI region. Fixation counts (defined as any data point within a 35-pixel radius for a minimum duration of 100 ms) were calculated by averaging the number of fixations to the AOI regions. The proportion of looking time was calculated by dividing the looking time to the AOI region by the total looking time to face. Not assessed by Farzin et al. (2009, 2011), a proportion of valid looking variable was calculated to assess overall attention during the task in order to exclude participants who had minimal viewing time across the task. The proportion of valid looking was calculated by dividing the total looking time to anywhere on the screen for all the faces divided by the total stimulus presentation time across all faces. Participants were excluded if they had less than 35% valid looking data across the faces. This resulted in six ASD, one DD, and three TD participants to be excluded from the analyses. Two of the six ASD participants that were excluded for valid looking data were also included in the eight ASD participants that could not complete IQ testing. The final sample of participants for the analyses included: 36 individuals with ASD, 28 individuals with DD, and 59 TD individuals.

Pupil data were exported from Tobii Studio and manipulated in SPSS version 24.0 (IBM Corporation, Armonk, NY, USA). For each participant, their pupil data were averaged across both eyes and then filtered to remove any outlier values related to blinks, loss of tracking data, large changes in head movement or if the participant did not look at the preceding scramble face image for three or more consecutive 250 ms intervals. Mean pupil diameter was calculated for interval durations of 250 ms across the scramble (1-s) and face presentation (5-s) for a total of 24 intervals. Consistent with Farzin et al. (2009, 2011), face specific pupil reactivity was calculated by subtracting the mean pupil size during the preceding scrambled face from the mean pupil size during each interval ($n = 20$) of the face presentation, and then "standardized" by dividing by the mean pupil size during the scrambled faces. Further, pupil reactivity was averaged across trials of each face emotion for test-retest reliability analyses within the subset of ASD participants.

Statistical Tests

Data were examined for outliers, nonnormality, and homoscedasticity. Since age was significantly different between groups with a wide age range within each group, age was included in all models as a covariate to account for these differences. Preliminary and the first set of analyses were completed in SAS® 9.4 (SAS Institute Inc., Cary, NC, USA). A mixed model analysis of covariance (ANCOVA) with random subject effects using AOI region, emotion, and group as the independent variables and proportion of looking as the dependent variable was conducted. Since fixation count was not normally distributed, a Poisson regression model, accounting for over-dispersion, using AOI region, emotion, and the group as the independent variables and fixation count as the dependent variable was conducted. Further, repeated measures ANCOVA with interval, emotion, and the group as the independent variables and pupil reactivity as the dependent variable was conducted. Within each model, significant main effects and interactions were followed up with least-square means to acquire adjusted mean differences. False Discovery Rate (Benjamini and Hochberg, 1995) was utilized to control for family-wise error in the *post hoc* analyses. In addition, adjustments were made for denominator degrees of freedom for all models (Kenward and Roger, 1997).

For the second set of analyses, R version 3.5.1 (R Foundation for Statistical Computing, Vienna, Austria) was utilized. To assess the test-retest reliability of the emotional faces paradigm with a subset of the ASD sample, we computed intraclass correlation coefficients (ICCs) between the two testing sessions using a two-way random-effects model with absolute agreement (ICC 2, 1; Shrout and Fleiss, 1979). The random-effects model is ideal because it allows for systematic differences between the two testing sessions. Further, ICC's are better able to detect systematic differences between testing sessions in comparison to correlation coefficients (Weir, 2005). If participants performed similarly across the two testing sessions, their ICC will be closer to 1. Analyses focus on the ICCs for each AOI within fixation counts and proportion of looking. Pupil reactivity was averaged across intervals with ICCs reported on the different emotional faces that were presented. Definitive guidelines for interpreting ICC values have not been well justified; however there are a few documented guidelines like the tiered approach suggested by Cicchetti (1994): <0.40 = poor, 0.40–0.59 = fair, 0.60–0.74 = good, and 0.75–1.00 = excellent. Skinner et al. (2018) caution against using eye-tracking measures with reliability coefficients less than 0.60.

RESULTS

Preliminary Analyses

Cognitive Abilities

We examined the relationship of cognitive ability on total data contribution to the eye-tracking task given the large amount of variability within the present study's sample. Utilizing a median split for Full-Scale IQ to separate the entire sample, an independent measures *t*-test revealed a significant difference between groups in the proportion of attention to the eye-tracking task ($t_{(114)} = -2.71, p = 0.008$). Specifically, participants who had an IQ of >95 ($M = 76.82, SD = 12.26$) attended to the eye-tracking task more in comparison to those with an IQ ≤95 ($M = 69.88$, $SD = 15.17$). When looking within groups, these differences were minimized. In the TD sample, no significant differences were found in their proportion of attention to the task utilizing a median split of IQ ($t_{(57)} = 1.74, p = 0.088$). The TD participants who had an IQ of >103 ($M = 79.26, SD = 10.13$) attended to the task similar to those with an IQ ≤103 ($M = 73.81, SD = 13.67$). Within the DD group, there were no significant differences found utilizing a median split of IQ on proportion of attention to the task ($t_{(25)} = 0.73, p = 0.472$). The DD participants with an IQ of >76 ($M = 72.99, SD = 14.71$) attended to the task similar to those with an IQ ≤76 ($M = 69.09, SD = 13.01$). Within the ASD group, there were no significant differences found utilizing a median split of IQ on proportion of attention to the task ($t_{(28)} = 1.42$, $p = 0.166$). The ASD participants with an IQ of >86 ($M = 73.79$, $SD = 17.68$) attended the task similar to those with an IQ ≤86 ($M = 65.15, SD = 15.52$).

Age

We examined the relationship of age on total data contribution to the eye-tracking task given the large amount of variability within the present study's sample. Utilizing a median split for age to separate the entire sample, an independent measures *t*-test revealed a significant difference between groups in the proportion of attention to the eye-tracking task ($t_{(121)} = -2.24$, $p = 0.027$). Specifically, participants >12.32 years ($M = 75.54$, $SD = 15.07$) attended to the eye-tracking task more in comparison to ≤12.32 years old ($M = 69.69, SD = 13.93$). When looking within groups, these differences were minimized for the ASD and DD groups. In the TD sample, significant differences were found in their proportion of attention to the task utilizing a median split of age ($t_{(57)} = -2.59, p = 0.012$). The TD participants >11.12 years ($M = 80.64, SD = 9.08$) attended to the task more than those ≤11.12 years old ($M = 72.74, SD = 13.64$). Within the DD group, there were no significant differences found utilizing a median split of age on the proportion of attention to the task ($t_{(26)} = -1.41, p = 0.171$). The DD participants >9.94 years ($M = 74.65, SD = 12.87$) attended to the task similarly to ≤9.94 years old ($M = 67.59, SD = 13.64$). Within the ASD group, there were no significant differences found utilizing a median split of age on the proportion of attention to the task ($t_{(34)} = -0.67, p = 0.506$). The ASD participants >16.41 years

TABLE 2 | Results of mixed-model ANCOVA within-subjects effects for the proportion of looking.

Variable	F	p
Age	0.01	0.941
Group	0.00	0.999
Emotion	0.00	1.000
AOI	307.85	0.000*
Group × Emotion	0.00	1.000
Group × AOI	4.70	0.000*
Emotion × AOI	1.04	0.400
Group × Emotion × AOI	0.49	0.923

*Note. AOI, area of interest. *p < 0.05.*

(M = 69.36, SD = 19.31) attended to the task similarly to ≤16.4 years old (M = 65.36, SD = 16.19).

Proportion of Looking

A mixed model ANCOVA with AOI region, emotion, and the group as independent variables, age as a covariate, and proportion of looking as the dependent variable was conducted (**Table 2**). Results revealed a main effect of AOI region ($F_{(3,1439)}$ = 307.85, p = 0.000). This effect was qualified by a significant interaction between AOI region and group ($F_{(6,1439)}$ = 4.70, p = 0.001; **Figure 2**). Least squares mean differences revealed the TD participants (M = 48.82 SE = 1.17) spent significantly more time looking at the eyes in comparison to the DD participants ($t_{(1439)}$ = 4.13, p = 0.000; M = 40.34, SE = 1.69) and the ASD participants ($t_{(1439)}$ = 2.50, p = 0.013; M = 44.08, SE = 1.50). Further, the TD participants (M = 20.60, SE = 1.17) spent significantly less time looking at the nose in comparison to the DD participants ($t_{(1439)}$ = −2.56, p = 0.011; M = 25.60, SE = 1.69) but similarly to the ASD participants ($t_{(1439)}$ = −1.71, p = 0.087, M = 23.84, SE = 1.50). No other significant main effects or interactions emerged. See **Figure 3** for a heat map of the average duration of looking for a subgroup of participants within each clinical group for one of the neutral faces.

Fixation Count

A Poisson regression model with AOI region, emotion, and the group as the independent variables, age as a covariate, and fixation count as the dependent variable was conducted (**Table 3**). Results revealed a significant main effect of AOI region ($F_{(3,1317)}$ = 300.61, p = 0.000) and group ($F_{(2,151.7)}$ = 3.35, p = 0.038). These effects were qualified by a significant interaction between group and AOI region ($F_{(6,1317)}$ = 5.64, p = 0.000; **Figure 4**). Least square mean differences revealed the TD participants (M = 26.52, SE = 1.10) exhibited significantly more fixations on the eyes in comparison to the DD ($t_{(235.1)}$ = 3.37, p = 0.001; M = 20.53, SE = 1.32) and the ASD ($t_{(243.2)}$ = 5.48, p = 0.000; (M = 17.91, SE = 1.05) participants. No other significant main effects or interactions emerged.

Pupil Reactivity

A repeated measures ANCOVA with interval (n = 20), emotion, and group as independent variables, age as a covariate, and pupil reactivity as the dependent variable was conducted (**Table 4**). Results revealed a significant main effect of emotion ($F_{(2,11398)}$ = 15.36, p = 0.000) and interval ($F_{(19,11305)}$ = 2.28, p = 0.001). A marginally significant effect for group also emerged ($F_{(2,81.24)}$ = 2.67, p = 0.075). These effects were qualified by a significant interaction between group and emotion ($F_{(4,11398)}$ = 14.81, p = 0.000; **Figure 5**). Least square

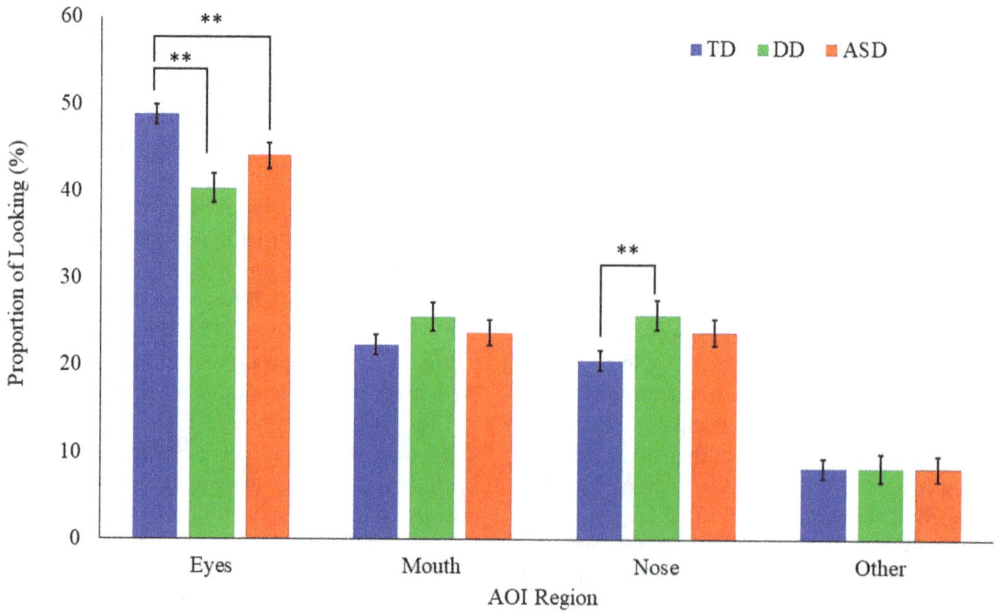

FIGURE 2 | Mean proportion of looking to each AOI region by group for all emotional faces. Proportion of looking is reported as percentages and error bars represent SEM. TD, typically developing; DD, developmentally delayed; ASD, autism spectrum disorder; **p < 0.05.

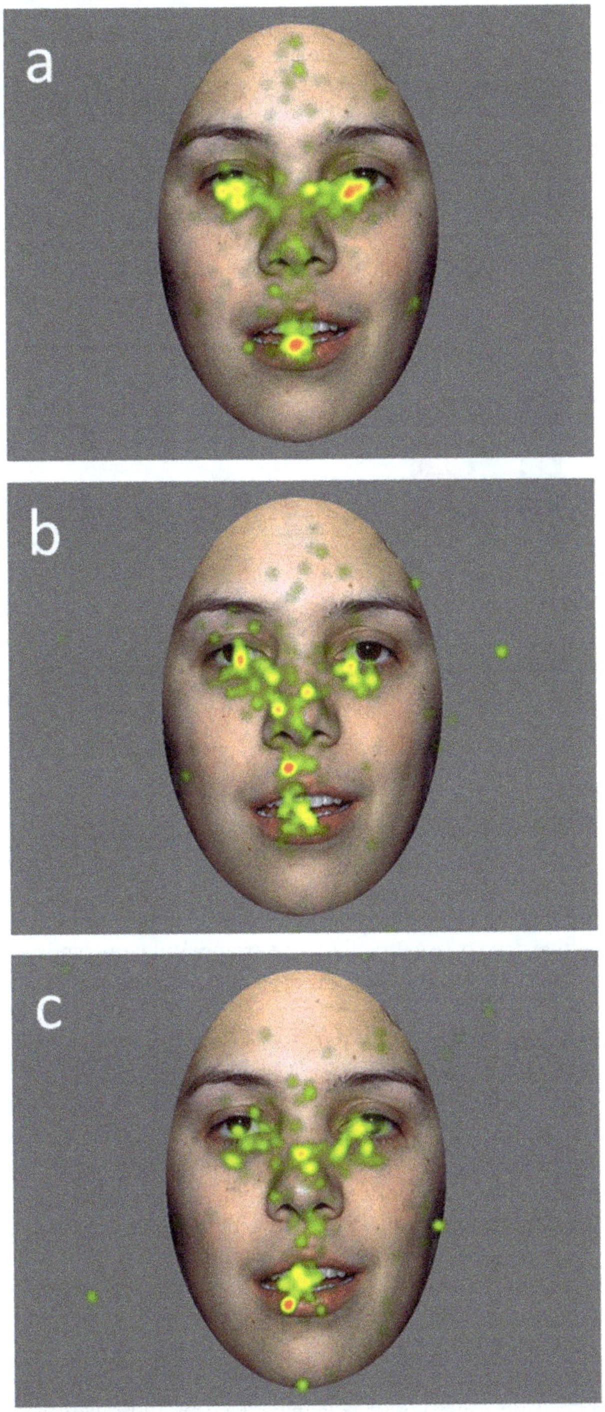

FIGURE 3 | Heat maps of average duration fixation on a calm face image for a subset of TD **(A)**, DD **(B)**, and ASD **(C)**, participants.

mean differences revealed the DD participants exhibited a significant reduction in pupil diameter during fearful faces in comparison to TD ($t_{(107.8)}$ = −3.88, p = 0.000) and ASD $t_{(107.8)}$ = 3.89, p = 0.000) participants. Additionally, the ASD participants exhibited a significant increase in pupil diameter during happy faces in comparison to TD participants ($t_{(104.3)}$ = 2.35, p = 0.021). Additionally, a marginally significant interaction emerged between diagnosis and interval ($F_{(38,11305)}$ = 1.35, p = 0.073). Least square mean differences revealed the interaction was being driven by the DD group on average exhibiting a significant reduction in pupil diameter across the last five intervals in comparison to the TD group (ps = 0.009–0.042). In contrast, the ASD group on average exhibited a significant increase in pupil reactivity across the last nine intervals in comparison to the DD group (ps = 0.011–0.047).

TABLE 3 | Results of Poisson regression for fixation count.

Variable	*F*	*p*
Age	14.33	0.001*
Group	3.35	0.037*
Emotion	1.83	0.162
AOI	300.61	0.000*
Group × Emotion	0.35	0.841
Group × AOI	5.64	0.000*
Emotion × AOI	1.36	0.228
Group × Emotion × AOI	0.65	0.803

Note. AOI, area of interest. $^{*}p < 0.05$.

Test-Retest Reliability in ASD

Test-retest reliability was assessed using ICCs between the two testing sessions for the ASD participants for fixation counts, the proportion of looking, and pupil reactivity (**Table 5**). A good degree of reliability was found for the majority of the AOIs based on the proportion of looking (ICCs = 0.62–0.68). The proportion of looking time at the nose fell in the fair range (ICC = 0.50). Within the AOIs for fixation counts, a fair degree of reliability was found for the nose, mouth, and scrambled regions (ICCs = 0.40–0.56) with the eye region exhibiting a poor degree of reliability (ICC = 0.39). Lastly, changes in pupil reactivity demonstrated poor to fair reliability across the different emotional faces that were presented. Pupil reactivity to the fear faces demonstrated the largest reliability coefficient (ICC = 0.54). Reliability coefficients for change in pupil reactivity within calm faces were not reported due to the variability within the testing sessions being greater than across sessions, resulting in a negative ICC value.

DISCUSSION

Social communication deficits are a hallmark characteristic of the ASD phenotype (American Psychiatric Association, 2013). More specifically, social attention deficits (e.g., reduced attention to social stimuli as a whole or atypical allocation of attention to social stimuli) within ASD have been hypothesized to have cascading effects on emotion recognition (Pelphrey et al., 2002; Wagner et al., 2013). With social attention deficits being a primary early biomarker for diagnostic outcomes in infancy (Jones and Klin, 2013; Elsabbagh et al., 2014; Jones et al., 2016), this is an ideal skill area for targeted assessment and treatment to potentially increase quality of life in individuals with ASD. Through precise, noninvasive measures like eye-tracking, the literature has shown promise in accurately identifying deficits

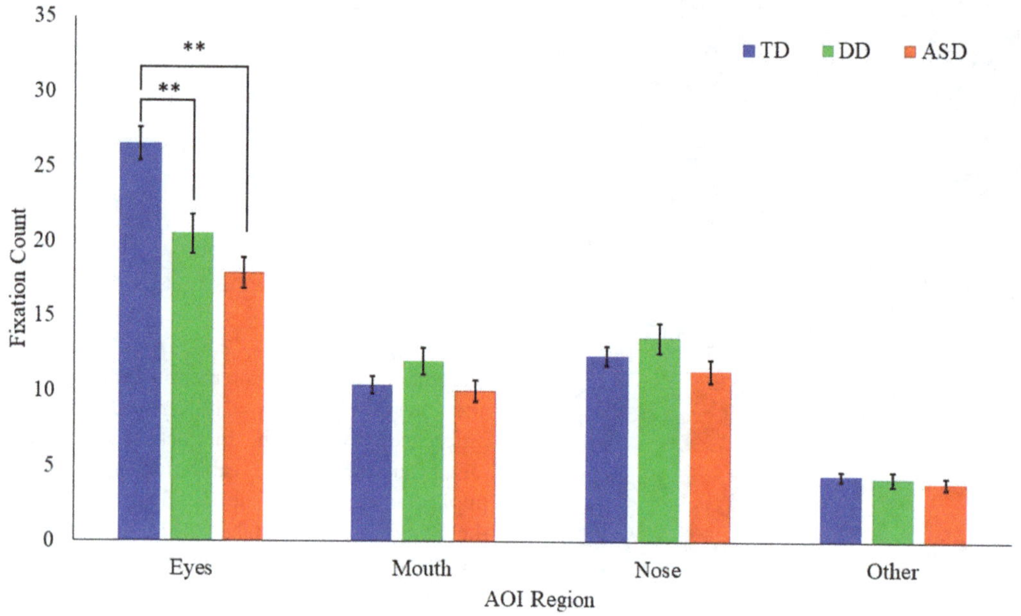

FIGURE 4 | Mean fixation count to each AOI region by group for all emotional faces. Error bars represent SEM. TD, typical developing; DD, developmentally delayed; ASD, autism spectrum disorder; $^{**}p < 0.05$.

TABLE 4 | Results of repeated-measures ANCOVA within-subjects effects for pupillary reactivity.

Variable	*F*	*p*
Age	2.21	0.141
Group	2.67	0.075
Emotion	15.36	0.000*
Interval	2.28	0.001*
Group × Emotion	14.81	0.000*
Group × Interval	1.35	0.073
Emotion × Interval	0.65	0.953
Group × Emotion × Interval	0.41	1.000

Note. AOI, area of interest. $^{*}p < 0.05$.

in social attention and emotion recognition, but the sensitivity of the mechanism for treatment outcomes remains uncertain (Bradshaw et al., 2015). The present study aimed to assess the utility of an eye-tracking paradigm to discriminate between clinical groups in social attention and emotion recognition through face scanning and pupillometry. The present study also assessed the reliability of this paradigm within the ASD sample to further our understanding of the utility of eye-tracking for future clinical trials.

As expected, our analyses align with previous research (Klin et al., 2002; Pelphrey et al., 2002; Corden et al., 2008; Riby and Hancock, 2008; Rice et al., 2012; Hanley et al., 2013; Auyeung et al., 2015) suggesting atypical attention allocation to social stimuli in ASD; however, these differences were not distinguishable by varying emotions based on face scanning patterns and were confined to one area of the face. Specifically, the ASD group spent less time and fixated less on the eye region across all emotions in comparison to the TD control group. Moreover, differences in attention to the eye region between the ASD and DD groups was unclear, leaving the question of whether these atypical social attention profiles are ASD specific or related to cognitive functioning. Previous research examining attention to faces in clinical populations with known cognitive deficits (e.g., fragile × syndrome, Williams syndrome, Angelman syndrome) have also found reduced attention to the eye region of faces (Farzin et al., 2009, 2011; Riby and Hancock, 2009; Hong et al., 2017); however, the use of idiopathic mental-age matched comparison groups in the current literature is scarce, adding to the uncertainty of these deficits being syndrome specific or related to cognitive functioning. Further, the proportion of looking time spent on the nose in the DD group emerged as a region of interest. In comparison to the TD control group, the DD group spent more time looking at the nose region. The social attention profile of reduced looking to eyes and increased looking to nose may be notable for those with low IQ. Since our ASD sample had a wide range of IQ scores, it's unclear in the current study if the visibly, but not statistically significant, elevated attention to the nose region in the ASD group is being driven by those with lower cognitive abilities. Although the preliminary analyses did not suggest differences in overall attention to the eye-tracking task based on IQ in the ASD group, it may be important in the future to examine if different social attention patterns emerge dependent on cognitive functioning. Notably, despite finding these subtle differences in social attention allocation for specific facial regions, the ASD group still exhibited a relatively similar social attention profile overall in comparison to the control groups (e.g., most time spent looking at eyes, less at nose, mouth, and other).

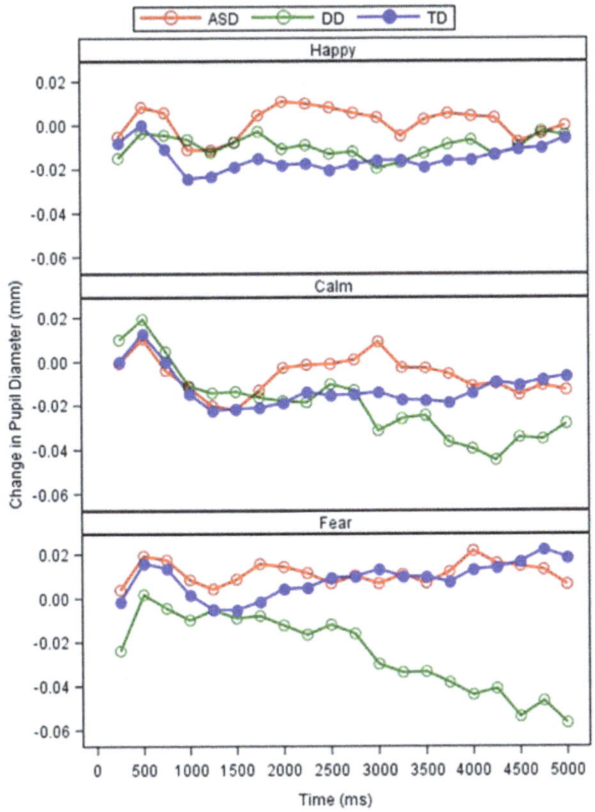

FIGURE 5 | Relative change in pupil diameter (mm) between scrambled face to calm, happy, and fearful faces across 250-ms intervals, by the group.

TABLE 5 | Test-retest reliability as measured by ICC calculations of eye-tracking measures between test sessions in ASD.

Variable	ICC (2, 1)	95% CI
Proportion of Looking		
Eyes	0.66	0.29–0.85
Nose	0.50	0.09–0.77
Mouth	0.68	0.35–0.86
Scramble	0.62	0.25–0.83
Fixation Count		
Eyes	0.39	−0.09–0.71
Nose	0.56	0.15–0.80
Mouth	0.45	0.02–0.74
Scramble	0.40	−0.07–0.72
Pupil Reactivity		
Calm	-	-
Happy	0.31	−0.18–0.71
Fear	0.54	0.00–0.85

Note. ICC (2,1), Interclass Correlation Coefficient using a two-way random-effects model with absolute agreement; ASD, autism spectrum disorder; CI, confidence interval; ICC values for calm were not reported due to significant variability resulting in negative values.

As anticipated, pupil reactivity was able to detect differences within the clinical groups based on the emotional faces that were presented. Unlike the findings presented by Sepeta et al. (2012), we found increased pupil reactivity in the ASD group when examining happy faces in comparison to the TD group. The TD group and DD group exhibited similar pupil reactivity profiles to the happy faces suggesting an ASD phenotype-specific response. Nonetheless, these findings conflict with the idea of abnormal social reward processing in ASD as measured through pupillometry. Based on the social motivation hypothesis, it is suggested that individuals with ASD will not attend to social stimuli because they do not form representations of the reward value of social stimuli (Dawson et al., 2005; Chevallier et al., 2012). Therefore, individuals with ASD will not seek out social stimuli because eye contact and faces are not intrinsically rewarding and may not be activating those cognitive reward systems appropriately. With the lack of facial scanning differences across emotions and increased pupil reactivity to the happy faces in the ASD group, additional work is needed to explore these findings and how they relate to emotion and social reward processing.

Unexpectedly, the ASD group exhibited similar pupil reactivity profiles to the calm and fear faces in comparison to the TD group. Unlike the findings presented by Nuske et al. (2014a), both the TD and ASD groups exhibited a slight increase in pupil diameter while viewing fearful faces. These findings may be explained by the lack of significant change in pupil diameter exhibited by our TD group that was found by Nuske et al. (2014a) as both the ASD and TD group in the present study partially resemble their ASD findings. Further, the paradigm that was utilized was slightly different as we did not strategically show neutral faces right before the fearful faces. However, our findings partially replicate previous work (Sepeta et al., 2012; Wagner et al., 2013) suggesting no group differences in pupil diameter in response to emotional faces. It is quite possible that emotion processing is better understood utilizing multiple mechanisms of autonomic activity. Bradley et al. (2008) utilized measures of pupillometry, heart rate, and skin conductance in a group of TD individuals who viewed emotional faces. Through these mechanisms, they were able to strongly support that pupil reactivity in response to emotionally-salient faces was moderated by the sympathetic system. Although many groups have been able to identify ASD specific emotion processing through pupillometry alone, a multimethod physiological approach may be warranted to delineate the mixed findings.

Aside from the group differences in social attention and emotion processing, the present study also examined the test-retest reliability of the emotional faces paradigm that was utilized in the ASD group. Test-retest reliability considers the variability between individuals' repeated measurements relative to the overall group variance (de Vet et al., 2006). Farzin et al. (2009, 2011) reported high reliability of an extended version of the paradigm in a small sample of FXS participants. Our reliability estimates were less promising based on the mechanism assessed while aligning with the known variability of the ASD phenotype and mixed literature supporting eye tracking as a reliable biomarker for treatment change. Specifically, our results found the highest reliability estimates through the proportion of looking time at the mouth or the eyes. The number of fixations across AOIs and pupil reactivity to the different emotions resulted in poor to fair reliability coefficients. The low ICCs found for some of the eye-tracking variables suggest they may not be appropriate for discriminative testing when comparing across groups and caution should be placed when interpreting the results of those specific AOIs. Of note, previous literature suggests higher reliability coefficients are more likely to occur from longer trial duration (Skinner et al., 2018). This may explain why our reliability estimates were not as strong as those reported by Farzin et al. (2011) because they administered more face trials than administered in the present study. The reliability estimates reported may have been boosted if the paradigm lasted longer and presented more faces; however, when working with individuals with neurodevelopmental disabilities, long eye-tracking tasks can be challenging to complete while still obtaining adequate and useable data.

In order to consider the validity of eye-tracking as a biomarker in ASD, we must also consider how the typical sample in the present study aligns with the current literature on social attention development. There is a robust amount of literature indicating that when TD individuals are presented with photos or videos of people, they are drawn to look at people rather than objects, with a particular focus on the eye region (e.g., for review, see Frischen et al., 2007; Birmingham and Kingstone, 2009). The facial scanning patterns of the present study's TD sample aligns with the current literature on social attention. Specifically, the TD sample predominantly attended to the eye region of faces as demonstrated through the overall proportion of looking time and fixation counts. As for pupillometry responses, there have been consistent findings in the TD literature indicating emotional stimuli, in comparison to neutral stimuli, produces greater pupillary responses (Henderson et al., 2014; Cohen et al., 2015). Although the focus of the present study was on group differences in pupillometry responses to emotional stimuli, resulting in the TD groups not being significantly different, our TD sample visually appears to demonstrate a slight increase in pupil size across the presentation of the different emotional faces. Specifically, the TD sample had a stronger reaction to fear faces compared to happy faces in comparison to calm faces. Therefore, the present study's findings within the TD sample align with previous literature on typical social attention profiles suggesting these findings build on the validity of the eye-tracking paradigm used, the interpretation of the findings within ASD and DD, and the utility of eye-tracking as a biomarker.

Overall, these findings continue to build on the promise of eye-tracking as a feasible and reliable biomarker for identifying social attention and emotion recognition deficits in ASD. This may be less apparent for detecting emotion recognition explicitly through facial scanning within ASD. However, the combined mechanisms of pupillometry and facial scanning provided more precision in the present study for understanding the social attention and emotion recognition profiles in a chronologically and cognitively diverse ASD group. Furthermore, the present study attempted to rule out the effects of IQ with the addition of an idiopathic mental-age matched control group. Unfortunately, an ASD specific social attention profile was not as clearly delineated given the lack of group differences between the mental-age matched control group and the ASD group. Notably, eight of our participants were not able to complete cognitive testing; however, six of the eight were able to complete the eye-tracking task with at least 35% valid looking data, which allowed for our sample to be cognitively diverse. Cognitive functioning did not present as a factor impairing overall attention during the task within the clinical groups. This suggests that regardless of cognitive functioning, these clinical groups were able to successfully complete the task and that there are potentially salient social attention profiles specific to cognitive abilities to be further explored rather than concerns with general attention in these clinical populations.

The utility of the emotional faces eye-tracking paradigm assessed in the present study should continue to be evaluated given the wide range of test-retest reliability coefficients reported, in addition to other eye-tracking paradigms that are widely used in the literature that have been shown to consistently distinguish between clinical groups. More recently, a clinical trial utilizing an extended version of the emotional faces paradigm suggested the paradigm was sensitive enough to detect increases in overall looking time, fixations, and pupil reactivity in adolescents and adults with FXS (Hessl et al., 2019). Since many individuals with FXS also receive a co-occurring diagnosis of ASD (Klusek et al., 2014; Talisa et al., 2014; Thurman et al., 2014), the emotional faces paradigm may be sensitive enough to detect a change in treatment trials targeting social and emotional impairments in idiopathic ASD. The specific mechanisms within the eye-tracking paradigm (e.g., proportion of looking vs. fixation counts) may be more or less viable for assessing treatment-specific outcomes that are lacking in the current literature.

Despite the many strengths of the present study, there are also limitations to consider when interpreting the findings. Specifically, age consistently presented as a significant variable in the analyses. Since our age range was quite wide (3–25 years), as well as IQ within the ASD sample, it may be important for future researchers to look at subgroup responses based on age and cognitive abilities as the paradigm utilized may be a better biomarker and outcome measure for certain subgroups within the different clinical groups. For example, differences in maturation in social attention within the clinical groups could be a driving factor of the group differences that emerged. Additionally, the reliability analyses were reported with a small subgroup of the ASD sample who had test-retest data available. Future work should continue to explore test-retest reliability in ASD utilizing a larger sample with a goal of identifying the ideal necessary length or amount of trials needed in an eye-tracking paradigm in this population. It would also be important to compare the test-retest reliability estimates across clinical groups as the reliability estimates reported in the present study could be specific to the variability in the ASD phenotype or the eye-tracking measure utilized. Future work should examine test-retest reliability within multiple clinical samples to further clarify these findings. Also, the present study utilized static photographs of faces to examine social attention and emotion recognition. The use of dynamic social stimuli that resemble real-life social situations could extend these findings. With the lack of differences between the emotions presented in the paradigm, as mentioned above, expanding the paradigm to included more faces may have provided additional power to find different social attention patterns for each of the emotions. Further, the present studies paradigm did not map onto the racial and ethnic diversity of the study's sample. Lastly, incorporating additional physiological (e.g., heart rate, skin conductance) or electrophysiological measures to assess social attention and emotion recognition from a biobehavioral perspective may provide a more sensitive model for assessing deficits and change across treatment while delineating some of the variability in the literature.

ETHICS STATEMENT

The studies involving humans were approved by the Cincinnati Children's Hospital Medical Center Institutional Review Board. Written informed consent was obtained from the patients/participants' legal guardian/next of kin. Standard Operating Procedures of the IRB were followed to evaluate if assent from participants was possible. This was carried out on a case by case basis, and was obtained where feasible.

AUTHOR CONTRIBUTIONS

CE, RS, KD, and EP contributed to study conceptualization and data collection. CE, RS, MH, and DR contributed to the manuscript preparation and revisions. DR led the writing of the manuscript. MH contributed to data extraction and preparation. DR and PH analyzed and interpreted the data.

FUNDING

This work was supported by an investigator-initiated grant from the Simons Foundation Autism Research Initiative (SFARI) to CE.

ACKNOWLEDGMENTS

We would like to thank Hilary Rosselot, Stephanie Booker, Kaela O'Brien, Shannon O'Connor, and Bridget Crippen for assistance with subject recruitment, data collection, data entry, and for regulatory support on this project. We would also like to thank the participants and their families who have contributed their time to make this research possible.

REFERENCES

Aman, M. G., Singh, N. N., Stewart, A. W., and Field, C. J. (1985). The aberrant behavior checklist: a behavior rating scale for the assessment of treatment effects. *Am. J. Ment. Defic.* 89, 485–491.

American Psychiatric Association. (2013). *Diagnostic and Statistical Manual of Mental Disorders (DSM-5®).* Washington, DC: American Psychiatric Publishing.

Anderson, C., Colombo, J., and Jill Shaddy, D. (2006). Visual scanning and pupillary responses in young children with autism spectrum disorder. *J. Clin. Exp. Neuropsychol.* 28, 1238–1256. doi: 10.1080/13803390500376790

Åsberg Johnels, J., Gillberg, C., Falck-Ytter, T., and Miniscalco, C. (2014). Face-viewing patterns in young children with autism spectrum disorders: speaking up for the role of language comprehension. *J. Speech Lang. Hear. Res.* 57, 2246–2252. doi: 10.1044/2014_jslhr-l-13-0268

Auyeung, B., Lombardo, M. V., Heinrichs, M., Chakrabarti, B., Sule, A., Deakin, J. B., et al. (2015). Oxytocin increases eye contact during a real-time, naturalistic social interaction in males with and without autism. *Transl. Psychiatry* 5:e507. doi: 10.1038/tp.2014.146

Benjamini, Y., and Hochberg, Y. (1995). Controlling the false discovery rate: a practical and powerful approach to multiple testing. *J. R. Stat. Soc. Series B* 57, 289–300. doi: 10.1111/j.2517-6161.1995.tb02031.x

Birmingham, E., Bischof, W. F., and Kingstone, A. (2008). Social attention and real-world scenes: the roles of action, competition and social content. *Q. J. Exp. Psychol.* 61, 986–998. doi: 10.1080/17470210701410375

Birmingham, E., and Kingstone, A. (2009). Human social attention. *Prog. Brain Res.* 176, 309–320. doi: 10.1016/s0079-6123(09)17618-5

Bolte, E. E., and Diehl, J. J. (2013). Measurement tools and target symptoms/skills used to assess treatment response for individuals with autism spectrum disorder. *J. Autism Dev. Disord.* 43, 2491–2501. doi: 10.1007/s10803-013-1798-7

Bradley, M. M., Miccoli, L., Escrig, M. A., and Lang, P. J. (2008). The pupil as a measure of emotional arousal and autonomic activation. *Psychophysiology* 45, 602–607. doi: 10.1111/j.1469-8986.2008.00654.x

Bradshaw, J. (1967). Pupil size as a measure of arousal during information processing. *Nature* 216, 515–516. doi: 10.1038/216515a0

Bradshaw, J., Shic, F., Holden, A. N., Horowitz, E. J., Barrett, A. C., German, T. C., et al. (2019). The use of eye tracking as a biomarker of treatment outcome in a pilot randomized clinical trial for young children with autism. *Autism Res.* 12, 779–793. doi: 10.1002/aur.2093

Bradshaw, J., Steiner, A. M., Gengoux, G., and Koegel, L. K. (2015). Feasibility and effectiveness of very early intervention for infants at-risk for autism spectrum disorder: a systematic review. *J. Autism Dev. Disord.* 45, 778–794. doi: 10.1007/s10803-014-2235-2

Chevallier, C., Kohls, G., Troiani, V., Brodkin, E. S., and Schultz, R. T. (2012). The social motivation theory of autism. *Trends Cogn. Sci.* 16, 231–239. doi: 10.1016/j.tics.2012.02.007

Chita-Tegmark, M. (2016). Attention allocation in ASD: a review and meta-analysis of eye-tracking studies. *Rev. J. Autism Dev. Disord.* 3, 209–223. doi: 10.1007/s40489-016-0077-x

Cicchetti, D. V. (1994). Guidelines, criteria and rules of thumb for evaluating normed and standardized assessment instruments in psychology. *Psychol. Assess.* 6, 284–290. doi: 10.1037/1040-3590.6.4.284

Cohen, N., Moyal, N., and Henik, A. (2015). Executive control suppresses pupillary responses to aversive stimuli. *Biol. Psychol.* 112, 1–11. doi: 10.1016/j.biopsycho.2015.09.006

Constantino, J. N., and Gruber, C. P. (2005). *Social Responsiveness Scale (SRS).* Los Angeles, CA: Western Psychological Services.

Corden, B., Chilvers, R., and Skuse, D. (2008). Avoidance of emotionally arousing stimuli predicts social-perceptual impairment in Asperger's syndrome. *Neuropsychologia* 46, 137–147. doi: 10.1016/j.neuropsychologia.2007.08.005

Dalton, K. M., Nacewicz, B. M., Johnstone, T., Schaefer, H. S., Gernsbacher, M. A., Goldsmith, H. H., et al. (2005). Gaze fixation and the neural circuitry of face processing in autism. *Nat. Neurosci.* 8, 519–526. doi: 10.1038/nn1421

Dawson, G., Webb, S. J., and McPartland, J. (2005). Understanding the nature of face processing impairment in autism: insights from behavioral and electrophysiological studies. *Dev. Neuropsychol.* 27, 403–424. doi: 10.1207/s15326942dn2703_6

de Vet, H. C. W., Terwee, C. B., Knol, D. L., and Bouter, L. M. (2006). When to use agreement versus reliability measures. *J. Clin. Epidemiol.* 59, 1033–1039. doi: 10.1016/j.jclinepi.2005.10.015

de Wit, T. C. J., Falck-Ytter, T., and von Hofsten, C. (2008). Young children with autism spectrum disorder look differently at positive versus negative emotional faces. *Res. Autism Spectr. Disord.* 2, 651–659. doi: 10.1016/j.rasd.2008.01.004

Eisenbarth, H., and Alpers, G. W. (2011). Happy mouth and sad eyes: scanning emotional facial expressions. *Emotion* 11, 860–865. doi: 10.1037/a0022758

Elliott, C. D. (2007). *Differential Ability Scales–Second edition (DAS-II).* San Antonio, TX: Harcourt Assessment.

Elsabbagh, M., Bedford, R., Senju, A., Charman, T., Pickles, A., Johnson, M. H., et al. (2014). What you see is what you get: contextual modulation of face scanning in typical and atypical development. *Soc. Cogn. Affect. Neurosci.* 9, 538–543. doi: 10.1093/scan/nst012

Falck-Ytter, T. (2008). Face inversion effects in autism: a combined looking time and pupillometric study. *Autism Res.* 1, 297–306. doi: 10.1002/aur.45

Farzin, F., Rivera, S. M., and Hessl, D. (2009). Visual processing of faces in individuals with fragile X syndrome: an eye tracking study. *J. Autism Dev. Disord.* 39, 946–952. doi: 10.1007/s10803-009-0744-1

Farzin, F., Scaggs, F., Hervey, C., Berry-Kravis, E., and Hessl, D. (2011). Reliability of eye tracking and pupillometry measures in individuals with fragile X syndrome. *J. Autism Dev. Disord.* 41, 1515–1522. doi: 10.1007/s10803-011-1176-2

Fletcher-Watson, S., and Hampton, S. (2018). The potential of eye-tracking as a sensitive measure of behavioural change in response to intervention. *Sci. Rep.* 8:14715. doi: 10.1038/s41598-018-32444-9

Frischen, A., Bayliss, A. P., and Tipper, S. P. (2007). Gaze cueing of attention: visual attention, social cognition, and individual differences. *Psychol. Bull.* 133, 694–724. doi: 10.1037/0033-2909.133.4.694

Gillespie-Smith, K., Doherty-Sneddon, G., Hancock, P. J. B., and Riby, D. M. (2014). That looks familiar: attention allocation to familiar and unfamiliar faces in children with autism spectrum disorder. *Cogn. Neuropsychiatry* 19, 554–569. doi: 10.1080/13546805.2014.943365

Guillon, Q., Hadjikhani, N., Baduel, S., Rogé, B., and Roge, B. (2014). Visual social attention in autism spectrum disorder: insights from eye tracking studies. *Neurosci. Biobehav. Rev.* 42, 279–297. doi: 10.1016/j.neubiorev.2014.03.013

Hanley, M., McPhillips, M., Mulhern, G., and Riby, D. M. (2013). Spontaneous attention to faces in Asperger syndrome using ecologically valid static stimuli. *Autism* 17, 754–761. doi: 10.1177/1362361312456746

Henderson, R. R., Bradley, M. M., and Lang, P. J. (2014). Modulation of the initial light reflex during affective picture viewing. *Psychophysiology* 51, 815–818. doi: 10.1111/psyp.12236

Hessl, D., Harvey, D., Sansone, S., Crestodina, C., Chin, J., Joshi, R., et al. (2019). Effects of mavoglurant on visual attention and pupil reactivity while viewing photographs of faces in fragile X Syndrome. *PLoS One* 14:e0209984. doi: 10.1371/journal.pone.0209984

Hong, M. P., Guilfoyle, J. L., Mooney, L. N., Wink, L. K., Pedapati, E. V., Shaffer, R. C., et al. (2017). Eye gaze and pupillary response in Angelman syndrome. *Res. Dev. Disabil.* 68, 88–94. doi: 10.1016/j.ridd.2017.06.011

Jones, W., and Klin, A. (2013). Attention to eyes is present but in decline in 2-6-month-old infants later diagnosed with autism. *Nature* 504, 427–431. doi: 10.1038/nature12715

Jones, E. J. H., Venema, K., Earl, R., Lowy, R., Barnes, K., Estes, A., et al. (2016). Reduced engagement with social stimuli in 6-month-old infants with later autism spectrum disorder: a longitudinal prospective study of infants at high familial risk. *J. Neurodev. Disord.* 8:7. doi: 10.1186/s11689-016-9139-8

Kenward, M. G., and Roger, J. H. (1997). Small sample inference for fixed effects from restricted maximum likelihood. *Biometrics* 53, 983–997. doi: 10.2307/2533558

Klin, A., Jones, W., Schultz, R., Volkmar, F., and Cohen, D. (2002). Visual fixation patterns during viewing of naturalistic social situations as predictors of social competence in individuals with autism. *Arch. Gen. Psychiatry* 59, 809–816. doi: 10.1001/archpsyc.59.9.809

Klusek, J., Martin, G. E., and Losh, M. (2014). Consistency between research and clinical diagnoses of autism among boys and girls with fragile X syndrome. *J. Intellect. Disabil. Res.* 58, 940–952. doi: 10.1111/jir.12121

Kret, M. E. (2015). Emotional expressions beyond facial muscle actions. A call for studying autonomic signals and their impact on social perception. *Front. Psychol.* 6:711. doi: 10.3389/fpsyg.2015.00711

Kwon, M.-K., Moore, A., Barnes, C. C., Cha, D., and Pierce, K. (2019). Typical levels of eye-region fixation in toddlers with ASD across multiple contexts. *J. Am. Acad. Child Adolesc. Psychiatry* 58, 1004–1015. doi: 10.1016/j.jaac.2018.12.011

Lord, C., Rutter, M., DiLavore, P., Risi, S., Gotham, K., and Bishop, S. (2012). *Autism Diagnostic Observation Schedule–2nd Edition (ADOS-2).* Los Angeles, CA: Western Psychological Corporation.

Messinger, D. S., Mattson, W. I., Mahoor, M. H., and Cohn, J. F. (2012). The eyes have it: making positive expressions more positive and negative expressions more negative. *Emotion* 12, 430–436. doi: 10.1037/a0026498

Murias, M., Major, S., Davlantis, K., Franz, L., Harris, A., Rardin, B., et al. (2018). Validation of eye-tracking measures of social attention as a potential biomarker for autism clinical trials. *Autism Res.* 11, 166–174. doi: 10.1002/aur.1894

Nuske, H. J., Vivanti, G., and Dissanayake, C. (2014a). Reactivity to fearful expressions of familiar and unfamiliar people in children with autism: an eye-tracking pupillometry study. *J. Neurodev. Disord.* 6:14. doi: 10.1186/1866-1955-6-14

Nuske, H. J., Vivanti, G., Hudry, K., and Dissanayake, C. (2014b). Pupillometry reveals reduced unconscious emotional reactivity in autism. *Biol. Psychol.* 101, 24–35. doi: 10.1016/j.biopsycho.2014.07.003

Pelphrey, K. A., Sasson, N. J., Reznick, J. S., Paul, G., Goldman, B. D., and Piven, J. (2002). Visual scanning of faces in autism. *J. Autism Dev. Disord.* 32, 249–261. doi: 10.1023/a:1016374617369

Riby, D. M., and Hancock, P. J. B. (2008). Viewing it differently: social scene perception in Williams syndrome and autism. *Neuropsychologia* 46, 2855–2860. doi: 10.1016/j.neuropsychologia.2008.05.003

Riby, D. M., and Hancock, P. J. B. (2009). Do faces capture the attention of individuals with Williams syndrome or autism? Evidence from tracking eye movements. *J. Autism Dev. Disord.* 39, 421–431. doi: 10.1007/s10803-008-0641-z

Rice, K., Moriuchi, J. M., Jones, W., and Klin, A. (2012). Parsing heterogeneity in autism spectrum disorders: visual scanning of dynamic social scenes in school-aged children. *J. Am. Acad. Child Adolesc. Psychiatry* 51, 238–248. doi: 10.1016/j.jaac.2011.12.017

Roid, G. H. (2003). *Stanford-Binet Intelligence Scales–Fifth Edition.* Itasca, IL: Riverside Publishing.

Rutter, M., Bailey, A., Lord, C., and Berument, S. (2003). *Social Communication Questionnaire (SCQ).* Los Angeles: Western Psychological Services.

Sawyer, A. C. P., Williamson, P., and Young, R. L. (2012). Can gaze avoidance explain why individuals with Asperger's syndrome can't recognise emotions from facial expressions? *J. Autism Dev. Disord.* 42, 606–618. doi: 10.1007/s10803-011-1283-0

Sepeta, L., Tsuchiya, N., Davies, M. S., Sigman, M., Bookheimer, S. Y., and Dapretto, M. (2012). Abnormal social reward processing in autism as indexed by pupillary responses to happy faces. *J. Neurodev. Disord.* 4:17. doi: 10.1186/1866-1955-4-17

Shrout, P. E., and Fleiss, J. L. (1979). Intraclass correlations: uses in assessing rater reliability. Available online at: https://pdfs.semanticscholar.org/b8d4/7b0c0b12dd77543e82e6bf6636ddd335cfea.pdf. Accessed April 19, 2019.

Skinner, I. W., Hübscher, M., Moseley, G. L., Lee, H., Wand, B. M., Traeger, A. C., et al. (2018). The reliability of eyetracking to assess attentional bias to threatening words in healthy individuals. *Behav. Res. Methods* 50, 1778–1792. doi: 10.3758/s13428-017-0946-y

Spezio, M. L., Adolphs, R., Hurley, R. S. E., and Piven, J. (2007a). Abnormal use of facial information in high-functioning autism. *J. Autism Dev. Disord.* 37, 929–939. doi: 10.1007/s10803-006-0232-9

Spezio, M. L., Adolphs, R., Hurley, R. S. E., and Piven, J. (2007b). Analysis of face gaze in autism using "Bubbles". *Neuropsychologia* 45, 144–151. doi: 10.1016/j.neuropsychologia.2006.04.027

Steinhauer, S. R., Siegle, G. J., Condray, R., and Pless, M. (2004). Sympathetic and parasympathetic innervation of pupillary dilation during sustained processing. *Int. J. Psychophysiol.* 52, 77–86. doi: 10.1016/j.ijpsycho.2003.12.005

Talisa, V. B., Boyle, L., Crafa, D., and Kaufmann, W. E. (2014). Autism and anxiety in males with fragile X syndrome: an exploratory analysis of neurobehavioral profiles from a parent survey. *Am. J. Med. Genet. A* 164, 1198–1203. doi: 10.1002/ajmg.a.36468

Thurman, A. J., McDuffie, A., Hagerman, R., and Abbeduto, L. (2014). Psychiatric symptoms in boys with fragile X syndrome: a comparison with nonsyndromic autism spectrum disorder. *Res. Dev. Disabil.* 35, 1072–1086. doi: 10.1016/j.ridd.2014.01.032

Tottenham, N., Borscheid, A., Ellertsen, K., Marcus, D. J., and Nelson, C. A. (2002). *Categorization of Facial Expressions in Children and Adults: Establishing a Larger Stimulus Set.* MIT Press FIVE CAMBRIDGE. Available online at: https://scholar.google.com/scholar?hl=en&as_sdt=0%2C36&q=tottenham+2002+facial+expressions&oq=Tottenham%2C+2002. Accessed April 17, 2019.

Wagner, J. B., Hirsch, S. B., Vogel-Farley, V. K., Redcay, E., and Nelson, C. A. (2013). Eye-tracking, autonomic, and electrophysiological correlates of emotional face processing in adolescents with autism spectrum disorder. *J. Autism Dev. Disord.* 43, 188–199. doi: 10.1007/s10803-012-1565-1

Weir, J. P. (2005). Quantifying test-retest reliability using the intraclass correlation coefficient and the SEM. *J. Strength Cond. Res.* 19, 231–240. doi: 10.1519/15184.1

Permissions

All chapters in this book were first published by Frontiers; hereby published with permission under the Creative Commons Attribution License or equivalent. Every chapter published in this book has been scrutinized by our experts. Their significance has been extensively debated. The topics covered herein carry significant findings which will fuel the growth of the discipline. They may even be implemented as practical applications or may be referred to as a beginning point for another development.

The contributors of this book come from diverse backgrounds, making this book a truly international effort. This book will bring forth new frontiers with its revolutionizing research information and detailed analysis of the nascent developments around the world.

We would like to thank all the contributing authors for lending their expertise to make the book truly unique. They have played a crucial role in the development of this book. Without their invaluable contributions this book wouldn't have been possible. They have made vital efforts to compile up to date information on the varied aspects of this subject to make this book a valuable addition to the collection of many professionals and students.

This book was conceptualized with the vision of imparting up-to-date information and advanced data in this field. To ensure the same, a matchless editorial board was set up. Every individual on the board went through rigorous rounds of assessment to prove their worth. After which they invested a large part of their time researching and compiling the most relevant data for our readers.

The editorial board has been involved in producing this book since its inception. They have spent rigorous hours researching and exploring the diverse topics which have resulted in the successful publishing of this book. They have passed on their knowledge of decades through this book. To expedite this challenging task, the publisher supported the team at every step. A small team of assistant editors was also appointed to further simplify the editing procedure and attain best results for the readers.

Apart from the editorial board, the designing team has also invested a significant amount of their time in understanding the subject and creating the most relevant covers. They scrutinized every image to scout for the most suitable representation of the subject and create an appropriate cover for the book.

The publishing team has been an ardent support to the editorial, designing and production team. Their endless efforts to recruit the best for this project, has resulted in the accomplishment of this book. They are a veteran in the field of academics and their pool of knowledge is as vast as their experience in printing. Their expertise and guidance has proved useful at every step. Their uncompromising quality standards have made this book an exceptional effort. Their encouragement from time to time has been an inspiration for everyone.

The publisher and the editorial board hope that this book will prove to be a valuable piece of knowledge for researchers, students, practitioners and scholars across the globe.

List of Contributors

Joshua B. Ewen
Department of Neurology and Developmental Medicine, Kennedy Krieger Institute, Baltimore, MD, United States
Department of Neurology, Johns Hopkins University School of Medicine, Baltimore, MD, United States
Department of Psychological and Brain Sciences, Johns Hopkins University, Baltimore, MD, United States

John A. Sweeney
Department of Psychiatry, University of Cincinnati, Cincinnati, OH, United States

William Z. Potter
National Institute of Mental Health, National Institutes of Health, Bethesda, MD, United States

Carla Caballero
Sports Research Center, Sports Sciences Department, Miguel Hernández University of Elche, Elche, Spain
Department of Psychology, Rutgers, The State University of New Jersey, Piscataway, NJ, United States

Sejal Mistry
Department of Mathematics, Rutgers, The State University of New Jersey, Piscataway, NJ, United States

Elizabeth B. Torres
Department of Psychology, Rutgers, The State University of New Jersey, Piscataway, NJ, United States
Computer Science, Center for Computational Biomedicine Imaging and Modeling, Rutgers, The State University of New Jersey, Piscataway, NJ, United States
Center for Cognitive Science, Rutgers, The State University of New Jersey, Piscataway, NJ, United States

Adam J. Naples, Katarzyna Chawarska and James C. McPartland
Child Study Center, School of Medicine, Yale University, New Haven, CT, United States

Sara J. Webb
Center for Child Health, Behavior, and Development, Seattle Children's Research Institute, Seattle, WA, United States

Raphael A. Bernier
Department of Psychiatry and Behavioral Sciences, University of Washington, Seattle, WA, United States

Shafali S. Jeste, Scott P. Johnson, Gerhard Hellemann, Damla Senturk and Catherine A. Sugar
University of California, Los Angeles, Los Angeles, CA, United States

Geraldine Dawson, Linmarie Sikich and Maura Sabatos-DeVito
Duke Center for Autism and Brain Development, Duke University, Durham, NC, United States

Susan Faja and April R. Levin
Boston Children's Hospital and Harvard Medical School, Boston, MA, United States Harvard University, Boston, MA, United States

Cynthia A. Brandt and James D. Dziura
Yale University, New Haven, CT, United States

Leon Rozenblit
Prometheus Research, LLC, New Haven, CT, United States

Michael Murias
Northwestern University, Chicago, IL, United States

Michael L. Platt
University of Pennsylvania, Philadelphia, PA, United

Frederick Shic
Center for Child Health, Behavior and Development, Seattle Children's Research Institute, Seattle Children's Hospital, Seattle, WA, United States
Department of Pediatrics, University of Washington School of Medicine, Seattle, WA, United States

Rachel Earl
Center on Human Development and Disability, University of Washington, Seattle, WA, United States

Joni N. Saby
Lurie Family Foundations MEG Imaging Center, Department of Radiology, The Children's Hospital of Philadelphia, Philadelphia, PA, United States

Timothy P. L. Roberts
Lurie Family Foundations MEG Imaging Center, Department of Radiology, The Children's Hospital of Philadelphia, Philadelphia, PA, United States
Department of Radiology, Perelman School of Medicine at the University of Pennsylvania, Philadelphia, PA, United States

Sarika U. Peters
Department of Pediatrics, Vanderbilt University Medical Center, Nashville, TN, United States

Charles A. Nelson
Laboratories of Cognitive Neuroscience, Division of Developmental Medicine, Boston Children's Hospital, Harvard Medical School, Boston, MA, United States

Eric D. Marsh
Division of Neurology and Pediatrics, Children's Hospital ofPhiladelphia, Philadelphia, PA, United States
Departments of Neurology and Pediatrics, Perelman School of Medicine at the University of Pennsylvania, Philadelphia, PA, United States

Melissa Tsuboyama and Harper Lee Kaye
Neuromodulation Program, Department of Neurology, Division of Epilepsy and Clinical Neurophysiology, Boston Children's Hospital, Boston, MA, United States
FM Kirby Neurobiology Center, Department of Neurology, Boston Children's Hospital, Boston, MA, United States

Alexander Rotenberg
Neuromodulation Program, Department of Neurology, Division of Epilepsy and Clinical Neurophysiology, Boston Children's Hospital, Boston, MA, United States
FM Kirby Neurobiology Center, Department of Neurology, Boston Children's Hospital, Boston, MA, United States
Berenson-Allen Center for Noninvasive Brain Stimulation, Beth Israel Deaconess Medical Center, Boston, MA, United States

Aaron Wolfe Scheffler
Department of Epidemiology and Biostatistics, University of California, San Francisco, San Francisco, CA, United States

Shafali Jeste
Department of Psychiatry and Biobehavioral Sciences, University of California, Los Angeles, Los Angeles, CA, United States

Damla Şentürk
Department of Biostatistics, University of California, Los Angeles, Los Angeles, CA, United States

Sara Jane Webb
Center on Child Health, Behavior, and Development, Seattle Children's Research Institute, Seattle, WA, United States
Department of Psychiatry and Behavioral Sciences, University of Washington School of Medicine, Seattle, WA, United States

Erin Barney, Heather Borland, Minah Kim and Megha Santhosh
Center on Child Health, Behavior, and Development, Seattle Children's Research Institute, Seattle, WA, United States

Scott Johnson
Department of Psychiatry and Biobehavioral Sciences, University of California, Los Angeles, Los Angeles, CA, United States

James Dziura and James McPartland
Yale Child Study Center, Yale University, New Haven, CT, United States

Walker S. McKinney, Shannon Kelly and Matthew W. Mosconi
Clinical Child Psychology Program, Life Span Institute and Kansas Center for Autism Research and Training (K-CART), University of Kansas, Lawrence, KS, United States

Zheng Wang
Department of Occupational Therapy, University of Florida, Gainesville, FL, United States

Pravin Khemani
Department of Neurology, Swedish Neuroscience Institute, Seattle, WA, United States

Su Lui
Department of Radiology, Huaxi Magnetic Resonance Research Center, West China Hospital of Sichuan University, Chengdu, China

Stormi P. White
Department of Pediatrics, Marcus Autism Center, Emory University School of Medicine, Atlanta, GA, United States

Victor Faundez and Meghan Wynne
Department of Cell Biology, Emory University, Atlanta, GA, United States

Amanda Crocker
Program in Neuroscience, Middlebury College, Middlebury, VT, United States

Daniel Tarquinio
Rare Neurological Diseases (Private Research Institution), Atlanta, GA, United States

Richard D. McLane
Division of Child and Adolescent Psychiatry, Cincinnati Children's Hospital Medical Center, Cincinnati, OH, United States

Lauren M. Schmitt
Division of Developmental and Behavioral Pediatrics, Cincinnati Children's Hospital Medical Center, Cincinnati, OH, United States

Ernest V. Pedapati
Division of Child and Adolescent Psychiatry, Cincinnati Children's Hospital Medical Center, Cincinnati, OH, United States
Division of Neurology, Cincinnati Children's Hospital Medical Center, Cincinnati, OH, United States
Department of Psychiatry and Behavioral Neuroscience, University of Cincinnati College of Medicine, Cincinnati, OH, United States

Rebecca C. Shaffer
Division of Developmental and Behavioral Pediatrics, Cincinnati Children's Hospital Medical Center, Cincinnati, OH, United States
Department of Pediatrics, University of Cincinnati College of Medicine, Cincinnati, OH, United States

Kelli C. Dominick and Craig A. Erickson
Division of Child and Adolescent Psychiatry, Cincinnati Children's Hospital Medical Center, Cincinnati, OH, United States
Department of Psychiatry and Behavioral Neuroscience, University of Cincinnati College of Medicine, Cincinnati, OH, United States

Paul S. Horn
Division of Neurology, Cincinnati Children's Hospital Medical Center, Cincinnati, OH, United States

Christina Gross
Division of Neurology, Cincinnati Children's Hospital Medical Center, Cincinnati, OH, United States
Department of Pediatrics, University of Cincinnati College of Medicine, Cincinnati, OH, United States

Ali Jannati, Gabrielle Block, Mary A. Ryan and Alexander Rotenberg
Neuromodulation Program and Division of Epilepsy and Clinical Neurophysiology, Department of Neurology, Boston Children's Hospital, Harvard Medical School, Boston, MA, United States
Berenson-Allen Center for Noninvasive Brain Stimulation and Division of Cognitive Neurolo gy, Department of Neurology, Beth Israel Deaconess Medical Center, Harvard Medical School, Boston, MA, United States

Harper L. Kaye
Neuromodulation Program and Division of Epilepsy and Clinical Neurophysiology, Department of Neurology, Boston Children's Hospital, Harvard Medical School, Boston, MA, United States

Fae B. Kayarian
Berenson-Allen Center for Noninvasive Brain Stimulation and Division of Cognitive Neurology, Department of Neurology, Beth Israel Deaconess Medical Center, Harvard Medical School, Boston, MA, United States

Shahid Bashir
Neuroscience Center, King Fahad Specialist Hospital Dammam, Dammam, Saudi Arabia

Lindsay M. Oberman
Neuroplasticity and Autism Spectrum Disorder Program, Department of Psychiatry and Human Behavior, E. P. Bradley Hospital, Warren Alpert Medical School, Brown University, East Providence, RI, United States

Alvaro Pascual-Leone
Berenson-Allen Center for Noninvasive Brain Stimulation and Division of Cognitive Neurology, Department of Neurology, Beth Israel Deaconess Medical Center, Harvard Medical School, Boston, MA, United States
Institut Guttman de Neurorehabilitació, Universitat Autónoma de Barcelona, Badalona, Spain

Luke Bloy, Matt Ku, Marissa Dipiero and J. Christopher Edgar
Lurie Family Foundations MEG Imaging Center, Department of Radiology, The Children's Hospital of Philadelphia, Philadelphia, PA, United States

Lisa Blaskey, Emily Kuschner, Leah Gaetz and Ayesha Anwar
Lurie Family Foundations MEG Imaging Center, Department of Radiology, The Children's Hospital of Philadelphia, Philadelphia, PA, United States
Center for Autism Research, Department of Pediatrics, The Children's Hospital of Philadelphia, Philadelphia, PA, United States

Amanda Bennett
Department of Pediatrics, The Children's Hospital of Philadelphia, Philadelphia, PA, United States

Carolyn Bridgemohan
Boston Children's Hospital, Boston, MA, United States
Harvard Medical School, Boston, MA, United States

David M. Cochran, Andrew W. Zimmerman and Roula Choueiri
University of Massachusetts Memorial Medical Center, Worcester, MA, United States
University of Massachusetts Medical School, Worcester, MA, United States

Yamini J. Howe and Ann M. Neumeyer
Harvard Medical School, Boston, MA, United States
Lurie Center for Autism, Massachusetts General Hospital for Children, Lexington, MA, United States

Katherine Pawlowski, Peter W. Forbes and Stephanie J. Brewster
Boston Children's Hospital, Boston, MA, United States

George M. Anderson
Child Study Center, Yale University School of Medicine, New Haven, CT, United States

Laura Sices
Boston University Medical Center, Boston, MA, United States
Boston University School of Medicine, Boston, MA, United States

Karen J. Miller and Monica Ultmann
Center for Children with Special Needs, Floating Children's Hospital at Tufts Medical Center, Boston, MA, United States
Tufts University School of Medicine, Boston, MA, United States

Jessica Helt
Lurie Center for Autism, Massachusetts General Hospital for Children, Lexington, MA, United States

Laura Farfel
Boston University Medical Center, Boston, MA, United States
Center for Children with Special Needs, Floating Children's Hospital at Tufts Medical Center, Boston, MA, United States
Autism Consortium at Harvard Medical School, Boston, MA, United States

Jean A. Frazier
University of Massachusetts Memorial Medical Center, Worcester, MA, United States
University of Massachusetts Medical School, Worcester, MA, United States
Eunice Kennedy Shriver Center, University of Massachusetts Medical School, Worcester, MA, United States

Anna K. Prohl, Benoit Scherrer, Xavier Tomas-Fernandez, Clemente Velasco-Annis, Sean Clancy and Simon K. Warfield
Computational Radiology Laboratory, Department of Radiology, Boston Children's Hospital, Harvard Medical School, Harvard University, Boston, MA, United States

Rajna Filip-Dhima, Kush Kapur, Erin Carmody, Meghan Dean and Molly Valle
Department of Neurology, Boston Children's Hospital, Harvard Medical School, Harvard University, Boston, MA, United States

Sanjay P. Prabhu
Division of Neuroradiology, Department of Radiology, Boston Children's Hospital, Harvard Medical School, Harvard University, Boston, MA, United States

Jurriaan M. Peters
Computational Radiology Laboratory, Department of Radiology, Boston Children's Hospital, Harvard Medical School, Harvard University, Boston, MA, United States
Department of Neurology, Boston Children's Hospital, Harvard Medical School, Harvard University, Boston, MA, United States

E. Martina Bebin
Department of Neurology, University of Alabama at Birmingham, Birmingham, AL, United States

Darcy A. Krueger
Department of Neurology and Rehabilitation Medicine, Cincinnati Children's Hospital Medical Center, Cincinnati, OH, United States

Hope Northrup
Department of Pediatrics, McGovern Medical School, University of Texas Health Science Center at Houston, Houston, TX, United States

Joyce Y. Wu
Division of Pediatric Neurology, UCLA Mattel Children's Hospital, David Geffen School of Medicine, University of California, Los Angeles, Los Angeles, CA, United States

Mustafa Sahin
Department of Neurology, Boston Children's Hospital, Harvard Medical School, Harvard University, Boston, MA, United States
F.M. Kirby Neurobiology Center, Boston Children's Hospital, Harvard Medical School, Harvard University, Boston, MA, United States

Amanda M. O'Brien
Program in Speech and Hearing Bioscience and Technology, Division of Medical Sciences, Harvard University, Cambridge, MA, United States

Laurie Bayet
Department of Psychology, American University, Washington, DC, United States

Katherine Riley
Laboratories of Cognitive Neuroscience, Division of Developmental Medicine, Boston Children's Hospital, Boston, MA, United States

Meera E. Modi
Translational Neuroscience Center, Boston Children's Hospital, Boston, MA, United States
Department of Neurology, Harvard Medical School, Boston, MA, United States

Nicholas E. Woodruff, Kara L. Brown and Morgan Tran
Department of Psychology, The University of Oklahoma, Norman, OK, United States

Jun Wang
Department of Psychology, Zhejiang Normal University, Jinhua, China

Ernest V. Pedapati
Department of Psychiatry and Behavioral Neuroscience, University of Cincinnati, Cincinnati, OH, United States
Division of Child and Adolescent Psychiatry, Cincinnati Children's Hospital Medical Center, Cincinnati, OH, United States
Division of Child Neurology, Cincinnati Children's Hospital Medical Center, Cincinnati, OH, United States

Debra L. Reisinger
Division of Developmental and Behavioral Pediatrics, Cincinnati Children's Hospital Medical Center, Cincinnati, OH, United States

Michael P. Hong
Department of Pediatrics, University of Cincinnati College of Medicine, Cincinnati, OH, United States

Index

www.ingramcontent.com/pod-product-compliance
Lightning Source LLC
LaVergne TN
LVHW082222200926
848484LV00008B/2291
9798887403045